Artificial Intelligence for Radiographers

Christina Malamateniou
Maryann Hardy • Karen M Knapp
Aarthi Ramlaul
Editors

Artificial Intelligence for Radiographers

Basic Principles, Clinical Applications and Implementation Considerations

Foreword by
Charlotte Beardmore, Edward H. T. Chan,
Kori L. Stewart, Patrick C. Brennan,
Samar El-Farra

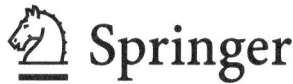 Springer

Editors
Christina Malamateniou
Division of Radiography, Department of
Allied Health Sciences, School of
Health and Medical Sciences, City St
George's University of London
London, UK

Karen M Knapp
Faculty of Health and Life Sciences
University of Exeter
Exeter, UK

Maryann Hardy
Faculty of Health Studies
University of Bradford
Bradford, UK

Aarthi Ramlaul 🆔
College of Health and Society
Buckinghamshire New University
High Wycombe, UK

Foreword Authors
Charlotte Beardmore
Executive Director of Professional
Policy, Society and College of
Radiographers
London, UK

Kori L. Stewart
Associate Professor of Diagnostic
Imaging & Director, Radiologic
Sciences Program, Quinnipiac
University
Hamden, CT, USA

Samar El-Farra
Vice President of RASE Emirates
Medical Society, Director – Institutional
Effectiveness and Accreditation
UODH, Dhaid, UAE

Edward H, T. Chan
President, Hong Kong College of
Radiographers and Radiation Therapists
Senior Lecturer, Hong Kong
Metropolitan University
Director of Professional Practice
International Society of Radiographers
and Radiological Technologists
Kowloon, Hong Kong

Patrick C. Brennan
Professor of Medical Imaging at
University of Sydney
Camperdown, NSW, Australia

ISBN 978-3-032-05079-3   ISBN 978-3-032-05080-9   (eBook)
https://doi.org/10.1007/978-3-032-05080-9

This Springer imprint is published by the registered company Springer Nature Switzerland AG
The registered company address is: Gewerbestrasse 11, 6330 Cham, Switzerland

If disposing of this product, please recycle the paper.

This book has been written with a lot of love, care, and mental effort, to reflect on what radiographers really need to know in relation to AI. The editors collectively dedicate this book to radiographers around the world. We hope the insights and guidance within these pages support you in your daily practice and help you embrace AI as a valuable tool to improve clinical service, research, and education, for patient, student, and practitioner benefit.

In addition, the editors would like to dedicate this text as follows:

Christina Malamateniou: *I would like to dedicate this work to Georgios, Katerina, Socratis, Christos, and Katerina, for teaching me every day the importance of love, learning, and love for learning. You are all my reasons.*

Maryann Hardy: *I would like to dedicate this work to all the future AI native radiographers…we had to start somewhere, and here is where we started.*

Karen M Knapp: *I would like to thank my family, friends, and the many mentors who have supported and believed in me over the years—thank you for always being there. To Christina, thank you for inviting me to be part of this project. It has been a truly rewarding experience, and I hope readers will enjoy this book as much as I have enjoyed contributing to it.*

Aarthi Ramlaul: *I would like to dedicate this work to my family for their unwavering support in all my publishing endeavours over the years. You are my inspiration.*

Foreword

It is both a privilege and an honour to write this Foreword for *Artificial Intelligence for Radiographers: Basic Principles, Clinical Applications and Implementation Considerations*. This landmark publication arrives at a time of unprecedented transformation for the medical imaging and radiotherapy professions. The integration of artificial intelligence (AI) into healthcare is no longer a distant prospect—it is an urgent, present reality that is reshaping the way we work, learn, and deliver care.

As radiographers, we stand at the intersection of technology, clinical practice, and patient-centred care. This role uniquely positions us to be more than just adopters of AI; we must be active participants in shaping its application, ethics, and integration into clinical workflows. Yet, for many practitioners, AI remains a complex and often misunderstood domain. This textbook provides a much-needed roadmap. It demystifies the core principles of AI, contextualises them within everyday radiographic practice, and offers practical, real-world case studies that highlight both the opportunities and challenges this technology presents.

The diversity of voices represented in this book—from radiographers, researchers, educators, vendors, policymakers, and patient advocates—makes it a uniquely valuable resource. The editors have ensured that the content is both academically rigorous and practically grounded, written not just for data scientists or engineers, but for the practising radiographer at the bedside, console, or classroom. Whether you are a student just beginning your career or a seasoned professional seeking to future-proof your skills, this book will equip you with the knowledge and confidence to engage meaningfully with AI.

From my perspective as President of the Hong Kong College of Radiographers and Radiation Therapists and as a Senior Lecturer at Hong Kong Metropolitan University, I see the growing demand for AI literacy among both students and practitioners. Across Asia and globally, AI is rapidly being embedded into radiology, radiotherapy, and imaging informatics. Educational institutions and professional bodies must ensure that the radiographic workforce is prepared—not only technically but also ethically and culturally—to thrive in an AI-enabled environment. This textbook makes a vital contribution to that mission.

Moreover, in my role as Director of Professional Practice at the International Society of Radiographers and Radiological Technologists (ISRRT), I am encouraged by the global collaboration that underpins this work. The book captures a truly international perspective, respecting regional diversity while promoting a shared vision: that radiographers, regardless of geography or role, can and should play a leading role in shaping the future of AI in healthcare. It reflects our profession's values—care, competence, integrity, and innovation.

I wholeheartedly commend the editors and contributors for their foresight, scholarship, and dedication. *Artificial Intelligence for Radiographers* is more than a textbook—it is a call to action. It invites all of us to engage with AI thoughtfully, critically, and with humanity at the centre. Let us rise to this challenge together, ensuring that AI serves not only the advancement of our profession but, most importantly, the wellbeing of the patients and communities we serve.

President, Hong Kong College of Radiographers   Edward H. T. Chan
and Radiation Therapists, Senior Lecturer
Hong Kong Metropolitan University
Director of Professional Practice
International Society of Radiographers
and Radiological Technologists
Kowloon, Hong Kong

Foreword

It is with great pride and anticipation that I introduce *Artificial Intelligence for Radiographers: Basic Principles, Clinical Applications and Implementation Considerations*. This textbook represents a landmark contribution to the field of radiography, offering a timely, comprehensive, and accessible exploration of Artificial Intelligence (AI) and its rapidly expanding role in imaging and radiation sciences. As AI continues to evolve and embed itself in clinical practice, education, and research, it is essential that radiography professionals everywhere are equipped with the understanding, confidence, and tools needed to harness its full potential. This book provides exactly that.

What sets this work apart is its unwavering focus on the real needs, voices, and contexts of radiographers worldwide. Rooted in radiographer-led research and guided by a collaborative spirit, it offers a roadmap for integrating AI thoughtfully and effectively into our daily professional lives. From foundational principles to cutting-edge applications, and from ethical considerations to implementation strategies, this textbook not only informs but empowers. It bridges disciplines, breaks down silos, and invites readers to become active participants in shaping the future of AI in healthcare.

The breadth of the renowned contributors—spanning continents, professions, and perspectives—is truly remarkable. Over 100 authors and collaborators, including clinicians, researchers, educators, patients, and industry partners, have shared their insights in a spirit of generosity and purpose. Their collective expertise weaves a rich tapestry of knowledge, and their diverse voices bring the AI ecosystem vividly to life. In an era where AI can either narrow or widen healthcare disparities, this book calls on us to co-design, critically engage, and advocate for technologies that serve people, enhance wellbeing, and respect the values of our profession.

At a time when healthcare systems are under immense pressure—grappling with workforce shortages, rising complexity, and the long shadows of the COVID-19 pandemic—AI presents both an opportunity and a challenge. As this textbook wisely acknowledges, AI is not a silver bullet, nor is it a distant threat. It is a powerful tool—one that can amplify clinical impact, improve decision-making, support resilience, and expand the reach of care. But only if we understand it. Only if we shape it. Only if we use it well.

I commend the editorial team for their visionary leadership, and I celebrate the fact that this book has been curated by a group of women in a domain where their voices are still underrepresented. The chapters are thoughtfully written, beautifully illustrated, and intentionally interconnected, reflecting years of pedagogical and practical experience. The use of real-world case studies, inclusive language, and a strong commitment to equity and patient-centred care makes this a truly groundbreaking resource.

Whether you are a student taking your first steps into the world of AI, an educator building curricula, a researcher exploring new frontiers, or a practitioner seeking clarity in a fast-changing landscape, this textbook will serve as your trusted companion. It marks a critical step forward for the radiography profession—not only in embracing technology but in leading its responsible, ethical, and meaningful integration into clinical care.

This is more than a textbook. It is a call to action, a collective voice of a global community, and a foundation upon which future scholarship and innovation will be built.

Vice President of RASE Emirates Medical Society   Samar El-Farra
Director – Institutional Effectiveness and Accreditation
UODH, Dhaid, UAE

Foreword

It is with tremendous enthusiasm that I celebrate this timely and essential textbook, *Artificial Intelligence for Radiographers: Basic Principles, Clinical Applications and Implementation Considerations*. As radiography enters a new era shaped by continued technological advancement, this work offers a much-needed foundation for comprehension, integration, and critical engagement with artificial intelligence (AI) in clinical practice.

The editors and contributors have curated a comprehensive and accessible resource that speaks directly to the evolving needs of radiographers. From foundational concepts in AI and radiomics to the ethical, governance, and implementation challenges we face, this textbook provides a roadmap for navigating the complexities of AI in medical imaging. Each chapter is thoughtfully constructed, offering both theoretical insights and practical applications across modalities including CT, MRI, ultrasound, nuclear medicine, and radiotherapy.

The inclusion of chapters on person-centred care, professional body perspectives, and future preparedness reflects a deep understanding that technology must serve, not replace, the compassionate, skilled, and patient-focused ethos of radiographic practice.

As an educator and researcher in medical imaging, health informatics, and patient-centred care, with a focus on emerging technologies, I am particularly encouraged by this book's commitment to empowering radiographers at all stages of their careers. Whether you are a student seeking to understand the basics, a healthcare professional exploring AI tools in your department, or a leader shaping policy and practice, this book will serve as a trusted guide.

I congratulate the editors and authors for their vision and dedication in bringing this important work to life. It is a significant contribution to the literature and will serve as a vital resource for the profession as we embrace the opportunities and responsibilities of AI in healthcare.

Associate Professor of Diagnostic   Kori L. Stewart
Imaging & Director
Radiologic Sciences Program
Quinnipiac University
Hamden, CT, USA

Foreword

Radiographers stand at the forefront of healthcare innovation, balancing advanced technology with the delivery of high-quality, compassionate, and personalised patient care. This textbook arrives at a pivotal moment for our profession, offering a timely and essential resource that explores the transformative role of Artificial Intelligence (AI) in imaging and oncology services. It is written for us, for clinicians, educators, researchers, and leaders who are navigating a rapidly evolving healthcare landscape and actively shaping its future.

AI is already influencing how we work, communicate, and deliver care. This book provides a clear, evidence-based overview of its integration into radiography, drawing on international expertise and real-world applications. It offers both practical insights and theoretical grounding, making it an invaluable guide for radiographers at every stage of their career.

More than a technical manual, this book is a call to action. Radiographers must lead the safe, ethical, and effective implementation of AI. Our expertise is vital in explaining AI to patients, supporting informed choices, and ensuring that technology enhances, not replaces, the human connection in care. Personalised care remains central to our practice. AI must complement clinical judgement, enabling tailored imaging and treatment pathways that meet individual needs.

The text highlights the importance of digital literacy, ethical decision-making, and leadership. It calls for new competencies within education and training programmes that reflect the changing demands of our profession. Whether you are a student building foundational skills or a practitioner driving service transformation, this book supports your journey.

Professional bodies and regulators play a crucial role in ensuring that education, training, and policy keep pace with technological, systemic, and personalised care advancements. The development of the entire radiography workforce is essential at all levels of practice and across all workplace settings. We must be equipped with the knowledge, skills, and attributes to lead service developments, contribute to research, and shape policy using our clinical insight.

A consistent theme throughout the book is the importance of robust AI governance. Structured knowledge sharing, collaboration across disciplines, and early involvement in research are critical. Radiographers must be active members of multiprofessional teams, applying human judgement and empathy to ensure safe, efficient, and evidence-based services.

This textbook also advocates for increased funding to support radiography-led research in AI, imaging, and oncology. It encourages publication in peer-reviewed journals and the sharing of expertise across the profession. Radiographers are the bridge between advanced technology and patient care, and with the right support, we can, as the text states, hold the "healthcare ecosystem together".

In summary, this book inspires, informs, and empowers radiographers to develop their skills, knowledge, and competence to safely embrace AI with confidence and clarity. By engaging with education leaders and acknowledging that ongoing skills development will be essential, we can lead innovation that strengthens our profession and improves patient outcomes. The book encourages us to move forward together as a radiography community, collaborating, adapting, and championing safe and effective evidence-based AI that supports innovation in care, and to enable the radiography profession to continue to enhance care delivered with empathy, expertise, and commitment to the people we serve.

CBE, FCR, Hon DSc, Hon MRCR,   Charlotte Beardmore
MBA (Open) DMS,
BSc(Hons) DCR (R) & (T),
Executive Director of Professional Policy
Society and College of Radiographers,
London, UK

Foreword

Artificial Intelligence (AI) is redefining the landscape of healthcare, presenting unprecedented opportunities and challenges for the radiography profession. As we stand at the intersection of tradition and technology, radiographers find themselves not only as implementers but increasingly as critical thinkers, innovators, and collaborators in the age of AI. The journey toward adoption is complex: it demands an open mind, a willingness to learn, and the continued courage to question.

Artificial Intelligence for Radiographers: Basic Principles, Clinical Applications and Implementation Considerations arrives at a pivotal moment. Around the globe, radiographers are navigating growing clinical demands and complexity, workforce shortages, and intensified burnout, all heightened by the lingering impacts of the COVID-19 pandemic. In this pressured environment, the promise of AI to bolster diagnostic accuracy, streamline workflows, and lessen the daily burden cannot be overstated. Yet, equally pressing are the new risks: widened healthcare inequities, potential for error, erosion of trust, and ethical dilemmas when technology is adopted uncritically or without the nuanced insight of frontline practitioners.

This textbook is both timely and necessary. Born from radiographer-led academic and clinical research, brought together by four world-class editors, and crafted by leading contributors spanning clinical, technical, academic, and professional communities, this body of work embodies the collective intelligence of the real-world AI ecosystem. Its creation was fuelled by a simple, urgent conviction: learning about AI from its basic principles through to its complex clinical applications and thorny implementation challenges is the key to harnessing its benefits and preventing its pitfalls within radiography. All the key modalities are covered.

What sets this book apart is its unwavering focus on practical understanding and collaboration. From professional and industry perspectives to organisational efficiencies and staff wellbeing, every chapter signposts actionable knowledge grounded in research and the lived realities of our profession. The book welcomes readers into the diverse languages of AI, from familiar clinical terminology to the innovative discourses of computer science, data ethics, biomedical engineering, and more. The sheer diversity of perspectives strengthens the message: successful AI is people-centred, not technology-centred.

As you engage with these pages, you are invited not just to learn, but to participate, question, critique, and contribute to the evolving field. Whether you feel AI is a familiar tool or a challenging new frontier, this book is your companion in shaping a future where technology truly empowers radiographers and supports exceptional, compassionate patient care. If there is a criticism it is that the title does not reflect the value of this text to those beyond the radiography profession. This is an immense book that will support all those with any involvement with medical imaging.

May this work inspire you to lead, innovate, and ensure that the future of radiography and indeed medical imaging enhanced by AI remains person-centred, safe, and rooted in the values of our professions.

Professor of Medical Imaging   Patrick C. Brennan
at University of Sydney
Camperdown, NSW, Australia

Prologue

Artificial intelligence (AI) as a notion has been around since the early 1940s, and has undergone many phases of development and refinement, trying to imitate human intelligence and human learning processes. In the 1980s it has even experienced the so-called "AI winter", where experts gave up the idea that AI would ever produce a meaningful impact for the improvement of human life, because it was impractical and too complex to work with. The development of faster computer processors, the big data revolution, the increasing understanding of how the human brain learns thanks to neuroscience developments, and the advent of deep learning in the early 2000s, all these have contributed to increasing confidence that AI can "jump" from the computer labs to the clinic.

In the last decade, since the early 2010s, AI has slowly but surely started to be integrated into clinical workflows. Medical Imaging, Radiology, and Radiography have been early adopters for different reasons. Medical imaging produces masses of data and AI needs that data to train models and identify patterns, from which it learns and can automate processes like image analysis. Medical imaging has also been one of the first clinical services to be digitalised, which helped data transfer and facilitated data analysis for early testing of AI models. Furthermore, radiologists and radiographers, as a workforce, are accustomed to rapid technological changes of software and hardware, and they are amongst the most technologically adept professions. All of these have made medical imaging the ideal testing ground for AI before other clinical disciplines, which now grow at pace.

AI has started to dominate radiographer professional discussions in the late 2010s, initially as a concern about future job security because of the speed tasks could be automated at. Different radiographer professional societies around the world have started to issue statements or conduct workforce surveys to understand this new "phenomenon", that was different from any other technological revolution recently experienced by healthcare professionals, to better understand it and support their members. AI is now being increasingly used to optimise medical imaging appointments and workflows, image acquisition and patient care, image postprocessing and reporting of scans.

The more we learn about AI, the more we understand not only its full transformative power but also potential risks, resulting from bias during the AI product lifecycle. If deployed correctly, AI can truly reimagine and reshape our healthcare systems, including radiography, and make them fairer, more inclusive, and improve both accuracy and efficiency for patient and staff benefit. It will, however, most certainly impact the ways we work with each other and with our patients. This will require a global rethink of how and what we learn as professionals, to deliver safe, efficient, and effective clinical services.

From early academic and clinical research, it has become evident that learning about AI, its strengths and limitations, will not only help us better accept it but will also enable us to codesign it for patient benefit, organisational improvement, and staff wellbeing. Learning about AI can help us shape it in a way that works for us and our patients. There is immense knowledge, talent, and ambition in radiography professionals around the world. So, we have written this AI textbook based on the findings of radiographer-led research in the field, to help everyone harness AI benefits, mitigate its risks, and help it reach its full potential within Radiography. We have never been too sceptical as a profession about new technology; why should this change now? AI is just another tool, a very powerful one indeed, that can help us navigate the increasingly challenging clinical cases we experience, address workforce shortages, minimise healthcare inefficiencies, improve staff wellbeing, and address burnout, which has only intensified after the COVID-19 pandemic, and brought many healthcare systems to their knees. If we learn about AI, we will use it appropriately. This is exactly why this textbook was created, and this is the rationale and vision it was written by; with the hope that knowledge and reflections stemming from reading it will help radiography practitioners embrace AI and work with it for a better, person-centred, future.

We hope you will enjoy the chapters lying ahead, from the introductory ones on AI history and AI methods (Chaps. 1 and 2), AI ethics and implementation considerations (Chaps. 3 and 4), person-centred care implications (Chap. 12) to the modality specific chapters (Chaps. 5, 6, 7, 8, 9, 10 and 11), and the chapters for the AI ecosystem (Chaps. 13 and 14). The final one (Chap. 15) considers everything and offers a perspective for the future of radiography with AI. We hope we can use these chapters to inform and advance your learning, as well as develop the learning of others, whether teaching in clinical practice or in an academic institution. We also hope this textbook highlights the many areas that radiography research needs to focus into the future, to ensure it not only develops the necessary evidence base but also expands our understanding of how we can harness this new technology to better serve our patients and students.

Preface

Early academic and clinical research in the field of AI led by radiographers has shown considerable gaps in our understanding of and confidence in working with AI. It has also highlighted that learning about AI, its strengths and limitations, and getting hands-on experience with it will not only help us better accept and integrate it but will also enable us to codesign it for patient and student benefit, organisational improvement, and staff wellbeing. Learning about AI can help us shape it in a way that works for us. There is immense knowledge, talent, and ambition in radiography professionals around the world. AI is another tool, that could help us navigate the increasingly challenging clinical cases we experience, address workforce shortages, minimise healthcare inefficiencies, improve staff wellbeing, and address burnout. AI can also magnify healthcare gaps, increase staff burnout—if adopted in a conveyor-belt style clinical model—spread misinformation, and even harm humans, if used incorrectly. Therefore, it is imperative we learn about AI, to use it appropriately.

Every chapter is connected to the rest of the textbook with direct signposting. A multitude of authors (more than 100, if we take into account the professional society and industry representatives who contributed Chaps. 13 and 14) of different professional backgrounds have painstakingly worked on it, everyone sharing their extensive expertise on paper and bringing their perspective from practice. It is this collective perspective that we would like to share with you all, and it is this collective intelligence of the real AI ecosystem that becomes alive through the pages of our textbook that we feel will help you learn the new "language" and the new ways that AI brings in healthcare and radiography. Some of these "languages", terms, and terminologies will feel acutely familiar to radiographers; this is because certain sections of the textbook were written by radiographers, radiologists, other clinical practitioners, or even public contributors and patient representatives, as relevant for the patient-centred care chapter, for instance. Other "languages", terms, or terminologies will require significant mental stretching; these might be the parts written by computer scientists, mathematicians, biomedical engineers, informaticians and IT consultants, business and management leaders, ethicists, AI governance and regulation specialists, lawyers, medical physicists, organisational management experts, or implementation scientists. We are grateful to them all for making the effort to make their writing more attuned to clinical practitioners without losing their unique identity and culture. We built a glossary to help you with this mental stretching and understanding of the different terms, to create a bridge across all different "tribes" of the AI ecosystem in medical imaging and radiotherapy, enough to be able to safely carry you to the "other side", and help you engage in new discussions, enquiries, learning, and growth.

This is a book with a global audience and authors coming from different parts of the world: Europe, North America, Asia, Africa, and Australia. We used the term radiographer as a simplification, but it was a much-needed convention given the area the editors and most of the chapter authors work and operate at. We appreciate that for parts of North America, Asia and some parts of Europe the term medical radiation technologist (MRT) is used instead. In other parts of the world the term medical radiation scientist (MRS) is employed. Within these there is a multitude of other more specialised terms to signify the radiography professional: sonographer, mammographer, radiotherapist, dosimetrist, radiation engineer, radiology nurse, nuclear medicine technologist, and many more, too many to be able to capture here. We do hope that despite this choice of using the term radiographer to represent all of the above, and the variation of educational cultures, clinical contexts, and national strategies for health, you will still be able to find yourself represented here, have your "aha moment" and recognise yourselves in the scenarios, case studies, enquiries, or calls for action we raise in this textbook.

We tried to make the book inclusive, diverse, and representative of the workforce globally. There are 24 male and 23 female primary authors. The four editors are all women and for a textbook on AI this is a unique reason for celebration, in a domain where only 22% of the recognised leaders are women. It is also about embracing the amazing contributions that each one of us can offer, because we can be better if we work together in unison, for the same cause. Interestingly, the chapter on patient-centred care was led by a man, and the chapter on AI methods was led by a woman: talking about breaking stereotypes here! We can all do anything with appropriate education and mentorship. We hope the newly qualified radiographers will feel inspired and help minimise this leadership gap in AI, working together for a better future that will be more inclusive and, most certainly, technology-enabled.

We are grateful to our chapter authors and the many contributors who helped bring together all this expertise and knowledge, which will more clearly define the body of evidence for AI in radiography. We hope this textbook can become the primary reading material for radiographers globally when it comes to understanding how AI works, how it can be applied, what its impacts are on clinical practice and workflows, what its benefits and risks are, and how we can shape it to work for us and our patients. Although our writing reflects on the fast pace of AI developments, so the book can be read comfortably for the next few years, we also appreciate AI changes fast, faster perhaps than any other technology we have so far experienced and faster than any book or written form of knowledge can really map out or fully grasp. We are confident, though, that this work will leave a permanent imprint on how AI started for radiography and other editors or authors in the future can build upon it to update it, and bring in the latest research and practice evidence. We like to see it as a timestamp, that puts radiography on the map of AI transformation and AI scholarship.

Each chapter was written with special effort to make it stand out as a unique piece of work, connected to the rest of the textbook. All chapters have the main text and associated images, and some include case studies, which are a way to bring to you real-life examples of AI to make complex notions simpler, more graspable, and hopefully, less abstract. Except for Chaps. 3 and 12, on ethics and patient-centred care, respectively, all case studies have a standard form, starting from the clinical challenge that is addressed with the respective AI solution, followed by the benefits and (if applicable) challenges stemming from it, and ways forward. Some of these case studies also include images to make their point, as required. Although we tried to optimise the writing to read as "one single voice", we quickly realised that this is neither feasible nor desirable; the different voices, tones, hopes, and concerns of clinical practitioners, scientists, professional body representatives, patients, and industry were retained, to ensure you can experience the authentic AI ecosystem, as it currently stands, and this is part of the learning.

The format and delivery of the textbook drew upon many years of educational, academic, research, and clinical experience of the editors and the rough structure of its content was based on the 7 years of teaching of AI and interacting with radiographer practitioners at the seminal "Introduction to AI for radiographers" CPD module at City St George's University of London, established and ran by the lead editor since 2019. The interaction, reflections, questions, and debates shaped the content, to make it relevant for and usable in radiography practice.

Some chapters are introductory or more generic, like 1, 2, 3, 4, and 12, and others are more specific, such as the modality Chaps. 5, 6, 7, 8, 9, 10 and 11. The following paragraphs will explain what each chapter is about.

Chapter 1 attempts to offer some history of AI and how we moved from symbolic AI to deep learning. Much of the historical elements explain why AI has taken the direction we see today. It also offers a rough introduction to artificial neural networks, the most commonly used AI models in current practice. Finally, it makes the important distinction of what is and what isn't AI, necessary in a world where everyone claims to be doing "a bit of" AI.

Chapter 2 is a chapter that gives you all the necessary theoretical underpinnings of AI and its little cousin, radiomics. This is a chapter we expect to be used a lot, because it can help provide seminal teaching notes for educators and support student learning for AI methods and principles. It includes different AI models and architectures, complemented with beautifully curated graphs so they are easy to understand and provide visual representations to complex topics. It also provides some insights into performance evaluation metrics for AI tools and discusses future approaches, including large language models and generative AI, which could revolutionise everything we know or do with AI.

Chapter 3 discusses the ethical challenges and potential solutions around AI use. It emphasises the importance of integrating both medical ethical principles (beneficence, non-maleficence, respect for autonomy, and justice) and specific AI-related ethical principles, from recent research in the field of radiography. Based on this information, the chapter also highlights the impact on professional identity and future competencies required for radiographers, for safe and effective clinical practice with AI.

Chapter 4 is an overview of AI in practice. It is necessary to read this chapter before reading any of the other modality-specific chapters in the textbook as it connects them all. It is also advisable to read it before you start implementing AI in your clinical setting, as it offers you a "one-stop-shop" for AI deployment. It provides unique insights on AI current use in radiography, the drivers, challenges, enablers, and impact of AI deployment in this field, the role of multidisciplinary teams and education in successful AI implementation and expands on related regulation and governance, with specific examples for different countries and geographies. It further discusses sustainability, reimbursement from the clinician's perspective, AI tool evaluation, including post-market surveillance, explainability, and introduces the idea of the limitations of AI, all necessary knowledge for optimal human-AI collaboration during deployment. There is a mix of theory and practice in this chapter, bringing the academic perspective and that of early adopters, as required, for a balanced view.

Chapters 5, 6, 7, 8, 9, 10 and 11 are the modality-specific chapters which take us through the current AI applications in the respective modality, following the patient journey: from appointments and booking, to image acquisition and optimisation, image analysis, post-processing, reporting, and quality assurance/quality control. The modality-specific chapters assume some basic modality expertise and knowledge. We do not discuss medical physics or processes from scratch, so please read them with this in mind. These chapters also discuss the benefits, challenges, and future uses of AI in projectional imaging (including plain X-ray and mammography), computed tomography (CT), magnetic resonance imaging (MRI), interventional radiography (including cardiology and medical imaging), ultrasound, nuclear medicine (and hybrid imaging), and radiotherapy (including, but not limited to, treatment planning). Each of these chapters uses carefully selected case studies, making specific effort to refer to a multitude of AI vendors for plurality and diversity of examples and optimal reader learning.

Chapter 12 might come as a surprise to some people, as they might feel that patient and person-centred care does not belong in an AI textbook. We feel it gives a holistic view of how AI can be used and implemented with human benefit at its heart. This chapter was co-authored by academic experts and people with lived experiences and was often led by the latter. It discusses principles of person-centred care, the challenges of patient care in an AI-enabled world and considers the importance of values-based practice and of coproduction techniques to elevate patient voice and choice. Finally, it brings together examples of four different case studies of AI deployment in patient care, underlining the perspectives of the patients themselves, their hopes but also concerns.

Chapter 13 may also be seen as unconventional, but we consider necessary for you all to meet the authentic AI ecosystem. We asked AI vendors to offer their perspectives of AI implementation in radiography, the advantages and disadvantages, and what needs to change to maintain the momentum of AI innovation despite the convoluted regulatory requirements, the lack of funding or robust reimbursement schemes, and complex clinical scenarios. The authors of this chapter come from an organisation that brings different vendors together, the AXREM (which stands for Association of Healthcare Technology Providers for Imaging, Radiotherapy and Care), and we felt this was a more balanced view that enabled diversity of perspectives whilst avoiding favouritism of some companies over others. They discussed innovation and commercialisation routes of AI and offered two distinct case studies to showcase how these could be materialised through academic or vendor-led initiatives. We hope this chapter will inspire all aspiring entrepreneurs amongst you to innovate with AI and help solve real clinical problems in radiography. Radiographers are uniquely suited and skilled to do this!

Chapter 14 brings together the global radiography community by integrating the current education, professional practice, and research initiatives led by the respective radiographer professional societies at a global level. There are links and signposting, as required and available, that demonstrate the increasing awareness of radiography professionals around the world about the big change that AI brings upon them, their practice, and expanding the knowledge base. We are excited and very grateful to all authors of the respective professional bodies and learned societies for sharing this expertise with us and with you, but also for their work to constantly support their members in this ever-changing, technology-enabled world.

Finally, Chap. 15 discusses the future of AI in radiography education, clinical practice, research, and the importance of partnerships and collaborations to navigate this challenging space with success and safety. It builds on the different chapters' discussions and on the expertise of the editors, offering a bold outlook for the future.

A *glossary* is also included in this textbook, to support you and the learning of the new language of AI, that will enable you to be part of the discussions and, hopefully, actions. A list of abbreviations is also provided.

We hope this textbook will enable you to rethink your radiography practice, design radiography research to improve AI use, teach others, innovate, be part of the future decision-making and healthcare solutions provision, for the benefit of the patients we care for, for the healthcare systems we serve, and for personal wellbeing and continued job satisfaction and pride in this AI-enabled work.

London, UK   Christina Malamateniou
Bradford, UK   Maryann Hardy
Exeter, UK   Karen M Knapp
High Wycombe, UK   Aarthi Ramlaul

Acknowledgements

- The Editors would like to thank the following people for providing the required images with permissions for various chapters:
  - Fiona Gray, Chris Wright, Dr. Alistair Piggot from Siemens Healthineers
  - Dr. Matthew Clemence, Jonathan Coupland, Robert Horner, Frederica Spalding from Philips Healthcare
  - Dr. Ilias Zapantis from UCL partners
  - Dr. Tim Horton and the Health Foundation
  - Dr. Dhruv Sahai from Carpl.ai
  - Drs. Clayton Taylor, Natasha Monga, and Mitva Patel from Ohio State University Medical Centre
  - Dr. Frank Pfister and Dr. Julia Moosbauer from deepc.ai
- The authors of Chap. 3, "Ethics of AI in radiography practice", would like to extend their heartfelt thanks to the colleagues from the ethics Work Package (WP) of the ELSA AI Lab Northern Netherlands for their invaluable contribution to this chapter. Their insights and expertise have greatly enriched our work.
- The authors of Chap. 4, "AI Governance and Implementation in radiography practice", would like to acknowledge the crucial support and contributions of graphs, images, tables, and know-how of the following people, who ensured the chapter was fully up-to-date: Dr. Kicky van Leeuwen, Stephan Romeijn, Dr. Hugh Harvey, Michael Pogose, Mélanie Champendal, and Professor Susan Shelmerdine.
- Shamie Kumar and Surabhi Srivastava of Qure.ai are thanked for offering the case study on lung cancer screening for Chap. 6.
- Koninklijke Philips N.V. is thanked for the use of Fig. 6.1 in Chap. 6.
- The authors of Chap. 12 would like to thank the following service user groups and named individuals for their contribution. The chapter was written in direct consultation with:
  - Service user groups: Health Voices Group, University of Suffolk, and Experts by Experience, University of Bradford
  - Named individuals: Adrian Radcliffe, Carol Johnson, Michael Andrews, Jean Gallagher, Shafiq Hussain-Ali, and Molly Kenyon
- Prof. Kevin Blythe, University of Glasgow, is thanked for the use of Fig. 13.2 in Chap. 13.
- We would like to thank the representatives from all the professional bodies who contributed to Chap. 14 and all named authors in that chapter for

helping disseminate the news of this textbook to their membership for maximum impact. We appreciate and value your input.

- The editors would like to thank the following people for their support in creating the further reading list to ensure the supplementary resources of the textbook were the most up-to-date in sync with the latest developments: Dr. Mike Klontzas, Dr. Burak Koçak, Dr. Renato Cuocolo, Dr. Elmar Kotter, Dr. Daniel Pinto dos Santos, Dr. Merel Huisman, Dr. Tugba Akinci D'Antonoli, Dr. Kicky van Leeuwen, Professor Susan Shelmerdine.
- The lead editor would like to thank
  - Collaborators from the CRRAG research group at City St George's University of London and Head of Department, Chris O'Sullivan, for practical support with flexibly managed workloads to ensure the timely completion of this textbook.
  - All students who attended the Introduction to AI for radiographers course since 2020 who inspired the learning outcomes, content, and writing style of this textbook.
  - All professional societies of radiographers and radiation technologists worldwide for embracing this effort practically, by contributing to Chap. 14, but also strategically, by disseminating the learnings of this textbook to a truly global audience.

Contents

Abbreviations

18F-FDG	Fluorodeoxyglucose (18F)
2D	Two Dimensional
3D	Three Dimensional
AAPM	American Association of Physicists in Medicine
ACS	AI-Assisted Compressed Sensing
AECs	Automatic Exposure Control
AI	Artificial Intelligence
AKI	Acute Kidney Injury
AIaMD	AI as a Medical Device
ALARA	As Low As Reasonably Achievable
ALARP	As Low As Reasonably Practicable
ANN	Artificial Neural Network
AR	Augmented Reality
ASD	Average Surface Distance
ASMIRT	Australian Society of Medical Imaging and Radiation Therapy
ASRT	American Society of Radiation Technologists
AUC	Area Under the Curve
AUROC	Area Under the Receiver Operating Characteristic Curve
AUTOMAP	Automated Transform by Manifold Approximation
BIR	British Institute of Radiology
CAD	Computer-Aided Detection/Diagnosis
CAD	Coronary Artery Disease
CADRA	Canadian Artificial Intelligence and Data in Radiotherapy Alliance
CAMRT	Canadian Association of Medical Radiation Technologists
CARO	Canadian Association of Radiation Oncology
CBCT	Cone Beam Computed Tomography
CDSS	Clinical Decision Support System
CE	Customer Engagement
cGycm	Gray-Centimetres Squared
CMR	Cardiac Magnetic Resonance (imaging)
CNNs	Convolutional Neural Networks
CNR	Contrast-to-Noise Ratio
COMP	Canadian Organisation of Medical Physicists
COPD	Chronic Obstructive Pulmonary Disease

COR	Clinical Outcomes Research
CORE	Clinical Outcomes in Routine Evaluation
CS	Compressed Sensing
CT	Computed Tomography
CTCA	Computed Tomography Coronary Arteries
CTI	Cap Thickness Index
CTO	Chronic Total Occlusions
DA	Discriminant Analysis
DCR	Dynamic Coronary Roadmap
DKD	Diabetic Kidney Damage
DL	Deep Learning
DLIR	Deep Learning-Based Image Reconstruction
DL-MAR	Deep Learning-Based Metal Artefact Reduction
DLR	Deep Learning Reconstruction
DNA	Deoxyribonucleic Acid
DRLs	Diagnostic Reference Levels
DSA	Digital Subtraction Angiography
DSC	Dice Score Coefficient
ECH	Electrocardiogram
ED	Emergency Department
EFRS	European Federation of Radiographer Societies
eGFR	Estimated Glomerular Filtration Rate
EHR	Electronic Health Records
EID-CT	Energy-Integrating Detector Computed Tomography
EL	Ensemble Learning
EU	European Union
EusoMII	European Society of Medical Imaging Informatics
FAST	Focused Assessment with Sonography in Trauma
FBP	Filtered Back Projection
FFR	Fractional Flow Reserve
FFR-CT	Fractional Flow Reserve Computed Tomography
FL	Federated Learning
FN	False Negative
FP	False Positive
FM	Foundation Model
FPR	False Positive Rate
FSI	Fluid–Structure Interaction
GAN	Generative Adversarial Networks
GMM	Gaussian Mixture Model
GPU	Graphical Processing Unit
GRAPPA	Generalised Auto-calibrated Partially Parallel Acquisition
GSPS	Grayscale Softcopy Presentation State
HCPs	Healthcare Professionals
HIT	Health Information Technology
HU	Hounsfield Units
ICA	Independent Component Analysis
iDL	Interpretable Deep Learning

iFR	Instantaneous Wave-Free Ratio
IGRT	Image-Guided Radiotherapy
IIRRT	Irish Institute of Radiography and Radiation Therapy
iMAR	Iterative Reconstruction/Algorithm for Metal Artefact Reduction
IMRT	Intensity Modulated Radiotherapy
ILD	Interstitial Lung Disease
IoU	Intersection over Union
IR	Iterative Reconstruction
ISO	International Organisation for Standardisation
ISRRT	International Society of Radiographers and Radiological Technologists
IT	Information Technology
IVUS	Intravascular Ultrasound
KBP	Knowledge-Based Planning
k-NN	k-Nearest Neighbours
LDCT	Low Dose Computed Tomography
LIME	Local Interpretable Model-Agnostic Explanations
Linac	Linear Accelerator
LLM/s	Large Language Model/s
LMMs	Large Multi-model Models
LPI	Lipid Percentage Index
LVMs	Large Vision Models
MAE	Mean Absolute Error
mCRPC	Metastatic Castration-Resistant Prostate Cancer
MDR	Medical Device Regulation
mGy	Milligray
MHRA	Medicines and Healthcare Products Regulatory Agency
MIRD	Medical Internal Radiation Dosimetry
ML	Machine Learning
ML (algorithms)	Machine Learning Algorithms
MLP/s	Multilayer Perceptron/s
MP	Myocardial Perfusion
MPVI	Morphological Plaque Vulnerability Index
MR	Mixed Reality
MRI	Magnetic Resonance Imaging
MRMC	Multi-reader Multi-case
MSA	Minimal Stent Area
MSE	Mean Squared Error
NCCTH	Non-contrast Computed Tomography Head
NET	Neuroendocrine tumours
NHS	National Health Service
NLM	National Library of Medicine
NM	Nuclear Medicine
NNs	Neural Networks
non-KBP	Non-knowledge Based Planning
O3	Operational Ontology for Oncology
OCT	Optical Coherence Tomography

O-MAR	Orthopaedic Metal Artefact Reduction
PACS	Picture Archiving and Communication System
PCA	Principal Component Analysis
PCC	Person Centred Care
PCD-CT	Photon-Counting Detector Computed Tomography
PCI	Percutaneous Coronary Intervention
PDP	Parallel Distributed Processing
PET/CT	Positron Emission Tomography/Computed Tomography
PET/MR	Photon Emission Tomography/Magnetic Resonance
PGMI	Perfect, Good, Moderate, Inadequate
PI	Parallel Imaging
PPV	Positive Predictive Value
PRO	Patient Reported Outcomes
PROST	Robotic System for Prostate Biopsy
PSNR	Peak Signal-to-Noise Ratio
qDESS	Quantitative Double-Echo Steady-State
RAKI	Robust Artificial Neural Networks for k-Space Interpolation
RASE	Radiographers Society of Emirates
RELAINCE	Recommendations for EvaLuation of AI for NuClear medicinE
ReLU	Rectified Linear Unit
RF	Random Forest
RIS	Radiology Information System
RMSE	Root Mean Squared Error
RNI	Radionuclide Imaging
RNNs	Recurrent Neural Networks
ROC	Receiver Operating Characteristic
ROI/s	Region/s of Interest
ROIS	Radiation Oncology Information System
R-PCI	Robotic-Assisted Percutaneous Coronary Intervention
RT	Radiotherapy
RUSS	Robotic Ultrasound Systems
SaMD	Software As a Medical Device
SC	Secondary Capture
sCT	Synthetic Computed Tomography
SENSE	Sensitivity Encoding
SHAP	SHAPley Additive Explanations
SLM	Small Language Models
SM	Statistical Modelling
SoPs	Standard Operating Procedures
SoR	Society of Radiographers
SORSA	Society of Radiographers of South Africa
SPECT	Single-Photon Emission Computed Tomography
SSIM	Structural Similarity Index
SURE	Stein's Unbiased Risk Estimator
SUV	Standardised Uptake Value
SVM	Support Vector Machine

T1w	T1 Weighted
T2w	T2 Weighted
TAT	Turnaround Time
TB	Tuberculosis
TCFA	Thin-Cap Fibroatheromas
TGA	Therapeutic Goods Administration
TID	Template ID
TN	True Negative
TOF	Time-of-Flight
TP	True Positive
T-PCI	Traditional Percutaneous Coronary Intervention
TPR	True Positive Rate
TTE	Trans-Thoracic Echocardiography
UI	User Interface
UNESCO	United Nations Educational, Scientific and Cultural Organisation
US	Ultrasound
VAEs	Variational Autoencoders
VBP	Values-Based Practice
VNA	Vendor Neural Archives
V-Net	V-Net, a volumetric network
VOI	Volume of Interest
VR	Virtual Reality
WBCT	Weight-Bearing Computed Tomography
WL	Window Level
WW	Window Width
XAI	Explainable AI
XOFF	Transmit Off
XON	Transmit On
XOR	Exclusive OR
XR	Extended Reality
ZTE	Zero-Echo Time

AI History and Basics: From Symbolism to Neural Networks

Constantino Carlos Reyes-Aldasoro
and Eduardo Alonso

1.1 Introduction

Artificial Intelligence (AI) is a multi-disciplinary research area that includes mathematics, computer science and engineering, psychology, neuroscience, philosophy and ethics. As such, it is difficult, even counterproductive, to try to define it categorically. Russell and Norvig [1] outline the main AI topics, namely, problem solving and search, knowledge representation and reasoning, and machine learning, along with applications such as computer vision, natural language processing and robotics. That is, machine learning (ML) is just one of the subfields of AI. In turn, deep learning (DL) is a special type of ML. To understand how they relate to each other, it is worth taking a brief look at the history of modern AI.

1.2 History of AI

Originally, the main approach to AI was what we call *symbolic*. Symbolic AI focuses on representing knowledge in a formal language (say, propositional or first-order logic), the axioms of the system, to which rules are applied to derive conclusions. Newell and Simon's Physical Symbol System Hypothesis [2], which posits that a physical symbol system has the necessary and sufficient means for general intelligent action, defined the symbolic approach in the first decades of AI, between the 1950s and the 1970s. It became clear soon, however, that most problems other than those applied to micro-worlds were intractable. To reduce the number of steps needed to calculate a solution, sophisticated heuristics were proposed; complementarily, machine learning algorithms were implemented to decrease computational complexity by finding patterns in the input. Notwithstanding the relative merits of such attempts, most AI problems remained (computationally) hard to solve. It was in the 1980s when a new, connectionist approach to building AI systems took shape—rather than manipulating symbols using pre-established 'if-then' rules to deduce new knowledge; such knowledge would emerge in a bottom-up manner through the interaction of networks of simple units. That is, rather than reproducing syllogistic reasoning, the emphasis was now on mimicking how the brain learns.

on behalf of Association of Healthcare Technology Providers for Imaging, Radiotherapy and Care (AXREM)

C. C. Reyes-Aldasoro (✉)
City St George's, University of London, London, UK
e-mail: Constantino-Carlos.Reyes-Aldasoro@city.ac.uk

E. Alonso
Artificial Intelligence Research Centre (CitAI), City St George's, University of London, London, UK
e-mail: E.Alonso@citystgeorges.ac.uk

© The Author(s), under exclusive license to Springer Nature Switzerland AG 2026
C. Malamateniou et al. (eds.), *Artificial Intelligence for Radiographers*,
https://doi.org/10.1007/978-3-032-05080-9_1

At this point, it is worth emphasising that 'symbolism' is still one of the main approaches in AI. Having said that, connectionist AI models are the tools prominently used in medical imaging and radiology, and hence, for the purpose of this textbook, we are proceeding with a cursory introduction of the fundamental concepts they are based on. Of course, there are other AI techniques, instantiated in expert systems and Large Language Models (LLMs) for conversational agents, for instance, that support clinicians as well.

However, before proceeding, let us advance a cautionary note: We tend to identify AI with technology. This is an oversimplification. Broadly speaking, there are four types of AI, which are differentiated by their respective goals and their relation to 'intelligence': (1) as simulation of intelligence, AI focuses on reproducing overt intelligent behaviour—epitomised by the Turing Test[1]; this is the approach followed by AI corporations that claim to outperform human competence in games, from IBM's Deep Blue to DeepMind's AlphaGo[2]; (2) AI serves also as models of intelligence, bridging the gap between reductionist neurophysics and pure associationism and positing computation as a valid representation of mental states and processes; (3) it is also a theory of intelligence, in that AI proposes mechanisms of 'thinking' (e.g. Universal Turing Machines[3]) irrespective of how humans do in fact think; and (4) finally, AI technology is just an efficient way of executing computational tasks that would require some sort of intelligence if performed by a human being (but is not inspired by nor tries to reproduce human intelligence). Such technologies can in turn be employed to solve problems in different sectors, for instance, health, transport, defence, energy or finances, and such applications do have huge socioeconomic impact, as well as posing ethical and legal challenges. However, they are not AI technology per se. In that respect, it is interesting to note the paradox that DL models of natural language processing simulate intelligent behaviour with no correlation to intelligent processing, whereas computer vision algorithms simulate intelligent processing of non-intelligent behaviour.

1.3   Artificial Neural Networks

Artificial Neural Networks (NNs) are a type of ML architecture that processes information through a 'hidden' layer and whose outputs are compared against a target. The goal of the NN is to minimise the error (loss function, also known as cost or objective function) between the output and the target for all training examples (Fig. 1.1). Once trained, the accuracy of the NN is assessed against unseen test datasets. More detailed information about other AI models and AI methods can be found in Chap. 2 of this textbook.

---

[1]Inspired in a Victorian parlour game, the 'imitation game' known as the Turing Test conjectures that if a human cannot determine via exchanging messages in a computer console whether they are interacting with another human or a machine, they must acknowledge that, be it a machine, the machine would be intelligent.

[2]Deep Blue was an IBM supercomputer that beat chess world champion Garry Kasparov in a six-game match in 1996. At the time, it was considered a milestone in the history of AI despite AI experts warning that Deep Blue's performance was due to massive parallelism and human feedback rather than by the computer's alleged 'intelligence'. In 2015, AlphaGo beat a human professional Go player. In this case, the achievement was uncontested: AlphaGo was a self-taught AI system, which, in addition, showed creativity in executing completely unexcepted winning movements. In must be noted that Go is much more complex than chess. At the opening move in chess there are 20 possible moves. In Go the first player has 361 possible moves.

[3]A Turing Machine (TM) is an abstract, hypothetical machine (not a physical computer) that serves as a model of computation: it consists of an infinite tape where symbols of a language are represented in cells; and a 'head' with instructions that manipulate such symbols along the tape, step by step. We can design a TM for a given function. In turn, we can simulate a TM, say TM1, with another TM, TM2, that would take as input TM1. Following the argument, we can build a Universal Turing Machine (UTM) that can simulate any TM. The Church–Turing thesis hypothesises that no human computer, or machine that mimics a human computer, can out-compute a UTM.

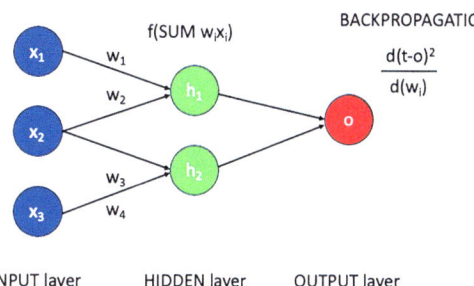

Fig. 1.1 A 'shallow' NN: A layer of normalised inputs is connected to a hidden layer. A non-linear activation function is applied to their weighted sum, and the result is fed to the output layer. The error between the outcome and the ground truth is backpropagated, the weights are adjusted using an optimisation algorithm and the process is iterated until they match

NNs like those depicted in Fig. 1.1 and other ML architectures, such as support vector machines or decision trees, are limited to well-constrained problems. Crucially, the drawbacks [3], namely, Perceptrons were unable to learn a specific type of mathematical functions, called XOR functions, were overcome by Hornik's proof that deep NNs could act as universal approximators [4] and the work on parallel distributed processing by the parallel distributed processing (PDP) Research Group [5]. Since then, increasing computational power provided mainly by Graphical Processing Units (GPUs), accessibility to large datasets and advanced learning techniques (ReLU functions, dropouts) have made DL very popular.

DL models [6] add multiple layers to simpler NNs (with one single hidden layer), enhancing their representational power. Rather than using hand-crafted features, DL defines hierarchies of layers that learn data at different levels of abstraction. For instance, from an unstructured dataset of pixels, a DL algorithm can learn first low-level features such as curves or shadows, then categories of increasing complexity, e.g. face, leg, tail and finally the concept itself, like 'CAT' or 'DOG'.

Most applications of DL to computer vision and thus medical imaging are based on a specific NN architecture: *Convolutional Neural Networks*

(CNNs) [7]. CNNs learn to extract relevant information in a similar way that we humans learn to group elements to make sense of visual input. CNNs are biologically inspired networks of convolutional and subsampling layers, including feature extraction (receptive fields that filter local features), feature mapping (weight sharing, which forces invariance) and subsampling (pooling). Using such techniques, CNNs exploit local correlation and enforce local connectivity patterns between neurons of adjacent layers. As a result, they transform low-level features (raw input) into compressed high-level representations. Figures 1.2 and 1.3 illustrate the basic steps in a CNN with a simple example taken from the analysis of two-dimensional data, such as image classification.

CNNs form the basis of Generative Adversarial Networks [8], which have become the standard DL architecture in many medical imaging applications. In short, a GAN is a generator model that is trained to generate new, increasingly convincing examples; and a discriminator model that tries to classify examples as either real (from the domain) or fake (generated), that is, it tries to distinguish candidates produced by the generator from the true data distribution. The two models are trained together in an adversarial (zero-sum) game until the discriminator model is fooled, meaning that the generator model is generating plausible examples. The generator is typically a deconvolutional neural network, and the discriminator is a convolutional neural network. Figure 1.4 depicts the process.

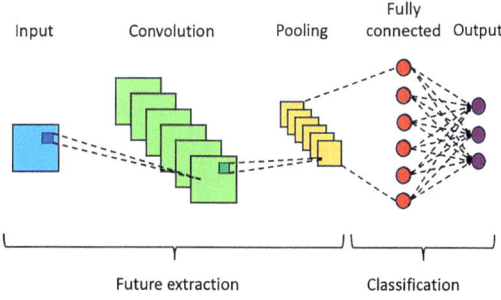

Fig. 1.2 A CNN architecture

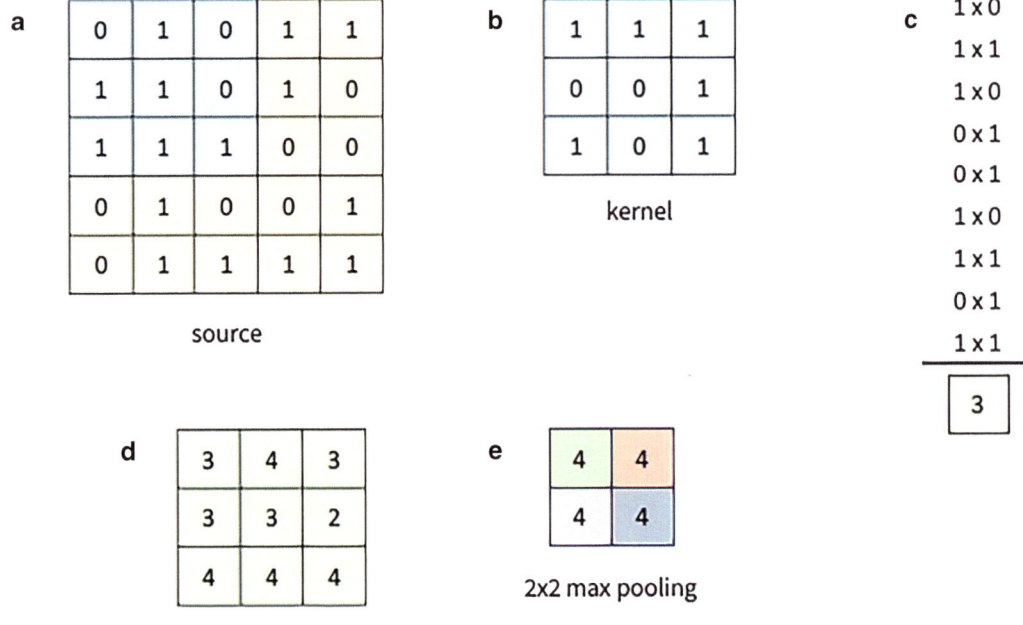

Fig. 1.3 Illustration of the computation process: (**a**) input data; (**b**) a 3 × 3 kernel (feature detector); (**c**) the kernel applied to the source, multiplying values element-wise and summing the result; (**d**) the resulting feature map obtained by sliding the kernel with a stride of 1; and (**e**) max pooling with a 2 × 2 stride to reduce dimensionality. A CNN is basically a network of multiple layers of convolving and pooling layers

Fig. 1.4 A GAN, where the generator learns to minimise its loss function via the feedback received from the discriminator. Technically, the generator learns to map from a latent space to a data distribution of interest until the discriminator thinks the novel candidates are not synthesised

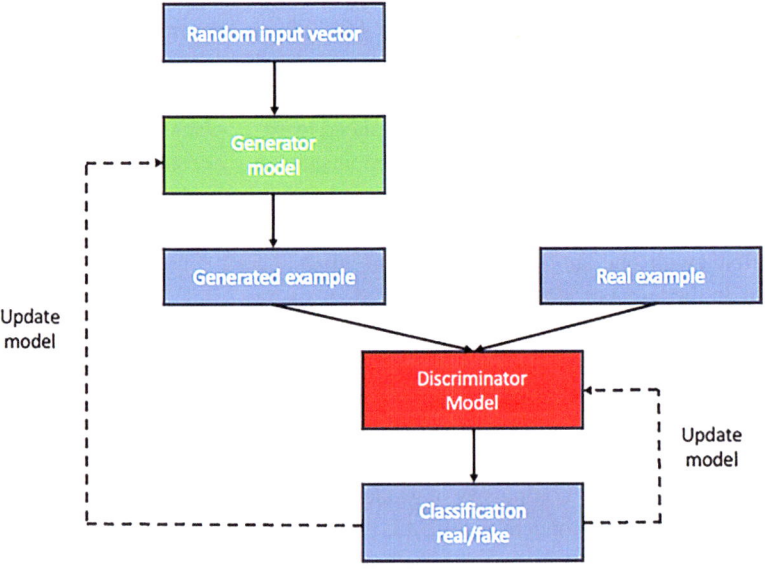

1.4   What Is and What Is Not AI

A key difference between AI and traditional techniques is the use of data to train architectures instead of a human-designed algorithm to process the data. For AI, a relatively large number of examples of the data to process, say X-rays of wrist fractures [9], are required in addition to a complementary set of 'labels'. Those labels are normally provided by a human expert, i.e. radiologists, radiographers and pathologists, and contain a decision or ground truth that will be used to train the architectures to reach a decision on new, unseen data. Since the images correspond to human patients, it is common practice to anonymise the datasets so that no individuals can be identified from the datasets. The case where the data and annotated labels exist is normally referred to as 'supervised learning' as there is an assumption that the annotations have been generated by experts in the area, say segmenting tumours [10] or classifying an X-ray into fracture or normal [11] and thus a 'supervision' of the process has taken place. The opposite situation, when there are no labels and no input from experts, is considered a case of 'unsupervised learning'. These cases tend to be more complicated as they will require extra steps, such as clustering or anomaly detection [12].

It is worth mentioning that within the context of medical imaging, computer-aided diagnosis or computer-aided detection (CAD) has existed for a long time and has been received with mixed results [13–15]. CAD refers to systems or tools that assist doctors in the interpretation of data with the purpose of increasing accuracy and consistency [16]. The methods underpinning CAD systems are diverse, ranging from traditional statistical techniques, pattern matching and probability theory [17] to, more recently, AI-based approaches [18–22].

1.5   The Future Trends of AI in Radiography and Radiology Through Data Mining

To identify the presence of AI in radiology and radiography, a mining of the National Library of Medicine's (NLM) bibliographic database Medline through the search engine PubMed (https://pubmed.ncbi.nlm.nih.gov/) was performed, as it has been previously described [23, 24]. PubMed was mined with a series of queries that combined keywords related to AI techniques, years of publication and the words Radiology or Radiography to ensure that the entries were specific to the area.

The specific keywords used were 'Artificial intelligence', 'ChatGPT', 'Computer vision', 'Convolutional neural', 'Deep learning', 'Expert systems', 'Generative adversarial', 'Machine learning' and 'Natural language processing'. It should be noted that the keywords are not exhaustive, and there could be others (e.g. *reinforcement learning*), but the ones selected are sufficient for an initial analysis of the area and trends. It should also be noted that some keywords only include two words when three or more are sometimes used, like convolutional neural networks or CNNs. However, when mining, any entry with the three words in that sequence would be retrieved with just those two, and these are specific enough and are words that are not used in the common language. Finally, it should also be noted that the entries may be retrieved with more than one of the keywords, so there will be duplicate counting of some entries.

The number of entries in PubMed for the keywords is shown in Fig. 1.5. During the period of study (1990–2023), the most frequently used keywords in the context of Radiology and Radiography were deep learning, followed by machine learning, artificial intelligence, convolu-

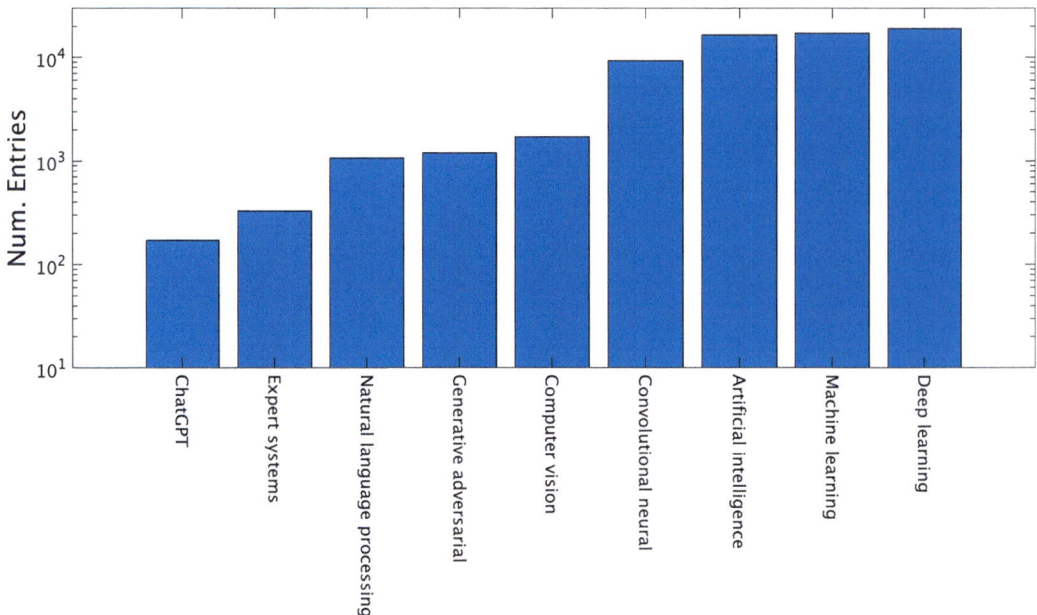

Fig. 1.5 Number of radiology/radiography-related entries and AI-specific keywords listed in increasing order (covering the 1990–2023 period)

tional neural, computer vision, generative adversarial, expert systems and ChatGPT. It should be noted that the vertical scale of the graph is logarithmic.

The analysis per year shows very interesting results, which are shown in Fig. 1.6. Here, the time is shown on the horizontal axis, and the entries related to each keyword are shown as a coloured ribbon. It is clear how some techniques have been associated with Radiology and Radiography entries in PubMed since the 1990s, and, with the exception of expert systems that have slightly decreased with time, all the others have increased, as would be expected. Notably, the increase in the frequency of deep learning,

convolutional neural and generative adversarial is much steeper than all others. The case of ChatGPT is also very interesting; even when it just appeared in the past year, it has grown incredibly fast. Whilst entries where natural language processing appeared since the 1990s, those that include ChatGPT will soon overtake many other keywords at the rate it has been growing.

Thus, from the trends shown in the graphs, it is clear that the future will include a variety of artificial intelligence tools, with possible combinations of those that focus on the radiographical images, like convolutional neural networks, and those that focus on language, like ChatGPT.

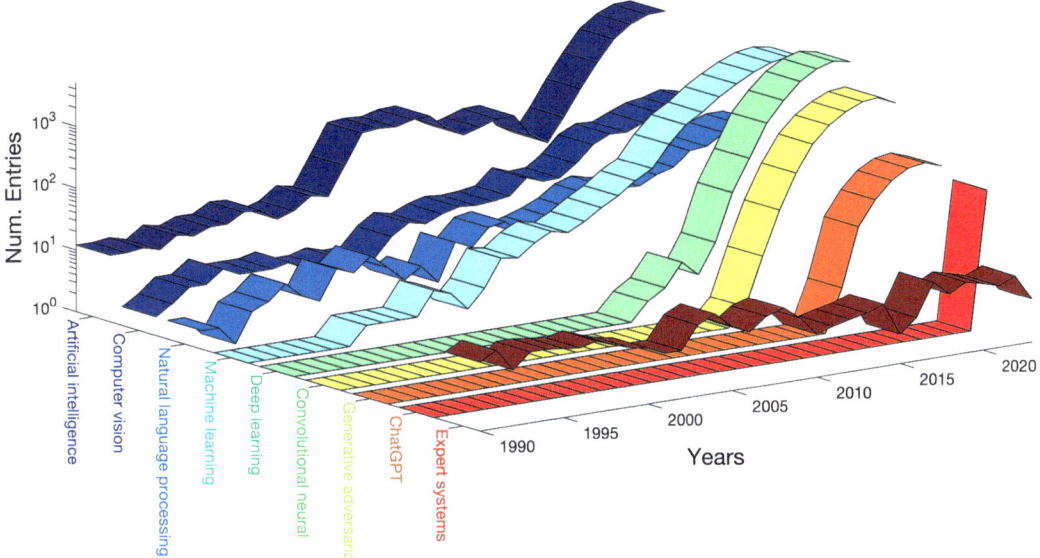

Fig. 1.6 Number of Radiology/Radiography-related entries and AI-specific keywords shown as yearly trends. Each ribbon corresponds to one keyword. 'Expert systems' is the only keyword that shows a slight decrease over time, whilst all others show an increase. Artificial Intelligence, Computer Vision, Natural Language pro-cessing and Machine learning have entries since the 1990s. The entries related to Deep Learning, Convolutional Neural, Generative Adversarial and ChatGPT are more recent and show a very rapid growth, suggesting that in future years, these will dominate the entries in PubMed. It should be noticed that the vertical axis is logarithmic

1.6 Chapter Summary

The presence of Artificial Intelligence is evident in many aspects of everyday life, from new mobile phones to AI-enabled image editing software. Thus, it should be no surprise that the fields of radiography and radiology will be strongly impacted by AI. Radiographers will need to engage with these AI-enabled tools, and therefore it is important to be, if not an expert, familiar and fluent with AI and many of its aspects.

References

1. Russell S, Norvig P. Artificial intelligence: a modern approach (4th edition) [Internet]. Pearson; 2020. Available from: http://aima.cs.berkeley.edu/.
2. Newell A, Simon HA. Computer science as empirical inquiry: symbols and search. Commun ACM. 1976;19(3):113–26.
3. Minsky M, Papert S. Perceptrons: an introduction to computational geometry. Cambridge, MA: MIT Press; 1969.
4. Hornik K, Stinchcombe M, White H. Multilayer feedforward networks are universal approximators. Neural Netw. 1989;2(5):359–66.
5. Rumelhart DE, Hinton GE, Williams RJ. Learning internal representations by error propagation. In: Rumelhart DE, Mcclelland JL, editors. Parallel distributed processing: explorations in the microstructure of cognition, volume 1: foundations. Cambridge, MA: MIT Press; 1986. p. 318–62.
6. Goodfellow I, Bengio Y, Courville A. Deep Learning [Internet]. The MIT Press; 2016 [cited 2023 Nov 30]. 800 p. Available from: https://mitpress.mit.edu/9780262035613/deep-learning/.
7. Goodfellow I, Pouget-Abadie J, Mirza M, Xu B, Warde-Farley D, Ozair S, et al. Generative adversarial nets. In: Advances in neural information processing systems [Internet]. Curran Associates, Inc.; 2014 [cited 2023 Nov 30]. Available from: https://papers.nips.cc/paper_files/paper/2014/hash/5ca3e9b122f61f8f06494c97b1afccf3-Abstract.html.
8. LeCun Y, Boser B, Denker JS, Henderson D, Howard RE, Hubbard W, et al. Backpropagation applied to handwritten zip code recognition. Neural Comput. 1989;1(4):541–51.
9. Reyes-Aldasoro CC, Ngan KH, Ananda A, d'Avila Garcez A, Appelboam A, Knapp KM. Geometric semi-automatic analysis of radiographs of Colles' fractures. PLoS One. 2020;15(9):e0238926.

10. Soltaninejad M, Yang G, Lambrou T, Allinson N, Jones TL, Barrick TR, et al. Supervised learning based multimodal MRI brain tumour segmentation using texture features from supervoxels. Comput Methods Prog Biomed. 2018;157:69–84.

11. Ananda A, Ngan KH, Karabağ C, Ter-Sarkisov A, Alonso E, Reyes-Aldasoro CC. Classification and visualisation of normal and abnormal radiographs; a comparison between eleven convolutional neural network architectures. Sensors (Basel). 2021;21(16):5381.

12. Marimont SN, Tarroni G. Anomaly detection through latent space restoration using vector quantized variational autoencoders. In: 2021 IEEE 18th international symposium on biomedical imaging (ISBI) [Internet]. 2021 [cited 2024 Sep 24]. p. 1764–7. Available from: https://ieeexplore.ieee.org/abstract/document/9433778.

13. Steward D. What is computer-aided diagnosis? Semin Vet Med Surg Small Anim. 1996;11(2):74–84.

14. Sutton GC. Computer-aided diagnosis: a review. Br J Surg. 1989;76(1):82–5.

15. Takahashi R, Kajikawa Y. Computer-aided diagnosis: a survey with bibliometric analysis. Int J Med Inform. 2017;101:58–67.

16. Doi K, MacMahon H, Katsuragawa S, Nishikawa RM, Jiang Y. Computer-aided diagnosis in radiology: potential and pitfalls. Eur J Radiol. 1999;31(2):97–109.

17. Yanase J, Triantaphyllou E. A systematic survey of computer-aided diagnosis in medicine: past and present developments. Expert Syst Appl. 2019;138:112821.

18. Chan HP, Hadjiiski LM, Samala RK. Computer-aided diagnosis in the era of deep learning. Med Phys. 2020;47(5):e218–27.

19. Kim EE. Artificial intelligence and computer-aided diagnosis in medicine. Curr Med Imaging Rev. 2020;16(1):1.

20. Malamateniou C, Knapp KM, Pergola M, Woznitza N, Hardy M. Artificial intelligence in radiography: where are we now and what does the future hold? Radiography. 2021;27:S58–62.

21. Mitsala A, Tsalikidis C, Pitiakoudis M, Simopoulos C, Tsaroucha AK. Artificial intelligence in colorectal cancer screening, diagnosis and treatment. A new era. Curr Oncol. 2021;28(3):1581–607.

22. Niazi MKK, Parwani AV, Gurcan MN. Digital pathology and artificial intelligence. Lancet Oncol. 2019;20(5):e253–61.

23. Reyes-Aldasoro CC. Modelling the tumour microenvironment, but what exactly do we mean by "model"? Cancer. 2023;15(15):3796.

24. Reyes-Aldasoro CC. The proportion of cancer-related entries in PubMed has increased considerably; is cancer truly "the emperor of all maladies"? PLoS One. 2017;12(3):e0173671.

Dr. Constantino Carlos Reyes-Aldasoro (MEng Mechanical and Electrical Engineering, UNAM, Mexico, MSc in Electrical Engineering, Imperial College, UK, PhD in Computer Science, Warwick, UK) is an interdisciplinary scientist with interest in Computer Science, Engineering and Life Sciences, in particular, to improve human health through the application of computational algorithms and imaging techniques to analyse biomedical data. He is the author of one book (Biomedical Image Analysis Recipes in Matlab, Wiley, 2015) and more than 80 peer-reviewed journal papers and numerous conferences. He is academic editor of *PLOS ONE, Journal of Imaging, ImmunoInformatics* and has served in the executive committees of the British Association for Cancer Research, Institute of Engineering and Technology Vision and Imaging Network, Royal Microscopical Society, Digital Analysis in Imaging.

Professor Eduardo Alonso is a professor in Artificial Intelligence and Director of the Artificial Intelligence Research Centre (CitAI) at City St George's, University of London. He has published over 100 peer-reviewed papers in top journals and contributed to several AI books (e.g. *The Cambridge Handbook of Artificial Intelligence*). He has been member of the Organizing and Programme Committees of the most reputed AI events, such as the International Joint Conferences on Artificial Intelligence (IJCAI) and the International Conference on Autonomous Agents and Multiagent Systems (AAMAS). He acted as vice-chair of the British Society for the Study of Artificial Intelligence and the Simulation of Behaviour (AISB). He is a member of the UK Engineering and Physical Sciences Research Council Peer Review College.

AI Methods: Understanding AI Models, Radiomic Analysis and Performance Metrics in Medical Imaging

2

Irina Grigorescu, Nouf A. Mushari, Charalampos Tsoumpas, and Maria Deprez

2.1 Introduction

Artificial Intelligence (AI) is one of the most cutting-edge fields in science and technology today. While there is no universally accepted definition of the term *artificial intelligence* [1, 2], most definitions converge on the idea of developing computer systems capable of performing tasks that traditionally require human intelligence, such as problem-solving, decision-making, and pattern recognition [3]. Originally coined in 1956 by a team of scientists led by John McCarthy [1, 4, 5], AI has since become ubiquitous, transforming industries such as healthcare, finance, transporta-

tion, and entertainment, by analysing large amounts of data, uncovering patterns, and leveraging these insights to make predictions, automate actions, and offer solutions [1, 3].

When reading about AI in news articles or research publications, it is common to encounter the terms Machine Learning (ML) and Deep Learning (DL). These terms are often used interchangeably with AI, despite referring to different concepts. Understanding the relationship between AI, ML, and DL is important, as they describe different levels of complexity and specialisation within the broader field of *artificial intelligence*.

AI is the broadest of these concepts (see Fig. 2.1). It refers to any computer system or algorithm capable of performing tasks that would normally require human intelligence. More generally, Russell et al. [1] define AI as "*the quest for the best agent program on a given architecture*", shifting focus away from mimicking human intelligence to emphasising the ability of an AI system to act as though it were intelligent (i.e. simulate intelligence). As such, tasks like problem-solving, decision-making, speech recognition, autonomous driving, image analysis, and recommendation systems all fall under the umbrella of AI.

ML, on the other hand, is a subset of AI. Originally coined in 1959 by Arthur Samuel [6], ML refers to the method of teaching computers to learn from data without being explicitly programmed for every task. In traditional programming, humans provide the logic or rules for

on behalf of Association of Healthcare Technology Providers for Imaging, Radiotherapy and Care (AXREM)

I. Grigorescu (✉) · M. Deprez
King's College London, London, UK
e-mail: irina.grigorescu@kcl.ac.uk;
maria.deprez@kcl.ac.uk

N. A. Mushari
Leeds Institute of Cardiovascular and Metabolic Medicine, University of Leeds, Leeds, UK

Radiological Sciences Department, Taif University, Taif, Saudi Arabia
e-mail: namushari@tu.edu.sa

C. Tsoumpas
Leeds Institute of Cardiovascular and Metabolic Medicine, University of Leeds, Leeds, UK

University Medical Center Groningen, University of Groningen, Groningen, The Netherlands
e-mail: c.tsoumpas@umcg.nl

© The Author(s), under exclusive license to Springer Nature Switzerland AG 2026
C. Malamateniou et al. (eds.), *Artificial Intelligence for Radiographers*,
https://doi.org/10.1007/978-3-032-05080-9_2

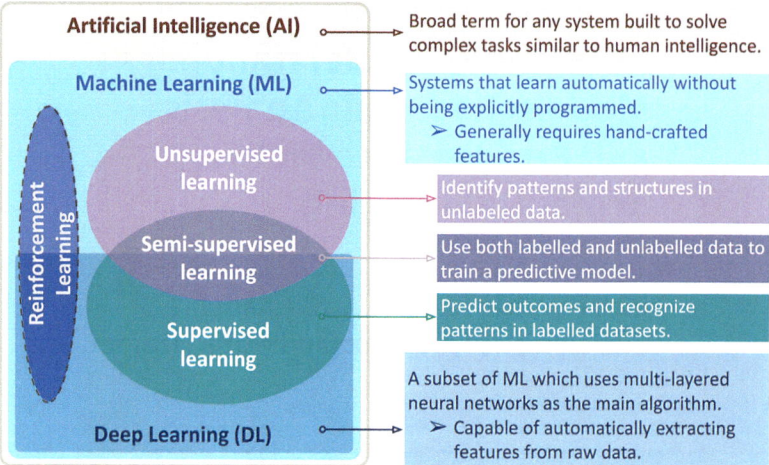

Fig. 2.1 Diagram illustrating the relationships between Artificial Intelligence (AI), Machine Learning (ML), and Deep Learning (DL). DL is shown as a specialised subset of ML, which in turn is a subset of AI. The diagram also highlights how the three main types of learning paradigms (supervised/unsupervised/semi-supervised) are integral to both ML and DL. A separate learning strategy called Reinforcement Learning (RL) is also included for the sake of completeness; however, its outline is dotted to indicate that it will not be covered in this chapter

solving a problem, but in ML, the system learns the rules and patterns from the data itself.

Finally, DL is a specialised subset of ML that uses multi-layered artificial neural networks (ANNs) to model and analyse complex patterns in data. They are called "deep" because of the multiple layers (input, hidden, and output) of nodes within these networks, each layer transforming data to extract increasingly complex representations for specific tasks [7]. Unlike traditional ML algorithms, which often require separate steps for feature extraction, DL models can automatically learn features from raw data, making them particularly effective for advanced tasks such as image recognition and natural language processing (see Fig. 2.2). The term "deep learning" was coined in 2006 by Geoffrey Hinton, who is often referred to as one of the "Godfathers

of Deep Learning" [8], and it is often behind modern breakthroughs in AI like AlphaFold [9] and ChatGPT[1] [10].

The key differences between Artificial Intelligence (AI), Machine Learning (ML), and Deep Learning (DL) are summarised in Fig. 2.1. For the remainder of this chapter, the focus will primarily be on ML and DL, examining the primary learning paradigms, exploring the most commonly used algorithms and models, and highlighting some of the cutting-edge approaches currently being researched and developed. For a more comprehensive understanding of ML and DL, we advise the readers to consult the following resources [11–13].

---

[1]https://openai.com/blog/chatgpt/

TRADITIONAL MACHINE LEARNING

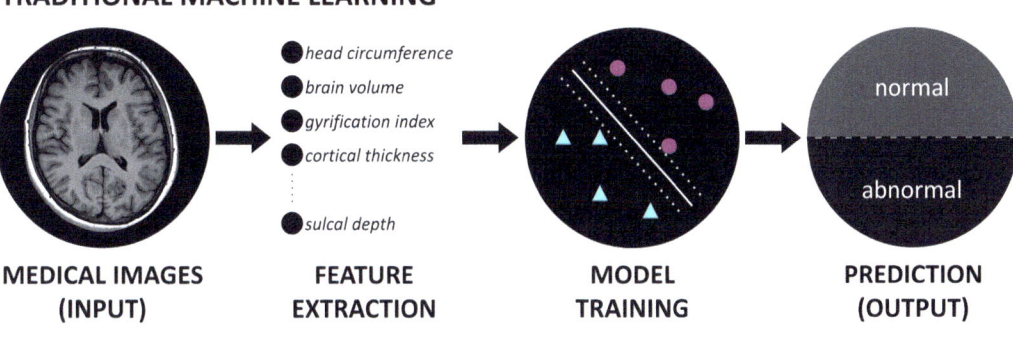

| MEDICAL IMAGES (INPUT) | FEATURE EXTRACTION | MODEL TRAINING | PREDICTION (OUTPUT) |

DEEP LEARNING

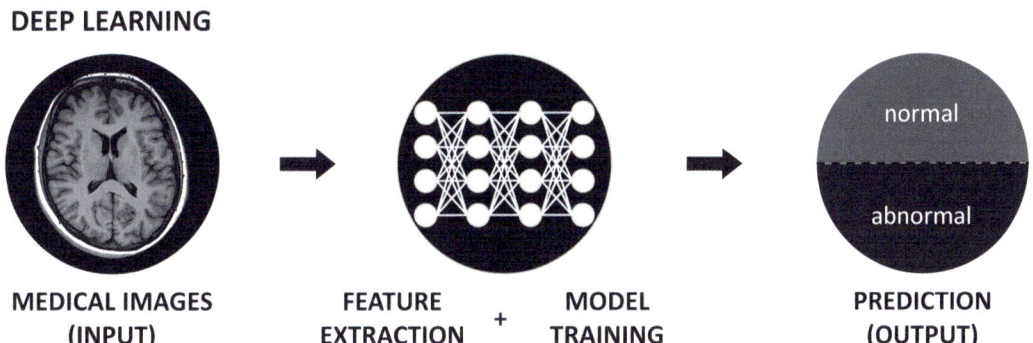

| MEDICAL IMAGES (INPUT) | FEATURE EXTRACTION + MODEL TRAINING | PREDICTION (OUTPUT) |

Fig. 2.2 Traditional ML algorithms (top) often require separate steps for feature extraction, while DL models can automatically learn features from raw data (bottom)

2.2 Types of Learning Methods

A common taxonomy for both ML and DL models is to group them by the type of learning method. Broadly speaking, there are four main categories (supervised, unsupervised, semi-supervised, and reinforcement learning), which we discuss here (see Fig. 2.3).

In supervised learning, the algorithm learns from a labelled dataset, meaning that each input has a corresponding output (the "correct" answer). The goal is for the model to make predictions based on this training data. Specifically, a machine or deep learning model trained in a supervised way aims to approximate the functional relationship between the provided data (features) and its corresponding labels (target values). Two of the fundamental tasks of supervised learning are regression and classification. In regression, the goal is to predict a continuous

numerical value based on some features, such as predicting brain volume from a neonate's gestational age at scan [14, 15]. In classification, the aim is to predict a discrete category (or class) based on some input data. Examples of this include diagnosing a tumour as benign or malignant [16], or classifying a computed tomography (CT) scan as normal or abnormal [17, 18]. Segmentation models can be seen as specialised classification models that extend traditional classification tasks to operate at the pixel (voxel) level, assigning a class label to each pixel (voxel) in an image [19]. For example, segmentation models can be used to delineate different tissue types or identify lesions in brain MRI [20, 21].

Supervised learning algorithms can produce highly accurate results given sufficient labelled data and can be continuously updated with new data to enhance performance over time [22]. However, supervised learning has its limitations,

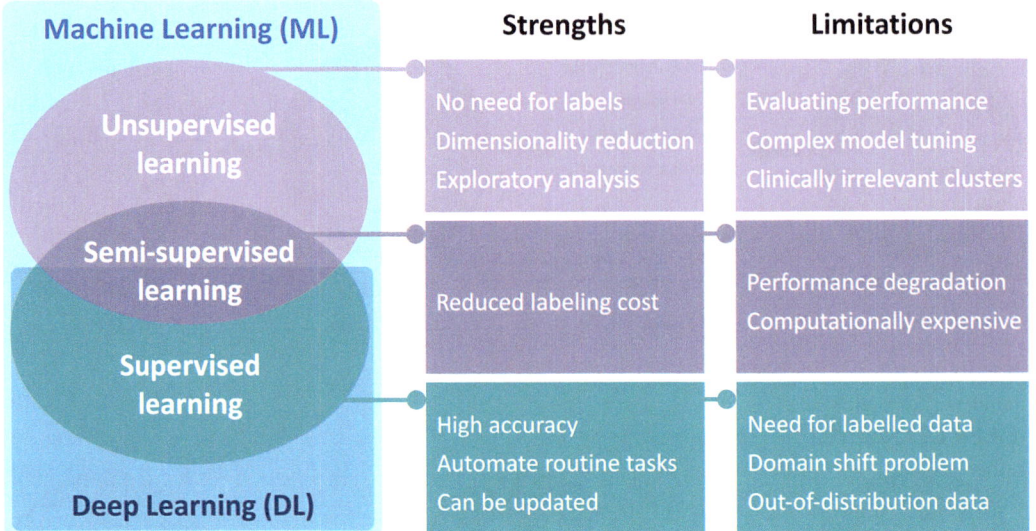

Fig. 2.3 Strengths and limitations of supervised, unsupervised, and semi-supervised models

such as the time-consuming task of obtaining accurate, reliable, and high-quality labels required for training [23]. Moreover, these models are generally susceptible to performance degradation when the test data differs significantly from the training data (e.g. if the model was trained on T2-weighted (T2w) brain MRI, it will not perform well when applied on a T1-weighted (T1w) contrast) [24].

In unsupervised learning, the algorithm is given data without explicit labels. The model must find patterns, structures, or relationships in the data on its own, without being told what the "correct" output should be. Specifically, in unsupervised problems, the training data is still characterised by a set of features, but as the outputs are not known, the model looks for hidden patterns or structures in the data. Some common approaches include clustering and dimensionality reduction.

In clustering, the aim is to partition the data into a predefined number of groups based on a criterion, such that there is good internal cohesion within the clusters, while also having good separation between the clusters [14]. An example of this is brain MRI segmentation, where the algorithm clusters voxel intensities based on similarity, grouping voxels of the same tissue type

(e.g. grey matter) together while distinguishing them from those of other tissue types, such as white matter or cerebrospinal fluid [25]. Dimensionality reduction aims to reduce the number of features in high-dimensional ML tasks, while preserving important characteristics of the data. It can be used for improving visualisation, reducing computational cost, or as a preprocessing step for other ML tasks [14].

Unsupervised learning algorithms have some limitations, one of which is the difficulty in validating their predictions due to the lack of labelled data. Additionally, these algorithms often depend on the selection of certain input parameters (hyperparameters), such as determining the number of clusters to group the data into. This can be time-consuming and challenging, especially in the absence of clear criteria for making these decisions.

Semi-supervised learning is an approach that combines both labelled and unlabelled data to train machine learning models. In this method, only a small portion of the dataset is annotated with ground truth (e.g. manually segmented medical scans), while the majority remains unlabelled. This strategy is particularly valuable in medical imaging, where obtaining labelled data is time-consuming and costly [26]. However, its effectiveness depends on the quality and representativeness of the unlabelled data, i.e. if the distribution of unlabelled samples differs significantly from the labelled ones, model performance can degrade [27]. Moreover, semi-supervised learning often requires careful algorithmic tuning and assumptions about the structure of the data, which can be particularly challenging in complex medical imaging applications [26, 28].

Finally, reinforcement learning is a unique paradigm within ML and DL whose goal is to achieve the maximum expected cumulative reward through interaction with the environment rather than from labelled datasets or patterns. Reinforcement learning is out of scope for this chapter, but for interested readers the following resources can be consulted [29, 30].

2.3 The Machine Learning Workflow

Developing an ML or DL solution for medical imaging applications requires a well-defined workflow. This is to ensure that the final algorithm is accurate and reliable and can be applied to real-world clinical scenarios. In this section, we outline an eight-step process that one may need to go through to produce a successful solution [31]. These steps are summarised in Fig. 2.4.

First, the objective needs to be clearly defined, as well as its clinical relevance. For example, predicting the age at birth of a neonate from brain MRI scans calls for a regression task, while predicting whether the neonate was born on term or preterm requires a classification-type algorithm. Moreover, as for every research project, the per-

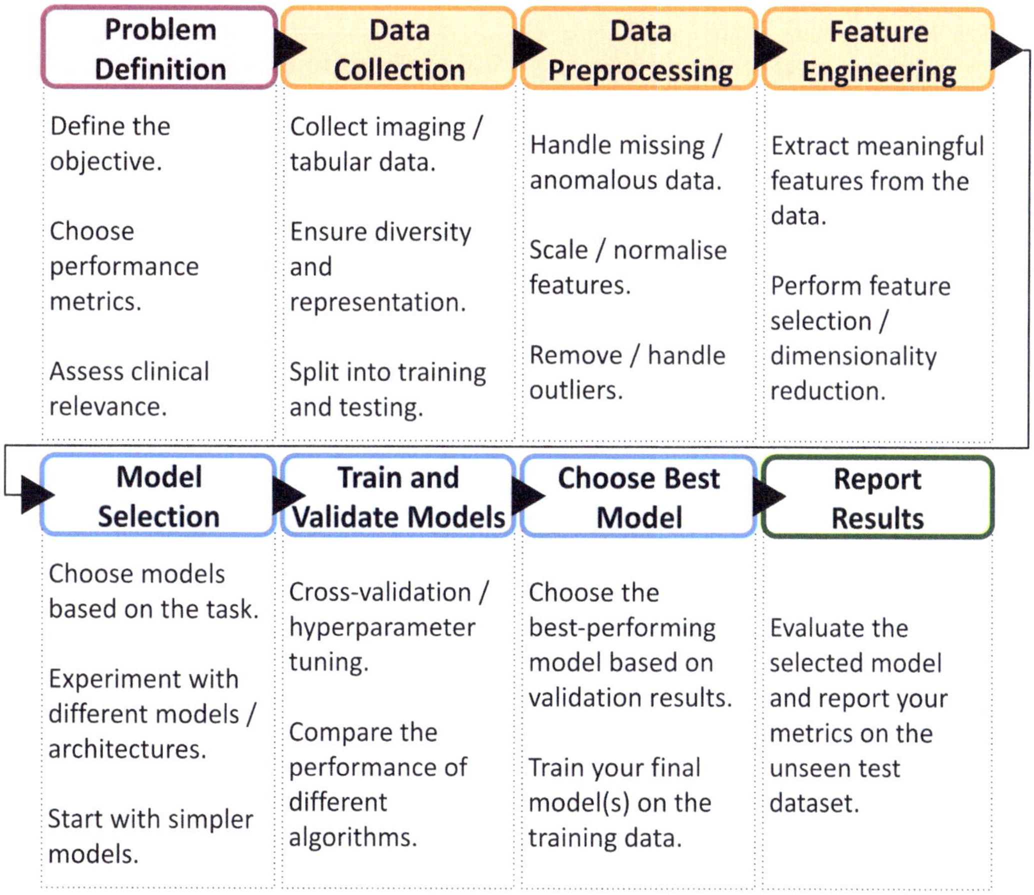

Problem Definition	Data Collection	Data Preprocessing	Feature Engineering
Define the objective.	Collect imaging / tabular data.	Handle missing / anomalous data.	Extract meaningful features from the data.
Choose performance metrics.	Ensure diversity and representation.	Scale / normalise features.	Perform feature selection / dimensionality reduction.
Assess clinical relevance.	Split into training and testing.	Remove / handle outliers.	

Model Selection	Train and Validate Models	Choose Best Model	Report Results
Choose models based on the task.	Cross-validation / hyperparameter tuning.	Choose the best-performing model based on validation results.	Evaluate the selected model and report your metrics on the unseen test dataset.
Experiment with different models / architectures.	Compare the performance of different algorithms.	Train your final model(s) on the training data.	
Start with simpler models.			

Fig. 2.4 The machine learning workflow

formance metrics should be chosen in accordance with the task [31].

Once the problem has been defined, the data collection should commence. Often, these two first steps are swapped or intertwined, but it is important to note that for a successful ML project the type of data will dictate what algorithm should be chosen (e.g. tabular data vs. imaging data vs. time-series data), while its diversity will ensure the models will be able to generalise well and not overfit to a sub-sample of the population (this occurs when a model learns the noise and specific details of the training data rather than the underlying pattern, at the expense of its ability to generalise to unseen data) [32]. At this step, it is also important to split the data into training and testing. All of the subsequent model training and validation should be done only on the training data, while the final model results should be reported on the test dataset [33].

Most ML algorithms require some form of data preparation, such as handling missing [34] or outlier data points, scaling and normalising, and standardising image resolution, intensity, and orientation. For more traditional ML algorithms (see Fig. 2.2), feature engineering is also required. This could entail extracting meaningful features from the data, either through derived/summary statistics or by using pre-existing feature extractors. Feature selection can also be used here to reduce dimensionality of the data and extract the most important features or dimensions.

Once the data is prepared, we can start looking into choosing the most appropriate ML algorithms, based on the task (regression vs. classification, image vs. tabular data) [33]. Experiment with simpler models first (e.g. linear/logistic regression for tabular data, convolutional neural networks (CNNs) for imaging data) to establish a baseline before moving to more complex methods, then try different algorithms and architectures of neural networks [31].

When training ML models, it is important to avoid overfitting, and this is commonly achieved by using a separate validation set, extracted from the training data, to evaluate performance and guide decisions such as hyperparameter tuning (parameters set before training, such as the num-

ber of layers in a neural network or the amount of regularisation) or model selection. Additionally, data augmentation is widely used as a regularisation technique to further improve generalisation. By generating new training instances through transformations such as adding noise, adjusting image intensity (e.g. brightness, saturation, contrast), or applying random affine transformations (e.g. rotation, translation, scaling, shearing), data augmentation effectively increases dataset diversity without requiring additional labelled data [35, 36].

Once the best-performing model and its hyperparameters have been chosen, it is trained on the entire training dataset, incorporating data augmentation as needed to enhance robustness. Finally, the selected model is evaluated on the test dataset to assess its performance on unseen data [31, 33].

2.4   Traditional Machine Learning Algorithms

In this section, we discuss machine learning algorithms which fall under the traditional ML umbrella (see Fig. 2.2, top), where feature extraction is done a priori to applying the models [37, 38]. We split the algorithms by the supervised vs. unsupervised taxonomy. The models described here are summarised in Table 2.1 and Fig. 2.5.

2.4.1   Supervised ML Models

In supervised learning, the model aims to approximate a functional relationship between input data (features) and known ("ground truth") output data (targets) [37]. Some of the most common algorithms for achieving this are explained here.

Linear models assume a linear relationship between input features and target variables and are often used as baselines due to their simplicity and interpretability [39]. Linear regression predicts continuous outcomes, while logistic regression handles classification tasks [40]. Regularisation techniques like ridge regression (L2 penalty) and lasso regression (L1 penalty)

Table 2.1 Popular ML algorithms grouped by the type of learning (supervised vs. unsupervised)

	Algorithm		Task	Advantages	Disadvantages
Supervised ML models	Linear models	*Logistic regression*	C	Simple to implement and interpret	Assumes a linear relationship
		Linear regression	R		
		Ridge regression	R	Helps mitigate multicollinearity	Does not perform variable selection
		Lasso regression		Performs feature selection	Can become unstable when there are highly correlated features
	Support Vector Machines (SVM)		R+C	Effective in high-dimensional spaces	Sensitive to the choice of kernel and hyperparameters
	Decision Trees		R+C	Easy to understand and interpret	Can easily overfit the training data
	Ensemble Methods		R+C	Reduces the risk of overfitting compared to individual decision trees	Requires more computational resources for training and prediction
	K-Nearest Neighbours (kNN)		C	Simple to implement and intuitive	Sensitive to the choice of K and distance metric
Unsupervised ML models	K-Means Clustering		CL	Simple to implement and efficient for large datasets	Assumes clusters are convex and isotropic, sensitive to initialisation
	Gaussian Mixture Models (GMM)		CL	Can model clusters with different shapes and sizes	Sensitive to initialisation
	Principal Component Analysis (PCA)		DR	Reduces the number of features while retaining most of the variance	Assumes linear relationships among features
	Independent Component Analysis (ICA)		DR	Effective in separating mixed signals	Sensitive to noise and requires careful pre-processing of data

R regression, *C* classification, *CL* clustering, *DR* dimensionality reduction

are applied to prevent overfitting by penalising large coefficients. Ridge regression shrinks coefficients to mitigate multicollinearity [41], while lasso can perform feature selection by reducing some coefficients to zero [42]. However, these models assume linearity, which may not always hold, and lasso regression can be unstable with highly correlated features [43].

A more complex linear model, the support vector machine (SVM), is a versatile supervised ML algorithm used for classification and regression tasks [44]. In classification, it aims to identify the optimal hyperplane (decision boundary) that maximises the margin between two classes [45], ensuring the largest possible separation between the closest data points (support vectors) while minimising misclassified points (margin violations). For regression tasks, instead of maximising the margin between classes, it tries to fit as many data points as possible within

a defined margin around the hyperplane [46]. Additionally, the "kernel trick" enables mapping input features into higher dimensions, allowing SVMs to solve complex, non-linear problems effectively [12]. Different kernel functions are designed to capture different types of relationships in the data. Although sensitive to the choice of hyperparameters and kernel, by selecting an appropriate kernel and tuning its parameters, SVMs can handle complex, non-linear decision boundaries.

A decision tree is a supervised machine learning algorithm for classification and regression [47]. It splits the data into subsets based on feature values, forming a tree structure where nodes represent features, branches represent decisions, and leaves represent outcomes. Decision trees are interpretable and can handle both categorical and numerical data, capturing non-linear relationships with minimal preprocessing [48]. However,

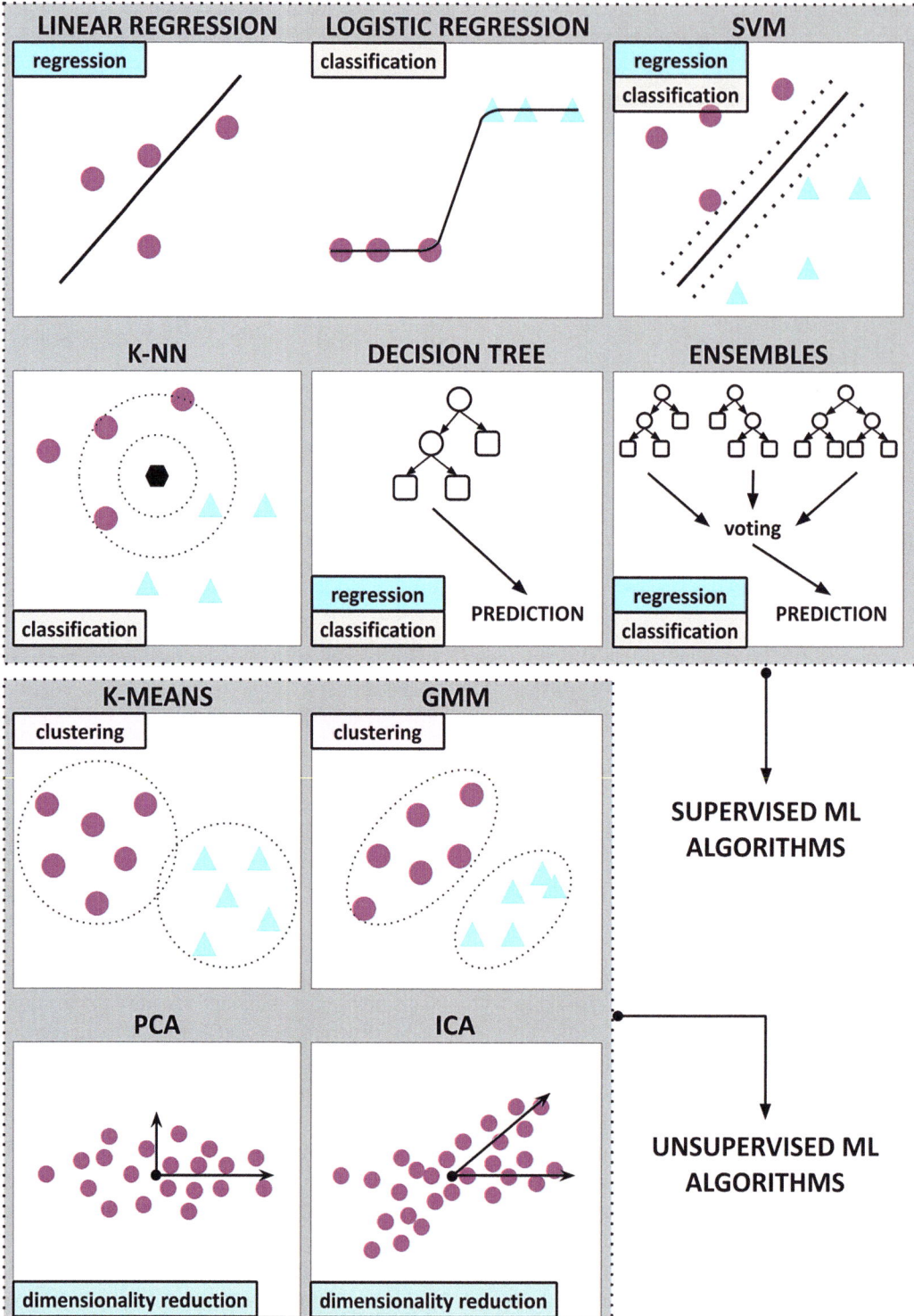

Fig. 2.5 Summary of ML algorithms and their main task (regression/classification/clustering/dimensionality reduction)

they can be prone to overfitting, especially when the tree becomes too deep, memorising the training data rather than generalising well to unseen examples [48].

To improve their robustness and performance, decision trees are often combined into ensemble methods like Random Forests [49, 50]. These methods aggregate predictions from multiple trees, reducing the risk of overfitting and improving accuracy [51]. In fact, ensemble learning is a machine learning technique that combines multiple learners, such as regression models, SVMs, or neural networks, to improve predictive performance [52]. By aggregating the outputs of individual models, ensemble methods can produce more accurate and robust predictions than a single model alone. However, ensemble methods typically require more computational resources for training and prediction, balancing their advantages with increased complexity [49, 53].

Finally, the k-Nearest Neighbours (k-NN) algorithm is a simple, yet effective supervised machine learning method for classification [54]. Instead of training a model, k-NN predicts outcomes based on the similarity of new data points to their nearest neighbours in feature space [55]. The number of neighbours, k, is a key hyperparameter that determines how many of the closest data points are considered when making a prediction. One advantage of k-NN is its simplicity and ability to adapt to new data without requiring extensive training [55, 56]. However, it struggles with high-dimensional data such as raw image pixels, as distances between points become less meaningful when the number of dimensions increases [57].

2.4.2 Unsupervised ML Models

k-Means Clustering is an unsupervised algorithm that partitions data into k clusters by minimising intra-cluster variance [58]. It assigns points to the nearest cluster centroid, recalculates centroids, and iterates until assignments stabilise [59]. Its simplicity and speed make it useful for preprocessing or initial analysis [60]. However, k-means assumes spherical, evenly sized clusters, struggles with complex data, is sensitive to outliers, and can be sensitive to the initialisation of the k hyperparameter [61].

A Gaussian Mixture Model (GMM) offers a more flexible approach by assuming data is generated from a mixture of Gaussian distributions [62]. Unlike the hard cluster assignments of k-means, GMMs provide soft clustering, assigning probabilities for each data point to belong to a cluster. This allows GMMs to model clusters with varying shapes and densities more effectively [63]. Similar to k-means, GMMs can also lead to suboptimal solutions with poor initialisation of parameters and are sensitive to outliers.

Principal Component Analysis (PCA) is a dimensionality reduction technique that projects high-dimensional data into a lower-dimensional space while preserving as much variance as possible. It identifies principal components that capture the largest variance in the data [64]. Moreover, it can be used for visualisation purposes by projecting complex imaging data into a 2D or 3D feature space. However, PCA assumes linear relationships between features, which may not always apply, and it is sensitive to data scale and often requires normalisation or standardisation [14].

Independent Component Analysis (ICA) is a dimensionality reduction technique that separates multivariate signals into additive, independent non-Gaussian components [65]. Unlike PCA, which maximises variance, ICA focuses on identifying statistically independent sources in the data. In medical imaging, ICA is used for fMRI data analysis to identify brain networks and separate noise from signal [66]. ICA's advantages include uncovering independent sources and effectively removing noise. However, it is computationally intensive, and its results depend on initialisation and algorithm choice [14].

2.5 Deep Learning

Deep learning is a subset of machine learning and artificial intelligence that uses neural networks with multiple processing layers to learn hierarchical representations of data [67]. Since its

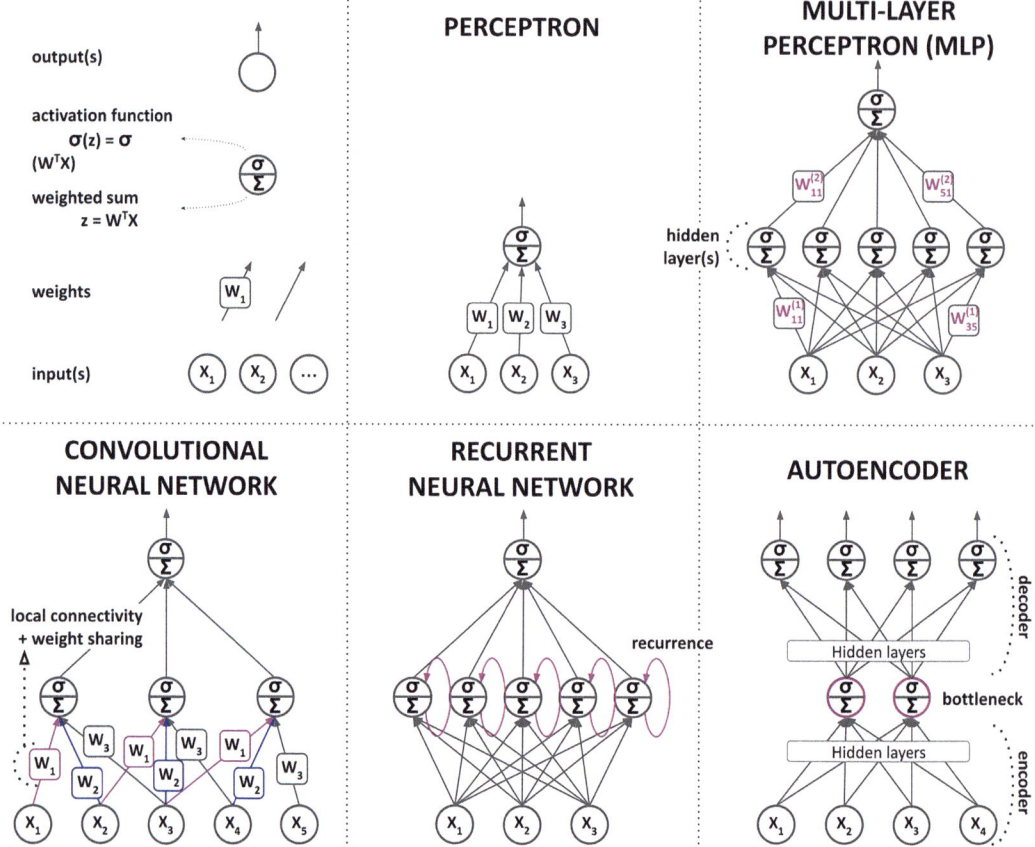

Fig. 2.6 Foundational neural network architectures

recent ground-breaking success in computer vision and speech recognition, deep learning has become a dominant trend in medical image analysis [68]. This section focuses on the theory behind artificial neural networks (ANNs), with a summary of the most common neural network architectures.

2.5.1 Artificial Neural Networks

The main component for any deep learning framework is the *perceptron* (see Fig. 2.6), introduced in 1958 by Frank Rosenblatt [69]. When stacking multiple perceptrons together, we arrive at the general architecture for any artificial neural network, the multilayer perceptron (MLP). MLPs

are made of an input layer, one or more fully connected hidden layers, and one output layer. Connections between pairs of neurons from adjacent layers have a weight attached to them, signifying the strength of those connections. Information flows from the input to the output layers, with the input neurons relaying the data without modifying it, while the neurons in the hidden layers apply an activation function to the weighted sum of incoming values. While many neural network architectures have been developed [70], this section focuses on the key building blocks that underpin more advanced models. Table 2.2 organises these models based on the supervised vs. unsupervised taxonomy, while Fig. 2.6 illustrates some of the most important neural network architectures.

Table 2.2 Popular DL algorithms grouped by the type of learning (supervised vs. unsupervised)

	Algorithm	Task	Advantages	Disadvantages
Supervised DL models	MLP	R+C	Can perform well on tabular data or extracted features from the images	Struggles with high-dimensional data like images because it lacks spatial awareness (cannot recognise patterns like edges, shapes)
	CNN	R+C	Designed to capture spatial patterns and have a reduced number of parameters compared to MLPs	Require large amounts of labelled data to perform well
	RNN	R+C	Good for analysing sequential/temporal data	Computationally expensive for long sequences
Unsupervised DL models	Autoencoder	AD DN DR	Can reduce high-dimensional image data into a lower-dimensional space. Can be used to remove noise from medical images. Can be used for anomaly detection	The quality of the reconstructed images can sometimes suffer. The latent representations learned by autoencoders are often difficult to interpret
	Variational Autoencoder	AD IG	Can be used for anomaly detection and to provide uncertainty estimation. Can generate new samples by sampling from the learned latent space	More complex to train than traditional autoencoders, and their probabilistic nature introduces additional challenges in terms of model tuning and convergence
	GAN	IG DN	Can generate realistic medical images, which can help with data augmentation and training of other models. Can be used for denoising applications	Challenging to train. May suffer from mode collapse. Require large amounts of training data
	Diffusion	IG DN	Remarkable performance in generating high-quality and realistic images	Computationally expensive and relatively slow generation process

R regression, *C* classification, *DR* dimensionality reduction, *AD* anomaly detection, *DN* denoising, *IG* image generation

2.5.2 Convolutional Neural Networks

The most popular type of neural network for analysing images is the convolutional neural network (CNN) [71]. Proposed by LeCun et al. in 1989 [72], CNNs introduce the convolutional kernel, a small filter that slides across an input layer and which enables two key features: local receptive field and parameter sharing. Unlike MLPs, where each connection has a unique weight, CNNs maintain fixed weights within the convolutional kernels as they move across the image. This reduces the number of parameters, making the network more efficient and less prone to overfitting compared to MLPs. However, CNNs typically require large amounts of labelled data to

perform well [73, 74] and are often viewed as a *"black box"* (or difficult to interpret), which can be a limitation in clinical settings. Efforts are underway to develop techniques that make CNNs more interpretable [75, 76].

The building block of a CNN is therefore the convolutional kernel, which is generally a small matrix of weights that slides across an input layer producing a feature (activation) map [77]. Some key hyperparameters for a convolutional filter are (1) its dimensions, (2) the stride (i.e. the number of steps it skips when sliding across the input), (3) the padding amount (i.e. how many extra values (usually zeros) are added around the input to control the output dimensions), and (4) dilation (i.e. controls the amount of gap between kernel elements to expand its receptive field without

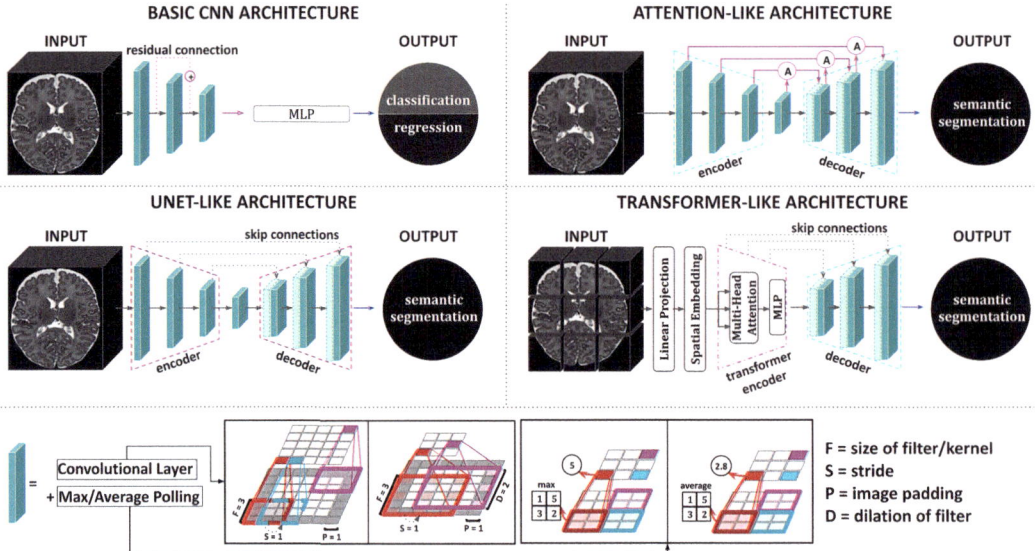

Fig. 2.7 Common CNN architectures (top and middle row). The bottom row shows example convolutional layers (with different filter sizes F, stride S, padding P and dilation rate D), followed by max and average pooling layers for a 2 × 2 kernel size

increasing the number of parameters) [78]. An example of two convolutional filters is shown in the bottom row of Fig. 2.7. Another common layer found in a CNN is the pooling layer [77]. It down-samples the feature maps by either selecting the maximum value within a patch (max pooling) or computing the average value (average pooling), effectively reducing spatial dimensions while retaining important features. An example of a max pooling and an average pooling layer is shown in the bottom row of Fig. 2.7.

2.5.3   Recurrent Neural Networks

Recurrent Neural Networks (RNNs) are neural networks that are designed to handle sequential data, with connections that allow them to retain memory of previous inputs [67]. They are particularly effective for time-series or sequential data processing, such as analysing dynamic imaging modalities or disease progression modelling [79]. However, RNNs, especially when used on long sequences or large datasets, can be more computationally intensive and harder to train than feed-

forward networks like CNNs [80, 81]. Figure 2.6 illustrates schematically this type of neural network architecture.

2.5.4   Autoencoders

Autoencoders are a type of unsupervised neural network designed to learn a compressed representation (encoding) of input data and then reconstruct the data from this representation [82]. They consist of an encoder that projects the data into a lower-dimensional latent space (bottleneck) and a decoder that reconstructs the original input. Autoencoders can reduce high-dimensional image data into a lower-dimensional latent space, which is useful for feature extraction and visualisation, and are often used for denoising and image enhancement [83]. However, the latent representations learned by autoencoders are often difficult to interpret, which can be a challenge in clinical applications where explainability is important [84]. The bottom-right corner of Fig. 2.6 illustrates schematically this type of neural network architecture.

2.6 Neural Network Architectures

A typical neural network topology is composed of convolutional layers, activation functions, max- or average-pooling layers, and sometimes fully connected layers [70]. Here we describe some of the more commonly used CNN architectures, as well as two of their more advanced variants. For a more comprehensive survey of recent architectures of deep CNNs, we refer our readers to [85].

2.6.1 Classic CNN Architectures

Some of the first CNNs to demonstrate the power of deep learning on large-scale datasets were AlexNet [86] and VGGNet [87]. Both networks are seminal, shaping modern deep learning research and neural network designs, and revolutionised deep learning and computer vision by winning the ImageNet competition [88]. In terms of architectural design, both networks consist of convolutional layers (5 for AlexNet and 16–18 for VGGNet), followed by fully connected layers (see Fig. 2.7, top left). Later, ResNet [89] addressed challenges in training very deep networks, such as vanishing gradients and performance degradation, by introducing residual connections. These shortcuts bypass one or more layers (see Fig. 2.7, top left), enabling better gradient flow and efficient training of ultra-deep networks.

For image segmentation tasks, one of the most widely used CNN architectures today [90] is the U-Net [91, 92], named for its symmetric encoder-decoder shape (see Fig. 2.7, bottom left). The encoder (contracting path) uses convolutional layers with increasing filter numbers and max pooling to reduce spatial dimensions. The decoder (expansive path) combines up-sampling layers with convolutions and incorporates skip connections, linking encoder feature maps to the corresponding decoder layers. These skip connections enhance feature representation and gradient flow, improving segmentation performance [90]. The final decoder layer maps feature vectors to the desired number of classes, making

U-Net highly effective for segmentation tasks. These pioneering CNNs (Fig. 2.7, first column) have become benchmarks for comparison, and inspirations for modern neural network innovations [93].

2.6.2 Advanced CNN Architectures

In this section, we explore two advanced adaptations of the U-Net that incorporate cutting-edge attention mechanisms to enhance their functionality. Attention mechanisms in deep learning have become a key area of research, improving performance by generating probability maps over input data, features, or channels, and thus allowing models to focus on relevant aspects of various tasks [94]. Attention is applied to pixels in images, words in sentences [95], and nodes in graphs [96], and is central to the Transformer architecture [95, 97], which revolutionised modern deep learning.

Attention U-Net [98] is an enhanced version of the classic U-Net, incorporating attention [99] to focus on relevant regions while suppressing irrelevant ones. In this architecture, attention gates replace the traditional skip connections. These gates use both encoder and corresponding decoder features to generate attention maps. Rather than directly concatenating the encoder feature maps through skip connections, the maps are first scaled using the attention maps before being combined with the decoder features. An example of this type of U-Net architecture is shown in Fig. 2.7, top right.

U-Net Transformers [100] also introduce attention by adapting the transformer architecture [97] and replacing the traditional U-Net encoder with a transformer-based encoder. This change allows the model to capture global contextual information more effectively through the attention mechanism, compared to local convolutions. Instead of processing the entire image or volume at once, the image is divided into smaller, non-overlapping patches. Each patch is treated as an individual unit, with the transformer using self-attention [99] to focus on relationships between patches both locally and globally. This enables the model to learn connections between distant areas of the image, crucial for segmentation tasks where global context helps inform local predictions.

2.7 Performance Evaluation Metrics

An important step of any ML or DL algorithm is measuring its performance. This section presents the most commonly used metrics for assessing regression, image comparison, classification, and segmentation tasks, covering error-based, similarity-based, overlap-based, and surface-based evaluation methods, as summarised in Table 2.3.

2.7.1 Regression Tasks

The R^2 score is a statistical measure used to assess the performance of a linear regression model as the proportion of variance in the data explained by the model [14]. In medical image analysis, R^2 is often employed to evaluate the explanatory power of a regression model [15, 101, 102]. However, R^2 can be misleading in cases where the data contains outliers, as these can influence the score and give an inaccurate measure of model performance. Additionally, variations to the R^2 score exist, such as adjusted R^2, which is often preferred when comparing models with different numbers of predictors [103].

Table 2.3 Common evaluation performance metrics grouped by the type of task (regression vs. classification)

	Metric	Definition
Regression metrics	R^2	Quantifies how well a model explains the variance in medical imaging data. **$R^2 = 1$** → perfect prediction
	RMSE	Measures the root mean squared error between expected and predicted values; it has the same units as the target variable. **RMSE = 0** → perfect prediction
Image comparison metrics	PSNR	Quantifies the quality of an image reconstruction as the ratio between the maximum possible intensity range of the images and the mean squared error between reconstructed and target images. **PSNR ↑** → better image quality
	SSIM	Evaluates the structural similarity between two images rather than just pixel-wise differences. **SSIM = 1** → perfect similarity
Classification metrics	Accuracy	The ratio of the number of correct predictions to the total number of input samples. It can be misleading for imbalanced datasets. **Acc = 100%** → correctly classified 100% of the data
	Precision (PPV)	The fraction of relevant instances among the retrieved instances. **PPV ↑** → fewer false positives
	Recall (TPR)	The fraction of correctly identified positive cases. **TPR ↑** → fewer false negatives
	AUC	It quantifies the ability of a model to distinguish between 2 classes, and it is used as a summary of the ROC curve. The ROC graphically evaluates the performance of the model by plotting the true-positive rate (recall) against the false-positive rate at varying threshold values. **AUC = 1** → perfect classification
Segmentation metrics	IoU	Defined as the intersection between the predicted and ground truth classes over their union. **IoU = 1** → perfect overlap
	DSC	Defined as two times the area of intersection between the predicted and ground truth classes, normalised by the sum of their areas. **DSC = 1** → perfect overlap
	HD	Measures the difference between the predicted boundary and the ground truth boundary. **HD = 0** → perfect overlap

Another way to measure the performance of regression models is by using the root mean squared error (RMSE) between predicted and expected target values [14]. RMSE measures the average magnitude of the prediction error in units of the target values, making it interpretable for medical image analysis [104]. Additionally, the mean absolute error (MAE) is also often reported in literature as it calculates the average of absolute differences between predicted and actual values, reducing sensitivity to outliers [105, 106].

2.7.2 Image Comparison Tasks

Derived from Mean Squared Error (MSE), peak signal-to-noise ratio (PSNR) is commonly used to assess image quality, especially in image super-resolution and denoising tasks [107, 108]. PSNR focuses on pixel-wise differences and may not effectively capture structural similarities important in medical images [109].

The structural similarity index (SSIM), on the other hand, is a perceptual metric that evaluates the similarity between two images while considering local structures rather than pixel-wise differences, thus making it more robust to small pixel shifts or intensity changes [110]. It is particularly useful for perceptual quality assessment, ensuring that fine anatomical details are preserved [111]. However, SSIM may exhibit instabilities in regions with low contrast or near edges [112].

2.7.3 Classification Tasks

In classification tasks, accuracy is often one of the most common measures reported, as it calculates the overall proportion of correctly classified instances out of all predictions. It is a measure that takes into account both the true positives and negatives (TPs and TNs), as well as the false positives and negatives (FPs and FNs). In cases where the two classes are imbalanced, accuracy can be misleading and should not be the only measure reported (i.e. a model that predicts the majority class most of the time will appear to have high accuracy but will fail to identify the minority class).

For these reasons, the two most important metrics to be reported are precision and recall [113]. The positive predicted value (PPV), also known as precision, is the fraction of relevant instances (TP) among the retrieved instances (TP + FP), while the true-positive rate (TPR), also known as sensitivity or recall, is defined as the fraction of correctly classified positive classes (TP) out of the total number of actual positive instances (TP + FN) [113, 114]. High precision means fewer false positives, while high recall, often used as a complementary measure to precision, means fewer false negatives [114].

The predictive ability of a classifier is typically measured using a fixed threshold, meaning that when the threshold is set to 0.5, a prediction with a probability of 0.6 will be treated the same as one with a probability of 0.99 [115]. This approach ignores the probability or confidence of class predictions, treating all correct predictions equally regardless of their certainty. A more comprehensive analysis can be achieved by evaluating performance across a range of thresholds, which allows for a deeper understanding of model predictive power [115]. One such metric used for this purpose is the Receiver Operating Characteristic (ROC) curve, which plots the true-positive rate (TPR) against the false-positive rate (FPR) across different thresholds [116]. The Area Under the Curve (AUC) provides a summary of the performance of the ROC curve. Unlike accuracy, this metric is useful even for imbalanced datasets, and it is often used to compare multiple models for better classification performance [11, 115].

2.7.4 Segmentation Tasks

For image segmentation models, two spatial overlap metrics are often used. First, the Intersection over Union (IoU), also known as the Jaccard index, is defined as the intersection between the predicted and ground truth class over their union [113]. However, the most prevalent metric in the literature is the Dice score coefficient

(DSC), also known as the F1 score or the harmonic mean of the precision and recall [117]. It is defined as two times the area of intersection between the predicted and ground truth classes, normalised by the sum of their areas [113, 117]. IoU and DSC are related, meaning that in practice, only one of them should be reported as a validation metric [113].

Finally, when the boundary (contour) is of importance, surface-based metrics such as the Hausdorff distance (HD) are often used [113, 117]. HD measures the maximum difference between the predicted boundary and the ground truth boundary, but it can be sensitive to noise and outliers. It is therefore recommended to use the 95th quantile of distances instead of the maximum [118]. The average surface distance (ASD), also known as the average Hausdorff distance, is the surface distance averaged over all points [113]. It is often reported as an image segmentation validation measure, as it is less sensitive to outliers than HD. For a more comprehensive investigation of medical image segmentation metrics, we refer the reader to the review paper by Taha et al. [113]

2.8 Modern DL Approaches

In recent years, deep learning has evolved beyond traditional CNNs. Modern deep learning paradigms have introduced advanced techniques that address challenges such as data efficiency, adaptability, model explainability, and uncertainty [23]. This section mentions several key advancements that are shaping the future of deep learning, particularly in complex tasks like medical imaging.

2.8.1 Advanced Learning Paradigms

Recent advancements in medical imaging have focused on enhancing model performance with limited labelled data through transfer learning [28], improving generalisation to new domains through domain adaptation [24], enabling

privacy-preserving decentralised learning with federated learning [119], and leveraging large datasets and billion-parameter AI models to tackle a wide range of downstream analysis tasks.

Transfer learning (or *knowledge transfer*) addresses the challenge of acquiring high-quality labelled medical imaging datasets [120]. By using pre-trained models, it enables improved performance on tasks with limited or noisy labels [28]. Thus, a model trained on one task where there is abundant annotated data can be adapted and reused for a different but related task. Typically, some model weights from the original training are preserved, while only a few layers are retrained for the new task. For example, a model pre-trained on large-scale generic computer vision datasets can be fine-tuned for segmenting medical images [121].

Domain adaptation is a subfield of transfer learning focused on adapting a model trained on data from one domain (the source domain) to perform well in a different, but related, domain (the target domain) [24]. Specifically, domain adaptation techniques assume that both the source and target domains share the same feature space (e.g. both datasets consist of neonatal brain MRI scans), but the data distributions differ (e.g. there are variations in the imaging protocol, scanners, or hospitals) [23, 122]. The goal is therefore to train models that generalise better by accounting for these shifts in imaging equipment or data distributions [24]. One approach is to generate synthetic data that bridges the gap between domains. For example, generative models like Cycle-GANs [123] can be used to translate images from the source to the target domain, enabling the main predictor (e.g. a segmentation model) to be trained on realistically adapted synthetic images while preserving the original data's labels [124, 125]. At inference, the generator is discarded as the model can now be applied directly to target data [24].

Building on the concept of transferring knowledge between tasks or domains, federated learning advances this by enabling model training across multiple decentralised devices or institutions without the need to share sensitive data [119]. This approach allows models to learn from data stored locally on various devices, ensuring privacy and security while benefiting from diverse datasets [126]. Federated learning is especially valuable in healthcare settings, where patient data must remain private. For example, multiple hospitals could collaborate to train a shared model on their MRI datasets without exchanging patient data [127].

Finally, a major focus of recent deep learning research has been the development of large AI models, commonly known as foundation models [128]. These models are trained on vast, diverse datasets, allowing them to perform a wide range of downstream tasks with minimal fine-tuning. By serving as general-purpose foundations for various applications, they offer remarkable versatility in AI research and deployment [129]. Qiu et al. [130] categorise foundation models into three groups based on their pretraining data: (1) Large Language Models (LLMs)—trained on language data and used for natural language processing tasks (e.g. ChatGPT—a transformer-based generative LLM that predicts the next word in a sentence using autoregressive learning [131]); (2) Large Vision Models (LVMs)—trained on vision data and applied to image-based tasks (e.g. the Segment Anything Model (SAM) for computer vision tasks [132] and MedSAM for medical images [133]); and (3) Large Multi-model Models (LMMs)—trained on multiple data types (e.g. language and vision) to handle both single- and multi-modal tasks.

2.8.2 Generative Models

Generative models enable the creation of new, high-quality data from existing datasets. These models have gained significant attention for their ability to generate realistic images, synthesise data for training, and improve tasks like data augmentation, denoising, and inpainting.

Variational autoencoders (VAEs) are a probabilistic extension of traditional autoencoders [134]. Intuitively, VAEs can be seen as autoencoders with regularised training [135] to ensure the latent space behaves in a way that supports a generative process (see Fig. 2.8, top). Specifically,

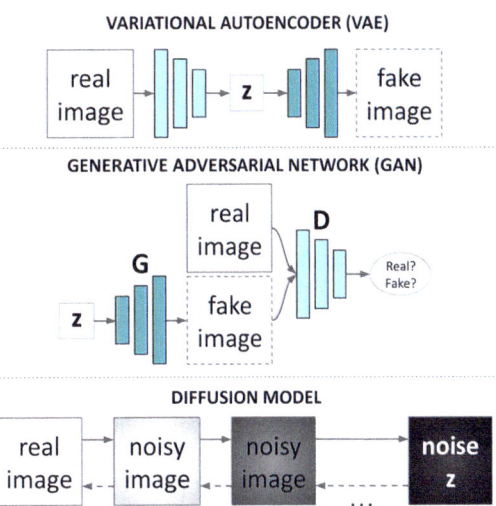

Fig. 2.8 Common types of generative DL models

VAEs encode the input data as a distribution over the latent space, sample from this distribution, and pass it through the decoder to reconstruct the data. VAEs are particularly useful for anomaly detection [136] (e.g. learning the distribution of normal MRIs and identifying deviations from it) and image generation [35] (e.g. sampling from the learned latent space to create new data). However, VAEs tend to produce blurrier reconstructions compared to standard autoencoders, as they prioritise capturing the overall data distribution rather than focusing on high-fidelity reconstructions [137]. Additionally, VAEs are generally more complex to train due to their probabilistic nature [135, 138].

Introduced in 2014, generative adversarial networks (GANs) [139] are a popular deep learning paradigm known for their ability to generate new data [140]. A GAN consists of two networks—a generator (G) and a discriminator (D)—competing in a zero-sum game [141], where the generator aims to produce realistic looking images, while the discriminator tries to differentiate between real and generated samples (see Fig. 2.8, middle). A key advantage of GANs is their effectiveness in data augmentation, particularly in medical imaging, by generating synthetic images to address the problem of limited labelled data [35]. However, GANs face challenges such as mode collapse, where the generator produces limited outputs despite a large input space, and they are notoriously difficult to train, requiring careful hyperparameter tuning and balance between the generator and discriminator [141, 142].

Recently, *diffusion models* have emerged as a powerful class of generative techniques, capable of creating high-quality synthetic data [143, 144]. These models work by adding noise to data and then learning to reverse the process, generating new samples (see Fig. 2.8, bottom) [35]. In medical imaging, diffusion models have applications in image synthesis and augmentation, denoising and super-resolution, as well as image segmentation and anomaly detection [145]. Compared to traditional generative models like GANs, diffusion models produce more detailed and realistic images, especially for complex textures and fine details [143, 146]. However, their training and inference require significant computational resources due to the iterative nature of the noise removal process [146, 147].

2.8.3 Radiomic Analysis

Radiomic analysis has emerged as a transformative and highly promising approach in the field of medical imaging, commonly known as radiomic features or radiomics. In recent years, the field of radiomics has garnered increasing attention and recognition due to its ability to extract a wealth of quantitative data from medical images [148]. Unlike traditional qualitative assessments, radiomic analysis delves deep into the pixel-level intricacies of these images, generating an extensive array of quantitative features. This wealth of information encompasses not only fundamental parameters such as size, volume, and intensity but also intricate details regarding texture, shape, and spatial relationships within the imaged regions ([149], Fig. 2.9). Such comprehensive data analysis offers significant potential for aiding in the diagnosis, prognosis, and treatment planning of various medical conditions.

The key applications of radiomics in medical imaging include cancer diagnosis and characterisation, treatment response assessment, prognosis and survival prediction, and neurological and cardiovascular disorders. Radiomics plays a pivotal role in oncology compared to other applications [150]. It can aid in distinguishing between benign and malignant lesions, assessing tumour heterogeneity, and predicting the aggressiveness of cancer. This not only facilitates early detection but also assists in tailoring personalised treatment plans. While in neuroimaging and cardiovascular imaging, radiomics has the potential to identify disease-specific biomarkers and help with early detection of conditions such as cardiac

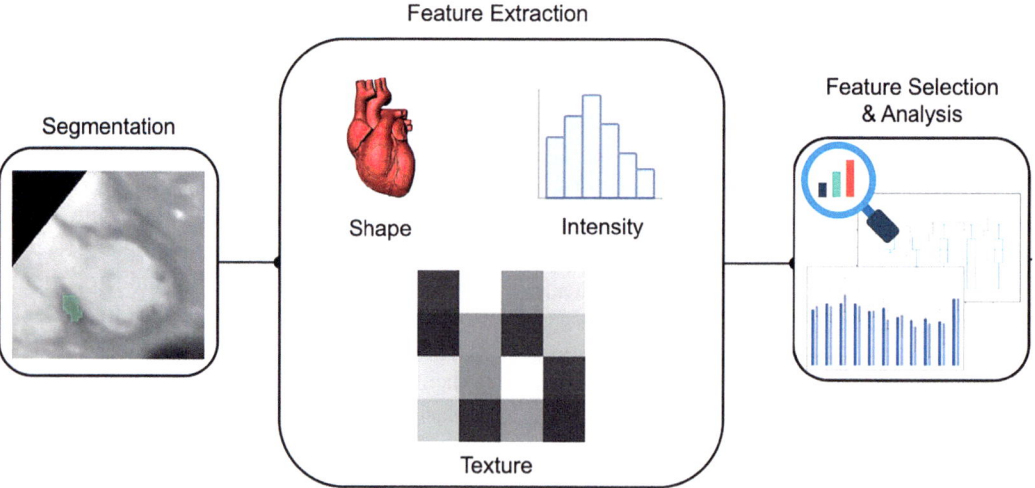

Fig. 2.9 Radiomic analysis workflow

disorders [151]. However, Rainey et al. [152] highlighted the necessity of structured education for healthcare practitioners in artificial intelligence to equip the current and future workforce for the imminent clinical integration of artificial intelligence in healthcare. Some educational institutions have initiated this incorporation to stay updated with the evolving landscape [153].

2.8.3.1 Factors Affecting Radiomic Analysis

The processes prior to feature extraction play a crucial role in modifying the input image and should not be underestimated. These include image acquisition (with all scanner settings), correction for attenuation and scatter, image reconstruction, and image segmentation. Often, these steps have been fine-tuned for visual interpretation, which may not necessarily yield the most favourable radiomic outcomes [154]. Nevertheless, the imperative for maintaining consistent methodologies dictates that these visually optimised images must be employed.

2.8.3.2 Feature Selection and Analysis

Feature selection is a crucial step in machine learning and data analysis, aimed at identifying the most relevant and informative features from a given dataset and eliminating noise or irrelevant information. The goal is to reduce the dimensionality of the data while retaining the most discriminative features, which can lead to improved computational efficiency and reduced model complexity, thereby improving model performance and interpretability. In addition, feature selection can mitigate the risk of overfitting by reducing the chances of the model learning from random or spurious correlations within the data as well as minimise the risk of Type I errors (i.e. rejecting a null hypothesis when it is true) [155].

There are various methods and techniques available for feature selection, ranging from simple statistical measures to more advanced algorithms. These methods can be broadly categorised into filter, wrapper, and embedded approaches [155]. The choice of feature selection method depends on various factors, such as the dataset size, dimensionality, and the specific problem. It is essential to carefully evaluate the trade-offs between computational cost, model performance, and interpretability when selecting a feature selection technique. Furthermore, it is crucial to validate the selected features and assess their stability and generalisability using appropriate evaluation metrics and validation strategies. Cross-validation and independent test datasets can help ensure the robustness and reliability of the selected features, improving the credibility of the results. However, it is suggested not to split small datasets into separate training and testing sets. Instead, it is advised to utilise the entire small dataset for model development and training with some form of cross-validation [156]. This helps estimate the generalisability of the selected features and reduce the risk of selecting features that are specific to the training set.

After reducing the radiomic feature dataset, the next step involves evaluating the diagnostic and predictive value of the remaining extracted features. This evaluation might be conducted alongside the feature selection process or separately. Traditionally, statistical analysis techniques have been employed for this purpose. However, there has been a rise in the popularity of machine learning classifiers for these tasks, like linear or logistic regression. These classifiers, along with others, have gained widespread acceptance in constructing diagnostic or predictive models. Machine learning classifiers offer a versatile and powerful toolset for analysing radiomic features and their relationship with clinical data. They encompass regression analysis, clustering, and decision tree-based approaches, enabling comprehensive exploration and interpretation of the data, as can be seen in Fig. 2.10.

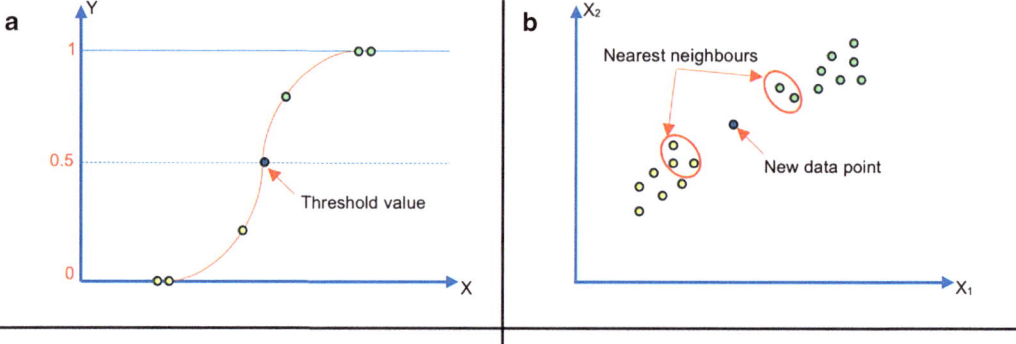

Fig. 2.10 An example of regression and clustering approaches. (**a**) Logistic regression predicts the output of a categorical dependent variable, but instead of giving the exact value as 0 and 1, it gives the probabilistic values that lie between 0 and 1 ("S" shaped logistic function), (**b**) K-neighbours (K nearest neighbours) defines clusters based on training data and then assigns new inputs to a cluster

2.9   Interpretability and Uncertainty

As deep learning models are increasingly used in high-stakes fields like healthcare, interpretability [157] and uncertainty quantification [158] have recently become crucial areas of research. Gaining insight into model decisions and measuring prediction uncertainty are key to enhancing trust and ensuring reliable real-world deployment.

Interpretable deep learning (iDL) seeks to address the opacity of deep learning models [33, 157] by providing explanations that highlight important features in the input data (e.g. relevant brain regions influencing predictions [75]). It can also facilitate model debugging, helping practitioners identify cases where a model arrives at the correct decision for the wrong reasons [159]. Broadly speaking, iDL methods can be categorised as post-hoc or intrinsic: post-hoc approaches generate explanations after training, while intrinsic methods integrate interpretability into the model's design from the outset [160]. Some post-hoc methods, such as Grad-CAM [161], Guided Backpropagation [162], and SmoothGrad [163] produce heatmaps that visualise which regions of an input image contributed most to a model's decision [164]. An example of interpretable DL techniques is shown in Fig. 2.11 (Figure adapted from Munroe et al. [75]).

Uncertainty estimation and quantification have become critical aspects of deep learning model deployment, particularly for assessing the reliability of models utilised in healthcare [158]. By providing a measure of confidence in model predictions, uncertainty quantification enhances trust in AI-driven decisions and supports more informed clinical interpretations [165]. There are two types of uncertainty: aleatoric uncertainty, which refers to the inherent noise in the data that cannot be reduced but can be modelled probabilistically, and epistemic uncertainty, which accounts for uncertainty in the model and can be reduced with more data [166]. Common techniques include ensemble methods, which aggregate predictions from multiple models to improve robustness [167], and Bayesian Neural Networks, where weights are treated as probability distributions rather than fixed values [168], allowing them to quantify uncertainty in predictions by sampling from these distributions [166, 169].

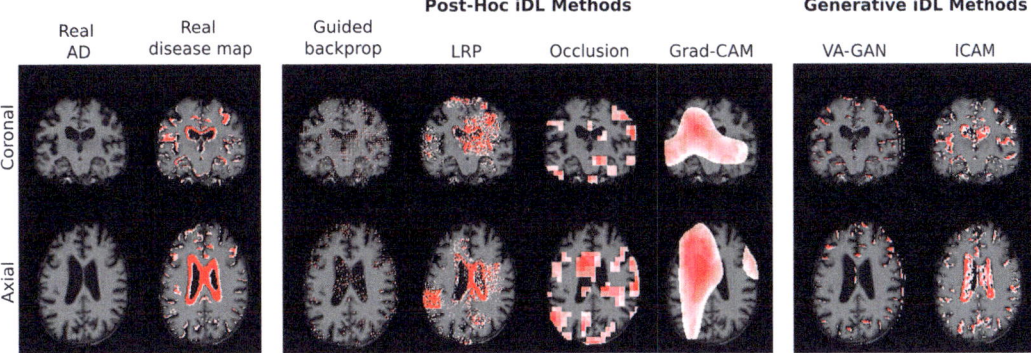

Fig. 2.11 Comparison of post-hoc interpretability maps and generative interpretability methods (shown here as colour heatmaps) applied to the classification of Alzheimer's disease (AD) versus mild cognitive impair-ment (MCI) in brain MRI volumes. The real disease map is the "ground-truth" shown for comparison. (Figure adapted from Bass et al. [170] and Munroe et al. [75])

2.10   Chapter Summary

Different AI models have been developed and applied for use in medical imaging, with more expected to be developed in the coming years. The actual use and implementation of these models in clinical practice depends on clinical need, governance, and acceptability by healthcare professionals, with AI literacy playing a huge role in this topic. The following chapters will explore the ethics (Chap. 3) and governance of AI (Chap. 4) and the use of some of these AI models in different medical imaging modalities (Chaps. 5, 6, 7, 8, 9, 10, and 11).

References

1. Russell SJ, Norvig P. Artificial intelligence: a modern approach. London: Pearson; 2016.
2. Hans Korteling JE, van de Boer-Visschedijk GC, RAM B, Boonekamp RC, Eikelboom AR. Human-versus artificial intelligence. Front Artif Intell. 2021;4:622364.
3. Helm JM, Swiergoss AM, Haeberle HS, Karnuta JM, Schaffer JL, Krebs VE, et al. Machine learning and artificial intelligence: definitions, applications, and future directions. Curr Rev Musculoskelet Med. 2020;13:69–76.
4. Jaakkola H, Henno J, Mäkelä J, Thalheim B. Artificial intelligence yesterday, today and tomorrow. In: 2019 42nd International Convention on Information and Communication Technology, Electronics and Microelectronics (MIPRO). IEEE; 2019. p. 860–7.
5. Rajaraman V. JohnMcCarthy—Father of artificial intelligence. Resonance. 2014;19:198–207.
6. Samuel AL. Some studies in machine learning using the game of checkers. IBM J Res Dev. 1959;3(3):210–29.
7. Hinton GE, Osindero S, Teh YW. A fast learning algorithm for deep belief nets. Neural Comput. 2006;18(7):1527–54.
8. Ranosa T. Godfathers of AI win this Y'ar's Turing Award and $1 Mill" on. Tech Times. 2019.
9. Jumper J, Evans R, Pritsel A, Green T, Figurnov M, Ronneberger O, et al. Highly accurate protein structure prediction with AlphaFold. Nature 2021;596(7873):583–589. Available from: https://doi.org/10.1038/s41586-021-03819-2.
10. Achiam J, Adler S, Agarwal S, Ahmad L, Akkaya I, Aleman FL, et al. Gpt-4 technical report. arXiv preprint arXiv:230308774. 2023.
11. Hastie T, Tibshirani R, Friedman J. The elements of statistical learning: data mining, inference, and prediction. New York: Springer; 2017.
12. Bishop CM. Pattern recognition and machine learning, vol. 2. New York: Springer; 2006. p. 1122–8.
13. Goodfellow I. Deep learning. Cambridge, MA: MIT press; 2016.
14. Depres M, Robinson EC. Machine learning for biomedical applications: with Scikit-learn and PyTorch. Academic; 2023.
15. Taoudi-Benchekroun Y, Christiaens D, Grigorescu I, Gale-Grant O, Schuh A, Pietsch M, et al. Predicting age and clinical risk from the neonatal connectome. NeuroImage. 2022;257:119319.
16. Kalaiyarasi M, Dhanasekar R, Ram SS, Vaishnavi P. Classification of benign or malignant tumor using machine learning. In: IOP conference series: materials science and engineering. Bristol: IOP Publishing; 2020. p. 12028.

17. Kandhasamy JP, Balamurali S. Performance analysis of classifier models to predict diabetes mellitus. Procedia Comput Sci. 2015;47:45–51.

18. Pande NA, Pusadekar R, Mitra K. Classification of lung CT scan images using machine learning. In: 2022 International Conference on Futuristic Technologies (INCOFT). IEEE; 2022. p. 1–4.

19. Jiang H, Diao S, Shi T, Shou Y, Wang F, Hu W, et al. A review of deep learning-based multiple-lesion recognition from medical images: classification, detection and segmentation. Comput Biol Med. 2023;157:106726.

20. Khalili N, Lessmann N, Turk E, Claessens N, de Heus R, Kolk T, et al. Automatic brain tissue segmentation in fetal MRI using convolutional neural networks. Magn Reson Imaging. 2019;64:77–89.

21. Pereira S, Pinto A, Alves V, Silva CA. Brain tumor segmentation using convolutional neural networks in MRI images. IEEE Trans Med Imaging. 2016;35(5):1240–51.

22. Aljuaid A, Anwar M. Survey of supervised learning for medical image processing. SN Comput Sci. 2022;3(4):292.

23. Shou SK, Greenspan H, Davatsikos C, Duncan JS, Van Ginneken B, Madabhushi A, et al. A review of deep learning in medical imaging: imaging traits, technology trends, case studies with progress highlights, and future promises. Proc IEEE. 2021;109(5):820–38.

24. Guan H, Liu M. Domain adaptation for medical image analysis: a survey. IEEE Trans Biomed Eng. 2021;69(3):1173–85.

25. Sulaiman SN, Non NA, Isa IS, Hamsah N. Segmentation of brain MRI image based on clustering algorithm. In: 2014 IEEE Symposium on Industrial Electronics & Applications (ISIEA). IEEE; 2014. p. 60–5.

26. Jiao R, Shang Y, Ding L, Xue B, Shang J, Cai R, et al. Learning with limited annotations: a survey on deep semi-supervised learning for medical image segmentation. Comput Biol Med. 2023;169:107840.

27. Lee DH. Pseudo-label: the simple and efficient semi-supervised learning method for deep neural networks. In: Workshop on challenges in representation learning, ICML. Atlanta; 2013. p. 896.

28. Cheplygina V, De Bruijne M, Pluim JPW. Not-so-supervised: a survey of semi-supervised, multi-instance, and transfer learning in medical image analysis. Med Image Anal. 2019;54:280–96.

29. Hu M, Shang J, Matkovic L, Liu T, Yang X. Reinforcement learning in medical image analysis: concepts, applications, challenges, and future directions. J Appl Clin Med Phys. 2023;24(2):e13898.

30. Shou SK, Le HN, Luu K, Nguyen HV, Ayache N. Deep reinforcement learning in medical imaging: a literature review. Med Image Anal. 2021;73:102193.

31. Aurélien G. Hands-on machine learning with scikit-learn & tensorflow. Geron Aurelien. 2017;134:145–50.

32. Willemink MJ, Kossek WA, Hardell C, Wu J, Fleischmann D, Harvey H, et al. Preparing medical imaging data for machine learning. Radiology. 2020;295(1):4–15.

33. Castiglioni I, Rundo L, Codari M, Di Leo G, Salvatore C, Interlenghi M, et al. AI applications to medical images: from machine learning to deep learning. Phys Med. 2021;83:9–24.

34. Emmanuel T, Maupong T, Mpoeleng D, Semong T, Mphago B, Tabona O. A survey on missing data in machine learning. J Big Data. 2021;8:1–37.

35. Kebaili A, Lapuyade-Lahorgue J, Ruan S. Deep learning approaches for data augmentation in medical imaging: a review. J Imaging. 2023;9(4):81.

36. Chlap P, Min H, Vandenberg N, Dowling J, Holloway L, Haworth A. A review of medical image data augmentation techniques for deep learning applications. J Med Imaging Radiat Oncol. 2021;65(5):545–63.

37. Barragán-Montero A, Javaid U, Valdés G, Nguyen D, Desbordes P, Macq B, et al. Artificial intelligence and machine learning for medical imaging: a technology review. Phys Med. 2021;83:242–56.

38. Rahmani AM, Yousefpoor E, Yousefpoor MS, Mehmood S, Haider A, Hosseinsadeh M, et al. Machine learning (ML) in medicine: review, applications, and challenges. Mathematics. 2021;9(22):2970.

39. Worster A, Fan J, Ismaila A. Understanding linear and logistic regression analyses. Can J Emerg Med. 2007;9(2):111–3.

40. Tripepi G, Jager KJ, Dekker FW, Soccali C. Linear and logistic regression analysis. Kidney Int. 2008;73(7):806–10.

41. Montgomery DC, Peck EA, Vining GG. Introduction to linear regression analysis. Hoboken: Wiley; 2021.

42. Kumarage PM, Yogarajah B, Ratnarajah N. Efficient feature selection for prediction of diabetic using LASSO. In: 2019 19th International conference on advances in ICT for emerging regions (ICTer). IEEE; 2019. p. 1–7.

43. Tibshirani R. Regression shrinkage and selection via the lasso. J R Stat Soc Series B Stat Methodol. 1996;58(1):267–88.

44. Vapnik V. The nature of statistical learning theory. Berlin: Springer; 2013.

45. Chandra MA, Bedi SS. Survey on SVM and their application in image classification. Int J Inf Technol. 2021;13(5):1–11.

46. Awad M, Khanna R. Support vector regression BT—efficient learning machines: theories, concepts, and applications for engineers and system designers. In: Awad M, Khanna R, editors. Berkeley: Apress; 2015. p. 67–80. Available from: https://doi.org/10.1007/978-1-4302-5990-9_4.

47. Breiman L, Friedman JH, Olsen RA, Stone CJ. Classification and regression trees by Leo Breiman. Chapter 7. 1984.

48. Kingsford C, Salsberg SL. What are decision trees? Nat Biotechnol 2008;26(9):1011–1013. Available from: https://doi.org/10.1038/nbt0908-1011.

49. Konukoglu E, Glocker B. Random forests in medical image computing. In: Handbook of medical image computing and computer assisted intervention. Academic; 2019.

50. Criminisi A, Shotton J, Konukoglu E. Decision forests: a unified framework for classification, regression, density estimation, manifold learning and semi-supervised learning. Found Trends Comput Graph Vis. 2011;7:81–227.

51. Nedjati-Gilani GL, Schneider T, Hall MG, Cawley N, Hill I, Ciccarelli O, et al. Machine learning based compartment models with permeability for white matter microstructure imaging. NeuroImage. 2017;150:119–35.

52. Kunapuli G. Ensemble methods for machine learning. New York: Simon and Schuster; 2023.

53. Breiman L. Random forests. In: Machine Learning. Springer; 2001.

54. Kramer O. K-nearest neighbors BT—dimensionality reduction with unsupervised nearest neighbors. In: Kramer O, editor. Berlin: Springer; 2013. p. 13–23. Available from: https://doi.org/10.1007/978-3-642-38652-7_2.

55. Ramteke RJ, Monali KY. Automatic medical image classification and abnormality detection using k-nearest neighbour. Int J Adv Comput Res. 2012;2(4):190.

56. Xie X. A k-nearest neighbor technique for brain tumor segmentation using Minkowski distance. J Med Imaging Health Inf. 2018;8(2):180–5.

57. Halder RK, Uddin MN, Uddin MA, Aryal S, Khraisat A. Enhancing k-nearest neighbor algorithm: a comprehensive review and performance analysis of modifications. J Big Data 2024;11(1):113. Available from: https://doi.org/10.1186/s40537-024-00973-y.

58. Ng HP, Ong SH, Foong KWC, Goh PS, Nowinski WL. Medical image segmentation using k-means clustering and improved watershed algorithm. In: Proceedings of the IEEE Southwest symposium on image analysis and interpretation. 2006.

59. MacQueen J. Some methods for classification and analysis of multivariate observations. In: Proceedings of the fifth Berkeley symposium on mathematical statistics and probability. 1967.

60. Chen CW, Luo J, Parker KJ. Image segmentation via adaptive K-mean clustering and knowledge-based morphological operations with biomedical applications. IEEE Trans Image Process. 1998;7(12):1673–83.

61. Qing X, Sheng S. A new method for initialising the K-means clustering algorithm. In: 2009 2nd International symposium on knowledge acquisition and modeling, KAM 2009. 2009.

62. Greenspan H, Ruf A, Goldberger J. Constrained Gaussian mixture model framework for automatic segmentation of MR brain images. IEEE Trans Med Imaging. 2006;25(9):1233–45.

63. Makropoulos A, Gousias IS, Ledig C, Aljabar P, Serag A, Hajnal JV, et al. Automatic whole brain MRI segmentation of the developing neonatal brain. IEEE Trans Med Imaging. 2014;33(9):1818–31.

64. Omucheni DL, Kaduki KA, Bulimo WD, Angeyo HK. Application of principal component analysis to multispectral-multimodal optical image analysis for malaria diagnostics. Malar J. 2014;13(1):485.

65. McKeown MJ, Jung TP, Makeig S, Brown G, Kindermann SS, Lee TW, et al. Spatially independent activity patterns in functional MRI data during the Stroop color-naming task. Proc Natl Acad Sci USA. 1998;95(3):803–10.

66. McKeown MJ, Hansen LK, Sejnowsk TJ. Independent component analysis of functional MRI: what is signal and what is noise? Curr Opin Neurobiol. 2003;13:620–9.

67. LeCun Y, Bengio Y, Hinton G. Deep learning. Nature. 2015;521(7553):436–44.

68. Shen D, Wu G, Suk HI. Deep learning in medical image analysis. Annu Rev Biomed Eng. 2017;19(1):221–48.

69. Rosenblatt F. The perceptron: a probabilistic model for information storage and organisation in the brain. Psychol Rev. 1958;65(6):386–408.

70. Leijnen S, van Veen F. The neural network zoo. In: Proceedings. MDPI; 2020. p. 9.

71. Abdou MA. Literature review: efficient deep neural networks techniques for medical image analysis. Neural Comput & Applic. 2022;34(8):5791–812.

72. LeCun Y, Boser B, Denker JS, Henderson D, Howard RE, Hubbard W, et al. Backpropagation applied to handwritten sip code recognition. Neural Comput. 1989;1(4):541–51.

73. Sarvamangala DR, Kulkarni RV. Convolutional neural networks in medical image understanding: a survey. Evol Intell. 2022;15(1):1–22.

74. Shang H, Qie Y. Applying deep learning to medical imaging: a review. Appl Sci. 2023;13(18):10521.

75. Munroe L, da Silva M, Heidari F, Grigorescu I, Dahan S, Robinson EC, et al. Applications of interpretable deep learning in neuroimaging: a comprehensive review. Imaging Neurosci. 2024;2:1–37.

76. Li X, Xiong H, Li X, Wu X, Shang X, Liu J, et al. Interpretable deep learning: interpretation, interpretability, trustworthiness, and beyond. Knowl Inf Syst. 2022;64(12):3197–234.

77. Wang J, Shu H, Wang SH, Shang YD. A review of deep learning on medical image analysis. Mobile Networks Appl. 2021;26(1):351–80.

78. Pacal I, Karaboga D, Basturk A, Akay B, Nalbantoglu U. A comprehensive review of deep learning in colon cancer. Comput Biol Med. 2020;126:104003.

79. Li M, Jiang Y, Shang Y, Shu H. Medical image analysis using deep learning algorithms. Front Public Health. 2023;11:1273253.

80. Orvieto A, Smith SL, Gu A, Fernando A, Gulcehre C, Pascanu R, et al. Resurrecting recurrent neural networks for long sequences. In: International conference on machine learning. PMLR; 2023. p. 26670–98.

81. Banerjee I, Ling Y, Chen MC, Hasan SA, Langlots CP, Moradsadeh N, et al. Comparative effectiveness of convolutional neural network (CNN) and recurrent neural network (RNN) architectures for radiology text report classification. Artif Intell Med. 2019;97:79–88.

82. Shai J, Shang S, Chen J, He Q. Autoencoder and its various variants. In: 2018 IEEE international conference on systems, man, and cybernetics (SMC). IEEE; 2018. p. 415–9.

83. Gondara L. Medical image denoising using convolutional denoising autoencoders. In: 2016 IEEE 16th international conference on data mining workshops (ICDMW). IEEE; 2016. p. 241–6.

84. Chushig-Muso D, Soguero-Ruis C, de Miguel-Bohoyo P, Mora-Jiménes I. Interpreting clinical latent representations using autoencoders and probabilistic models. Artif Intell Med. 2021;122:102211.

85. Khan A, Sohail A, Sahoora U, Qureshi AS. A survey of the recent architectures of deep convolutional neural networks. Artif Intell Rev. 2020;53:5455–516.

86. Krishevsky A, Sutskever I, Hinton GE. Imagenet classification with deep convolutional neural networks. Adv Neural Inf Proces Syst. 2012;25:38.

87. Simonyan K, Sisserman A. Very deep convolutional networks for large-scale image recognition. arXiv preprint arXiv:14091556. 2014.

88. Mishkin D, Sergievskiy N, Matas J. Systematic evaluation of convolution neural network advances on the imagenet. Comput Vis Image Underst. 2017;161:11–9.

89. He K, Shang X, Ren S, Sun J. Deep residual learning for image recognition. In: Proceedings of the IEEE conference on computer vision and pattern recognition. 2016. p. 770–778.

90. Asad R, Aghdam EK, Rauland A, Jia Y, Avval AH, Bosorgpour A, et al. Medical image segmentation review: the success of U-net. IEEE Trans Pattern Anal Mach Intell. 2024;46:10076–95.

91. Ronneberger O, Fischer P, Brox T. U-net: convolutional networks for biomedical image segmentation. In: Medical image computing and computer-assisted intervention–MICCAI 2015: 18th international conference, Munich, Germany, October 5–9, 2015, proceedings, part III 18. Springer; 2015. p. 234–41.

92. Çiçek Ö, Abdulkadir A, Lienkamp SS, Brox T, Ronneberger O. 3D U-Net: learning dense volumetric segmentation from sparse annotation. In: Medical Image Computing and Computer-Assisted Intervention–MICCAI 2016: 19th International Conference, Athens, Greece, October 17–21, 2016, Proceedings, Part II 19. Springer; 2016. p. 424–32.

93. Swapna M, Sharma YK, Prasadh BMG. CNN Architectures: Alex Net, Le Net, VGG, Google Net, Res Net. Int J Recent Technol Eng. 2020;8(6):953–60.

94. Bahdanau D. Neural machine translation by jointly learning to align and translate. arXiv preprint arXiv:14090473. 2014.

95. Vaswani A. Attention is all you need. Adv Neural Inf Proces Syst. 2017;30:261–72.

96. Velickovic P, Cucurull G, Casanova A, Romero A, Lio P, Bengio Y. Graph attention networks. Stat. 2017;1050(20):10–48550.

97. Dosovitskiy A. An image is worth 16x16 words: Transformers for image recognition at scale. arXiv preprint arXiv:201011929. 2020.

98. Oktay O. Attention u-net: Learning where to look for the pancreas. arXiv preprint arXiv:180403999. 2018.

99. Niu S, Shong G, Yu H. A review on the attention mechanism of deep learning. Neurocomputing. 2021;452:48–62.

100. Hatamisadeh A, Tang Y, Nath V, Yang D, Myronenko A, Landman B, et al. Unetr: transformers for 3d medical image segmentation. In: Proceedings of the IEEE/CVF winter conference on applications of computer vision. 2022. p. 574–584.

101. Camirand Lemyre F, Chalifoux K, Desharnais B, Mireault P. Squaring things up with R2: what it is and what it can (and cannot) tell you. J Anal Toxicol. 2022;46(4):443–8.

102. Gupta A, Stead TS, Ganti L. Determining a meaningful R-squared value in clinical medicine. Acad Med Surg. 2024.

103. Akossou AYJ, Palm R. Impact of data structure on the estimators R-square and adjusted R-square in linear regression. Int J Math Comput. 2013;20(3):84–93.

104. Kaur R, Kaur S. Comparison of contrast enhancement techniques for medical image. In: 2016 conference on emerging devices and smart systems (ICEDSS). IEEE; 2016. p. 155–9.

105. Paulo A, Filho F, Olegário T, Pinto B, Loureiro R, Ribeiro G, et al. Brain age prediction based on head computed tomography segmentation. In: International workshop on machine learning in clinical neuroimaging. Springer; 2023. p. 112–22.

106. Willmott CJ, Matsuura K. Advantages of the mean absolute error (MAE) over the root mean square error (RMSE) in assessing average model performance. Clim Res. 2005;30(1):79–82.

107. Chow LS, Paramesran R. Review of medical image quality assessment. Biomed Signal Process Control. 2016;27:145–54.

108. Diwakar M, Kumar M. A review on CT image noise and its denoising. Biomed Signal Process Control. 2018;42:73–88.

109. Shiao YH, Chen TJ, Chuang KS, Lin CH, Chuang CC. Quality of compressed medical images. J Digit Imaging. 2007;20:149–59.

110. Wang S, Bovik AC. A universal image quality index. IEEE Signal Process Lett. 2002;9(3):81–4.

111. Brunet D, Vrscay ER, Wang S. On the mathematical properties of the structural similarity index. IEEE Trans Image Process. 2011;21(4):1488–99.

112. Pambrun JF, Noumeir R. Limitations of the SSIM quality metric in the context of diagnostic imaging. In: 2015 IEEE international conference on image processing (ICIP). IEEE; 2015. p. 2960–3.

113. Taha AA, Hanbury A. Metrics for evaluating 3D medical image segmentation: analysis, selection, and tool. BMC Med Imaging. 2015;15:1–28.

114. Hicks SA, Strümke I, Thambawita V, Hammou M, Riegler MA, Halvorsen P, et al. On evaluation metrics for medical applications of artificial intelligence. Sci Rep. 2022;12(1):5979.

115. Huang J, Ling CX. Using AUC and accuracy in evaluating learning algorithms. IEEE Trans Knowl Data Eng. 2005;17(3):299–310.

116. Green DM, Swets JA. Signal detection theory and psychophysics. Vol. 1. New York: Wiley; 1966.

117. Jiao R, Shang Y, Ding L, Xue B, Shang J, Cai R, et al. Learning with limited annotations: a survey on deep semi-supervised learning for medical image segmentation. Comput Biol Med. 2024;169:107840.

118. Huttenlocher DP, Klanderman GA, Rucklidge WJ. Comparing images using the Hausdorff distance. IEEE Trans Pattern Anal Mach Intell. 1993;15(9):850–63.

119. Guan H, Yap PT, Bosoki A, Liu M. Federated learning for medical image analysis: a survey. Pattern Recognit. 2024;151:110424.

120. Pan SJ, Yang Q. A survey on transfer learning. IEEE Trans Knowl Data Eng. 2009;22(10):1345–59.

121. Bar Y, Diamant I, Wolf L, Lieberman S, Konen E, Greenspan H. Chest pathology detection using deep learning with non-medical training. In: 2015 IEEE 12th international symposium on biomedical imaging (ISBI). IEEE; 2015. p. 294–7.

122. Grigorescu I, Vanes L, Uus A, Batalle D, Cordero-Grande L, Nosarti C, et al. Harmonised segmentation of neonatal brain MRI. Front Neurosci. 2021;15:662005.

123. Shu JY, Park T, Isola P, Efros AA. Unpaired image-to-image translation using cycle-consistent adversarial networks. In: Proceedings of the IEEE international conference on computer vision. 2017. p. 2223–2232.

124. Mahmood F, Chen R, Durr NJ. Unsupervised reverse domain adaptation for synthetic medical images via adversarial training. IEEE Trans Med Imaging. 2018;37(12):2572–81.

125. Gholami A, Subramanian S, Shenoy V, Himthani N, Yue X, Shao S, et al. A novel domain adaptation framework for medical image segmentation. In: Brainlesion: glioma, multiple sclerosis, stroke and traumatic brain injuries: 4th International Workshop, BrainLes 2018, Held in Conjunction with MICCAI 2018, Granada, Spain, September 16, 2018, Revised Selected Papers, Part II 4. Springer; 2019. p. 289–98.

126. Yang Q, Liu Y, Chen T, Tong Y. Federated machine learning: concept and applications. ACM Trans Intell Syst Technol. 2019;10(2):1–19.

127. Sheller MJ, Reina GA, Edwards B, Martin J, Bakas S. Multi-institutional deep learning modeling without sharing patient data: a feasibility study on brain tumor segmentation. In: Brainlesion: glioma, multiple sclerosis, stroke and traumatic brain injuries: 4th International workshop, BrainLes 2018, held in conjunction with MICCAI 2018, Granada, Spain, September 16, 2018, Revised selected papers, Part I 4. Springer; 2019. p. 92–104.

128. Shi P, Qiu J, Abaxi SMD, Wei H, Lo FPW, Yuan W. Generalist vision foundation models for medical imaging: a case study of segment anything model on zero-shot medical segmentation. Diagnostics. 2023;13(11):1947.

129. Shang S, Metaxas D. On the challenges and perspectives of foundation models for medical image analysis. Med Image Anal. 2024;91:102996.

130. Qiu J, Li L, Sun J, Peng J, Shi P, Shang R, et al. Large AI models in health informatics: applications, challenges, and the future. IEEE J Biomed Health Inform. 2023;27:6074–87.

131. Shou C, Li Q, Li C, Yu J, Liu Y, Wang G, et al. A comprehensive survey on pretrained foundation models: a history from bert to chatgpt. Int J Mach Learn Cybern. 2024:1–65.

132. Kirillov A, Mintun E, Ravi N, Mao H, Rolland C, Gustafson L, et al. Segment anything. In: Proceedings of the IEEE/CVF International conference on computer vision; 2023. p. 4015–26.

133. Ma J, He Y, Li F, Han L, You C, Wang B. Segment anything in medical images. Nat Commun. 2024;15(1):654.

134. Kingma DP. Auto-encoding variational bayes. arXiv preprint arXiv:13126114. 2013.

135. Rivera M. How to train your VAE. In: 2024 IEEE International Conference on Image Processing (ICIP). IEEE; 2024. p. 3882–8.

136. Shou L, Deng W, Wu X. Unsupervised anomaly localisation using VAE and beta-VAE. arXiv preprint arXiv:200510686. 2020.

137. Kwon G, Han C, Kim D, shik. Generation of 3D brain MRI using auto-encoding generative adversarial networks. In: International conference on medical image computing and computer-assisted intervention. Springer; 2019. p. 118–26.

138. Wang Y, Blei D, Cunningham JP. Posterior collapse and latent variable non-identifiability. Adv Neural Inf Proces Syst. 2021;34:5443–55.

139. Goodfellow I, Pouget-Abadie J, Mirsa M, Xu B, Warde-Farley D, Osair S, et al. Generative adversarial networks. Commun ACM. 2020;63(11):139–44.

140. Yi X, Walia E, Babyn P. Generative adversarial network in medical imaging: a review. Med Image Anal. 2019;58:101552.

141. Gui J, Sun S, Wen Y, Tao D, Ye J. A review on generative adversarial networks: algorithms, theory, and applications. IEEE Trans Knowl Data Eng. 2021;35(4):3313–32.

142. Kaseminia S, Baur C, Kuijper A, van Ginneken B, Navab N, Albarqouni S, et al. GANs for medical image analysis. Artif Intell Med. 2020;109:101938.

143. Ho J, Jain A, Abbeel P. Denoising diffusion probabilistic models. Adv Neural Inf Proces Syst. 2020;33:6840–51.

144. Sohl-Dickstein J, Weiss E, Maheswaranathan N, Ganguli S. Deep unsupervised learning using non-

equilibrium thermodynamics. In: International conference on machine learning. PMLR; 2015. p. 2256–65.

145. Kazerouni A, Aghdam EK, Heidari M, Asad R, Fayyas M, Hacihaliloglu I, et al. Diffusion models in medical imaging: a comprehensive survey. Med Image Anal. 2023;88:102846.

146. Croitoru FA, Hondru V, Ionescu RT, Shah M. Diffusion models in vision: a survey. IEEE Trans Pattern Anal Mach Intell. 2023;45(9):10850–69.

147. Cao H, Tan C, Gao S, Xu Y, Chen G, Heng PA, et al. A survey on generative diffusion models. IEEE Trans Knowl Data Eng. 2024;36:2814–30.

148. Shur JD, Doran SJ, Kumar S, Ap Dafydd D, Downey K, O'Connor JP, Papanikolaou N, Messiou C, Koh D-M, Orton MR. Radiomics in oncology: a practical guide. Radiographics. 2021;41(6):1717–32.

149. Risso S, Botta F, Raimondi S, Origgi D, Fanciullo C, Morganti AG, Bellomi M. Radiomics: the facts and the challenges of image analysis. Eur Radio Exp. 2018;2(1):1–8.

150. Gillies RJ, Kinahan PE, Hricak H. Radiomics: images are more than pictures, they are data. Radiology. 2016;278(2):563–77.

151. Polidori T, De Santis D, Rucci C, Tremamunno G, Piccini G, Pugliese L, Serunian M, Guido G, Pucciarelli F, Bracci B. Radiomics applications in cardiac imaging: a comprehensive review. Radiol Med. 2023;128:1–12.

152. Rainey C, O'Regan T, Matthew J, Skelton E, Wosnitsa N, Chu K-Y, Goodman S, McConnell J, Hughes C, Bond R, McFadden S, Malamateniou C. Beauty is in the AI of the beholder: are we ready for the clinical integration of artificial intelligence in radiography? An exploratory analysis of perceived AI knowledge, skills, confidence, and education perspectives of UK radiographers. Front Digital Health. 2021;3:739327.

153. Malamateniou C, Knapp K, Pergola M, Wosnitsa N, Hardy M. Artificial intelligence in radiography: where are we now and what does the future hold? Radiography. 2021;27:S58–62.

154. Hatt M, Le Rest CC, Tixier F, Badic B, Schick U, Visvikis D. Radiomics: data are also images. J Nucl Med. 2019;60(Supplement 2):38S–44S.

155. Remeseiro B, Bolon-Canedo V. A review of feature selection methods in medical applications. Comput Biol Med. 2019;112:103375.

156. Steyerberg EW. Validation in prediction research: the waste by data splitting. J Clin Epidemiol. 2018;103:131–3.

157. Sadeghi S, Alisadehsani R, Cifci MA, Kausar S, Rehman R, Mahanta P, et al. A review of explainable artificial intelligence in healthcare. Comput Electr Eng. 2024;118:109370.

158. Nemani V, Biggio L, Huan X, Hu S, Fink O, Tran A, et al. Uncertainty quantification in machine learning for engineering design and health prognostics: a tutorial. Mech Syst Signal Process. 2023;205:110796.

159. Lapuschkin S, Wäldchen S, Binder A, Montavon G, Samek W, Müller KR. Unmasking Clever Hans predictors and assessing what machines really learn. Nat Commun. 2019;10(1):1096.

160. Singh A, Sengupta S, Lakshminarayanan V. Explainable deep learning models in medical image analysis. J Imaging. 2020;6(6):52.

161. Selvaraju RR, Cogswell M, Das A, Vedantam R, Parikh D, Batra D. Grad-CAM: visual explanations from deep networks via gradient-based localisation. In: 2017 IEEE International Conference on Computer Vision (ICCV); 2017. p. 618–26.

162. Springenberg JT, Dosovitskiy A, Brox T, Riedmiller M. Striving for simplicity: The all convolutional net. arXiv preprint arXiv:14126806. 2014.

163. Smilkov D, Thorat N, Kim B, Viégas F, Wattenberg M. Smoothgrad: removing noise by adding noise. arXiv preprint arXiv:170603825. 2017.

164. Seineldin RA, Karar ME, Elshaer S, Coburger J, Wirts CR, Burgert O, et al. Explainability of deep neural networks for MRI analysis of brain tumors. Int J Comput Assist Radiol Surg. 2022;17(9):1673–83.

165. Lambert B, Forbes F, Doyle S, Dehaene H, Dojat M. Trustworthy clinical AI solutions: a unified review of uncertainty quantification in deep learning models for medical image analysis. Artif Intell Med. 2024;150:102830.

166. Huang L, Ruan S, Xing Y, Feng M. A review of uncertainty quantification in medical image analysis: probabilistic and non-probabilistic methods. Med Image Anal. 2024;97:103223.

167. Lakshminarayanan B, Pritsel A, Blundell C. Simple and scalable predictive uncertainty estimation using deep ensembles. Adv Neural Inf Proces Syst. 2017;30:13.

168. Barbano R, Shang C, Arridge S, Jin B. Quantifying model uncertainty in inverse problems via Bayesian deep gradient descent. In: In: 2020 25th International Conference on Pattern Recognition (ICPR). IEEE; 2021. p. 1392–9.

169. Gawlikowski J, Tassi CRN, Ali M, Lee J, Humt M, Feng J, et al. A survey of uncertainty in deep neural networks. Artif Intell Rev. 2023;56(Suppl 1):1513–89.

170. Bass C, Da Silva M, Sudre C, Williams LZ, Sousa HS, Tudosiu PD, Alfaro-Almagro F, Fitzgibbon SP, Glasser MF, Smith SM, Robinson EC. Icamreg: Interpretable classification and regression with feature attribution for mapping neurological phenotypes in individual scans. IEEE transactions on medical imaging. 2022;42(4):959–70.

Dr. Irina Grigorescu is a research associate at King's College London, based in the Department of Early Life Imaging. She specializes in deep learning-based analysis of foetal and neonatal brain and body imaging, focusing on the development of computational tools for medical image registration and segmentation, as well as techniques for interpretable deep learning and domain adaptation.

Dr. Nouf A. Mushari is an assistant professor in the Department of Radiological Sciences at Taif University. She holds a Ph.D. from the University of Leeds, where her research focused on the application of radiomics analysis and artificial intelligence (AI) in PET/MR imaging. Her work contributes to advancing diagnostic imaging techniques by integrating AI-driven approaches for more accurate and personalized assessments. Dr. Mushari's research interests include medical imaging technologies, AI applications in healthcare, and the development of novel imaging biomarkers. She has presented her work at national and international conferences and is actively involved in interdisciplinary research projects.

Professor Charalampos Tsoumpas is a full professor on Quantification in Molecular Diagnostics and Radionuclide Therapy at the Department of Nuclear Medicine & Molecular Imaging, University of Groningen. He is a physicist (2002, bachelor, National Kapodistrian University of Athens) and Biomedical Engineer (2004, masters, National Technical University of Athens) and received his PhD from Imperial College in 2008. His academic training and experience include positions at King's College London and University of Leeds and throughout his career has supervised 25 PhD theses. He is a Fellow of IOP, Fellow of IPEM, and IEEE Senior Member.

Dr. Maria Deprez is a senior lecturer at King's College London, based in the Department of Early Life Imaging. She has over 20 years of experience in image analysis of foetal, neonatal and paediatric MRI and US. She and her group have contributed novel techniques for image segmentation, registration, reconstruction, and modelling of growth and development during early life, including classical and deep learning approaches.

Ethics of AI in Radiography Practice

3

Hendrik Erenstein, Mirjam Plantinga, and Peter M. A. van Ooijen

3.1 Introduction

The application of AI in healthcare comes with many opportunities but also presents ethical challenges [1]. Given that technology, including AI, is developed and implemented by people, the influence and impact of technology on human behaviour and practice will depend on how it is directed and controlled. Consequently, it is crucial that we recognise and comprehend the ethical challenges that come with the development and implementation of AI in healthcare.

Ethics is about norms and values, about what is right and what is wrong. It is about critically discussing and reflecting on the morality of choices and decisions from different perspectives.

on behalf of Association of Healthcare Technology Providers for Imaging, Radiotherapy and Care (AXREM)

H. Erenstein
Hanze University of Applied Sciences, Groningen, The Netherlands
e-mail: h.erenstein@pl.hanze.nl

M. Plantinga · P. M. A. van Ooijen (✉)
Department of Genetics and Data Science Center in Health, University of Groningen, University Medical Center Groningen, Groningen, The Netherlands

Department of Radiotherapy and Data Science Center in Health (DASH), University of Groningen, University Medical Center Groningen, Groningen, The Netherlands
e-mail: m.plantinga@umcg.nl;
p.m.a.van.ooijen@umcg.nl

However, do not expect answers to be clear cut about when, where, or how to use AI or whether it is ethically acceptable. An ethical reflection involves careful consideration and weighing up of different, and sometimes conflicting, norms and values. The weighing of these norms and values can also vary depending on the specific decision or action and context in which they are made.

The purpose for which you intend to apply AI, whether to assist in healthcare diagnostics, or in choosing which movie to watch or music to listen to, alters the context of decisions and impacts ethical reflection. In healthcare, patients are in a vulnerable position, and good care is essential. Trust between patients and healthcare professionals (HCPs) is vital, and values such as safety, quality of care, and trustworthiness significantly impact this trust. As a result, errors in AI-informed healthcare decisions are less acceptable, and potentially more dangerous, compared to mistakes in music selection or movie suggestions.

The aim of this chapter is to create awareness of some of the ethical issues that need to be considered in the context of the use of AI in radiography. When focusing on the use of AI in healthcare, both *medical ethical principles* and general *ethical AI principles* need to be considered. Beneficence, non-maleficence, respect for autonomy, and justice have long been the specific principles in medical ethics [2]. Regarding general ethical AI principles, many different frameworks and guidelines exist. In this chapter, we

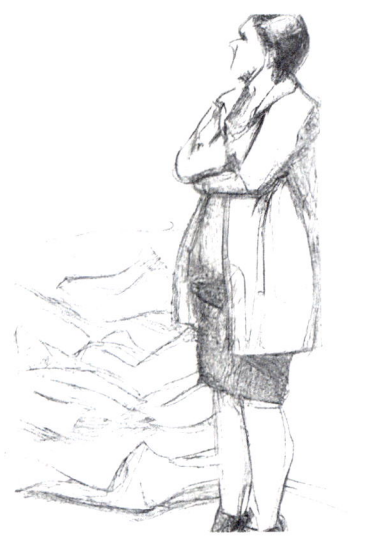

Fig. 3.1 Case study 1: Discuss around the ethics of data collection and use. Since there is no AI without data, considerations of the ethics of AI always need to include discussions regarding the ethics of data collection and use

will use the six ethical principles formulated by the World Health Organisation (WHO) [3]. These principles are: Protect autonomy; Promote human well-being, human safety, and the public interest; Ensure transparency, explainability, and intelligibility; Foster responsibility and accountability; Ensure inclusiveness and equity; and Promote AI that is responsive and sustainable. We will refer to these principles as *the six WHO principles.*

The six WHO principles overlap largely with ethical principles brought forward on ethical use of AI in radiography and healthcare and with general principles in medical ethics [2, 4–14]. Using these principles, we will reflect on what the introduction of AI in radiography means in terms of adherence and compliance and discuss the use of AI in fulfilling different tasks, or roles, in the context of radiography, starting with image acquisition and image processing, followed by patient interaction. The chapter will finish with a reflection on the impact of the use of AI on professional identity and requirements for the development of key competencies for radiographers to address the AI ethics requirements. Additionally, case studies have been included throughout the chapter to highlight related topics to prompt further discussions. The first case study is presented in Fig. 3.1.

3.2 Image Acquisition and Processing

The use of AI in image acquisition and processing in medical imaging has played an increasing role for at least two decades. One example is auto-positioning in radiography, a rule-based implementation of AI (if x then y, else z). In recent years, more complex techniques have been developed, such as those aimed at recognising and diagnosing images. However, AI can also play a role in the steps leading up to, and following, image acquisition. A simplified scheme of these steps is shown in Fig. 3.2. More information about automatic positioning can be found in Chaps. 5, 6, and 7 for AI applications in projectional and cross-sectional radiography, respectively (CT and MRI).

Most radiographers will be able to recall examination referrals that were irrelevant, incorrect (e.g. examination of the wrong extremity or wrong anatomical side (right or left)) requested, with the patient complaining, or referrals that were plainly unnecessary. AI tools could be trained to support and facilitate this part of the process. However, because an incorrect imaging referral and the potential subsequent delay in imaging examination may have profound consequences for patient experience, departmental workflow, and clinical outcomes, the responsible use of AI in this context is paramount. This entails paying attention to the six WHO principles and focusing on the use of AI as a tool that aids the radiographer in conducting the task faster, reliably, and equally well or better than before AI was used (WHO principle 2). In doing so, radiographers should maintain autonomy and responsibility, and AI should not be leading the examination referral, but the process should always keep the human-in-the-loop (WHO principles 1 and 4).

To achieve responsible use of AI by healthcare professionals, it is necessary to further consider the principle of explainability (WHO principle 3) [10]. Five conditions necessary for fostering trust are brought forward; one of these

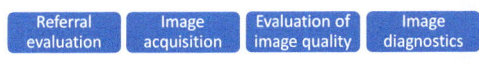

Fig. 3.2 Simplified scheme of the imaging process as used in this chapter. As noted throughout this paragraph, AI has the potential to support radiographers at every step

is Trust by healthcare professionals, which requires professionals to have sufficient reasons to believe that the AI output is reliable and advocates for a level of knowledge and understanding of the process that generates the AI output [10]. The AI 'black box', which is the lack of knowledge of the development, training, testing, and validation steps of AI algorithms in healthcare, can be a challenge for AI use and an obstacle to AI implementation in clinical practice; it often prevents the full understanding of these processes by healthcare practitioners and limits their knowledge to the bare essentials, in the pretext of preserving intellectual property and protecting commercial secrets. Explainability of AI is regarded as a factor that enhances understanding. Many research and implementation projects are focussing on ways to increase explainability [9–11]. On the other hand, discussion is taking place on whether explainability could, and should, be regarded as a key legal requirement for responsible AI use in the future, and whether this requirement is necessary, or even possible, in all contexts and decisions [15]. More on AI explainability in the radiography context can be found in Chaps. 4 and 7.

In addition to explainability, transparency is often mentioned as a requirement for ethical healthcare (WHO principle 3). For example, transparency regarding input data and algorithm development is essential to identify potential biases in the data and/or model, assess a model's performance and efficacy ('does it do what it says on the tin?'), and communicate possible risks or harm of its use. One example is the establishment of a Foundation Model Transparency Index specifying 100 indicators ranging from data and labour to social impact [16]. This Index shows the importance, but also the complexity, of transparency. The complexity of transparency is further highlighted by others. A study investigating the transparency of AI-based radiography products offered and used across Europe found that transparency was limited [17]. For example, most products provided no information on the collection of training data or population characteristics, making it difficult to assess the possibility of algorithmic bias [17]. Furthermore, ethical requirements regarding the input data, such as the availability of consent, were rarely documented. Consequently, transparency and explainability are not always sufficiently employed in practice but are key factors to consider to responsibly develop and implement AI in healthcare and foster the necessary trust for the adoption of AI technologies by medical institutions and professionals.

In recent years, deep learning algorithms and 3D-cameras have been adopted to provide dynamic auto-positioning in conventional radiography, including, for example, auto-collimation (see Chap. 5 for more technical details on it). But it is not just conventional radiography where AI is complementing the image acquisition process. Auto-positioning has also been adopted within the CT environment where AI-enhanced 3D-cameras are able to identify the isocentre and position patients with an accuracy equalling experienced radiographers [18]. AI product implementation aimed at standardising examination positioning could potentially improve workflows, through reducing repeat examinations, improving image quality, and optimising patient dose. However, due to the increasing complexity of these techniques, the explainability of 'how' the scanner is making its positioning suggestion has become increasingly challenging.

As with image acquisition, AI has shown potential to provide support during the evaluation of image quality [19]. However, it is important to realise that rejection or acceptance of an image based on its quality and positioning provides an illusion of a binary choice. Clinical practice is rife with borderline cases, for example, a patient unable to fully inhale for a chest radiograph. The acquired image might be rejected by an AI model because of insufficient inspiration, suggesting a retake of the image is necessary. However, retaking an image of a patient who is unable to fully inhale will not generate a better image; it would rather put more unnecessary strain on the patient and impact their experience. Hence, input data used by the model should be transparent for radiographers to make a well-balanced and well-informed decision. Strictly adhering to the AI-based rejection of an image and excluding other information might also put patient safety at risk (WHO principle 2). Radiographers should use their own clinically informed knowledge and judgement based on education and years of expe-

rience, to determine the validity of the AI output and be aware of their autonomy, responsibility, and the risk of automation bias and the tendency towards over-reliance on technology without critical evaluation (WHO principles 1 and 4). Figure 3.3 demonstrates the ethical challenges associated with AI implementation in medical imaging and radiotherapy. Figure 3.4 presents the respective possible solutions, as discussed by clinical professionals in these fields [13].

Although some countries, like the UK and Denmark, are already familiar with the *reporting radiographer*, the advanced practice role where a radiographer performs image reading and interpretation, this *role* has not been globally adopted. However, it could be argued that AI might be used to augment the performance of a reporting radiographer for specific diagnostic tasks,

AI ethical challenges

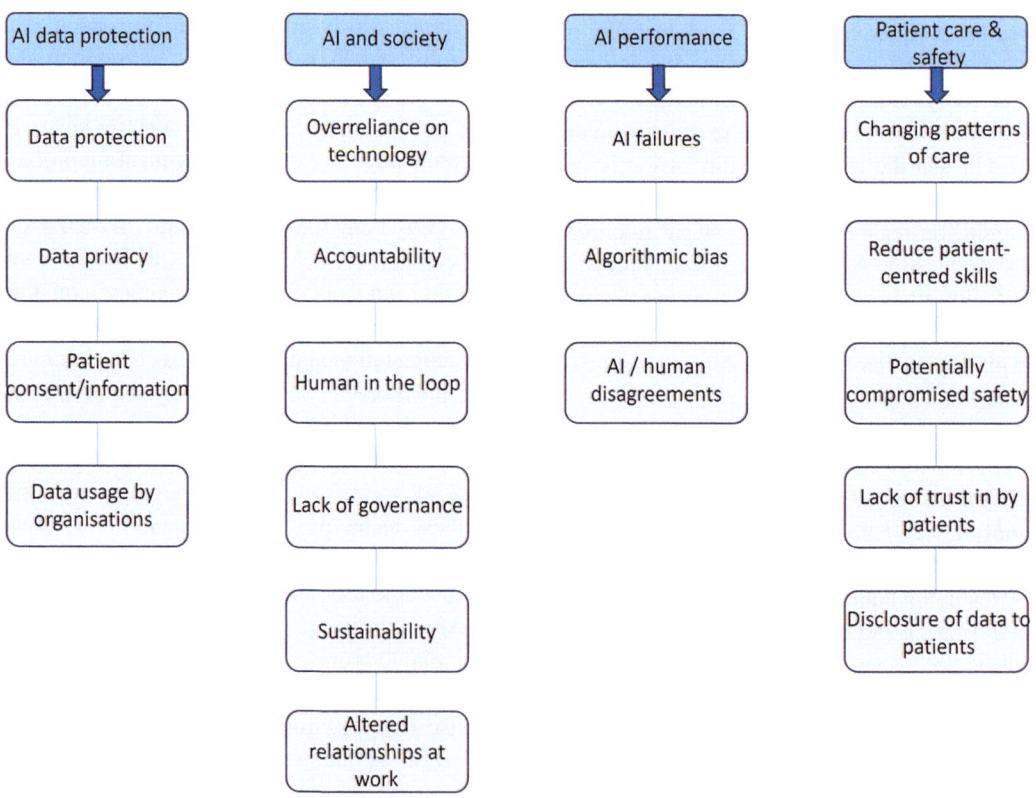

Fig. 3.3 Ethical challenges stemming from the use of AI in medical imaging and radiotherapy as discussed by respective professionals [13]

Potential solutions to ethical challenges

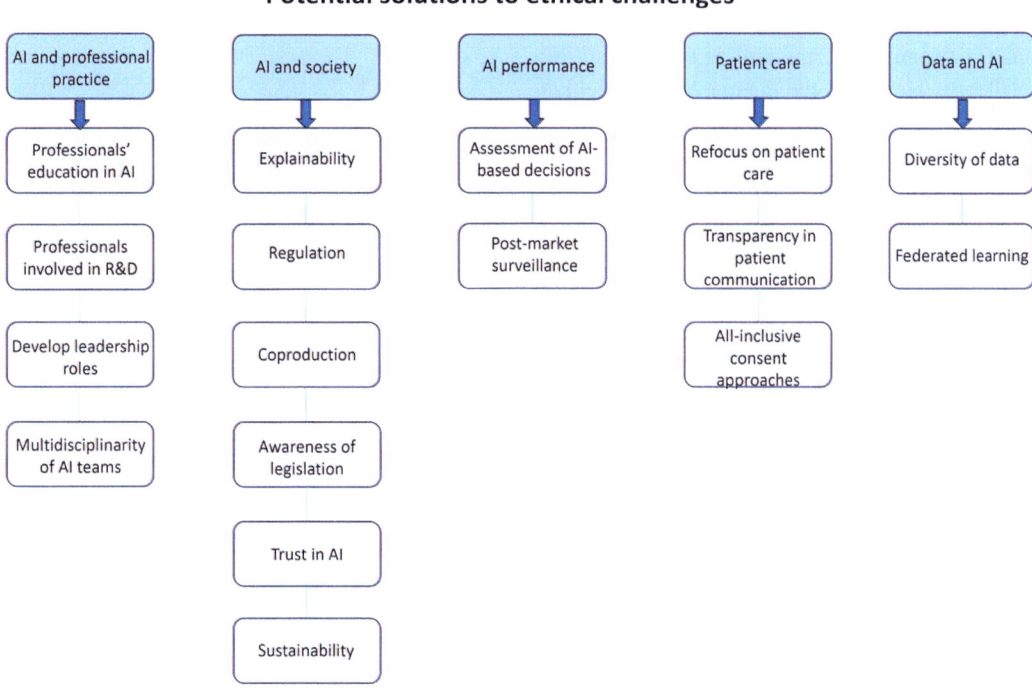

Fig. 3.4 Suggested solutions to AI ethical challenges stemming from the use of AI in medical imaging and radiotherapy as discussed by respective professionals [13]

although most studies currently present data on the role of AI as a decision support tool for triage, detection, and diagnosis for radiologists only (see Chap. 5 for more information on this topic). For instance, conventional chest imaging plays a pivotal role in tuberculosis (TB) screening and triage in Africa [20, 21]. According to the WHO, a scarcity of radiologists is a valid reason why the application of AI could improve public well-being by increasing TB diagnosis and, consequently, improve treatability and health outcomes for people impacted by it (WHO principle 2) [21]. It is possible that radiographers, supported by AI, could provide an on-site TB triage and abnormality reporting service without direct consultation with a radiologist. A comparable example could be seen at AI-supported triaging in emergency departments. Introduction of AI-triaging might improve time-to-diagnosis and patient well-being, while providing radiographers with a chance to expand their clinical contribution and roles; a similar set-up is already being trialled in some London hospitals in the

UK for same-day CT scans if a reporting radiographer, supported by AI, has identified a suspicious finding in their chest X-rays. That data will be published in late 2025, before the threshold of inclusion in this textbook, but it is important to see how things evolve in this very active domain that will transform radiographer responsibilities, accountability, and the way they interact with patients. Similar schemes could simultaneously alleviate radiologist workload by assessing (semi-)automated ER-referrals [22]. However, improvement for public well-being is only viable if the decisions made are transparent (WHO principle 3).

AI plays a huge role in shaping radiography practice and the profession. Nonetheless, aside from the already noted ethical challenges, there is also the concept of deskilling, which is the loss of necessary skills to deliver a safe and effective clinical service. As technology has augmented radiography in the past, the profession and practices moved with it and certain skills were inevitably lost, with new skills developed. The new generation of radiographers lacks the skills of developing analogue films, but, given the abundance of digital systems, this is rarely seen as a challenge. However, the far-reaching implementation of AI might have a bigger impact. Losing the ability to perform proper patient positioning due to a dependency on a highly dynamic automatic positioning system could severely limit radiographer autonomy in situations unsupported by AI, e.g. in patients with special or complex needs or paediatric patients, who might be able to stay still for the AI-enabled positioning to work. While it is difficult to pinpoint the exact risks of deskilling, it certainly challenges the six WHO key principles.

In a time where healthcare is under sustained pressure by complex causes (e.g. increasing population age, decreasing workforce, the aftermath of COVID-19), AI may provide relief by increasing workflow efficiency (e.g. through automatic scheduling of appointments or auto-positioning technologies) or improve patient safety by minimising human errors (e.g. acting as a second reader). However, this could also challenge the complex balance between access to healthcare and maintaining the knowledge and skills of healthcare professionals [22–24].

While initially the use of AI in image acquisition and processing was based on basic, rule-based (e.g. if x then y, else z) algorithms through programming, AI models and algorithms are now more complex and based on machine learning and deep learning techniques (see more about the history of AI in Chap. 1 where this discrimination is made). This not only provides opportunities for clinical practice development but also requires a consideration of ethical principles. Having reflected on the principles of transparency and explainability as explained above, have a look at case study 2 and Fig. 3.5, and consider the importance of the other WHO principles when using AI in the context of image acquisition and processing.

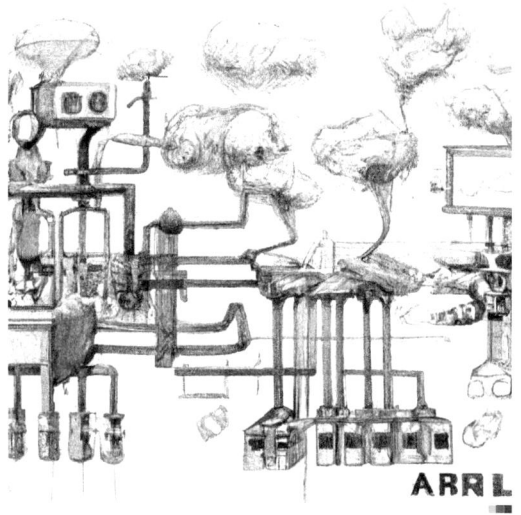

Fig. 3.5 Case study 2: Considering the impact of the WHO principles when AI is used for image acquisition and processing, reflect on how transparent and explainable these processes are for you and how this impacts your learning and your practice. Also reflect on the role of sustainability; training AI models can cost a lot of energy; however, it might improve workflow and decrease energy per examination

3.3 Patient Interaction

While AI in image acquisition and processing is well established, the use of AI in the context of patient interaction is a more recent development and one currently under exploration. Although language-based AI has been a research topic for decades, its adoption into healthcare has been hindered by limited reliability and a lack of accessibility. However, with the release of ChatGPT and related AI models, known as Large Language Models (LLMs), significant steps towards the adoption of language-based AI have been made. Such models have the advantage of being able to increase accessibility of information as end-users can prompt LLMs to rewrite and rephrase information, for instance, radiography reports, to make them easier to understand [25]. This would apply, for instance, to a case where a radiological report, where scientific jargon is used, could be changed into a report where lay language is used, to ensure the information is accessible to patients.

Many see the increase in the use of AI, including LLMs, as a possibility to increase efficiency and to address the already existing and increasing shortages on the healthcare labour market. The broad availability of LLMs, such as ChatGPT, Deepseek, Llama, and other branded names, has made it accessible to everyone, and it is currently used by people searching for different types of healthcare-related information, e.g. adding their symptoms and asking for a potential diagnosis. However, patients and radiographers alike should be aware that LLMs are text-generating models based on statistical probabilities, not able to understand the full content, context, or correctness of the information that is provided. They are also, in their majority, not accredited, so strictly speaking they cannot and should not be used for any medical-related enquiry (more about this is discussed in Chap. 4 under regulation). As a result, the AI answers provided could be factually incorrect and could lead to unnecessary stress and anxiety for patients and dangerous practice for healthcare professionals, if relying heavily on them. Currently, LLMs are being implemented in healthcare to provide concept answers to patient questions or to generate patient summaries. Even with these tools, healthcare practitioners (HCPs) remain responsible for patient care, for safeguarding the promotion of human well-being, human safety, and the public interest (WHO principle 2), and for providing reliable and accessible information to patients. Additionally, HCPs are also responsible for evaluating the output of the AI models used in their patients' care, and for querying the correctness (or not!) of information produced by these models. Consequently, in the context of healthcare, a *human in the loop* is therefore required to ensure responsibility and accountability (WHO principle 4).

Given the lack of transparency and explainability of the output of most AI models, as discussed above, assessing the validity of information provided by LLMs can often be challenging. Users should be aware of their responsibility to critically assess the information provided and ensure that their professional autonomy or decision-making will not be undermined by automation bias (WHO principles 1 and 4) [4, 7].

It is important to realise that the limitations of LLM-generated information are not restricted to factual correctness; cultural attunement also plays a huge role as a central element of societal norms. In the initial stages of public LLM releases, most data and parties involved were from the USA and China and, although some models were fine-tuned by renowned academic groups in the field, these new models rarely reached mainstream audiences [26, 27]. The information provided by LLM models is likely to be influenced by the socio-demographic context (people, practices, processes) in which these were developed, frequently and often inadvertently, reproducing stereotypes which might be irrelevant or offensive in another context or audience [28–31]. Therefore, when AI algorithms are implemented in a narrow scope, it is vital to be aware of culturally sensitive topics, such as religion, alcohol use, or gender equality (WHO principle 5), which could be impacted in the way they are analysed, presented, or interpreted by these models. Hence, when implementing LLMs for different audiences, local cultural norms and values should be respected and prioritised in favour of well-being, to avoid controversy, conflict, division, or misinformation (WHO principle 2). Conversely, if an AI model is integrated into and used by a multicultural context, then its training, testing, and external validation should include diverse data, representative of the population this model is intended to be used on.

Interaction with patients is the cornerstone of healthcare communication and service delivery; therefore, the impact of currently available LLMs on the communication between patients and HCPs should be carefully considered and weighed before their use. On the one hand, it is expected and hoped that the use of LLMs will lessen the administrative burden, such as history taking and data input, for HCPs, including radiographers, and give them more time to interact with patients. On the other hand, advancing technologies can speed up image acquisition processes and shorten the duration of radiography appointments, decreasing the opportunity for radiographer–patient interaction. Additionally, as AI models will be increasingly employed to collate patient data from various digital sources, HCPs may be required to spend more time interacting with their computer screen to facilitate and evaluate this process (in the form of quality assurance/quality control), rather than with the patient. Furthermore, recent studies have shown that, although AI may not express authentic empathy or share other people's suffering, it can show compassion in different interactions with humans through its facilitation of active support. It was so convincing that third-party evaluators perceived it as being better than skilled humans [32]. What the future interaction of radiographers with patients will look like is hard to predict. But no matter what direction this might take us into, the radiographers remain responsible and accountable (WHO principle 4) for providing safety and quality of the clinical service and delivering patient care (WHO principle 2). Professionals and professional associations, together with patients and academics, will also play a crucial role in determining the standards of patient care and produce guidance for optimal interaction of HCPs with technology and the patients [4, 7, 12]. The Society and College of Radiographers issued specific guidance in 2021 with emphasis on education, research, clinical practice, and partnerships, highlighting potential ethical issues and suggesting solutions [12]. This guidance is now being updated to include LLMs and will be published later in 2025 or early 2026. Moving from a clinical governance structure onto an AI governance unified framework in medical imaging and radiotherapy requires emphasis on seven pillars, as presented in Fig. 3.6: (a) AI research and innovation; (b) public, patient, and practitioner involvement; (c) training of staff; (d) regulation,

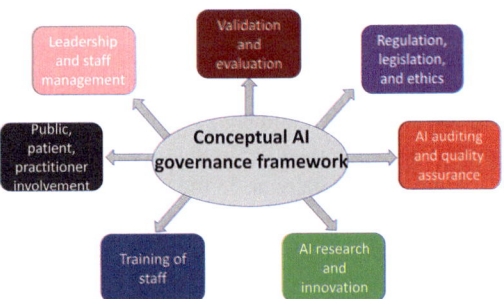

Fig. 3.6 The seven pillars of AI governance as produced by a scoping review of the medical imaging and radiotherapy literature [14]

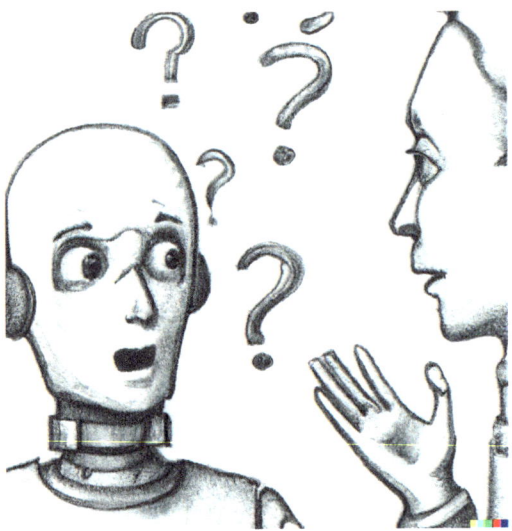

Fig. 3.7 Case study 3: Considering the changes of AI technologies and the six WHO principles, imagine how radiographer–patient interactions can be mediated and altered by AI in the future

legislation, and ethics; (e) validation and evaluation; (f) AI auditing and quality assurance; and (g) leadership and staff management [14].

In this section, the use of AI in the context of patient interaction has been reflected upon. However, while it is purported that LLMs may address accessibility and inclusion, low literacy skills or language barriers can hinder the use of these AI technologies. Consider case study 3 highlighted using Fig. 3.7 and articulate your thoughts about the accessibility of recent technologies taking the WHO principles into consideration.

3.4 Professional Identity and Required Competencies

Ever since the advent of radiography with Wilhelm Conrad Röntgen's discovery of X-rays in 1895, the role of the radiographer has been developing and changing. Comparable to the introduction of MRI, CT, and ultrasound technologies in the past, the introduction of AI requires new competencies while also allowing radiographers to let go of others. For example, the introduction of computed radiography reduced dependency on analogue film development but increased the relevance of knowledge in digital postprocessing. This adjustment in competencies may not only impact professional tasks and roles, but also the professional identity a person holds. This, in turn, impacts their willingness to adopt AI technologies in practice [33]. A recent European study of more than 2200 radiographers reported that, despite general optimism for a future with AI, radiographers are concerned about changing patterns in patient care and technology competencies. They worry about how this digital transformation will impact their careers, job satisfaction, and professional identity, which has traditionally balanced on the interface between patients and technology [34].

To drive responsible development and implementation of AI, HCPs need to develop the knowledge, skills, and competences to ask the right questions when interacting with AI, whether they are users or stakeholders in a process of AI development or procurement [35]. In the UNESCO recommendation on the Ethics of Artificial Intelligence (2021), the promotion of awareness and understanding of AI technologies, including digital skills and AI ethics training, is highlighted [36]. Many other organisations, professional bodies, and regulatory agencies make a call for increasing digital literacy not as an option, but rather as a professional responsibility. More details on the requirements of digital literacy and AI education are discussed in Chaps. 4

and 15, looking into the future of radiography, as it will coexist with AI. The UNESCO report also highlights the principle of 'multi-stakeholder and adaptive governance and collaboration'. This principle underscores the importance of involving various stakeholders, including patients, throughout the AI system lifecycle to promote inclusiveness, coproduction, and usability (WHO principle 5). Chapter. 12 on person-centred care elaborates on the principles required to engage key stakeholders in the coproduction of AI tools.

Educators and academics should be aware of the undeniable role they have in the successful and responsible adoption of AI into radiography. They can do this as role models, by constantly learning and researching more about AI; they also need to be the champions of change, by creating educational provisions for their students, to keep up to date with recent technological developments, and by gathering and expanding the evidence base for the profession around AI through research and scholarship. This textbook is trying to achieve exactly that! A recent paper on responsible AI highlights the importance of training and governance as key to safe and effective AI implementation [6]. The more specific elements of responsible AI can be seen in Fig. 3.8. This figure and other research work confirm that the availability of ethical guidelines for AI development alone does not suffice to ensure responsible AI development and implementation, but that people also need to be empowered and educated to be able to act responsibly [6, 35]. The recently published European AI Act therefore also requires organisations to develop 'AI literacy' among their employees [37]. Responsible development and implementation of AI thus requires the development of new competencies among the different stakeholders, not only in a technical sense but also in a moral sense [6, 33]. Although educational programs for radiographers vary, a dedicated section of education should be devoted to ethical challenges. As highlighted in this chapter, these ethical challenges play a key role in the responsible development and implementation of AI in healthcare. Knowledge of the ethical challenges also provides a footing to critically assess and use AI and

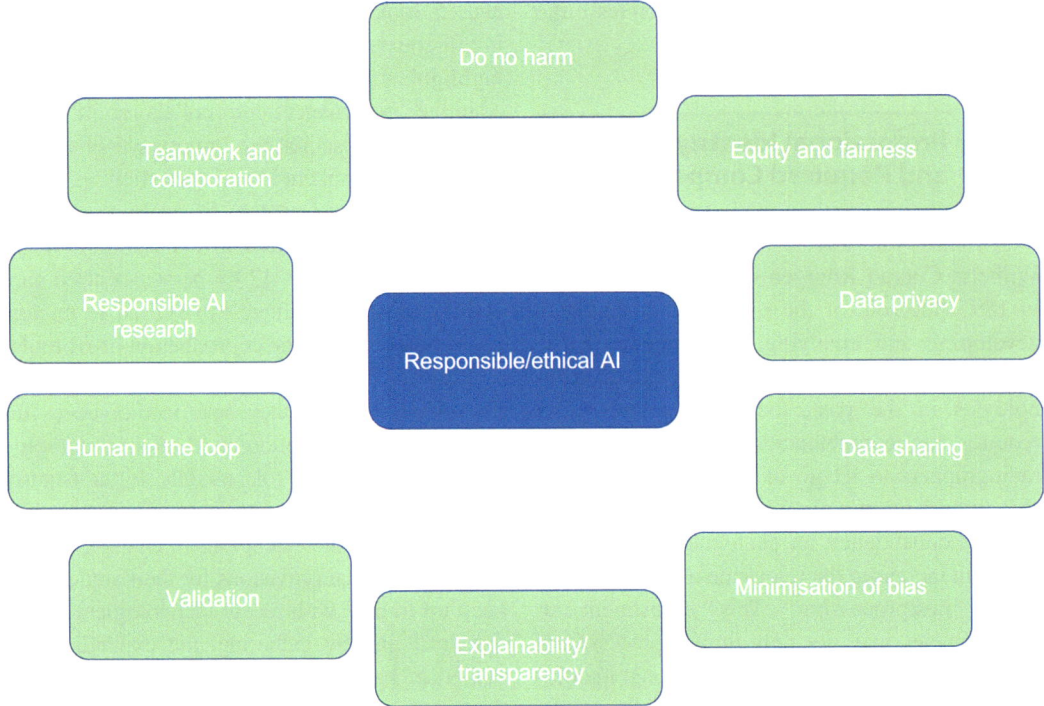

Fig. 3.8 Responsible AI practice requires both robust governance and AI training [6]. Training on the key ethics elements seen in this figure is vital for safe and effective AI implementation in radiography and healthcare in general

shape professional expectations on how to act responsibly and be held accountable (WHO principle 4). In addition, as Maheshwari et al. (2024) argue, with respect to the WHO principles, professionals do not only require information themselves, but they also have a responsibility for explaining the use and functioning of the tools they use, including AI, to their patients [10].

This closing section highlights the professional challenges and new responsibilities to current and future radiographers posed by the introduction of AI. Critical reflection on the required skills to maintain the quality of care is needed by both clinical practitioners and educators. Consider case study 4 in Fig. 3.9 and discuss which skills should be maintained and which, if any, radiographers can let go. As part of this, the current skillset used and the new skills that will be relevant in the years to come will need to be reflected upon. Understand the ethical principles related to AI in radiography, including both medical ethics (beneficence, non-maleficence, respect for autonomy, and justice) and the WHO's ethical AI principles (Protecting autonomy; Promoting human well-being, safety, and public interest; Ensuring transparency, explainability, and intelligibility; Fostering responsibility and accountability; Ensuring inclusiveness and equity; and Promoting responsive and sustainable AI). Recognise the ethical challenges posed by AI in radiography, which extend beyond imaging to include issues such as data privacy, algorithmic bias, and the impact on patient care and professional practice. Identify and suggest future com-

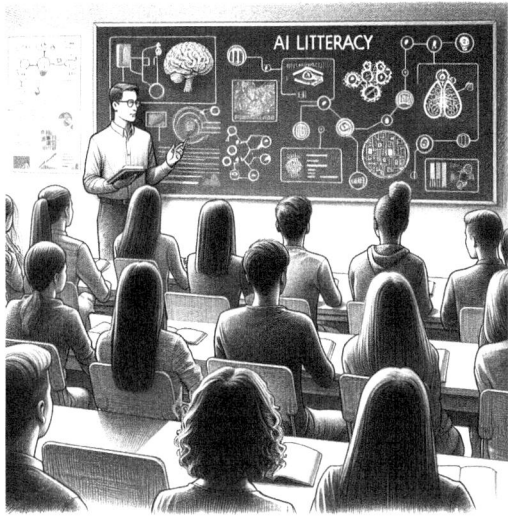

Fig. 3.9 Case study 4: Discuss what knowledge can stay and what needs to go to ensure radiographers are equipped for a digital future. Please note the word literacy is misspelled due to the known confabulations (also known as hallucinations) of LLMs

petencies needed for radiographers, such as proficiency in AI technologies, ethical decision-making skills, and the ability to navigate the evolving landscape of AI in healthcare.

3.5   Chapter Summary

This chapter has introduced the ethical challenges that come with the introduction of AI in the field of radiography and wider healthcare. The topic of ethics is vast, and whole books have been written about the underlying themes of autonomy, public interest, equality, and safety. The references provided offer opportunities for further reading and sources of information that may be beneficial for the interested learner. Please note that the references mentioned in the text are more accessible and not strictly academic [38–44].

Acknowledgments We extend our heartfelt thanks to the colleagues from the ethics Work Package (WP) of the ELSA AI Lab Northern Netherlands for their invaluable contribution to this chapter. Their insights and expertise have greatly enriched our work.

References

1. European parliament. Artificial intelligence in healthcare. Applications, risks, and ethical and societal impacts. 2022.
2. Beauchamp TL, Childress JF. Principles of biomedical ethics. New York: Oxford; 1979.
3. World Health Organisation. Ethics and governance of artificial intelligence for health: WHO guidance. 2021.
4. Geis JR, Brady AP, Wu CC, Spencer J, Ranschaert E, Jaremko JL, et al. Ethics of artificial intelligence in radiography: summary of the joint European and North American multisociety statement. Radiography. 2019;293(2):436–40.
5. Goisauf M, Cano AM. Ethics of AI in radiography: a review of Ethical and societal implications. Front Big Data. 2022;5:850383.
6. Walsh G, Stogiannos N, van de Venter R, Rainey C, Tam W, McFadden S, et al. Responsible AI practice and AI education are central to AI implementation: a rapid review for all medical imaging professionals in Europe. BJR Open. 2023;5(1):20230033.
7. Brady AP. Radiography AI in the real world: commentary on "Developing, purchasing, implementing and monitoring AI tools in radiography: practical considerations. A multi-society statement from the ACR, CAR, ESR, RANZCR & RSNA". Eur Radiol. 2024;34(8):5077–9.
8. Morley J, Machado CCV, Burr C, Cowls J, Joshi I, Taddeo M, et al. The ethics of AI in health care: a mapping review. Soc Sci Med. 2020;260:113172.
9. Baker S, Xiang W. Explainable AI is responsible AI: how explainability creates trustworthy and socially responsible artificial intelligence. arXiv (Cornell University). 2023.
10. Maheshwari K, Jedan C, Christiaans I, van Gijn M, Maeckelberghe E, Plantinga M. AI-inclusivity in healthcare: motivating an institutional epistemic trust perspective. Camb Q Healthc Ethics. 2024;34:1–15.
11. Dias R, Torkamani A. Artificial intelligence in clinical and genomic diagnostics. Genome Med. 2019;11(1):70–12.
12. Malamateniou C, McFadden S, McQuinlan Y, England A, Woznitza N, Goldsworthy S, Currie C, Skelton E, Chu KY, Alware N, Matthews P, Hawkesford R, Tucker R, Town W, Matthew J, Kalinka C, O'Regan T. Artificial intelligence: guidance for clinical imaging and therapeutic radiography professionals, a summary by the Society of Radiographers AI working group. Radiography (Lond). 2021;27(4):1192–202.
13. Stogiannos N, Georgiadou E, Rarri N, Malamateniou C, Ethical AI. A qualitative study exploring ethical challenges and solutions on the use of AI in medical imaging. Eur J Radiol Artif Intell. 2025;1:100006.
14. Stogiannos N, Malik R, Kumar A, Barnes A, Pogose M, Harvey H, McEntee MF, Malamateniou C. Black box no more: a scoping review of AI governance

frameworks to guide procurement and adoption of AI in medical imaging and radiotherapy in the UK. Br J Radiol. 2023;96(1152):20221157.

15. Robbins S. A misdirected principle with a catch: explicability for AI. Mind Mach. 2019;29(4):495–514.

16. Bommasani R, Klyman K, Kapoor S, Longpre S, Xiong B, Maslej N, et al. The foundation model transparency index v1.1. 2024.

17. Fehr J, Citro B, Malpani R, Lippert C, Madai VI. A trustworthy AI reality-check: the lack of transparency of artificial intelligence products in healthcare. Front Digital Health. 2024;6:1267290.

18. Booij R, Budde RPJ, Dijkshoorn ML, van Straten M. Accuracy of automated patient positioning in CT using a 3D camera for body contour detection. Eur Radiol. 2019;29(4):2079–88.

19. Nousiainen K, Mäkelä T, Piilonen A, Peltonen JI. Automating chest radiograph imaging quality control. Phys Med. 2021;83:138–45.

20. World Health Organisation. Regional Office for Africa. Tuberculosis in the WHO African Region: 2023 progress update. 2023.

21. World Health Organisation. WHO consolidated guidelines on tuberculosis: module 2: screening: systematic screening for tuberculosis disease. 2021.

22. Katzman BD, van der Pol CB, Soyer P, Patlas MN. Artificial intelligence in emergency radiography: a review of applications and possibilities. Diagn Interv Imaging. 2023;104(1):6–10.

23. Aquino YSJ, Rogers WA, Braunack-Mayer A, Frazer H, Win KT, Houssami N, et al. Utopia versus dystopia: professional perspectives on the impact of healthcare artificial intelligence on clinical roles and skills. Int J Med Inform. 2023;169:104903.

24. Chen Y, Stavropoulou C, Narasinkan R, Baker A, Scarbrough H. Professionals' responses to the introduction of AI innovations in radiography and their implications for future adoption: a qualitative study. BMC Health Serv Res. 2021;21(1):1–813.

25. Amin K, Khosla P, Doshi R, Chheang S, Forman HP. Artificial intelligence to improve patient understanding of radiography reports. Yale J Biol Med. 2023;96(3):407–17.

26. Humza Naveed, Khan AU, Qiu S, Saqib M, Anwar S, Usman M, et al. A comprehensive overview of large language models. arXiv.org. 2024.

27. Zhao WX, Zhou K, Li J, Tang T, Wang X, Hou Y, et al. A survey of large language models. arXiv (Cornell University). 2023.

28. Naous T, Ryan MJ, Ritter A, Xu W. Having beer after prayer? Measuring cultural bias in large language models. arXiv (Cornell University). 2023.

29. Kotek H, Dockum R, Sun D. Gender bias and stereotypes in large language models. New York: ACM; 2023.

30. Levy S, Adler WD, Karver TS, Dredze M, Kaufman MR. Gender bias in decision-making with large language models: a study of relationship conflicts. 2024.

31. UNESCO I. Challenging systematic prejudices: an investigation into gender bias in large language models. 2024.

32. Ovsyannikova D, de Mello VO, Inzlicht M. Third-party evaluators perceive AI as more compassionate than expert humans. Commun Psychol. 2025;3(1):4.

33. Lambert SI, Madi M, Sopka S, Lenes A, Stange H, Buszello C, et al. An integrative review on the acceptance of artificial intelligence among healthcare professionals in hospitals. NPJ Digit Med. 2023;6(1):111.

34. Stogiannos N, Walsh G, Ohene-Botwe B, McHugh K, Potts B, Tam W, O'Sullivan C, Quinsten AS, Gibson C, Gorga RG, Sipos D, Dybeli E, Zanardo M, Sá Dos Reis C, Mekis N, Buissink C, England A, Beardmore C, Cunha A, Goodall A, John-Matthews JS, McEntee M, Kyratsis Y, Malamateniou C. R-AI-diographers: a European survey on perceived impact of AI on professional identity, careers, and radiographers' roles. Insights Imaging. 2025;16(1):43.

35. Hagendorff T. The ethics of AI ethics: an evaluation of guidelines. Mind Mach. 2020;30(1):99–120.

36. UNESCO. Recommendation on the ethics of artificial intelligence. Paris: United Nations Educational, Scientific and Cultural Organization; 2022.

37. EU Parliament. European Union Artificial Intelligence Act. 2024. https://artificialintelligenceact.eu/.

38. Topol EJ. Deep medicine. 1st ed. New York: Basic Books; 2019.

39. Fry H. Hello world. London/New York/Toronto/Sydney/Auckland: Doubleday; 2018.

40. Crawford K. Atlas of AI: power, politics, and the planetary costs of artificial intelligence. 1st ed. New Haven: Yale University Press; 2021.

41. Beaulieu A, Leonelli S. Data and society: a critical introduction: [hardback]. Washington, DC: SAGE; 2022.

42. Kantayya S. Coded bias. 2020.

43. Jacobs B, Popma J. Medical research, big data and the need for privacy by design. Big Data Soc. 2019;6(1):2053951718824352.

44. Bak M, Madai VI, Fritzsche M, Mayrhofer MT, McLennan S. You can't have AI both ways: balancing health data privacy and access fairly. Front Genet. 2022;13:929453.

Hendrik Erenstein is a committed lecturer and researcher at the Medical Imaging and Radiation Therapy department of Hanze University of Applied Sciences in Groningen. Specializing in radiography, radiation safety, and artificial intelligence, Hendrik is dedicated to advancing the field through both research and teaching. He is passionate about fostering the professional growth of current and future healthcare professionals, ensuring they possess the necessary knowledge and skills for their careers. With support from the Hanze UAS, EFRS, and EuSoMII, he strives to contribute to the adoption of artificial intelligence in healthcare, emphasising both technical advancements and ethical considerations.

Mirjam Plantinga is an associate professor on responsible data-driven innovation in healthcare at the departments of genetics and Data Science Center in Health (DASH) of the University Medical Center Groningen (UMCG) in the Netherlands. She has a background in economics, philosophy, and sociology and leads the ELSA AI Lab Northern Netherlands, which mission is to foster responsible AI in health, prevention, and care by investigating the ELSA (ethical, legal, and societal aspects) of the use of AI in Healthcare and translating this knowledge to practice. Her research interests include responsible data-driven research, responsible healthcare innovation, and public and patient involvement.

Professor Peter M. A. van Ooijen is a full professor on AI in Radiotherapy at the UMCG, Groningen, the Netherlands. With his team, he works on the implementation of AI into radiotherapy to move towards fully adaptive radiotherapy by automatic segmentation of targets and organs at risk and the prediction of outcome and toxicity of treatment. In this work, responsible AI is central with topics like explainability and uncertainty visualisation. He (co)authored over 230 PubMed listed papers and numerous book chapters. He is a senior member of IEEE, past-president of EuSoMII and active in AI related committees of the European Society of Radiology (ESR), European Society for Radiotherapy and Oncology (ESTRO), and European Society of AI in Health (ESAIH).

AI Governance and Implementation in Radiography Practice

4

Christina Malamateniou, Amrita Kumar, Gerald Lip, Robin Pierce, and Yiannis Kyratsis

4.1 Introduction

The natural continuum of the AI product lifecycle brings it from inception and evaluation to deployment in clinical practice. Implementation of AI tools into a clinical workflow is where the novelty of AI technologies is really put to the test with unseen data to explore their impact on patient outcomes, patient and staff experiences, workflows and effective and efficient use of resources. Figure 4.1 demonstrates the different stages of implementation across the AI tool life-

cycle [1]. Whole books have been written already about AI implementation in medical imaging [2]. This chapter will attempt to give a concise overview of perhaps the most important step in making AI jump from the lab to the clinic, with emphasis and contextualisation on radiography practice, as required.

The term "implementation" is often used interchangeably with "integration" and "deployment." Implementing AI requires a solid clinical challenge that needs addressing, a well-trained and tested AI tool, an organically connected team of experts, a robust business plan and seamless infrastructure for deployment and evaluation [2]. The notion and practice of AI implementation have been shown to be also impacted by different factors: the presence of robust AI governance [3–7], the existence of evidence-based, customised AI literacy educational provisions [8–14], the use of rigorous and longitudinal product evaluation techniques (this is where post-market surveillance, intended to assure continuing safety, effectiveness and cybersecurity of the AI, plays a huge role) [2, 4, 7, 8, 10, 15, 16], acceptability and trust by patients and staff, and the understanding of the multifaceted impact of AI on clinical outcomes, workflows, society, cost of service provision and future workforce development [3, 4, 10, 12, 15, 17]. This chapter will attempt to touch upon some of these topics within the context of radiography and medical imaging, as pertinent to those who consider deploying AI locally. It will provide both theoretical underpinnings as

on behalf of Association of Healthcare Technology Providers for Imaging, Radiotherapy and Care (AXREM)

C. Malamateniou (✉)
Division of Radiography, Department of Allied Health Sciences, School of Health and Medical Sciences, CRRAG Research Group at City St George's, University of London, London, UK
e-mail: christina.malamateniou@city.ac.uk

A. Kumar
Frimley Health NHS Foundation Trust, Maidenhead, UK

G. Lip
NHS Grampian, Aberdeen, Scotland

R. Pierce
University of Exeter, Exeter, UK

Y. Kyratsis
Chair Sustainable Healthcare Workforce, Erasmus University Rotterdam, Erasmus School of Health Policy & Management, Rotterdam, The Netherlands

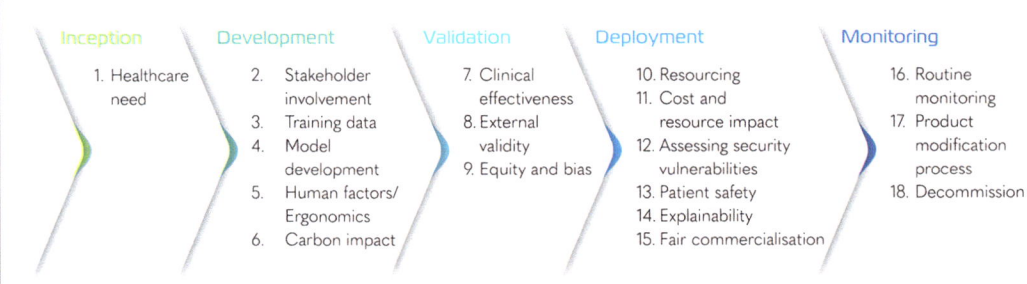

Fig. 4.1 The lifecycle of an AI tool from inception to monitoring, all important steps to be considered toward fully integrated clinical implementation [1]. Names of different phases might change over time, as terminology becomes adjusted to better reflect practice and policy

outlined by academic and research scholarship and practice advice on AI implementation by early adopters.

4.2 AI Implementation: A Fast-Changing World in Radiography and Medical Imaging

Medical imaging is one of the fastest areas of growth for AI models and it has quickly become the reference point for AI use in other healthcare disciplines, such as ophthalmology, pathology, cardiology and dermatology. AI uptake varies massively across different imaging modalities, with MRI and CT holding the lion's share when it comes to AI applications [18], mainly due to the complexity of the tasks involved and the amount of data they create annually. Practical knowledge from AI implementation use demonstrates that the variability of AI implementation diffusion is largely governed by data availability, local patient demographics (and incidence of pathologies), healthcare needs and priorities (e.g. COVID-19 has triggered AI innovation to address the need for fast diagnosis [19]), industry interest (mediated by feasibility and cost/benefit analysis) and acceptability by healthcare professionals and patients [7, 20, 21]. Figure 4.2 shows the main drivers for AI deployment in UK healthcare settings (based on March 2025 data) [20]. The growth of AI innovation in medical imaging has skyrocketed in the last decade with some sign of slowing down in the last 2 years (2024–2025), which has been mainly attributed to more robust AI governance in different parts of the world and a more competitive market [22]. However, AI implementation in this field is still in its infancy, making any comments about its potential success or comprehensive impact a bit too premature. Early data from the UK show that AI implementation in healthcare is still occurring in a more ad-hoc manner, mainly led by one-off funding calls, free trials, emergence of a new AI tool or local AI champions. While many of the challenges faced are similar to the ones other innovations have experienced in the past, when it comes to AI, in particular, its fast pace of development, concerns about potential adverse effects and the complex nature of evaluation and post-market surveillance are highlighted as obstacles to deployment [20]. Facilitators for effective AI implementation continue to be the constants of AI literacy for all professionals involved, robust governance and guidance, a unified AI strategy to ensure funding is released for long-term plans and not short-term wins, and collaboration for structured knowledge sharing, to avoid duplication of effort and share expertise [20]. Many of these topics will be further analysed below.

Navigating the variety of solutions and innovation of AI in medical imaging can be challenging, but some platforms, either already available or under development can help address this com-

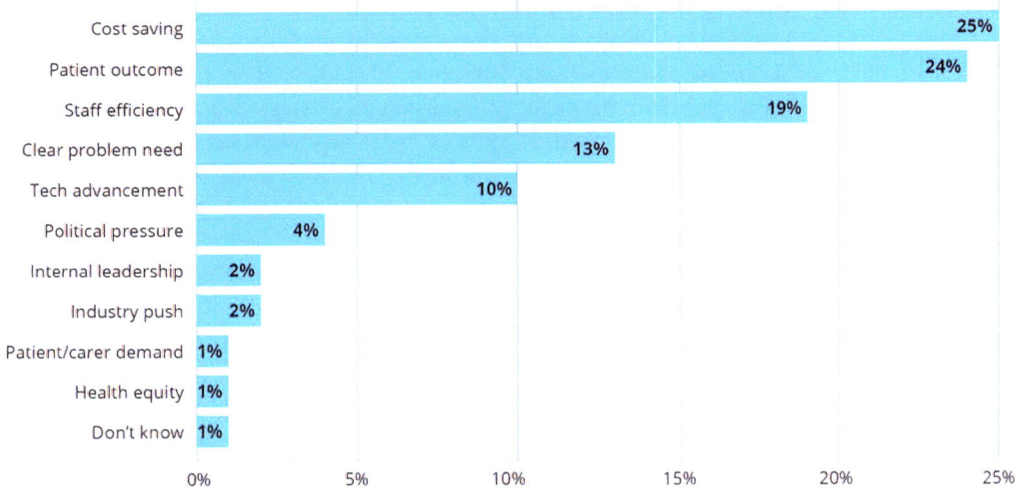

Fig. 4.2 The main drivers of AI deployment in UK healthcare settings. (Adapted from the Healthcare Foundation, March 2025 report [20])

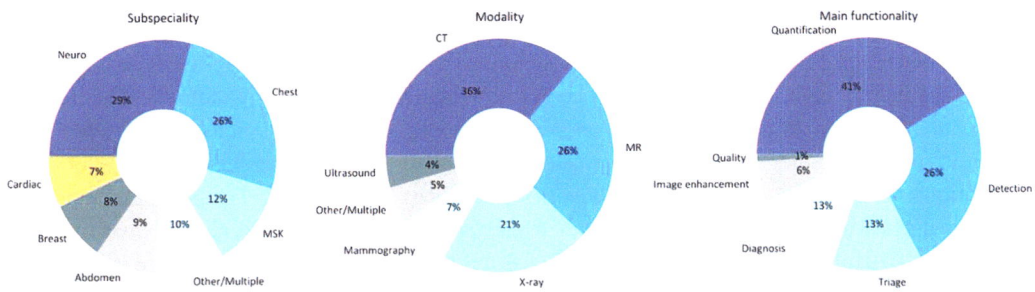

Fig. 4.3 The variety of CE marked products presented by anatomical area, imaging modality and functionality provided (data valid as of March 2025). (Image courtesy of Romion Health [24])

plexity, guide decision-making and foster meaningful collaborations. There is a variety of AI tools now available for different modalities of medical imaging and anatomical areas, providing different functionalities [23] (Fig. 4.3) and marketed by different companies globally. Chapters 5, 6, 7, 8, 9, 10 and 11 will provide unique insights into how AI implementation materialises in tasks traditionally performed by radiographers across different medical imaging and radiotherapy modalities. The different AI applications can be searched for in different websites, the most, perhaps, well known and well used being the Radiology Health AI register [23, 25], which is regularly updated and curated by Romion Health

[24] This website, which is searchable for different anatomical areas, modalities and certifications and includes published evidence to support industry claims of effectiveness and efficiency of a product, has enabled more transparency and accessibility for medical imaging solution in the AI field.

Furthermore, a first version of the UK AI registry, for mapping out the landscape of different AI implementation efforts in medical imaging/radiology in the UK, has recently been launched under the auspices of the Royal College of Radiologists [26]. Finally, a new project, endorsed by the European Society of Medical Imaging Informatics (EuSoMII) and the

European Federation of Radiographer Societies (EFRS) has developed an online database to gather all AI educational provisions for medical imaging professionals in Europe and make them more accessible and searchable by academic discipline (radiographer, radiologist, physicist, etc.), language of the course and mode of delivery (onsite or online). This project, called AIMIROE (*AI* education for *M*edical *I*maging and *R*adiotherapy in *E*urope) will launch its searchable database in the second half of 2025 under the EuSoMII website [27].

4.3 Which Areas of Radiography Practice Does AI Implementation Really Impact?

Contrary to radiology, where the majority of currently published research evidence in AI implementation touches upon the different levels of image interpretation (triage, detection and/or diagnosis) [28], in radiography the majority of applications relate to key operational aspects of the clinical service (Fig. 4.4), such as workflow management, patient safety (radiation dose reduction, MRI safety checks), patient preparation and positioning, image acquisition and optimisation (including slice positioning, contrast administration, image quality), image post-processing (registration, segmentation and quantification) [10, 29–31]. A small number of AI applications, in countries like the UK and Denmark, where radiographers also perform reporting, are currently being explored [31, 32]. There is more space for further research and exploration in this area for radiographers (medical radiation technologists or medical radiation scientists, as called in different parts of the world), as necessary to create the evidence base required to facilitate safe and effective AI-enabled radiography practice. Thus, the potential (and long-promised!) benefits of AI in radiography practice, relating to efficiency, efficacy/quality of service, patient care and staff well-being [7, 10], can be tested against real clinical scenarios. Similar to radiology, radiography practice could equally be impacted by automation bias and over-reliance/over-trust on technology, deskilling (hence the need for re-skilling!), challenges in interfaces where human-AI interaction is required, lack of transparency, in what remains a predominantly "black-box' culture, and, subse-

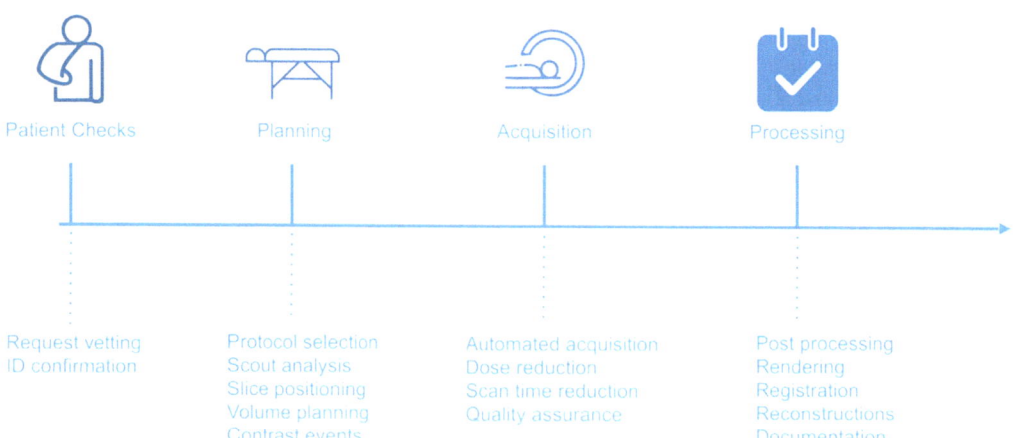

Fig. 4.4 Indicative areas of anticipated impact of AI in the cross-sectional radiographic workflow [29]. This list is expected to grow and expand as more radiographers engage with research, education and gain expertise in clinical practice in this area

quent lack of acceptability and trust by humans (whether patients or professionals) [33, 34]. The Society and College of Radiographers, in anticipation of the magnitude of the impact of AI on radiography practice, has published a comprehensive AI guidance document for clinical imaging and radiotherapy professionals, outlining priorities for clinical practice, education, research and the importance of forging strong partnerships with other healthcare professionals to safely navigate this space [10].

4.4 The Role of Multidisciplinary and Multiagency Collaboration for the Success of AI Implementation in Medical Imaging and Radiotherapy

Collaborations have always been vital in the medical imaging and radiotherapy disciplines. These were important to uphold patient safety and the "do no harm" principles, warrant service quality, but also to optimise efficiency, use of resources and ensure staff well-being and job satisfaction [10, 35]. The medical imaging and radiotherapy ecosystems are expected to experience seismic changes because of AI implementation, which could change the ways people learn, work, communicate, progress and help each other [7, 36]. The native AI ecosystems in medical imaging and radiotherapy include professionals from all different disciplines: radiographers, radiologists, oncologists, referring consultants, nuclear medicine physicians, dosimetrists, medical physicists, clinical scientists, biomedical engineers, and increasingly now computer scientists, mathematicians and other scientists [7, 37]. The complexity of transitioning into a new era, in order to harmoniously co-exist with AI, means not only that new professionals will become part of this native ecosystem such as behavioural scientists, cognitive neuroscientists, healthcare psychologists, but also new professions will emerge, like the one of implementation scientists [38] and technical physicians [39], who can play a key

role in AI implementation due to their unique skill mix, lying between technical and clinical competencies. Radiographers, clinical scientists and other professionals have, by nurture and education, a dyadic professional identity on the interface between advanced technology and patient care, and could become, subject to customised AI literacy training, the necessary "bridges" and the "glue" that could keep this ecosystem together in the coming years of anticipated cataclysmic change. They could achieve this by ensuring seamless communication between professionals, timely escalation of patient concerns or of technological glitches to the experts, gatekeeping of quality of everyday clinical service and innovating AI solutions, as they are always in touch with the clinical realities, challenges and encounters that require optimisation. In their position on the boundary between clinical needs and technological advancements, they can address a leadership void and drive AI implementation forward.

While the ecosystem of clinical professionals is the one roughly described above, it does not represent all the agencies and functions that coexist in medical imaging and radiotherapy. These include the patients, at the centre of everything we do, the policy makers and regulators, who have a huge role in driving the AI agenda forward, the industry representatives, who are always eager for collaborations and contribute to innovation, the academics and educators, who have a huge role to play in reskilling and upskilling the workforce but also reimagining a fairer, more equitable and more effective healthcare. A team of about 50 different professionals and agencies, including patients, within medical imaging and radiotherapy have worked together to reaffirm the need for multidisciplinary and multiagency collaboration for the success of this gigantic societal effort to integrate AI. They have also imagined, as presented in Fig. 4.5, how this ecosystem could look like [37]. It is vital to appreciate that, despite professional boundaries, individual agendas and costs, regulatory changes and other policy implications, the patient stays always at the heart of healthcare service provision.

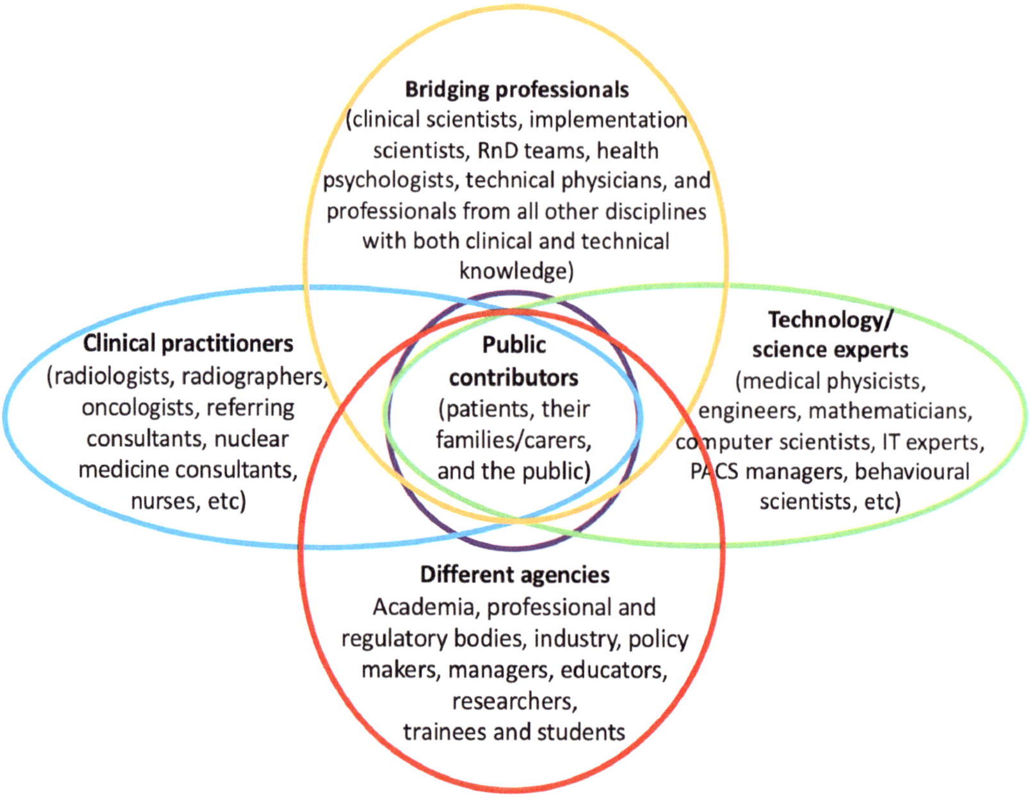

Fig. 4.5 The complex medical imaging and radiotherapy ecosystem, which includes the patients at its centre and around them multidisciplinary clinical and technical teams, educators and academics, industry and policy makers, to be in position to safely and effectively deploy AI in clinical practice [37]

4.5 Working Towards Holistic Person-Centred AI Implementation

There are different enablers, challenges and opportunities affecting different professionals in different ways as AI is integrated into clinical services, and some of these will be discussed in the below chapters. For example, while stroke consultants can see the real benefit of AI use in immediate confirmation of stroke from medical imaging, to inform quick provision of customised treatment, which saves lives [40], the way AI is sometimes implemented in MRI and CT radiology workflows and other areas, trying to minimise the long waiting lists for scans or other services, might create a conveyor-belt-like pipeline, accentuate staff burnout, moral injury and impact their well-being [41, 42], the opposite of what the inspirational quote of 'having more time to care' has promised [20, 43]. As staff well-being is central to the workforce, it must be prioritised at all costs and ensure AI implementation will be truly person-centred, including not just patient care but also caring for our healthcare systems most valuable resource: its people [20, 37]. Figure 4.6 below shows intended use of time from healthcare staff in the UK, if AI integration manages to improve healthcare efficiencies.

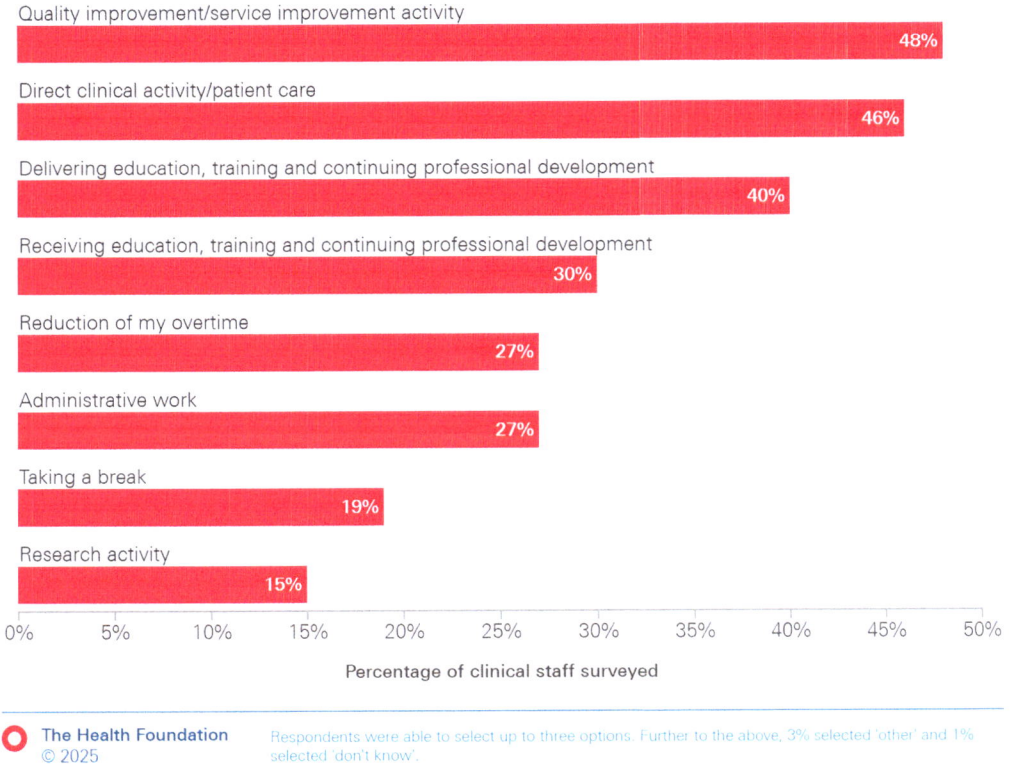

Fig. 4.6 Intended use of time freed up by AI technology, as reported by healthcare staff surveyed in the UK [44]

4.6 A Conceptual Framework for AI Implementation: Challenges and Enablers

Implementing AI systems and sustainably integrating them into existing workflows requires the consideration of both technical-technological and social-human aspects [45, 46]. A conceptual framework is outlined that integrates key challenges and enablers for successful AI implementation within healthcare organisations. The primary challenges in AI implementation, as detailed in Table 4.1, fall into three main interacting domains:

- *Technical challenges* involve data infrastructure limitations, interoperability issues, and dealing with variability in patient populations and clinical protocols.
- *Organisational barriers* include resistance from healthcare professionals, suboptimal organisational readiness for AI adoption and

Table 4.1 Challenges of AI implementation in healthcare

Technical challenges [45–49]	The lack of appropriate data infrastructure poses several challenges to the optimal training and validation of AI applications which hinders implementation:
	Efficiency Issues: wasted resources, increased development time, limited scalability
	Reliability Concerns: inconsistent data quality, difficulties in understanding the basis for AI model decisions, which reduces transparency and can undermine trust, limiting reproducibility
	The lack of interoperability between diverse AI platforms and vendors, legacy technology and data formats can result in:
	Data silos
	System and technology integration issues
	Workflow disruptions
	Barriers to collaboration.
	In the implementation of AI in healthcare, challenges also arise due to the limited generalisability across diverse patient populations:
	Biased algorithm training data introduce biases affecting the accuracy and fairness of clinical decisions and hindering effectiveness and clinical utility
	Variable image acquisition protocols can lead to inconsistencies in data quality and format. AI applications is highly varied in practice, making it hard to prove their value
	Inconsistent algorithm performance across diverse patient demographics and imaging conditions hinders AI deployment
	The heterogeneity of clinical protocols and variability in healthcare delivery pose additional significant challenges
Organisational challenges [50–54]	Healthcare organisations are pluralist social entities and AI-induced change may be contested. Resistance by healthcare professionals presents significant barriers to the implementation of AI in healthcare; reasons for such resistance include skills gap, suboptimal staff engagement in designing and deploying AI, fear of job displacement, algorithmic aversion, or lack of understanding of how AI can complement human expertise, AI disrupting established workflow routines and tasks
	There are also issues of AI interpretability and explainability. The "black box" nature of some AI algorithms can hinder their acceptance, as clinicians may be hesitant to trust results without understanding the underlying decision-making process
	Suboptimal technology-organisation-system alignment: the focus often is solely on the technology itself and NOT on how AI will be integrated, applied, and the motivations, constraints and specific clinical, policy and market contexts as well as financing and incentives systems that influence those applying AI and benefitting from AI
	Business challenges: lack of strategic plan for integrating AI, long-term and appropriate scale of investment, financing and reimbursement
Socio-Ethical and Legal challenges [55–57] (see also Chap. 3 and the regulation section of this chapter for further insight)	Accountability: healthcare professionals and organisations bear moral responsibility for patient safety and well-being. Coping with *exponential*, *disruptive* AI technology presents challenges in ensuring safety assurance to protect patients from harm
	Liability: as AI becomes more autonomous, determining liability for adverse outcomes due to unsafe or ineffective AI becomes increasingly complex
	Decision-making biases inherent in AI algorithms
	Privacy Concerns: without proper access control and data encryption there is increased risk of data breaches for sensitive patient information; also, increased difficulty in complying with regulations (i.e., Health Insurance Portability and Accountability Act (HIPAA) (USA) and the General Data Protection Regulation (GDPR) (UK and EU)) [58, 59]; fragmented data storage or lack of proper data governance impedes control over data use
	Security Concerns: increased vulnerability to cyberattacks, risk of data loss or corruption hampering AI development and use
	The absence of standardised protocols and guidelines hinders the validation and clinical evidence of AI models. There is a need for large-scale, well-designed studies to validate the performance of AI algorithms in real-world clinical settings

lack of alignment of technology with organisational goals, resulting in fragmented efforts.

- *Socio-ethical and legal* considerations encompass accountability concerns, decision-making biases and the necessity for standardised protocols and regulatory compliance.

Regarding enablers, the conceptual framework emphasises involving staff in co-designing AI applications; bridging stakeholders from the wider ecosystem, the private sector and AI vendors; developing risk management strategies and equipping staff with necessary AI skills, also, by fostering a culture of experimentation to address the challenges. The key enablers for successful AI implementation in healthcare (detailed in Table 4.2) involve the following overlapping processes:

Several AI-integrating processes enable responsible and impactful AI implementation:

- Co-creating AI applications through user engagement
- Bridging local and trans-local stakeholders
- Mitigating risk and adapting to socio-ethical issues
- Demystifying the opacity of AI applications
- Staff competence building and fostering a culture of experimentation

Figure 4.7 also demonstrates potential solutions to AI implementation challenges as proposed by clinical practitioners in the UK [20].

More enablers and challenges to AI implementation in radiology and radiography can be found in relevant literature [2, 33, 34, 46, 49, 63].

Table 4.2 Enablers of AI implementation in healthcare

Co-creating AI applications through user engagement [45, 57, 60]	Implementation needs to be the primary focus of efforts in co-designing and customising AI applications. This entails integrating valuable evidence and frontline adopter experiences by allocating time, space and resources for learning and role redefinition
Bridging local and trans-local designs and stakeholders [45, 57, 60]	Connecting localised adaptations of AI models to adaptable global designs involves codifying and sharing knowledge gained from implementation experiences in specific contexts. This bridging process occurs through interactions among various groups, including innovators, vendors, adopters, regulators, and implementers, across different levels—local, national, and European—spanning institutions and civil society. By developing ecosystems of skills, computing, data and applications, communities can engage actively, address local needs, tap into local creativity and knowledge and cultivate a human-centred, diverse, and socially driven approach to AI
Mitigating risk and adapting to socio-ethical issues [60]	Navigating socio-ethical challenges in AI implementation requires attention to public perceptions, professional dynamics, regulations and financial considerations. Organisations must establish comprehensive risk management strategies to tackle data privacy and security concerns. This involves implementing policies, procedures, and safeguards, including the adoption of "ethical-, privacy-, and secure-by-design" algorithms
Demystifying the opacity of AI applications [45, 61]	Balancing transparency with predictive power is crucial but difficult, as different stakeholders have varying requirements for understanding AI decisions. Achieving interpretability can enhance accountability and help identify and rectify biases. However, simplifying models for interpretability may reduce predictive accuracy, impacting overall utility. Interpretability ensures that decisions are precise and defensible, fostering trust among users and stakeholders. It is essential for ethical considerations, regulatory adherence and seamless integration of AI insights into decision-making processes
Staff competence building and fostering a *culture of experimentation* [62]	Provide comprehensive training to staff for effective understanding and utilisation of AI. This training should cover medical, technological, organisational-managerial, legal and ethical competencies

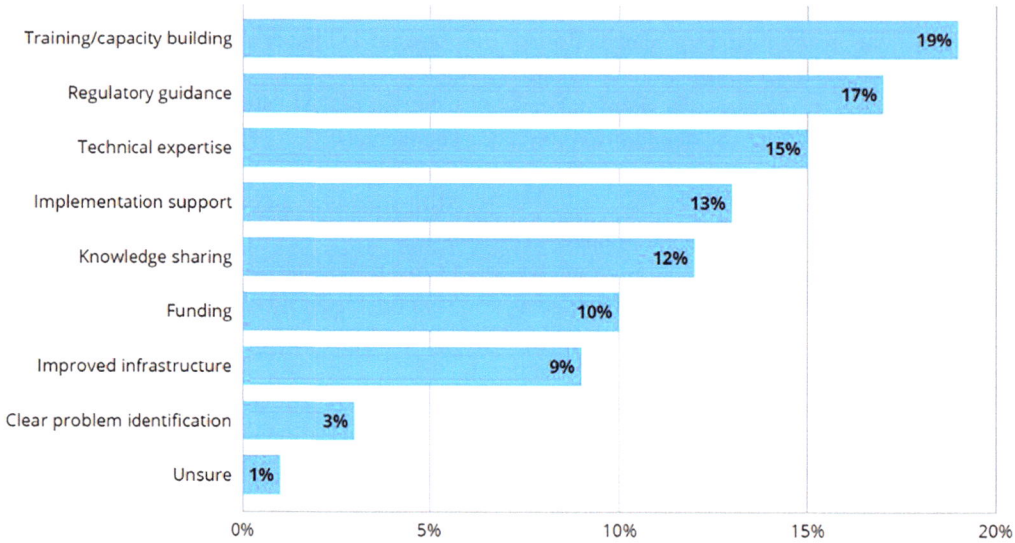

Fig. 4.7 The most potent support measures to overcome barriers in AI adoption, as proposed by UK-based clinical practitioners [20]

4.7 A Paradigm Shift on How Big Data Is Harnessed in Healthcare

Healthcare and medical imaging, much like other industries, is amidst a huge digital transformation on its journey from analogue to digital systems [64, 65]. Most hospitals have been digitised in the last 5–10 years but are still using multiple legacy technology systems that have been accumulating vast amounts of primarily unconnected, unorganised data [63].

The potential of this data is now being realised, by amalgamating the vast amounts of already available digital data with those that are becoming more readily accessible through wearable technologies. The potential to derive and create value from this big data is immense, as it can lead to more personalised, stratified approaches to

healthcare. This would enable a true longitudinal dataset, which could make healthcare a lot more continuous, and proactive instead of the reactive, episodic way we currently use it. AI has huge potential here to help derive value given its ability to synthesise big data in considerably less time than if applied by humans. This is just one of the areas that AI has the potential to revolutionise and transform the existing business process and delivery of healthcare and needs to be factored into the overall business strategy [66]. More about the potential of big data can be found also in Chap. 11.

Creating a robust business case is often the first step towards successful adoption [67, 68]. Section 4.7 and Table 4.3 expand this knowledge into a real-life AI deployment scenario in radiology in the UK, offering practical tips derived from this experience.

Table 4.3 A real-life scenario for AI implementation in medical imaging, including customised objectives, actions and key actors for the different stages of implementation

Stage of implementation	Measurable objective	Action items	Designated actors
1. Discovery and evaluation	Identify clinical priorities Define metrics of success and failure	Scoping document to align with existing vision and 5-year strategy	Executive team—CEO, medical director and hospital board
2. Build the team	Set up AI programme board	Buy-in from executive team	Clinicians, IG, R&D, procurement, contracts, HR, IT & digital teams
3. Identify opportunities and value	Build in-house dataset to leverage AI to create value from available data Buy evidenced models to address bottlenecks like cancer diagnosis delays	Hybrid approach to build vs buy	AI board members, clinical head of departments, analytics team
4. Project plan	Consider partnership with external vendors/academic institutions for help to implement	Bring in funding Gain implementation and evaluation expertise	Regional academic hubs, NHS Digital, NHSx
5. Build minimally viable machine (*minimally viable means a machine with features that will give a reasonable expectation that it will ultimately pass regulatory certification*)	Simple implementation testing Observe biases and mitigate Act-fast, fail-fast approach (*this can only be done in a non-clinical setting, or in a controlled, registered, premarket clinical investigation*)	Create scorecard for each study Modification from feedback loop generated from MVM	Liaise with team members in quality improvement/ digital transformation teams
6. Deploy and scale	Build a productive model and test intensively Observe any biases and mitigate accordingly	Present and publish initial results locally and nationally	AI board including analytics teams

4.8   How to Create a Robust Business Case for AI Implementation: Learning from Practical Experience

It is vital when writing the business case to discuss the main objective(s), the opportunities lying ahead and potential risks.

- *Objective*: Focus on system-wide strategic set-up of AI-enabled technology infrastructure including implementation and evaluation in hospitals creating value for patients, clinicians and providers.
- *Opportunity*: Set up a strategic business model for AI implementation for competitive advantage and delivery of value-based healthcare

[69]. Time has come to invest in AI and machine learning to transform healthcare in order to provide better healthcare delivery, improving patient health outcomes, and operational efficiencies. AI can be harnessed for health prevention/ promotion, improved diagnostics and treatment, as well as automating processes through system efficiencies.

- *Foreseeable risks of AI*: Safeguards will need to be fully assessed and put in place regarding making fair and safe use of the varied datasets, including transparency, robustness, and ethical issues around patient trust and consent. Developing the expertise to harness the potential of the data will also need to be considered— including recruitment and training. It will be important to develop trust with key stakehold-

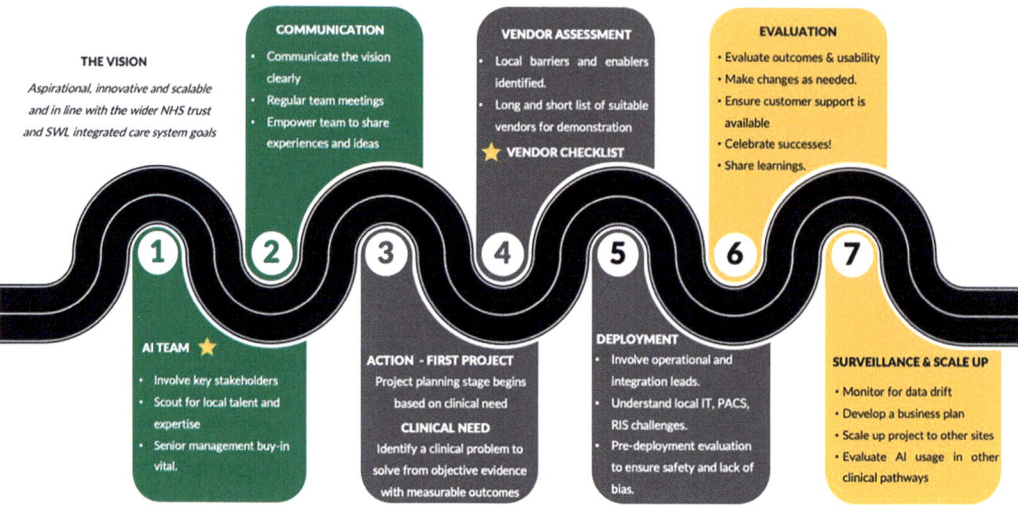

Fig. 4.8 The proposed different stages of AI implementation in radiology with emphasis on change management [70]

ers (clinicians, information governance teams, research and digital data teams) so that it can progress openly, in a transparent manner. More about ethics principles of AI implementation is discussed in Chap. 3.

Recommendations vital for the success of the business case:

1. Set up an AI Programme Board with clear leadership, aligned with local and national digital strategy and executive teams.
2. Bring together all relevant domain experts and clinical/ non-clinical stakeholders.
3. Partner with industry and academic institutions to include the required computational power and domain experts to process multiple datasets.
4. Engage in an agile, experimental approach to implement and evaluate AI-enabled technology that has potential for adoptability and scalability within healthcare.

Table 4.3 provides a step-by-step approach to a real-life scenario of a business model of AI implementation in medical imaging

Real-life AI implementation involves different stages that can be seen in Fig. 4.8 that presents a use case from radiology [70]. Regulation, in the next section, is one of the key areas requiring attention.

4.9 Regulation and Governance of AI in Healthcare: Beyond Ethics

Different regulations will be discussed in this section in relation to AI used as a medical device [71, 72]. In Chap. 3, the ethics of AI was addressed. As a differentiation and for purposes of definition, within this textbook ethics concerns the implicit aspect of governance that relates to thoughts, behaviours and actions employed without a legal requirement in place. In contrast, regulations relate to the explicit aspect of governance that relates to thoughts, behaviours and actions bound to legal requirements and formal guidance, standards and frameworks. This is the context within which we will use them in this textbook.

While regulation of technological innovation often lags behind the technology, the use of AI in medical imaging is largely governed much like other technologies used in the medical context. Generally viewed as medical devices, AI devices in medical imaging are largely regulated by agencies with oversight of medical devices. In 2024 and 2025, more regulation has been introduced or expected to be introduced in the European Union (EU) and the UK. The EU AI Act [73] was published at the end of 2024, with many aspects of it, though, still under development, negotiation or contemplation by the European Parliament.

Large geopolitical effects shape AI regulation and policy making. Similarly, in the UK, the UK AI Bill is (as of spring of 2025) currently under review by the different regulatory and policy-making agencies, having experienced a period of delays [74].

If we follow the example of the EU AI Act, we can see that the advent of overarching regulatory schemes for AI, such as the EU AI Act and others, will contain specific provisions for AI medical devices; AI medical devices are in effect a subset of Software as a Medical Device (SaMD) [75] and Software in a Medical Device (SiMD) [76]. While concerns exist about the impact of more regulation on innovation and the AI market growth, it is generally agreed that more regulation can accelerate implementation and ensure the safety of AI tools, so we can harness their benefits for everyone [77].

4.9.1 Medical Devices Regulations in the EU, UK and USA

Many AI-driven technologies used in radiology are generally classified as medical devices. The regulation of medical devices is risk based in several jurisdictions, including the EU, UK and USA. However, these jurisdictions differ in oversight bodies and the relevant regulatory instruments. In the EU, medical devices are regulated by the Medical Device Regulation 2017/745 (MDR) [71] and the *In vitro* Medical Device Regulation 2017/746 (IVDR) [78]; the IVDR tends to have less relevance to radiography and radiology than the MDR. The MDR's Annex VIII introduces 22 Rules to classify medical devices based on risk, ranging from Class I to Class III, with Class I referring to devices that pose almost no risk and Class III covering high-risk devices that include machinery that is important to patient health or sustaining the life of the patient. Software, including AI, is specifically covered in Rule 11, where it is stated that: 'Software intended to provide information which is used to take decisions with diagnosis or therapeutic purposes is classified as class IIa [71] except if such decisions have an impact that may cause:

- death or irreversible deterioration of a person's state of health, in which case it is in class III; or
- a serious deterioration of a person's state of health, or a surgical intervention, in which case it is classified in class IIb.

Software intended to monitor physiological processes is classified as Class IIa, except if it is intended for monitoring of vital physiological parameters, where the nature of variations of those parameters is such that it could result in immediate danger to the patient, in which case it is classified as class IIb'.

Figure 4.9 is a graph that shows how medical software is classified by risk, including some exceptions [79].

Different geographical locations employ different rules and regulations when it comes to AI used in healthcare, and these rules also apply to radiography and radiology. Figure 4.10 maps out the different standards and regulations for AI use globally.

The EU does not govern the regulation of medical devices through a centralised body, unlike for medicinal products that are governed through the European Medicines Agency (EMA) [80] but rather implements the MDR through approximately 40 Notified Bodies, commercial companies 'designated' by the European Commission to have the authority to issue a CE (Conformité Européenne) mark indicating EU market authorisation. The European Commission has developed EUDAMED [81], the IT system database to provide public access to information about devices and their associated *economic operators* (manufacturers, importers, distributors and authorised representatives) pertaining to Regulation (EU) 2017/745 (MDR) [71] and Regulation (EU) 2017/746 on IVD [78].

Since Brexit, the UK has shifted from continued use of EU processes and rules, including the MDR [71] and recognition of the CE mark [72] to developing its own regulations for medical devices [72, 82, 83]. However, the UK government has enacted legislation to extend acceptance of the CE mark on devices in Great Britain until 30 June 2030 [84], at the latest and is publicly

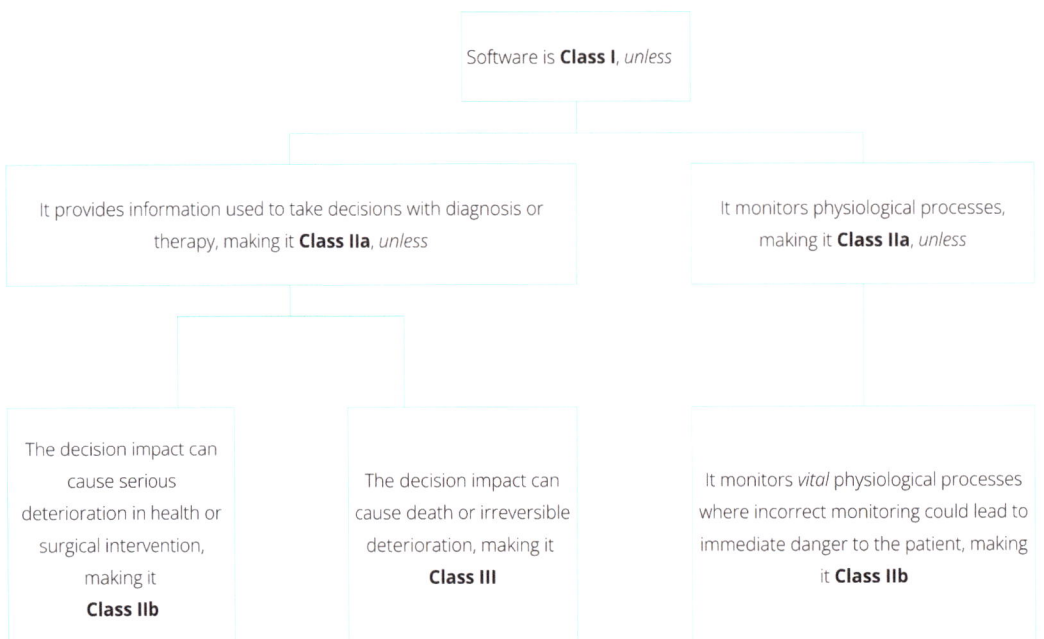

Fig. 4.9 A graph that summarises how medical software is classified by risk, including some exceptions. (Courtesy Hardian Health (2025), adapted from [79])

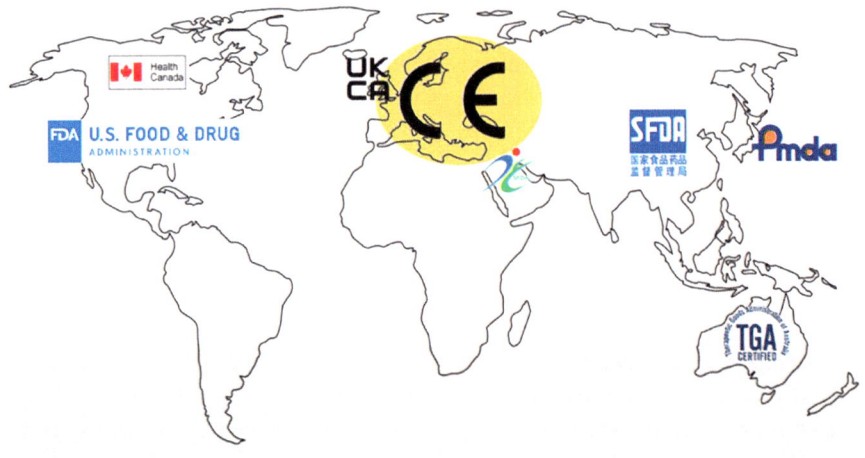

Fig. 4.10 A map of the different standards and regulations applied worldwide for medical devices, including AI, in healthcare and medical imaging. (Courtesy Romion Health [24] (2025))

consulting on a scheme of international reliance [85]. Nevertheless, several changes have been introduced through primary and secondary legislation [86, 87] indicating the process for placing medical devices on the market in Great Britain. Particularly notable is the introduction of the UKCA (UK Conformity Assessment) marking, which is a new route to market and product marking and is available for manufacturers wishing to place medical devices on the market in Great Britain. The UKCA marking came into use on 1 January 2021, and it is a product marking used for specific goods, such as medical devices that are placed on the market in Great Britain. To date, the UKCA marking is not recognised in the EU, EEA or Northern Ireland. In these markets, a CE mark will still be required [86]. The oversight agency for medical devices, in most instances, is the Medicines and Healthcare products Regulatory Agency (MHRA). The MHRA has the power to designate UK Approved Bodies to conduct conformity assessments for the evaluation of compliance with requirements for UKCA marking [88, 89]. The UK has introduced the Software and AI as a Medical Device Change Programme (SaMD)–Roadmap to ensure that regulatory requirements for software and AI adequately protect patients and are clear for manufacturers [75, 90]. Currently, software is not classified proportionate to the risk it can pose to patient and public safety under the amended Medical Device Regulations 2002 [90]. SaMD is responsible for ensuring that rules for classification that are developed impose adequate safety and performance requirements proportionate to the risk posed and, at the same time, ensure that rules for classification are sufficiently flexible such that the risk profile of novel devices can be addressed without unduly restricting innovation [91].

In the USA, the Federal Food and Drug Administration (FDA) regulates medical devices. Software with a medical intended purpose is generally regarded as a medical device and under the risk-based classification ranging from Class I (low risk) to Class III (high risk). AI software used in radiology is generally classified as moderate risk and, therefore, falls into Class II (in the USA, there is no Class IIa and IIb, just Class II). Many Class II devices are required to implement 'special controls' designed to ensure the safety and effectiveness of the device. Under the Food, Drug and Cosmetic Act, a novel device can be granted a 'de novo' request; alternatively, a device that is less novel may qualify for the 510(k) pathway for substantially equivalent devices following a 'predicate' device that has undergone de novo qualification [92]. For example, radiological computer-aided triage and notification software, Viz.ai, was granted de novo and paved the way for 30 subsequent devices that qualified for the 510(k) substantially equivalent pathway [93].

Figure 4.11 shows the FDA-cleared algorithms in healthcare, and most of them (76%) are deployed in radiology. This shows the growth of the domain, and also the urgent need to ensure robust regulation is in place to avoid patient and practitioner harm.

4.9.2 Standards and Guidance

Standards also play a role in the regulation of AI in radiology. In the UK, the British Standard BS 30440 was published in 2023 outlining the evidence required by technology developers to assess and validate products incorporating AI. This standard, entitled 'Validation Framework for the Use of AI in Healthcare' [1] complements a guidance document issued by the Society and College of Radiographers, 'Artificial Intelligence: Guidance for Clinical Imaging and Therapeutic Radiography Workforce Professionals'. This guidance provides recommendations for the development, testing, validation and implementation of AI solutions [10]. A standard for Health informatics, ISO 12052:2017, the DICOM standard (Digital Imaging and Communication in Medicine), has also been developed to address the 'exchange of digital images and information related to the production and management of

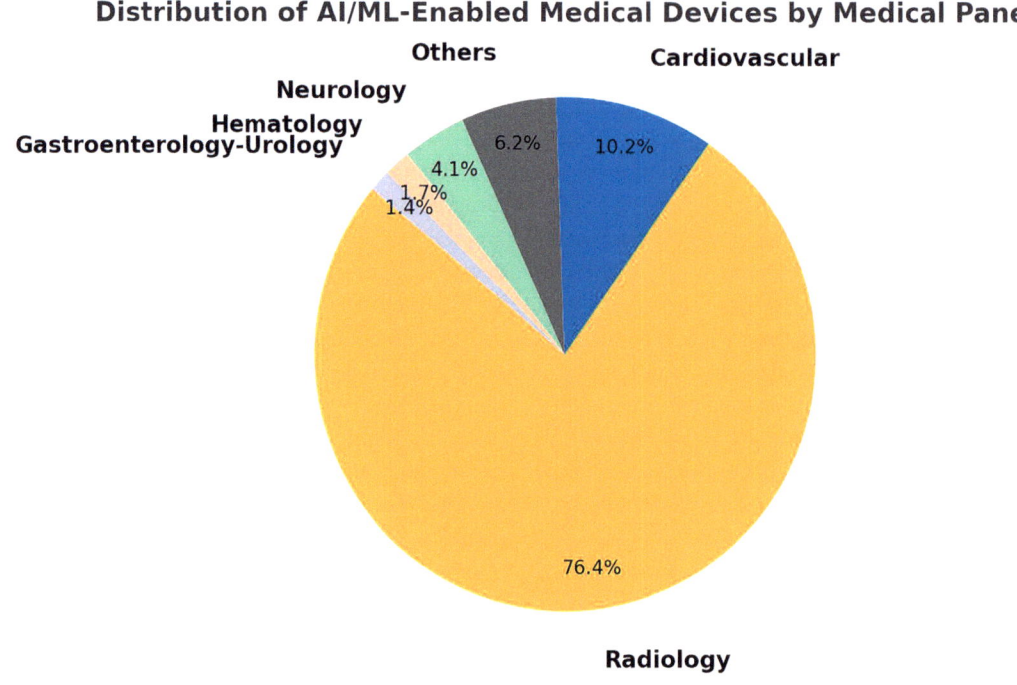

Fig. 4.11 Most AI algorithms cleared by the FDA (total *n* = 950) belong to radiology (76%). (Courtesy Romion Health [24] (2025))

Table 4.4 Pertinent regulatory frameworks for medical device patient safety and data protection/cybersecurity and AI in the UK, EU and USA

	Medical device patient safety	Data protection/ cybersecurity and AI

🇬🇧 UK	• Medicines and Medical Devices Act 2021
	• UK Medical Device Regulation 2002 (SI 2002 No. 618, as amended by Brexit)
	  ○ *July 2025 onwards: new postmarket regulation*
	  ○ *July 2026 onwards: new premarket regulation*
	• UK Health and Social Care Act 2012
	  ○ *Digital Clinical Safety (DCB 0129/ DCB 0160)*
		• Data Protection Act 2018
		• UK GDPR ⇔ EU GDPR

🇪🇺 EU	• EU 2017/745 Medical Device Regulation (MDR)	• EU 2016/679 General Data Protection Regulation (GDPR) • *EU AI Act*
🇺🇸 USA	• Food, Drug and Cosmetics Act (FDCA) • 21st Century Cures Act • FDA Title 21 regulations	• HIPAA (Federal Health Insurance Portability and Accountability Act) • CCPA (California Consumer Privacy Act)...

Courtesy Hardian Health [95] (2025). More regulatory updates are expected within 2025–2026, such as the European Health Data Space (EHDS) regulation and the European Health Technology Assessment (HTA) regulation

those images, between medical imaging equipment and management and communication systems'. This standard also facilitates interoperability of medical equipment [94]. More related standards, pertinent frameworks and regulations can be found summarised in Table 4.4 below.

4.9.3 Intended Use

The 'intended use' of AI as a medical device refers to the specific purpose and function for which the AI-powered device is designed, and it's crucial for regulatory compliance and safe, effective use in healthcare, especially concerning patient safety. When building medical software, writing a clear and well-thought-out intended use statement enables all the next steps in product development. The intended use statement needs to be short document that clearly outlines the device's intended purpose using ideally the following headings [96]:

A. *Intended medical indication*: what specific medical conditions are you targeting, and what clinical claims are you making?
B. *Intended patient population*: what specific patient group will your product benefit?
C. *Intended user groups*: who are the key user groups of your SaMD?
D. *Intended anatomy*: if your health-tech product has a physical component, does it come into contact with any part of the body?
E. *Use environment*: where exactly do you envision your software being used (e.g., on an app, cloud-based)
F. *Operating principle*: can you map out a step-by-step process that gives a simple overview of the patient journey (and information flow) when your software is in use? If you are using AI components, can you give a simple diagram of your algorithm architecture or pipeline?
G. *Foreseeable misuse*: how could your software be used in ways you don't intend? This is hard to imagine as people can use AI software in ways currently unimaginable, but an effort towards this direction is always useful.
H. *What are the technical risks?* Think about cybersecurity, denial of adversarial attacks, for instance.
I. *What are the clinical risks?* Think about the software being used in unsuitable clinical use cases or for different diseases than the ones originally intended [96].

It is vital for end-users of AI technology to comply with the intended use of the AI tool. Otherwise, accountability (and in legal terms, liability) in case of erroneous use or patient harm will weigh heavily on them, too, with all sanctions and implications stemming from product misuse.

As the use of AI in radiology continues to expand and novel products are introduced in the market, regulators and oversight bodies will need to ensure that regulatory frameworks are sufficient to the task of accurate assessment of risk profiles of innovative products and the kinds of controls, restrictions, and compliance requirements are in place. As such, it is reasonable to expect that the regulatory landscape will continue to be adapting and changing well into the next decade.

4.10 Evaluation of AI

There is a multitude of proposed frameworks to evaluate AI in healthcare and radiology/medical imaging, in particular [3, 72, 97–99]. The type of evaluation depends on what is evaluated and whether this is pre- or post-deployment [2].

4.10.1 Pre-Market Testing

For instance, in Chap. 2 (AI methods), a section on performance metrics presents the most commonly used metrics for assessing algorithmic performance, mainly regression, image comparison, classification and segmentation tasks, covering error-based, similarity-based, overlap-based and surface-based evaluation methods. There are though other types of evaluation, including economic evaluation and analysis [100], regulatory compliance (as in above section), evaluation of organisational workflow changes [101], evaluation of environmental sustainability achieved because of AI [102, 103], clinical evaluation on patient outcomes, evaluation of patient and staff experiences, societal impact, to name just a few [70]. Prospective evaluation studies are always more useful and insightful for clinicians, as they can fully control the study design, sample size, randomisation and stratification, inclusion and exclusion criteria and type of intervention studied, while controlling for other factors. Despite that, most real-world evaluations are currently retrospective, interventions might not be fully standardised, data may be skewed and sample sizes suboptimal. They do, however, provide unique insights to inform future prospective studies. Figure 4.12 presents how complex evaluation of AI can be.

4.10.2 Post-Market Surveillance

There is also increasing understanding that evaluation of AI is not a static measure; it changes as AI implementation changes. Initially positive or initially disappointing results should be viewed with caution. Comprehensive longitudinal evaluation is required to be able to see the bigger picture, not just a snapshot of one point in time. Post-market surveillance captures this need for ongoing monitoring, considering staff changes, equipment upgrades, AI model drifts and change of patient demographics for a given clinical setting. Over time, there is degradation of AI model performance known as drift, due to changes in the underlying population or images due to the

inherent dependence on data this is trained from [104]. More about this post-market surveillance is discussed just below.

A comprehensive evaluation like the one described here would need robust and longer-term research funding schemes, which are not currently widely available. For practical reasons, most researchers often must focus on one aspect of AI implementation to be able to study it closely and to ensure feasibility in the available budget and time horizon of their research project.

Post-market surveillance or continual evaluation of AI is an essential component of any AI deployment. The aim of monitoring is primarily to ensure that AI is performing safely.

As AI software is classified as a medical device, the developer has a legal responsibility to maintain the safety of their device which includes post-market surveillance. Any updates and changes to the AI model are required to be measured by law as per UKCA and CE marking. (Additionally, in the UK, the National Health Service Data Control Board standards DCB0160 and DCB0129 are required by primary legislation, the Health and Social Care Act, to be applied to all so-called health IT systems of which software as a medical device/ AI is a subset) [105]. Developers and organisations are also responsible for continuous evaluation as described above in this chapter.

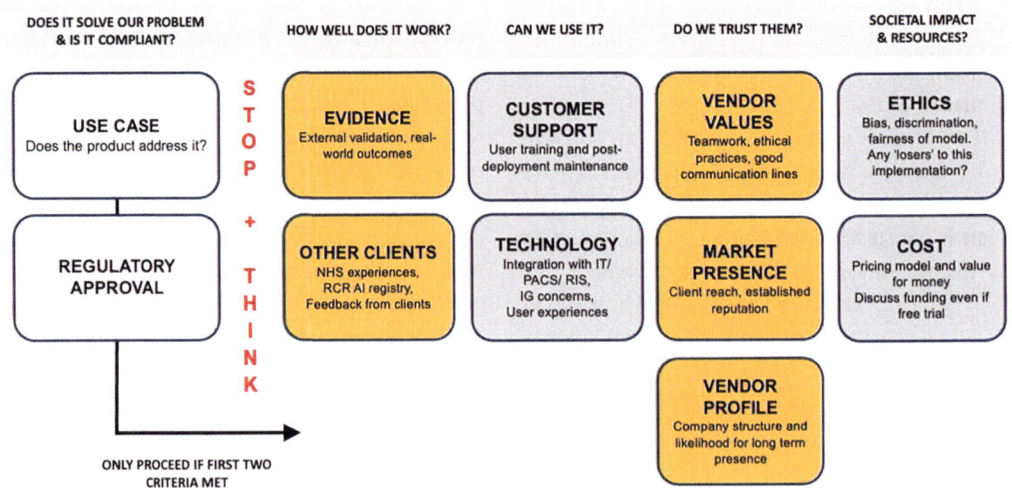

Fig. 4.12 A realistic framework presenting the complexity and diversity of AI evaluation in radiology, depending on the area studied. Clinical problem solving and safety need to be prioritised, as critical for product success [70]

The aim of monitoring and evaluation can be divided into clinical and non-clinical measures (Table 4.5) [4, 70]. Measures to ensure there is no accentuation of bias or inequality should be part of this process.

Post-market surveillance of AI requires appropriate quality assurance systems that have (1) a two-way process, where the hospital must have a method of sharing outcomes data (non-individualised), (2) a process for collecting information (feedback, audit), (3) analytical methods to assess collected data, (4) procedures to investigate the cause of safety concerns, escalating and implementing corrective action, (5) tools (a log) to trace and identify devices needing corrective action, as well as the course of action.

Further to this, regular testing of models with test sets is required to ensure continuing accuracy and consistency; this is another useful approach to ensure consistent software performance (Fig. 4.13).

Outcomes and variables that should be considered during this post-market monitoring include:

(i) Population characteristics—age, sex, ethnicity, disease prevalence, local demographics

(ii) AI software—version updates

(iii) Imaging characteristics—raw or post processed images, potential filters

4.10.3 Feedback Tools

These can range from basic tools, which are user-dependent and may result in over-reporting of false positives or sampling bias, with no capacity for two-way feedback. Tools like that exist in different AI platforms. Lately companies have developed semi-automated tools using natural language processing [107]. These tools can show the ground truth from the AI report via computer reading, using an extract and match tool in a semi-automated process. Cases of discordance are then flagged for review locally with recommendations for regular audit and test sets.

The case for automatic monitoring particularly applies when AI starts being deployed at scale. At that stage, simpler feedback tools will not be able to detect changes, bias or be sensitive enough to underlying drift or changes in performance. De Vries et al [108] describe retrospective analysis of a UK data set of 80,000 mammograms, where an update in software which affected the image parameters of a post-processed mammogram resulted in a significant change in performance of the AI model. In this paper, a recall rate jump was seen across four machines over a 3-year period from an average of 13% increased to about 40% due to a software change, affecting the images post-processed appearance, requiring recalibration of the AI tool.

Models can also deliver multiple findings and evaluation of multiple models with multiple findings should also be factored in. In this example from Venugopal et al. [109] and as shown in Fig. 4.14, there are three different AI models which encompass several chest X-ray findings. These show that the models demonstrated a consistent correlation with each other and of the separate multiple findings at a regular frequency, such as consolidation, pneumothorax, lung nodules but over a longer temporal period, an external event, e.g., COVID-19, changed the performance of the models which exhibited differences in performance.

Table 4.5 Proposed clinical and non-clinical measures for AI product evaluation

Non-clinical	Clinical
Technical connectivity	Clinical performance
Uptime—is the AI always on?	Sensitivity and specificity of the AI models using various tools as detailed in Chap. 2
Number analysed and rejected—is the AI reading all relevant cases?	
Communication alerts—are there any issues in connection to the RIS and PACS?	Agreement
	Feedback tools available to clinicians with an accept/reject analysis tool
Speed—preset agreed measures for transfer of AI results	Drift analysis
Metadata collection	Timely detection of variance from normal average with trigger points to allow for root cause analysis
Version control	
AI software versions	
Change of hardware or machine software in particular image settings	

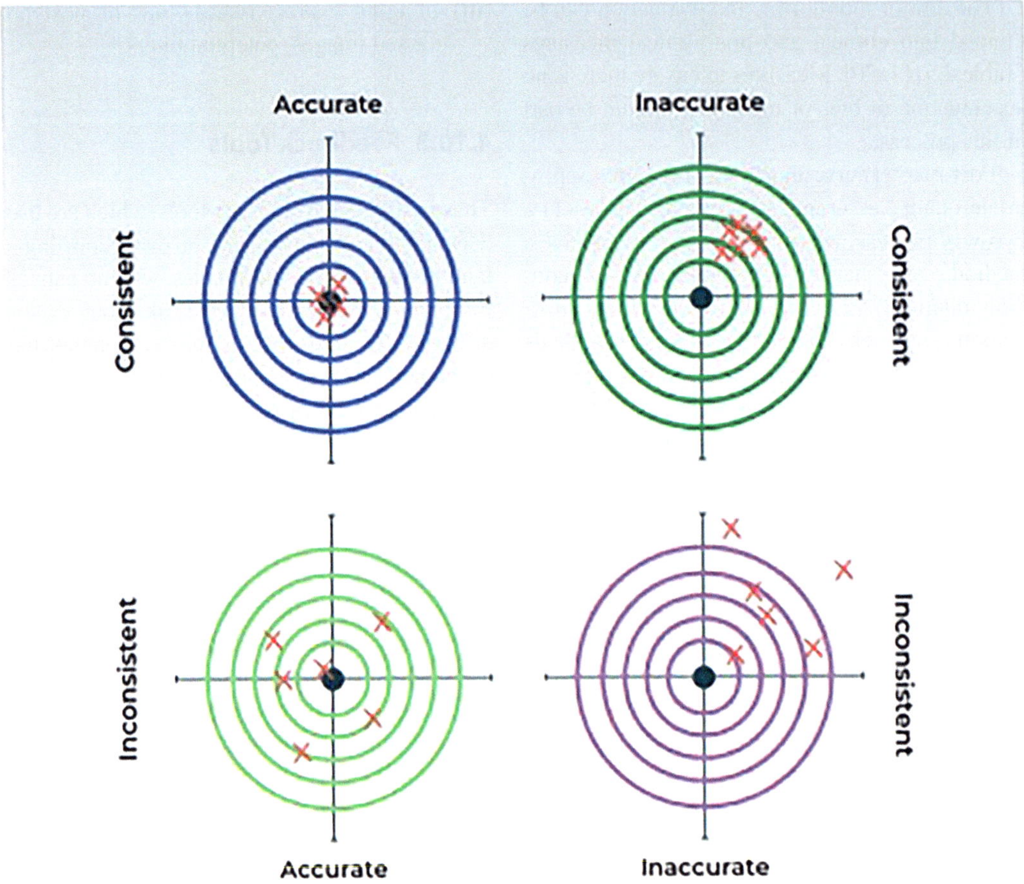

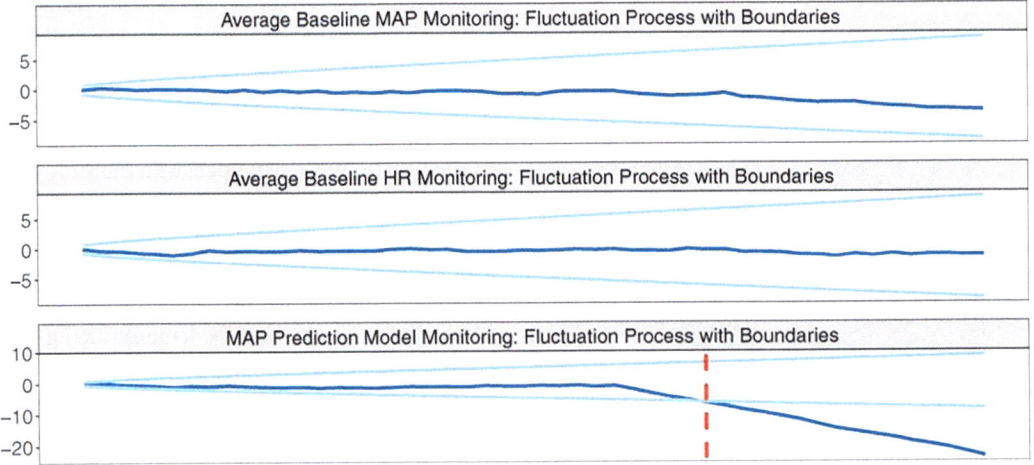

Fig. 4.13 Accuracy and consistency quadrants that depict the ideal and varied outcomes of AI predictions. (Courtesy of carpl.ai [106])

Fig. 4.14 Prediction model with threshold boundaries triggering an alert when an untoward event (in this case COVID19/red dotted line) changed the performance of the model [109]

Evaluation of AI performance is a requirement of medical device regulation. The increasing complexity of models, scale of use and integration into healthcare requires development of robust real-time monitoring systems [110]. A use of direct and indirect tools as well as defined control and alert limits will allow for safe real-time deployment. The EU AI act has dedicated two articles (article 34 and 72) to post-market surveillance as a key element of AI implementation in healthcare [4].

4.11 The Role of Training and Digital Literacy for AI Implementation

The Topol review in 2019 has highlighted AI training as a priority, so 'healthcare professionals can deliver the digital future' [43]. In a European survey (2025) of more than 2200 radiographers, funded by the Society and College of Radiographers (SCoR) and endorsed by the European Federation of Radiographer Societies (EFRS), lack of AI literacy, lower levels of radiography education and lack of theoretical or practical prior knowledge of AI all correlated very strongly with lack of trust and lower AI acceptability in clinical practice by medical imaging and radiotherapy professionals [111]. This is not a new finding. Other studies before this one, across different professions in one or more countries, have replicated it [111–118]. So, there is a real need for AI training and education of all key healthcare professionals to facilitate AI implementation and build trust. More recently this need became also a legal requirement, as different regulatory bodies require AI training for the safe use of AI tools in healthcare. For instance, since September 2023, the Health and Care Professions Council (HCPC) in the UK requires digital literacy as a key competency for radiographers to ensure they can remain registered and are fit for practice [119, 120]. More recently the EU AI Act in articles 3 and 4 support the 'development of training programs to empower both radiology personnel and patients with the knowledge and skills necessary for safe and effective

engagement with AI technologies in radiological practice' [4]. AI training is not a luxury anymore; it is our professional responsibility towards our patients. The content, delivery, format of AI education should be carefully customised to different professionals to ensure we maximise its impact and benefits [11–13, 121].

4.12 AI Explainability: An Enabler for AI Implementation and Legacy for Ongoing Success

Explainable artificial intelligence (XAI) in medical imaging aims to make AI-driven diagnostic decisions transparent and understandable for healthcare providers [122, 123]. The rapid adoption of deep learning in tasks like classification, prediction, segmentation and denoising highlights significant issues due to the opaque nature of these models. Despite their high accuracy, the inability of AI systems to clearly explain their reasoning, commonly called the 'black box' problem, raises important concerns about trust and reliability.

XAI addresses these concerns through a structured taxonomy based on stage (ante-hoc explanations embedded within models or post-hoc interpretations of existing models), scope (local explanations for specific predictions or global explanations clarifying overall model behaviour) and explanation format (visual, numerical, rule-based, textual, example-based and mixed methods). Visual methods like heatmaps (e.g. Grad-CAM) illustrate influential image areas; numerical explanations quantify feature importance; rule-based explanations use clear IF-THEN logic; textual methods provide explanations in plain language; example-based explanations compare predictions with similar or contrasting cases and counterfactual explanations identify minimal hypothetical changes that could alter model decisions. Mixed methods integrate multiple formats for deeper insights [124, 125]. However, standardised terminology remains limited, and the choice of explanation type should align with user preferences and clinical context [126].

The growth of XAI is driven by ethical, societal, and regulatory pressures, including GDPR's 'right to explanation' [127, 128]. Ultimately, XAI enhances clinical trust, patient safety and ethical accountability, underscoring the need for clear terminology and user-focused explanation methods [126].

4.13 Reimbursement and Financial Aspects for AI—The Clinician's Perspective

AI is rapidly transforming healthcare, promising faster diagnoses, improved patient outcomes, and cost-effectiveness. However, understanding how to reimburse and finance AI technologies is crucial for successful integration into routine clinical practice. The medical imaging AI market is forecast to reach almost $14 billion by 2032, increasing from $762 million in 2022 [129].

As AI technology becomes more prevalent in healthcare, there are challenges in terms of reimbursement. One of the main challenges is that traditional reimbursement models may not adequately cover the costs of implementing AI technology. For example, there may be upfront costs associated with purchasing and implementing AI systems, as well as ongoing costs for maintenance and training. These costs may not be fully reimbursed by payers, leading to financial challenges for healthcare providers. Another challenge is that current reimbursement models may not value the outcomes and efficiency gains that AI technology can provide. For example, AI-enabled diagnostic tools may be more accurate and efficient than traditional methods, leading to better patient outcomes and lower costs in the long run. However, if payers do not recognise the value of these outcomes, providers may not be adequately reimbursed for their use of AI technology.

The US Centres for Medicare & Medicaid Services (CMS) announced in 2021 a coverage provision for AI-specific Common Procedural Terminology (CPT) code and the creation of the first New Technology Add-On Payment (NTAP) for an AI device, which is a significant develop-

ment in the payment for AI-enabled services [130]. Currently the CMS reimburses the use of the following AI devices (Table 4.6). Beyond the USA, reimbursement and incentives for new AI-powered technologies have not been set. In Europe, there is a growing shortage of healthcare workers, so the need for AI may be greater. Japan does have reimbursement for some AI solutions, and in the UK, the National Health Service also pays separately for some AI applications. However, for most regions across Europe, and for most AI applications, incentives or reimbursement strategies for new technologies have not been formally established.

Reimbursement for AI applications is dependent on these solutions delivering improved outcomes for patients, backed by real-world clinical studies and budget-impact modelling that show the health economic benefit and return-on-investment (ROI) for providers. However, the number of such studies from vendors to date is limited; hence, there is little direct reimbursement. More recently there has been a publication of a framework that has proposed that radiology AI applications with clinical utility should be reimbursed separately, provided they have evidence demonstrating that improved diagnostic performance leads to improved outcomes from a societal perspective, or if improved outcomes can reasonably be anticipated based on clinical utility offered [131].

While there are challenges associated with reimbursement, there are also financial opportunities that AI technology presents. By developing a comprehensive business case, engaging with payers, and investing in training and development, providers can maximise the financial benefits of AI in healthcare. Ultimately, AI technology has the potential to transform healthcare delivery and improve patient outcomes, making it a valuable investment for providers.

More about how AI can be resourced and funded from an industry perspective can be found in the two case studies of Chap. 13, written by industry leaders. This is also an area of active and much needed development and research to overcome the obstacles in delivering first class, AI-enabled clinical service.

Table 4.6 Radiology software that is currently reimbursed by the CMS in radiology [131]

Pathway	Technology	Description	CMS decision
IPPS (NTAP)	Viz LVO (ContaCT)	Triage and notification software for stroke patients with suspected large vessel occlusion (LVO) in patients undergoing computed tomography (CT) angiography	NTAP status granted in 2020 and applicable until 2022
	Rapid ASPECTS	Software to calculate Alberta stroke programme early CT score (ASPECTS) from CT images in patients with stroke	Rejected in 2022
	Aidoc Briefcase for PE	Triage and notification software for pulmonary embolism (PE) in patients undergoing CT pulmonary angiography	Rejected in 2022
OPPS (APC)	HeartFlow	Software to quantify coronary flow from coronary CT images	New Technology APC granted in 2018; reassigned to clinical APC in 2022
	LiverMultiScan	Software to quantify liver pathology such as iron and fat content from liver magnetic resonance imaging (MRI)	New Technology APC granted from 2022
	Optellum Lung Cancer Prediction (LCP)	Software algorithm to produce a raw risk score for pulmonary nodules seen on chest CTs	New Technology APC granted from 2022
	MRCP+	Software to reconstruct biliary tree and quantify biliary obstruction from magnetic resonance cholangiopancreatography (MRCP)	New Technology APC granted from 2022
	Cleerly labs coronary analysis	Software application to determine the presence and extent of coronary atherosclerosis and stenosis from coronary CT angiography images	New Technology APC granted from 2023
MPFS	HeartFlow	Software to quantify coronary flow from coronary CT images	Included in the 2022 Medicare Physician Fee Schedule

4.14 Sustainable AI: What Does It Mean in the Context of Medical Imaging and Radiotherapy?

AI has emerged as a transformative force in healthcare and other industries, promising innovation, enhanced productivity and efficiency, and improved decision-making. However, the rapid development and deployment of AI raise critical questions about its sustainability, not just in terms of its environmental impact but also in its social, economic and ethical dimensions [102, 103].

4.14.1 Environmental Sustainability

The exponential growth of AI has ignited discussions on its environmental sustainability. Of particular concern is the significant energy consumption and carbon emissions associated with training AI models, especially those employing deep learning techniques [1] and, more recently, generative AI [132]. The processing demands of large-scale models, such as those used in natural language processing and image recognition, are typically met by data centres powered by non-renewable energy sources. Additionally, the disposal of electronic waste poses environmental challenges. Achieving sustainable AI entails a shift towards energy-efficient algorithms, optimisation of cloud infrastructure, reducing energy use by switching the equipment off when not in clinical use [102, 103, 133] and the integration of renewable energy sources in data centres. In particular, for environmental sustainability in medical imaging, many research studies have been recently published and the most recent European Congress of Radiology in 2025 was dedicated to environmental sustainability [134, 135].

4.14.2 Economic Sustainability

The economic dimension of sustainable AI encompasses accessibility and workforce implications. Automation facilitated by AI has the potential to displace jobs, necessitating measures to mitigate adverse economic impacts and promote workforce reskilling and upskilling. Balancing technological advancement with economic inclusivity is essential for sustainable AI applications.

4.14.3 Ethical and Social Implications

Ethical concerns surrounding AI sustainability revolve around bias, transparency, and accountability. Biased training data can perpetuate societal inequalities, emphasising the need for transparent AI decision-making processes and robust mechanisms for accountability. Prioritising fairness, transparency and inclusivity is paramount. Moreover, safeguarding data privacy and security is integral to sustaining public trust and protecting individual privacy in the era of extensive data utilisation for AI model training.

4.14.4 Responsible Innovation

Sustainable AI necessitates a paradigm shift towards responsible innovation, which entails interdisciplinary collaboration to consider the broader societal implications of AI deployment. Alignment with societal values and active stakeholder engagement are crucial to ensure that AI technologies adhere to ethical standards and contribute positively to societal well-being.

4.14.5 Regulatory Frameworks

Effective regulatory frameworks are imperative for addressing the multifaceted challenges of sustainable AI. Governments and international bodies must establish guidelines promoting responsible AI development and usage, encompassing environmental standards, ethical consid-erations, and economic inclusivity. A collaborative global effort is essential to establish coherent regulatory landscapes that foster responsible and sustainable AI advancement.

To sum up, the attainment of sustainable AI necessitates a multifaceted strategy that integrates technological innovation, ethical deliberations, economic inclusivity and regulatory governance. Striking a delicate balance between innovation and responsibility is paramount to fully harnessing AI's potential while safeguarding both our environment and societal well-being.

4.15 The Complex Impact of AI in Healthcare

AI presents exciting new prospects in medical imaging promising automation, optimisation and heightened efficiency. Yet, its implementation also raises a multitude of considerations spanning social, professional, economic, ethical, legal and cultural realms. Furthermore, impact of AI changes with time, as the organisation, team and equipment change or as the vision and mission get adjusted. Figure 4.15 shows the impact of AI in different UK clinical settings.

4.15.1 Social Impact

- *Improved patient care*: AI algorithms can analyse vast amounts of medical imaging data, potentially enabling earlier and more accurate diagnoses and fostering improved patient outcomes and treatment efficiency. Additionally, it can afford healthcare professionals more time for patient interaction, also empowering patients in their care journey.
- *Increasing access to care*: AI has the potential to mitigate workforce shortages in medical imaging, particularly in underserved areas, thereby expanding access to quality healthcare services.
- *Potential for bias*: Yet AI algorithms trained on biased datasets may also perpetuate existing inequalities in healthcare access and diagnosis [136].

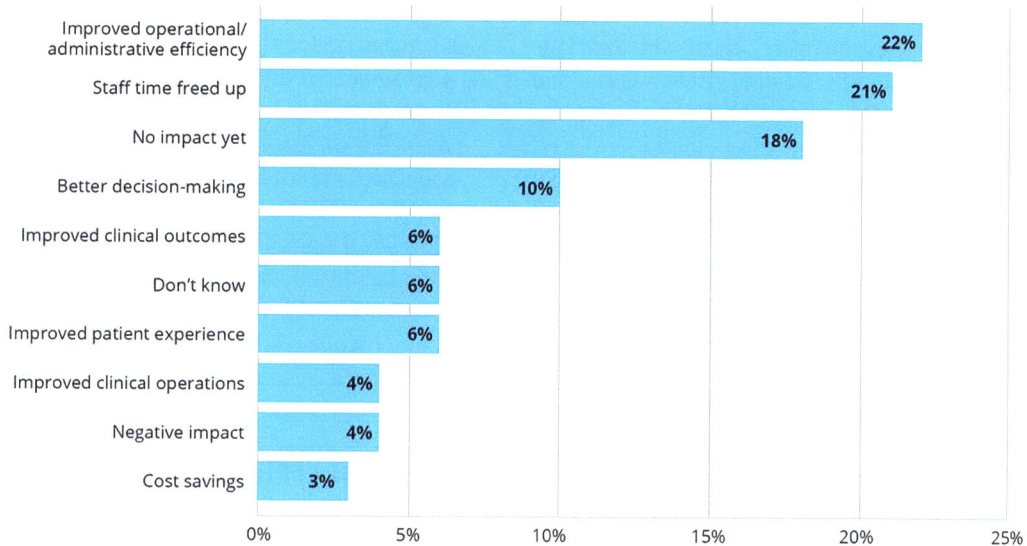

Fig. 4.15 Different types of impacts stemming from AI implementation in different healthcare settings in London, UK [20]

- *Patient trust*: Transparent communication regarding AI's role in diagnosis is crucial for maintaining patient trust and mitigating anxieties about over-reliance on technology [137].

4.15.2 Professional Impact

- *Role transformation*: AI automation of routine tasks can streamline patient care workflows, allowing professionals to focus on complex cases and patient interaction [138]. However, healthcare professionals may need additional training to leverage AI effectively and ensure patient safety, underscoring the necessity for ongoing upskilling [139]. While AI is unlikely to completely replace radiologists, it may reshape their roles, necessitating adaptation and lifelong learning [139, 140]. The role of radiographers may evolve from traditional image acquisition towards more analytical tasks in collaboration with AI systems [141].
- *Workforce well-being:* AI can potentially alleviate the burden of routine and time-consuming tasks, contributing to reduced stress and burnout and improving well-being among radiologists and radiographers

[141–143]. However, concerns related to job displacement and changing roles may also negatively impact emotional well-being among healthcare workers. For example, it was reported that radiographers may face anxiety and uncertainty about how AI will impact their roles and career progression [142].

4.15.3 Economic Impact

(a) *Cost Savings and Efficiency Gains:* Improved resource allocation is a key benefit of AI. By prioritising critical cases, AI can help optimising staffing and equipment usage, leading to significant cost savings [141]. Additionally, AI algorithms can identify suboptimal image quality, reducing the need for repeat scans and conserving valuable resources. Another area where AI can contribute to economic efficiency is in standardised reporting, ensuring consistency and reducing the time spent on documentation, ultimately leading to cost savings. However, it's important to acknowledge the upfront investments and ongoing costs associated with AI implementation and maintenance [139].

(b) *Balancing the value equation:* Cost-effectiveness analyses, deliverable from the discipline of Health Economics and Outcomes Research (HEOR), are necessary to evaluate whether the potential cost savings from AI outweigh the upfront investments and ongoing expenses. Furthermore, integrating AI into value-based care models can incentivise cost-effective use by rewarding positive patient outcomes rather than service volume [144]. This shift in approach aligns with the broader goals of delivering high-quality, efficient healthcare services.

(c) *Job market dynamics:* The implementation of AI may alter the job market dynamics in medical imaging, potentially creating new roles while transforming existing ones.

4.15.4 Cultural Impact

- *AI Legitimation*: Cultural factors influence the acceptance and trust in AI technologies, emphasising the need to establish trust among stakeholders. Cultural perspectives on ethics and privacy affect AI acceptance.

- *Shifting culture:* AI can contribute to a more data-driven approach to diagnosis, potentially influencing healthcare decision-making processes [145].

- *Importance of human expertise*: Despite AI's advancements, human expertise in radiology remains crucial for interpretation, clinical context, and patient communication [146].

4.15.5 Ethical and Legal Impact

(a) *Data privacy*: AI implementation raises ethical considerations related to patient data privacy and confidentiality. Ensuring patient data privacy and compliance with regulations like the Health Insurance Portability and Accountability Act (HIPAA) (USA) and the General Data Protection Regulation (GDPR)

(UK and EU) is paramount when using AI in healthcare [58, 59].

(b) *Algorithmic Bias*: Mitigating bias in AI development and deployment is crucial to avoid discrimination against certain patient populations [146].

(c) *Liability, Transparency and Explainability*: Clear legal frameworks are needed to determine liability in cases where AI contributes to diagnostic errors [147]. It is important to ensure explainability of AI decisions to maintain transparency and trust.

4.16 When AI Implementation Fails

AI is by no means a perfect tool. It is as good as the data we train it with and as good as the people (human intelligence) who use it. There are so many reasons where AI can and will fail: a) technical reasons of the AI model itself (including training, testing and pre-deployment evaluation), b) IT infrastructure, often related to connectivity, cloud performance and compatibility of different devices, c) and human factors, which is, perhaps, the most complex and more challenging to study and grasp of them all and includes trust, policy, culture, leadership and teamwork, amongst other aspects [34]. We cannot avoid over-reliance on technology, or even data bias, because real life is messy, patchy and imperfect. We can, though, accept that we live and work in an imperfect world and create a culture where errors and failures will be celebrated as a chance for improvement and learning opportunity. With the multitude of clinical contexts and complexity of clinical scenarios, it is very likely that, what works in one setting and set-up won't work in another. So, we will always need the human in the loop, to optimise, contextualise and deliver person-centred care. We do, however, have a responsibility to understand and teach these pitfalls, so our clinical practitioners will be prepared to remedy them and improve AI performance for the benefit of their patients and of the workforce [148].

4.17   Chapter Summary

AI implementation in medical imaging and radiotherapy is multifactorial, complex and contextual. It is also at its early stages, and this is perfect timing to understand more about its mechanisms, challenges and enablers, and help fine tune it for optimal outcomes and maximum impact. Robust governance, customised AI training, thorough evaluation and consideration of its impact on patients, practitioners, workflows, organisations and societies can help us optimise its performance and minimise potential risks. Working together is vital to ensure the native ecosystems harness opportunities from the collective expertise, and the change happening is organic and co-produced by all the consistent members of the ecosystem and different end-users.

References

1. Sujan M, Smith-Frazer C, Malamateniou C, Connor J, Gardner A, Unsworth H, Husain H. Validation framework for the use of AI in healthcare: overview of the new British standard BS30440. BMJ Health Care Inform. 2023;30(1):e100749.
2. Ranschaert E, Rezazade Mehrizi MH, Grootjans W, Cook TS. AI implementation in radiology, challenges and opportunities in clinical practice. Springer; 2024.
3. Geis JR, Brady A, Wu CC, Spencer J, Ranschaert E, Jaremko JL, Langer SG, Kitts AB, Birch J, Shields WF, van den Hoven van Genderen R, Kotter E, Gichoya JW, Cook TS, Morgan MB, Tang A, Safdar NM, Kohli M. Ethics of artificial intelligence in radiology: summary of the joint European and North American multisociety statement. Insights Imaging. 2019;10(1):101.
4. Kotter E, D'Antonoli TA, Cuocolo R, Hierath M, Huisman M, Klontzas ME, Martí-Bonmatí L, May MS, Neri E, Nikolaou K, Pinto Dos Santos D, Radzina M, Shelmerdine SC, Bellemo A, European Society of Radiology (ESR). Guiding AI in radiology: ESR's recommendations for effective implementation of the European AI Act. Insights Imag. 2025;16(1):33.
5. Stogiannos N, Malik R, Kumar A, Barnes A, Pogose M, Harvey H, McEntee MF, Malamateniou C. Black box no more: a scoping review of AI governance frameworks to guide procurement and adoption of AI in medical imaging and radiotherapy in the UK. Br J Radiol. 2023;96(1152):20221157.
6. Stogiannos N, O'Regan T, Scurr E, Litosseliti L, Pogose M, Harvey H, Kumar A, Malik R, Barnes A, McEntee MF, Malamateniou C. Lessons on AI implementation from senior clinical practitioners: an exploratory qualitative study in medical imaging and radiotherapy in the UK. J Med Imaging Radiat Sci. 2025;56(1):101797.
7. Stogiannos N, Litosseliti L, O'Regan T, Scurr E, Barnes A, Kumar A, Malik R, Pogose M, Harvey H, McEntee MF, Malamateniou C. Black box no more: a cross-sectional multi-disciplinary survey for exploring governance and guiding adoption of AI in medical imaging and radiotherapy in the UK. Int J Med Inform. 2024;186:105423.
8. European Society of Radiology (ESR). What the radiologist should know about artificial intelligence - an ESR white paper. Insights Imag. 2019;10(1):44.
9. Tejani AS, Elhalawani H, Moy L, Kohli M, Kahn CE Jr. Artificial intelligence and radiology education. Radiol Artif Intell. 2022;5(1):e220084.
10. Malamateniou C, McFadden S, McQuinlan Y, England A, Woznitza N, Goldsworthy S, Currie C, Skelton E, Chu KY, Alware N, Matthews P, Hawkesford R, Tucker R, Town W, Matthew J, Kalinka C, O'Regan T. Artificial intelligence: guidance for clinical imaging and therapeutic radiography professionals, a summary by the Society of Radiographers AI working group. Radiography (Lond). 2021;27(4):1192–202.
11. van de Venter R, Skelton E, Matthew J, Woznitza N, Tarroni G, Hirani SP, Kumar A, Malik R, Malamateniou C. Artificial intelligence education for radiographers, an evaluation of a UK postgraduate educational intervention using participatory action research: a pilot study. Insights Imaging. 2023;14(1):25.
12. Walsh G, Stogiannos N, van de Venter R, Rainey C, Tam W, McFadden S, McNulty JP, Mekis N, Lewis S, O'Regan T, Kumar A, Huisman M, Bisdas S, Kotter E, Pinto Dos Santos D, Sá Dos Reis C, van Ooijen P, Brady AP, Malamateniou C. Responsible AI practice and AI education are central to AI implementation: a rapid review for all medical imaging professionals in Europe. BJR Open. 2023;5(1):20230033.
13. Stogiannos N, Skelton E, Kumar S, Ahmed S, Amedu C, Vince C, Schiavottiello M, O'Sullivan C, Malamateniou C. Evaluation of a customised, AI-focused educational seminar delivered to final year undergraduate radiography students in the UK: a cross-sectional study. Radiography (Lond). 2025;31(3):102926.
14. Akudjedu TN, Torre S, Khine R, Katsifarakis D, Newman D, Malamateniou C. Knowledge, perceptions, and expectations of artificial intelligence in radiography practice: a global radiography workforce survey. J Med Imaging Radiat Sci. 2023;54(1):104–16. https://doi.org/10.1016/j.jmir.2022.11.016. Epub 2022 Dec 18. PMID: 36535859.

15. Brady AP, Allen B, Chong J, Kotter E, Kottler N, Mongan J, Oakden-Rayner L, Pinto Dos Santos D, Tang A, Wald C, Slavotinek J. Developing, purchasing, implementing and monitoring AI tools in radiology: practical considerations. A multisociety statement from the ACR, CAR, ESR, RANZCR & RSNA. J Med Imaging Radiat Oncol. 2024;68(1):7–26. https://doi.org/10.1111/1754-9485.13612. Epub 2024 Jan 23. PMID: 38259140.

16. van de Sande D, Van Genderen ME, Smit JM, Huiskens J, Visser JJ, Veen RER, van Unen E, Ba OH, Gommers D, Bommel JV. Developing, implementing and governing artificial intelligence in medicine: a step-by-step approach to prevent an artificial intelligence winter. BMJ Health Care Inform. 2022;29(1):e100495.

17. Bergquist M, Rolandsson B, Gryska E, Laesser M, Hoefling N, Heckemann R, Schneiderman JF, Björkman-Burtscher IM. Trust and stakeholder perspectives on the implementation of AI tools in clinical radiology. Eur Radiol. 2024;34(1):338–47.

18. van Leeuwen KG, de Rooij M, Schalekamp S, van Ginneken B, Rutten MJCM. Clinical use of artificial intelligence products for radiology in The Netherlands between 2020 and 2022. Eur Radiol. 2024;34(1):348–54.

19. Leslie D. Tackling COVID-19 through responsible AI innovation: five steps in the right direction. Harv Data Sci Rev. 2020. Retrieved from https://hdsr.mitpress.mit.edu/pub/as1p81um. Accessed 31st Mar 2025.

20. Lawrence A, Hardie T, Zapantis I, Ohenhen O, Hepworth J. AI in London healthcare: the reality behind the hype, UCL Partners and the Health Foundation report, available form https://uclpartners.com/wp-content/uploads/UCLP-AI-in-London-healthcare-03.25-final.pdf. 2025. Accessed 31st Mar 2025.

21. Hua D, Petrina N, Young N, Cho JG, Poon SK. Understanding the factors influencing acceptability of AI in medical imaging domains among healthcare professionals: a scoping review. Artif Intell Med. 2024;147:102698.

22. World Economic Forum. Balancing innovation and governance in the age of AI. https://www.weforum.org/stories/2024/11/balancing-innovation-and-governance-in-the-age-of-ai/#:~:text=In%20many%20cases%2C%20it%20will,the%20risks%20without%20stifling%20innovation. 2024. Accessed 31st Mar 2025.

23. van Leeuwen KG, Schalekamp S, Rutten MJCM, van Ginneken B, de Rooij M. Artificial intelligence in radiology: 100 commercially available products and their scientific evidence. Eur Radiol. 2021;31(6):3797–804.

24. Romion Health. Available via https://www.romion-health.com/. Accessed 31st Mar 2025.

25. Radiology AI Register. Available via https://radiology.healthairegister.com/. Accessed 31st Mar 2025.

26. Royal College of Radiologists, AI registry. Available from https://www.rcr.ac.uk/our-services/artificial-intelligence-ai/ai-registry/. Accessed 31st Mar 2025.

27. European Society of Medical Imaging Informatics (EuSoMII). Available form https://www.eusomii.org/. Accessed 31st Mar 2025.

28. Hosny A, Parmar C, Quackenbush J, Schwartz LH, Aerts HJWL. Artificial intelligence in radiology. Nat Rev Cancer. 2018;18(8):500–10.

29. Hardy M, Harvey H. Artificial intelligence in diagnostic imaging: impact on the radiography profession. Br J Radiol. 2020;93(1108):20190840.

30. Malamateniou C, O'Regan T, McFadden SL, Jackson M. Artificial intelligence (AI) in radiography practice, research and education: a review of contemporary developments and predictions for the future. Radiography (Lond). 2024;30(Suppl 2):56–9.

31. Rainey C, O'Regan T, Matthew J, Skelton E, Woznitza N, Chu KY, Goodman S, McConnell J, Hughes C, Bond R, Malamateniou C, McFadden S. UK reporting radiographers' perceptions of AI in radiographic image interpretation - current perspectives and future developments. Radiography (Lond). 2022;28(4):881–8.

32. Pedersen MRV, Jensen J, Gale N, Senior C, Woznitza N, Heales CJ. Reporting radiographers in Europe survey: support, role satisfaction, and advanced clinical practice within the European federation of radiographer society (EFRS) member countries. Radiography (Lond). 2024;30(1):87–94.

33. Stogiannos N, O'Regan T, Scurr E, Litosseliti L, Pogose M, Harvey H, Kumar A, Malik R, Barnes A, McEntee MF, Malamateniou C. AI implementation in the UK landscape: knowledge of AI governance, perceived challenges and opportunities, and ways forward for radiographers. Radiography (Lond). 2024;30(2):612–21. https://doi.org/10.1016/j.radi.2024.01.019. Epub 2024 Feb 7. PMID: 38325103.

34. Sujan M, Furniss D, Grundy K, Grundy H, Nelson D, Elliott M, White S, Habli I, Reynolds N. Human factors challenges for the safe use of artificial intelligence in patient care. BMJ Health Care Inform. 2019;26(1):e100081.

35. Johnson K, Martin P, McDonald D, McGrail M. Interprofessional education and collaborative practice with practicing radiographers: a mixed methods scoping review. Radiography (Lond). 2025;31(1):434–41.

36. Rainey C, O'Regan T, Matthew J, Skelton E, Woznitza N, Chu KY, Goodman S, McConnell J, Hughes C, Bond R, Malamateniou C, McFadden S. An insight into the current perceptions of UK radiographers on the future impact of AI on the profession: a cross-sectional survey. J Med Imag Radiat Sci. 2022;53(3):347–61.

37. Stogiannos N, Gillan C, Precht H, Reis CSD, Kumar A, O'Regan T, Ellis V, Barnes A, Meades R, Pogose M, Greggio J, Scurr E, Kumar S, King G, Rosewarne

D, Jones C, van Leeuwen KG, Hyde E, Beardmore C, Alliende JG, El-Farra S, Papathanasiou S, Beger J, Nash J, van Ooijen P, Zelenyanszki C, Koch B, Langmack KA, Tucker R, Goh V, Turmezei T, Lip G, Reyes-Aldasoro CC, Alonso E, Dean G, Hirani SP, Torre S, Akudjedu TN, Ohene-Botwe B, Khine R, O'Sullivan C, Kyratsis Y, McEntee M, Wheatstone P, Thackray Y, Cairns J, Jerome D, Scarsbrook A, Malamateniou C. A multidisciplinary team and multiagency approach for AI implementation: a commentary for medical imaging and radiotherapy key stakeholders. J Med Imaging Radiat Sci. 2024;55(4):101717.

38. Bauer MS, Kirchner J. Implementation science: what is it and why should I care? Psychiatry Res. 2020;283:112376.

39. Groenier M, Spijkerboer K, Venix L, Bannink L, Yperlaan S, Eyck Q, van Manen JG, Miedema HAT. Evaluation of the impact of technical physicians on improving individual patient care with technology. BMC Med Educ. 2023;23(1):181.

40. NHS England. How artificial intelligence is helping to speed up the diagnosis and treatment of stroke patients available via https://www.england.nhs.uk/blog/how-artificial-intelligence-is-helping-to-speed-up-the-diagnosis-and-treatment-of-stroke-patients/. 2024. Accessed 31st Mar 2025.

41. Liu H, Ding N, Li X, Chen Y, Sun H, Huang Y, Liu C, Ye P, Jin Z, Bao H, Xue H. Artificial intelligence and radiologist burnout. JAMA Netw Open. 2024;7(11):e2448714.

42. Kim BJ, Lee J. The mental health implications of artificial intelligence adoption: the crucial role of self-efficacy. Humanit Soc Sci Commun. 2024;11:1561.

43. Topol E. Preparing the healthcare workforce to deliver the digital future. Available via https://topol.hee.nhs.UK/the-topol-review/. 2019. Accessed 31st Mar 2025.

44. Moulds A, Horton T. How would clinicians use time freed up by technology? Report by The Health Foundation (2025). Available via https://www.health.org.uk/reports-and-analysis/briefings/how-would-clinicians-use-time-freed-up-by-technology. Accessed 25th June 2025.

45. Kyratsis Y, Scarbrough H, Begley A, Denis J-L. Digital health adoption: looking beyond the role of technology. Front Digital Health—Health Technol Implement. 2022;4 https://doi.org/10.3389/fdgth.2022.989003.

46. Greenhalgh T, Wherton J, Papoutsi C, Lynch J, Hughes G, A'Court C, Hinder S, Fahy N, Procter R, Shaw S. Beyond adoption: a new framework for theorizing and evaluating nonadoption, abandonment, and challenges to the scale-up, spread, and sustainability of health and care technologies. J Med Internet Res. 2017;19(11):e367. https://doi.org/10.2196/jmir.8775.

47. Topol EJ. High-performance medicine: the convergence of human and artificial intelligence. Nat Med. 2019;25(1):44–56.

48. Celi LA, Cellini J, Charpignon ML, Dee EC, Dernoncourt F, Eber R, Mitchell WG, Moukheiber L, Schirmer J, Situ J, Paguio J, Park J, Wawira JG, Yao S, Fraser HS. Sources of bias in artificial intelligence that perpetuate healthcare disparities - A global review. PLoS Digit Health. 2022;1(3):e0000022.

49. Strohm L, Hehakaya C, Ranschaert ER, et al. Implementation of artificial intelligence (AI) applications in radiology: hindering and facilitating factors. Eur Radiol. 2020;30:5525–32. https://doi.org/10.1007/s00330-020-06946-y.

50. Anthony C. When knowledge work and analytical technologies collide: the practices and consequences of black boxing algorithmic technologies. Adm Sci Q. 2021;66(4):1173–212. https://doi.org/10.1177/00018392211016755.

51. Alami H, Lehoux P, Denis JL, Motulsky A, Petitgand C, Savoldelli M, Rouquet R, Gagnon MP, Roy D, Fortin JP. Organizational readiness for artificial intelligence in health care: insights for decision-making and practice. J Health Organ Manag. 2020;3;ahead-of-print. https://doi.org/10.1108/JHOM-03-2020-0074.

52. Lebovitz S, Lifshitz-Assaf H, Levina N. To engage or not to engage with AI for critical judgments: how professionals deal with opacity when using AI for medical diagnosis. Org Sci. 2022;33(1):1–494. https://doi.org/10.1287/orsc.2021.1549.

53. Chowdhury S, Budhwar P, Dey PK, Joel-Edgar S, Abadie A. AI-employee. Collaboration and business performance: integrating knowledge-based view, sociotechnical systems and organisational socialisation framework. J Bus Res. 2022;144:31–49. https://doi.org/10.1016/j.jbusres.2022.01.069.

54. Hemmings N, Hutchings R, Castle-Clarke S, Palmer W. Achieving scale and spread. London: Nuffield Trust; 2020.

55. Rigby MJ. Ethical dimensions of using artificial intelligence in health care. AMA J Ethics. 2019;21(2):121–4.

56. Glikson E, Woolley AW. Human trust in artificial intelligence: review of empirical research. Acad Manag Ann. 2020;14(2):627–60. https://doi.org/10.5465/annals.2018.0057.

57. Scarbrough H, Kyratsis Y. From spreading to embedding innovation in healthcare: implications for theory and practice. Health Care Manag Rev. 2022;47(3):236–44.

58. US Department of Health and Human Services, Health Information Privacy, Summary of the HIPAA Privacy Rule. Available from https://www.hhs.gov/hipaa/for-professionals/privacy/laws-regulations/index.html. Accessed 31st Mar 2025.

59. European data protection regulation. General data protection regulation (GDPR). Available from https://gdpr-info.eu/. Accessed 31st Mar 2025.

60. Annoni A, Benczur P, Bertoldi P, Delipetrev B, De Prato G, Feijoo C, Fernandez Macias E, Gomez Gutierrez E, Iglesias Portela M, Junklewitz H, Lopez Cobo M, Martens B, Figueiredo Do

Nascimento S, Nativi S, Polvora A, Sanchez Martin JI, Tolan S, Tuomi I, Vesnic Alujevic L. In: Craglia M, editor. Artificial intelligence: a European perspective. Luxembourg. ISBN 978-92-79-97219-5. JRC113826.: EUR 29425 EN, Publications Office of the European Union; 2018. https://doi.org/10.2760/936974.

61. Amann J, Blasimme A, Vayena E, et al. Explainability for artificial intelligence in healthcare: a multidisciplinary perspective. BMC Med Inform Decis Mak. 2020;20:310. https://doi.org/10.1186/s12911-020-01332-6.

62. Phillips N. Digital leadership: meeting the challenge of leading in a digitally transformed world. J Financ Transform. 2021;52:8–15.

63. Blessing E, Hubert K. Technological infrastructure and challenges: integration challenges in implementing AI solutions in legacy systems. 2024. ⟨hal-04972070⟩.

64. Stoumpos AI, Kitsios F, Talias MA. Digital transformation in healthcare: technology acceptance and its applications. Int J Environ Res Public Health. 2023;20(4):3407.

65. NHS England digital transformation. Available from https://www.england.nhs.uk/digitaltechnology/. Accessed 31st March 2025.

66. Ahmed A, Xi R, Hou M, Shah SA, Hameed S. Harnessing big data analytics for healthcare: a comprehensive review of frameworks, implications, applications, and impacts. IEEE Access. 2023;11:112891–928. https://doi.org/10.1109/ACCESS.2023.3323574.

67. Health innovation Network. Writing your NHS business case. Available from: https://thehealth-innovationnetwork.co.uk/how-we-can-help-you/support-for-innovators/writing-your-nhs-business-case/#:~:text=There%20are%20core%20components%20of,and%20a%20capability%20to%20deliver. Accessed 31st March 2025.

68. Carter H. How to write a robust business case for service development. Nurs Times [online]s. 2017;113(7):25–8.

69. Hurst L, Mahtani K, Pluddemann A, Lewis S, Harvey K, Briggs A, Boylan A-M, Bajwa R, Haire K, Entwistle A, Handa A and Heneghan C. Defining value-based healthcare in the NHS: CEBM Report May 2019.

70. Shelmerdine SC, Togher D, Rickaby S, Dean G. Artificial intelligence (AI) implementation within the National Health Service (NHS): the South West London AI Working Group experience. Clin Radiol. 2024;79(9):665–72.

71. EU Medical Device Regulation (MDR) Regulation (EU) 2017/745 of the European Parliament and of the council (2017). (annex viii, 6.3. Rule 11).

72. NHSx: A Buyer's guide to AI in health and care. Available from https://transform.england.nhs.uk/media/documents/NHSX_A_Buyers_Guide_to_AI_in_Health_and_Care.pdf. 2020. Accessed 31st March 2025.

73. EU Artificial Intelligence act. Available from https://artificialintelligenceact.eu/ai-act-explorer/. 2024. Accessed 31st March 2025.

74. UK Parliament, Artificial Intelligence Rugulation (Bill). Available from: https://bills.parliament.uk/bills/3942. Accessed 31st March 2025.

75. Software as a medical device (SaMD). Available from https://www.fda.gov/medical-devices/digital-health-center-excellence/software-medical-device-samd. Accessed 31st March 2025.

76. Software in a medical device (SiMD) Available from https://www.imdrf.org/documents. Accessed 31st March 2025.

77. Wang X, Wu YC. Balancing innovation and regulation in the age of generative artificial intelligence. J Inf Policy. 2024;14:385–416.

78. In Vitro Device Regulation (IVDR). Available from https://euivdr.com/. Accessed 31st March 2025.

79. MDCG 2021-24 Guidance on classification of medical devices. Available from: https://health.ec.europa.eu/system/files/2021-10/mdcg_2021-24_en_0.pdf. Accessed 31 Mar 2025.

80. European Medicines Agency (EMA). Available from https://www.ema.europa.eu/en/homepage. Accessed 31st March 2025.

81. European Commission. EUDAMED—European Database on Medical Devices. Available from https://ec.europa.eu/tools/eudamed/#/screen/home. Accessed 31st March 2025.

82. Evidence Standards Framework (ESF) for digital health technologies. Available from https://www.nice.org.uk/about/what-we-do/our-programmes/evidence-standards-framework-for-digital-health-technologies. Accessed 31st Mar 2025.

83. Software and artificial intelligence (AI) as a medical device. Available from https://www.gov.uk/government/publications/software-and-artificial-intelligence-ai-as-a-medical-device/software-and-artificial-intelligence-ai-as-a-medical-device. Accessed 31st Mar 2025.

84. The Medical Devices (Amendment) (Great Britain) Regulations 2023. Available from https://www.legislation.gov.uk/ukdsi/2023/9780348247657/pdfs/ukdsi_9780348247657_en.pd. Accessed 31st Mar 2025.

85. MHRA. Available from https://www.gov.uk/government/news/the-mhra-seeks-views-on-pre-market-regulations-for-medical-devices-to-improve-patient-access-and-strengthen-patient-safety. 2024. Accessed 31 Mar 2025.

86. Gov.UK. Regulating medical devices in the UK: Guidance. UKCA mark and Conformity Assessment Bodies. Last updated 17 February 2025. Available from https://www.gov.uk/guidance/regulating-medical-devices-in-the-uk. Accessed 31 Mar 2025.

87. Medicines and Medical Devices Act 2021. Available from https://www.legislation.gov.uk/ukpga/2021/3/data.pdf. Accessed 31 Mar 2025.

88. MHRA Policy paper "Impact of AI on the regulation of medical products". Available from https://

www.gov.uk/government/publications/impact-of-ai-on-the-regulation-of-medical-products. Accessed 31 Mar 2025.

89. List of UK approved bodies for medical devices. Available from https://www.gov.uk/government/publications/medical-devices-uk-approved-bodies/uk-approved-bodies-for-medical-devices. Accessed 31 Mar 2025.

90. Medical Devices Regulations. SI 2002 No 618, amended). 2002. Available from https://www.legislation.gov.uk/uksi/2002/618/contents. Accessed 31 Mar 2025.

91. UK.GOV. Software and AI as a medical device change programme—roadmap: guidance. Last updated 14 June 2023. Available from https://www.gov.uk/government/publications/software-and-ai-as-a-medical-device-change-programme/software-and-ai-as-a-medical-device-change-programme-roadmap. Accessed 31 Mar 2025.

92. Federal Food Drug and Cosmetic Act. Title 21, Section 321. December 4 29, 2022. Available from https://www.govinfo.gov/content/pkg/USCODE-2022-title21/html/USCODE-2022-title21-chap9-subchapI-sec301.htm. Accessed 31 Mar 2025.

93. Hills JM, Visser JJ, Cliff ER, van der Geest-Aspers K, Bizzo BC, Dreyer KJ, Adams-Prassi J, Andriole KP. The lucent yet opaque challenge of regulating artificial intelligence in radiology. NPJ Digit Med. 2024;7(1):69.

94. DICOM standard (Digital Imaging and Communication in Medicine), ISO 12052:2017. Available from: https://www.iso.org/standard/72941.html#:~:text=ISO%2012052%3A2017%2C%20within%20the,and%20communication%20of%20that%20information. Accessed 31 Mar 2025.

95. Hardian Health. Available from https://www.hardianhealth.com/. Accessed 31 Mar 2025.

96. Premarket Intended use. Available from www.hardianhealth.com/regulatory/pre-market-intended-use. 2025. Accessed 31 Mar 2025.

97. Tanguay W, Acar P, Fine B, Abdolell M, Gong B, Cadrin-Chênevert A, Chartrand-Lefebvre C, Chalaoui J, Gorgos A, Chin AS, Prénovault J, Guilbert F, Létourneau-Guillon L, Chong J, Tang A. Assessment of Radiology artificial intelligence software: a validation and evaluation framework. Can Assoc Radiol J. 2023;74(2):326–33.

98. Park SH, Han K, Jang HY, Park JE, Lee JG, Kim DW, Choi J. Methods for clinical evaluation of artificial intelligence algorithms for medical diagnosis. Radiology. 2023;306(1):20–31.

99. Allen B, Dreyer K, Stibolt R Jr, Agarwal S, Coombs L, Treml C, Elkholy M, Brink L, Wald C. Evaluation and real-world performance monitoring of artificial intelligence models in clinical practice: try it, buy it, check it. J Am Coll Radiol. 2021;18(11):1489–96.

100. Bharadwaj P, Nicola L, Breau-Brunel M, Sensini F, Tanova-Yotova N, Atanasov P, Lobig F, Blankenburg M. Unlocking the value: quantifying the return on investment of hospital artificial intelligence. J Am Coll Radiol. 2024;21(10):1677–85.

101. Kim B, Romeijn S, van Buchem M, Mehrizi MHR, Grootjans W. A holistic approach to implementing artificial intelligence in radiology. Insights Imaging. 2024;15(1):22.

102. Doo FX, Vosshenrich J, Cook TS, Moy L, Almeida EPRP, Woolen SA, Gichoya JW, Heye T, Hanneman K. Environmental sustainability and AI in radiology: A double-edged sword. Radiology. 2024;310(2):e232030.

103. Rockall AG, Allen B, Brown MJ, El-Diasty T, Fletcher J, Gerson RF, Goergen S, González APM, Grist TM, Hanneman K, Hess CP, Ho ELM, Salama DH, Schoen J, Sheard S. Sustainability in radiology: position paper and call to action from ACR, AOSR, ASR, CAR, CIR, ESR, ESRNM, ISR, IS3R, RANZCR, and RSNA. Korean J Radiol. 2025;26(4):294–303.

104. Vela D, Sharp A, Zhang R, et al. Temporal quality degradation in AI models. Sci Rep. 2022;12:11654.

105. NHS England, Applicability of DCB 0129 and DCB 0160. Available at: https://digital.nhs.uk/services/clinical-safety/applicability-of-dcb-0129-and-dcb-0160. Accessed 31 Mar 2025.

106. Carpl.ai. Available from https://carpl.ai/. Accessed 31 Mar 2025.

107. Blackford. Available from https://blackfordanalysis.com/. Accessed 31 Mar 2025.

108. de Vries C, Colosimo S, Staff R, Dymiter J, Yearsley J, Dinneen D, et al. Impact of different mammography systems on artificial intelligence performance in breast cancer screening. Radiol: Artif Intell. 2023;5(3):e220146. Epub 2023 Mar 22. https://doi.org/10.1148/ryai.220146.

109. Venugopal V, Gupta S, Takhar R, Mahajan V. New Epochs in AI supervision: design and implementation of an autonomous radiology AI monitoring system. 2311.14305v1.pdf (arxiv.org)

110. Feng J, Phillips RV, Malenica I, et al. Clinical artificial intelligence quality improvement: towards continual monitoring and updating of AI algorithms in healthcare. npj Digit Med. 2022;5:66. https://doi.org/10.1038/s41746-022-00611-y.

111. Stogiannos N, Walsh G, Ohene-Botwe B, McHugh K, Potts B, Tam W, O'Sullivan C, Quinsten AS, Gibson C, Gorga RG, Sipos D, Dybeli E, Zanardo M, Sá Dos Reis C, Mekis N, Buissink C, England A, Beardmore C, Cunha A, Goodall A, John-Matthews JS, McEntee M, Kyratsis Y, Malamateniou C. R-AI-diographers: a European survey on perceived impact of AI on professional identity, careers, and radiographers' roles. Insights Imaging. 2025;16(1):43. https://doi.org/10.1186/s13244-025-01918-6.

112. Rainey C, O'Regan T, Matthew J, Skelton E, Woznitza N, Chu KY, Goodman S, McConnell J, Hughes C, Bond R, McFadden S, Malamateniou C. Beauty is in the AI of the beholder: are we ready for the clinical integration of artificial intelligence in radiography? An exploratory analysis of perceived

AI knowledge, skills, confidence, and education perspectives of UK radiographers. Front Digit Health. 2021;3:739327.

113. Huisman M, Ranschaert E, Parker W, Mastrodicasa D, Koci M, Pinto de Santos D, Coppola F, Morozov S, Zins M, Bohyn C, Koç U, Wu J, Veean S, Fleischmann D, Leiner T, Willemink MJ. An international survey on AI in radiology in 1041 radiologists and radiology residents part 2: expectations, hurdles to implementation, and education. Eur Radiol. 2021;31(11):8797–806.

114. Stogiannos N, Jennings M, George CS, Culbertson J, Salehi H, Furterer S, Pergola M, Culp MP, Malamateniou C. The American Society of Radiologic Technologists (ASRT) AI educator survey: a cross-sectional study to explore knowledge, experience, and use of AI within education. J Med Imaging Radiat Sci. 2024;55(4):101449.

115. Coakley S, Young R, Moore N, England A, O'Mahony A, O'Connor OJ, Maher M, McEntee MF. Radiographers' knowledge, attitudes and expectations of artificial intelligence in medical imaging. Radiography (Lond). 2022;28(4):943–8.

116. Pedersen MRV, Kusk MW, Lysdahlgaard S, Mork-Knudsen H, Malamateniou C, Jensen J. A Nordic survey on artificial intelligence in the radiography profession - is the profession ready for a culture change? Radiography (Lond). 2024;30(4):1106–15.

117. Abuzaid MM, Elshami W, McConnell J, Tekin HO. An extensive survey of radiographers from the Middle East and India on artificial intelligence integration in radiology practice. Health Technol (Berl). 2021;11(5):1045–50.

118. Champendal M, De Labouchère S, Ghotra SS, Gremion I, Sun Z, Torre S, Khine R, Marmy L, Malamateniou C, Dos Reis CS. Perspectives of medical imaging professionals about the impact of AI on Swiss radiographers. J Med Imaging Radiat Sci. 2024;55(4):101741.

119. HCPC, Digital skills and new technologies. Available from https://www.hcpc-uk.org/standards/standards-of-proficiency/revisions-to-the-standards-of-proficiency/digital-skills-and-new-technologies/. Accessed 31 Mar 2025.

120. HCPC, Standards of proficiency for radiographers. Available from https://www.hcpc-uk.org/standards/standards-of-proficiency/radiographers/. Accessed 31 Mar 2025.

121. Doherty G, McLaughlin L, Hughes C, McConnell J, Bond R, McFadden S. Radiographer education and learning in artificial intelligence (REAL-AI): a survey of radiographers, radiologists, and students' knowledge of and attitude to education on AI. Radiography (Lond). 2024;30(Suppl 2):79–87.

122. von Eschenbach WJ. Transparency and the black box problem: why we do not trust AI. Philos Technol. 2021;34:1607–22.

123. Reyes M, Meier R, Pereira S, Silva CA, Dahlweid FM, von Tengg-Kobligk H, et al. On the interpretability of artificial intelligence in radiology: challenges and opportunities. Radiol: Artif Intell. 2020;2

124. Adadi A, Berrada M. Peeking inside the black-box: A survey on explainable artificial intelligence (XAI). IEEE Access. 2018;6:52138–60.

125. Vilone G, Longo L. Explainable artificial intelligence: a systematic review. (arXiv). 2020. https://arxiv.org/abs/2006.00093.

126. Champendal M, Müller H, Prior JO, dos Reis CS. A scoping review of interpretability and explainability concerning artificial intelligence methods in medical imaging. Eur J Radiol. 2023;169(July):111159.

127. Binns R. Algorithmic accountability and public reason. Philos Technol. 2018;31:543–56.

128. Agarwal S, Kirrane S, Scharf J. Modelling the general data protection regulation. Jusletter IT. 2017;2014.

129. Managed Healthcare Executive. Available from: https://www.managedhealthcareexecutive.com/view/ai-in-medical-imaging-market-expected-to-increase-to-14-2-billion-by-2032. 2023. Accessed 31 Mar 2025.

130. Parikh RB, Helmchen LA. Paying for artificial intelligence in medicine. npj Digit Med. 2022;5:63.

131. Lobig F, Subramanian D, Blankenburg M, Sharma A, Variyar A, Butler O. To pay or not to pay for artificial intelligence applications in radiology. NPJ Digit Med. 2023;6(1):117.

132. MIT news. Explained: generative AI's environmental impact. 2025. Available from: https://news.mit.edu/2025/explained-generative-ai-environmental-impact-0117. Accessed 31 Mar 2025.

133. Heye T, Meyer MT, Merkle EM, Vosshenrich J. Turn it off! A simple method to save energy and CO_2 emissions in a hospital setting with focus on Radiology by monitoring nonproductive energy-consuming devices. Radiology. 2023;307(4):e230162.

134. Gross JS, Thiel CL. All specialties in radiology must address the climate crisis. Radiology. 2022;303(2):E24.

135. European Congress of Radiology. Available from: https://www.myesr.org/a-congress-with-a-conscience-ecr-2025-leads-the-way-in-sustainability-and-social-progress/. 2025. Accessed 31 Mar 2025.

136. Obermeyer Z, Biasotti F, Crum J, Mullachery J, Alvarez JM, Loo KH, et al. Explainable AI for bias in healthcare. Nat Med. 2019;25(1):138–46. https://doi.org/10.1038/s41591-018-0821-x.

137. Haque OS, Li H, Karhade S, Mandelblatt J, Monteleone M, Forman LP. Trust in artificial intelligence for healthcare. Nat Biomed Eng. 2020;4(5):369–77. https://doi.org/10.1038/s41551-020-0543-4.

138. Nasr-Esfahani E, Karimi-Mahabadi HA, Soroushmehr SM, Rezaei M. Deep learning for chest pathology detection: a comprehensive survey. J Med Imag Health Inform. 2018;10(7):1089–108. https://doi.org/10.1118/JMIH.18002.

139. Paiva SR, Nogueira RL, Amaro CO, Mendes RA, Santos TM, Paiva AC, Carvalho PC. The role of artificial intelligence in radiology. Eur J Radiol. 2020;130:109261. https://doi.org/10.1016/j.ejrad.2020.05.024.

140. McCall JB, Wolfson S, Mahmoodi M, Beane DB, Veeraraghavan S, Singh S. Artificial intelligence in radiology: a review of the literature and a call to action. Radiology. 2020;296(2):380–90. https://doi.org/10.1148/radiol.2020192277.

141. Egginton S, Jevon P, Metcalfe S. The impact of artificial intelligence in radiography. Radiography. 2020;26(4):380–5. https://doi.org/10.1016/j.radi.2020.03.002.

142. Ngiam YY, Klassen AL, Klassen JM, Wang Y. Can artificial intelligence reduce radiologist burnout? Am J Roentgenol. 2021;216(4):949–54. https://doi.org/10.2214/AJR.20.200776.

143. Fasterholdt I, Naghavi-Behzad M, Rasmussen BSB, et al. Value assessment of artificial intelligence in medical imaging: a scoping review. BMC Med Imaging. 2022;22:187. https://doi.org/10.1186/s12880-022-00918-y.

144. Lombi L, Rossero E. How artificial intelligence is reshaping the autonomy and boundary work of radiologists. A qualitative study. Sociol Health Illn. 2023;46(2):200–18. https://doi.org/10.1111/1467-9566.13702.

145. Joshi A, Wuttishapikul N, Fedrizzi M, Hsu J, Kuhn M, Rajpurkar A, et al. The state of healthcare artificial intelligence and machine learning. Nat Med. 2020;26(12):1805–17. https://doi.org/10.1038/s41591-020-01415-3.

146. Mittermaier M, Raza MM, Kvedar JC. Bias in AI-based models for medical applications: challenges and mitigation strategies. npj Digit Med. 2023;6:113.

147. Char DS, Shah NH, Magnus D. Implementing machine learning in health care—addressing ethical challenges. N Engl J Med. 2016;374(18):1744–8.

148. Li MD, Little BP. Appropriate reliance on artificial intelligence in radiology education. J Am Coll Radiol. 2023;20(11):1126–30.

Professor Christina Malamateniou is an associate professor of technology-enabled care in radiography and the director of the CRRAG research group at City St George's University of London. She had held many AI leadership positions at national and international level (EFRS, SCoR, ECR, EuSOMII). She is a well-published author with more than 100 papers in peer reviewed journals and 7 published national and international guidelines, including the first guidance on AI for radiographers, and has delivered more than 150 keynote lectures, 60 of them on AI, at a global audience. She has total research funding as PI and Co-I of more than £3.7mi and has supervised many master's and PhD students. She has been researching AI education, governance, implementation, leadership and the impact of AI on the profession of radiography and on professional identities. She has established the first AI course for radiographers since 2019, which was the inspiration for this textbook.

Dr. Amrita Kumar is a leading figure in healthcare AI implementation, named among 2023's Top 60 Influential Women in UK. As a nationally recognised clinician, she spearheads AI integration across five NHS hospital providers in Southeast England, conducting real-world trials in cancer pathways serving 6 million people. Her groundbreaking AI working group earned the 2024 NHS Parliamentary Award for establishing implementation and governance frameworks now adopted by multiple hospitals. Since 2022, she chairs the National AI & Innovation Special Interest Group at the British Institute of Radiology and serves as AI advisor to the Royal College of Radiologists and NHS England, shaping national healthcare AI strategy.

Professor Gerald Lip is the clinical director of Breast Screening in the North East of Scotland and is the Chief Investigator of the GEMINI project, a prospective evaluation of mammography AI in a UK population. He has published and researched in the field of AI with over 30 publications in the field. His most recent post is as the lead of Artificial Intelligence in the medical school of the University of Aberdeen continues his role in education of the next generation in this new and growing field.

Professor Robin Pierce is a Full Professor of AI and the Law at the University of Exeter. Her current research focuses on ethical, policy and regulatory approaches to the adoption and integration of digital technologies in health, medicine and the life sciences.

Dr. Yiannis Kyratsis, (PhD Imperial College London Business School) is Chair of Sustainable Healthcare and Workforce at Erasmus School of Health Policy and Management, Erasmus University Rotterdam. His research focuses on professional work, identity and role, the collaboration between professionals and AI, sustained innovation implementation, institutionalist accounts of organizational change. His research has been published in top management and medical journals, including *Academy of Management Journal, Academy of Management Perspectives,* and *Sociology of Health and Illness.* He has served as an associate editor in Academy of Management Perspectives, Health Care Management Review, BMC Public Health, Frontiers Digital Health, and Health Services Research

AI in Projectional Radiography

5

Ciara McNally, Clare Rainey, and Katy Szczepura

5.1   Introduction

Although many applications of AI in tasks associated with projectional radiography are in the early stages, there is steady growth in this field impacting different areas of the patient journey, some of which are demonstrated in Fig. 5.1.

Most AI-enabled applications in plain X-ray radiography currently relate to image interpretation, which would be relevant to both radiologists and reporting radiographers. These are the ones that have produced 80% of the scientific evidence base in this domain [1]. Other applications relating to operational aspects of X-ray radiography [2] are correct patient positioning (including completeness of anatomic coverage, correction of rotation and dynamic appraisal of

patient inspiration phase as in Fig. 5.2 [3]), protocol optimisation and automatic protocol retrieval (e.g. for adults, paediatric patients and bariatric patients) [4], image quality improvement (including contrast and resolution increase, reduction of motion artefacts and minimisation of image noise [2–7]), automatic image quality appraisal (for images from mobile X-ray units or erect ones) [8, 9], dose optimisation (including appropriate collimation, reduction of scatter radiation, reduction of recalls or repeat scans) [10–12], decision support (such as detection of lung cancer, pneumothorax, pneumonia, assessment of endotracheal tube positioning, as in Fig. 5.3, or establishing a breast cancer diagnosis) [1, 2, 13–17] and triage for workflow optimisation [2, 4, 18].

However, the usefulness of most of these applications on the patient journey, clinical outcomes and departmental workflows remains largely unexplored, lacking solid external evaluation data from prospective research studies led by clinical practitioners involved in the use of these products (in this case, radiographers). Some studies are still in the exploratory phase, without published academic outputs in peer-reviewed journals, with outputs submitted as preprints or as company promotional material. The true potential of this huge investment in AI-enabled technology in projectional radiography remains unverified while systematic prospective research is lacking. While this remains a

on behalf of Association of Healthcare Technology Providers for Imaging, Radiotherapy and Care (AXREM)

C. McNally (✉)
Diagnostic Radiography, University of Bradford, Bradford, UK
e-mail: c.mcnally@bradford.ac.uk

C. Rainey
Medical Imaging & Radiation Therapy, University of Cork, Cork, Ireland
e-mail: Clare.Rainey@ucc.ie

K. Szczepura
Medical Imaging Physics, University of Salford, Salford, UK
e-mail: k.szczepura@salford.ac.uk

© The Author(s), under exclusive license to Springer Nature Switzerland AG 2026
C. Malamateniou et al. (eds.), *Artificial Intelligence for Radiographers*,
https://doi.org/10.1007/978-3-032-05080-9_5

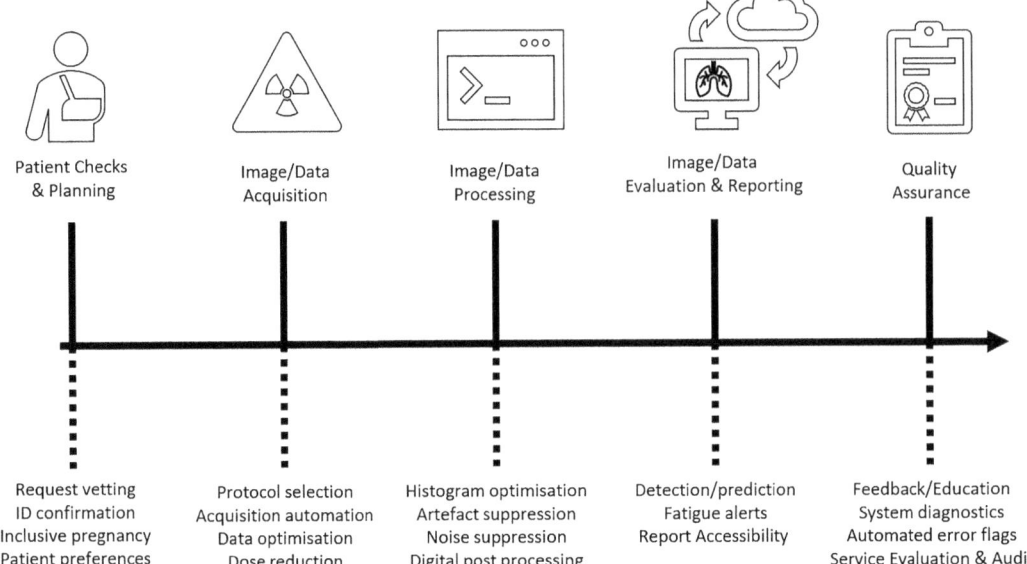

| Patient Checks & Planning | Image/Data Acquisition | Image/Data Processing | Image/Data Evaluation & Reporting | Quality Assurance |

Request vetting	Protocol selection	Histogram optimisation	Detection/prediction	Feedback/Education
ID confirmation	Acquisition automation	Artefact suppression	Fatigue alerts	System diagnostics
Inclusive pregnancy	Data optimisation	Noise suppression	Report Accessibility	Automated error flags
Patient preferences	Dose reduction	Digital post processing		Service Evaluation & Audit

Fig. 5.1 Opportunities and areas of impact of AI in the projectional radiography workflow. There are implications for AI implementation across the projectional radiography workflow. Benefits at the patient checks and planning stage include request vetting and confirmation of patient identification, pregnancy status and preferences. AI-facilitated optimisation of data acquisition and data processing can be achieved via protocol selection, acquisition automation, artefact suppression, noise suppression and post-processing whilst affording dose reduction. Data evaluation and reporting have been supported by bone fracture detection and lesion detection in recent years, with development in this area likely to advance as post-market surveillance of AI-assisted detection tools continues. There are opportunities for AI implementation in quality assurance tasks including system diagnostics, automated error flags and service evaluation and audit

challenge for the deployment of these tools in clinical practice, it also poses a great opportunity and a call for action for research radiographers and academic radiologists to create the necessary evidence base through well-planned and executed research projects in this field. Often the lack of robust data comes down to the lack of explainability of AI-enabled X-ray imaging and the need to preserve intellectual property or safeguard commercial innovation that prevents full-scale clinical studies or direct comparisons between different AI tools.

The clinical applications of AI in plain X-ray radiography relate mainly to projectional radiography of the chest and the musculoskeletal (MSK) system[1]. There is much less research and innovation reported in other clinical applications, where different imaging modalities might be more appropriate. When it comes to projectional radiography of the chest, there are many different AI-enabled products [19, 20] and clinical indications. For instance, in clinical practice, there are more than 120 AI products available, but most of the applications relate to triage, detection and diagnosis of lung cancer, assessment of viral pneumonia, establishing a COVID-19 diagnosis, pneumothorax, tuberculosis, heart health, cardiomegaly and other clinical conditions [21–25]. Similarly, in MSK imaging, AI applications mainly relate to trauma (e.g. fracture detection or classification), bone age estimation, grading or progression of osteoarthritis, differential diagnosis of bone and soft tissue tumours, and assessment, positioning, and long-

Provides instant guidance about three key factors for every PA chest X-ray exam

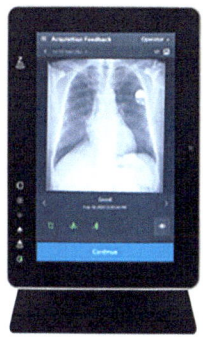
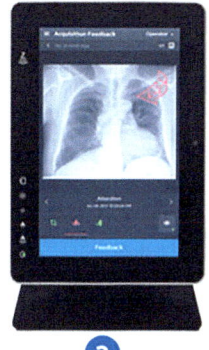
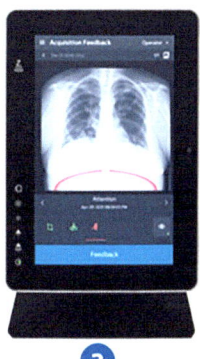

1 **2** **3**

Precise acquisition	Collimation	Rotation	Inhalation
Excellent result, with no adjustment required	Indicates that collimation is less than optimal.	Shows that adjustment in rotation was needed.	Calls out less-than-desirable breath-hold.

Individual statistics   **Acquisition dashboard**

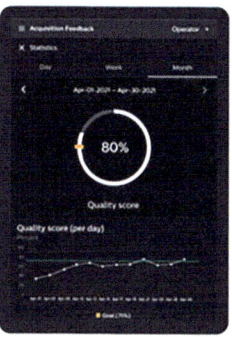

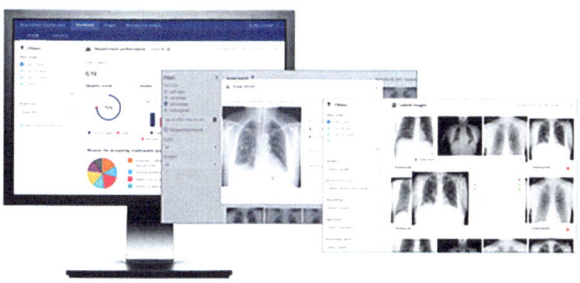

A department-level view with individual report generation provides administrators with valuable metrics to easily identify opportunities for improvement.

Individual acquisition data allows X-ray technologists to track their own statistics using the smart device so that they can very quickly see progress over time.

Fig. 5.2 Commercial AI tools available to assess and optimise collimation, rotation and inhalation (breathing) phase for the patient [3, 18]. (Image Credit: Koninklijke Philips N.V.)

term evaluation of orthopaedic implants [26–28] (Fig. 5.4). Many of these pathologies or conditions will require a diagnostic follow-up for further confirmation, such as computed tomography (CT) or magnetic resonance imaging (MRI), but the role of AI for triaging on projectional radiography cannot be underestimated. For more information on AI-enabled tools in CT and MRI,

please look further into Chaps. 6 and 7, respectively.

Mammography and breast imaging AI-enabled applications relate to either interpretative or non-interpretative tasks. For the former, AI has helped in triage, lesion detection, cancer diagnosis with increased sensitivity and specificity and monitoring of response to neoadjuvant therapy. For the

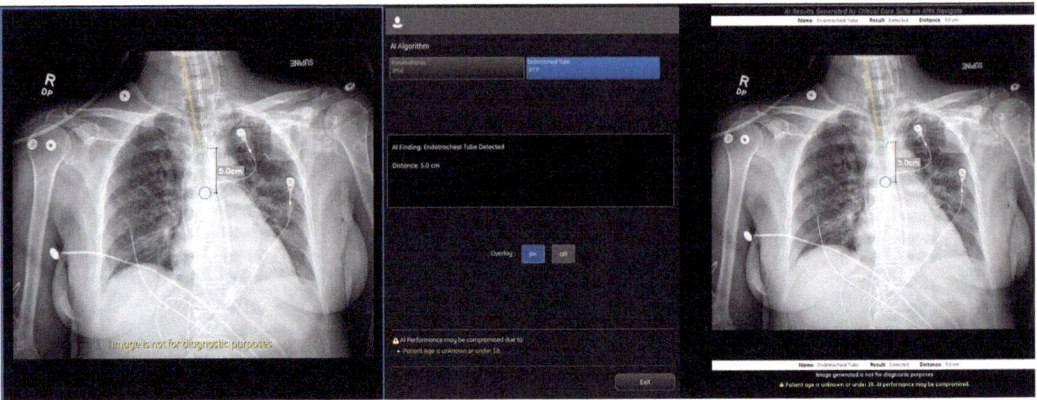

Fig. 5.3 Commercial AI-enabled software for assessment of endotracheal tube positioning [2, 4]

Clinical setting	Main clinical tasks	Imaging modalities	Examples from literature
Trauma	Fracture detection	Radiography/CT	Fractures around the hip [7], spine [8], multiple anatomic sites [9]
	Fracture classification	Radiography/CT	Fractures of the calcaneus [10], femur [11], humerus [12], spine [13], around the knee [14], and ankle [15]
	Detection of ligament or meniscal tears	MRI	Anterior cruciate ligament and meniscal tears [16]
Bone age	Bone age estimation	Radiography	BoneXpert [17] and VUNO Med-BoneAge [18] for hand radiographs
Osteoarthritis	Grading	Radiography	Grading of knee osteoarthritis [19]
	Cartilage lesion detection	MRI	Detection of knee cartilage lesions [20]
	Prediction of progression	Radiography	Progression of knee osteoarthritis [21]
Bone and soft-tissue tumors	Benign/malignant discrimination	Radiography/CT/MRI	Primary bone tumors [22]
	Grading	CT/MRI	Bone chondrosarcoma [23–25] and soft-tissue sarcomas [26]
	Prediction of outcomes (recurrence, survival, therapy response)	CT/MRI	Osteosarcoma [27–29] and soft-tissue sarcomas [30]
Orthopedic implants	Identification and classification	Radiography	Spinal hardware [31], knee [32] and shoulder [33] arthroplasty
	Implant positioning and measurements	Radiography	Acetabular component positioning after hip arthroplasty [34]
	Implant-related complications	Radiography/MRI	Knee or hip arthroplasty loosening [35]

Fig. 5.4 Overview of the AI-enabled clinical tasks in musculoskeletal imaging [26–28]

latter, AI has been involved in image acquisition optimisation, image quality assessment and enhancement, dose reduction, workflow triage, breast density quantification and cancer risk assessment [29–31]. The different AI-enabled tasks in breast imaging are both at different stages of digital maturity and at different phases of clinical availability to patients (Fig. 5.5). There are many factors responsible for the delay in the clinical implementation of these tools, such as the size of the resultant data from imaging, variation in breast positioning and compression related to patient body habitus and mammographer experience (despite standardisation of imaging techniques), variability of manufacturer specifications, and the quality and type of information provided in medical history [29]. Examples of different AI-enabled accredited products for breast imag-

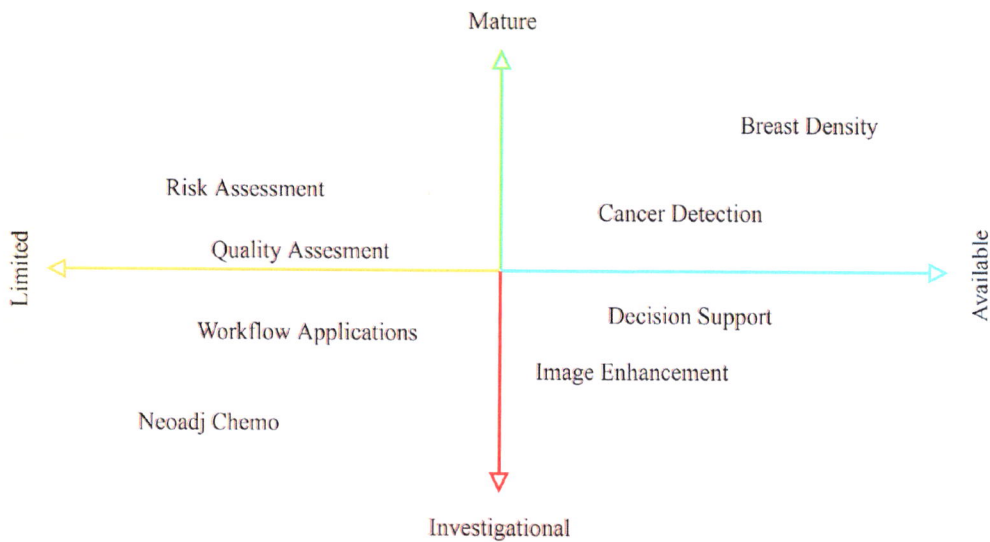

Mature

Breast Density

Risk Assessment

Cancer Detection

Limited   Quality Assesment   Available

Workflow Applications   Decision Support

Image Enhancement

Neoadj Chemo

Investigational

Fig. 5.5 Visual representation of maturity and availability of different AI applications for breast imaging [29]

ing can be seen in Fig. 5.6, organised by vendor, country of origin and imaging modality where they are used, the majority in mammography.

It is important to note that, while most of these AI-enabled tools in projectional imaging have the necessary approvals by the relevant regulatory bodies (please see Chaps. 4 and 13 for the regulation required before AI products for medical use are put on the market), there are still some products that are actively seeking accreditation for clinical use.

Radiographers are accustomed to using technology in the care of their patient; however, it is important to approach new technologies with a critical awareness of their own knowledge of the tools in use to ensure responsible engagement. This chapter aims to equip you with the knowl-

edge and skills required to oversee semi-automated AI-driven processes in projectional radiography, exploring the associated opportunities, challenges and barriers, from patient checks and planning through to image acquisition, processing, reporting and quality assurance.

The effective implementation of AI-assisted modification and automation of tasks in projectional radiography involves a multitude of considerations, which we have consolidated into one workstream following the patient journey. This will be contextualised and illustrated with case studies throughout the chapter. However, before we can explore these fully, we must first review the background to the nature of diagnostic imaging in projectional radiography in the digital age.

Product Name	Vendor	Country of Origin	Modality
Cancer Detection			
cmAssist®	CureMetrix	United States	Mammography
Genius AI™ Detection	Hologic®, Inc.	United States	Mammography and Tomosynthesis
Lunit INSIGHT MMG	Lunit	South Korea	Mammography
MammoScreen® 2.0	Therapixel	France	Mammography and Tomosynthesis
ProFound AI®	iCAD, Inc.	United States	Mammography and Tomosynthesis
Saige-Dx™	DeepHealth, Inc.	United States	Mammography
Transpara®	ScreenPoint Medical B.V.	Netherlands	Mammography and Tomosynthesis
Decision Support			
Koios DS™ Breast	Koios™ Medical, Inc.	United States	Ultrasound
QuantX™	Qlarity Imaging	United States	MRI
Density Quantification			
cmDensity™	CureMetrix, Inc.	United States	Mammography
IntelliMammo™ densityai™	Densitas®	Canada	Mammography
PowerLook® Density Assessment	iCAD, Inc.	United States	Mammography
Quantra™ 2.2	Hologic®, Inc.	United States	Mammography and Tomosynthesis
Saige-Density™	DeepHealth, Inc.	United States	Mammography and Tomosynthesis
Syngo.BreastCare	Siemens®	Germany	Mammography
Visage Breast Density	Visage Imaging, Inc.®	United States	Mammography
Volpara TruDensity®	Volpara Imaging	New Zealand	Mammography
WRDensity	Whiterabbit.ai	United States	Mammography
Triage			
cmTriage®	CureMetrix, Inc.	United States	Mammography
HealthMammo	Zebra Medical Vision	Israel	Mammography
Saige-Q™	DeepHealth, Inc.	United States	Mammography and Tomosynthesis
Syngo.BreastCare	Siemens®	Germany	Mammography

Fig. 5.6 Examples of different AI-enabled accredited products for breast imaging, organised by vendor, country of origin and imaging modality [29]

5.2 Nature of Diagnostic Imaging in the Digital Age

Before the introduction of digital radiography, film/screen technology served as the primary image receptor in projectional radiography. Image quality at that time was determined predominantly by the selection of exposure parameters and the response of the narrow latitude of the film to the exposure, known as 'speed'. There was a direct correlation between exposure and contrast, with suboptimal selection of exposure factors potentially resulting in unacceptable image quality and repeated imaging.

The introduction of computed radiography and digital image receptors altered this dependence by permitting some leniency in the acceptable exposure parameters with a wider exposure latitude than film/screen radiography [32, 33]. This is accomplished, in part, by the processing and post-processing technology available in digital radiography systems.

We are now aware that this led to additional problems, over time, where the increased image quality from increased exposure has been desirable, leading to an incremental increase in overall population dose. This is commonly known as 'dose creep' [34]. The understanding of the technology used in these systems may help mitigate against undesirable outcomes and allow the user to maximise the benefits of these systems and their impact on clinical practice, while mitigating associated risks.

There are several key processes involved in the production of the digital radiographic image, such as, automatic digitisation, signal sampling and computer processing. When X-rays are detected, an analogue electronic signal is generated. This can happen either indirectly via scintillation or directly through electron-hole pair production. The computer's bit depth plays a crucial role in sampling and digitising this analogue signal. As bit depth increases, grey scale also increases, therefore resulting in improved contrast resolution. Exposure field recognition and image histogram optimisation then determine the dynamic range and radiographic contrast [35].

With the increasing computer processing power and capabilities in medical imaging, digital image quality is improving, due in part to increased bit depth potential. Even minor variations in differential absorption, due to anatomical attenuation coefficients, are accounted for. This results in an enhanced detection power and an improved diagnostic display of anatomical information, almost irrespective of the input signal value. Consequently, issues such as overexposure, underexposure and over-penetration have become less significant in terms of image appearance [35].

While digital processing enhances the diagnostic appearance of images, a critical issue arises with the disconnect between exposure factors and data processing optimisation. As mentioned, this gap necessitates vigilance among radiographers to avoid the phenomenon known as 'dose creep'. Consequently, within this chapter, the term 'image optimisation' has been replaced with 'data optimisation' to better reflect the additional nuances, complexities, and challenges inherent in data-generating tasks. This change acknowledges that data manipulation often lacks transparency, making it crucial for professionals to remain attentive to these subtleties.

The subsequent chapter sections will follow the impact of AI and advanced technology-enabled innovations along the patient journey in relation to projectional radiography.

5.3 The Patient Journey

5.3.1 Patient Pre-scan Checks & Patient-Centred Planning

There are conflicting views on the impact of AI assistance in radiology on 'person-centred' care, with some suggesting that, while AI can help improve operational efficiencies and enable more 'time to care', others note that the use of AI may detract from the patient-healthcare professional relationship. However, patients may be comfortable with the use of automation in certain tasks to achieve an optimised, holistic and bespoke approach to service provision [36]. More insights into this topic can be found in Chap. 12 of this textbook.

Assistance with administrative tasks may be an area in which AI can prove beneficial to both the radiographer and the patient. The use of AI for this task is still in a very early stage, and many of the examples described here remain at the lab-based stage of development. For instance, authorisation of diagnostic imaging referrals via machine learning could permit the analysis of text data from patient databases and radiology information systems to verify the appropriateness of the requested modality, projection and transport mode based on clinical indications. Automatic verification of patient identification, assessment of needs and implementation of support may allow for increased efficiencies and standardisation of care for diverse patient populations [37, 38]. For example, the preferred pronouns for members of the LGBTQ+ community and other crucial aspects of patient individuality may be safely documented and integrated at the planning stage, providing the radiographer with the relevant and correct information to be in position to offer a truly person-centred imaging experience. This, if materialised, could help streamline equality, diversity and inclusion pipelines and increase accessibility within the radiology department.

AI may also be able to play a role in supporting patients living with dementia by documenting specific needs and allowing this information to be used to provide a clinical environment best suited to the patients' individual needs [39]. Other proposed benefits for the use of AI and advanced technologies in the care of patients with dementia include the minimisation of clinician subjectivity in diagnosis, assistance with the differentiation of types of dementia and upskilling the workforce in dementia awareness. That said, when considering the patient-facing aspects of the use of technology in this population, literature is divided, with studies suggesting that there may be differences in acceptance of AI in relation to the progression and stage of the patient's condition [40, 41]. Further up-to-date and 'live'

research is needed in this area to ensure that any technology used meets the needs of patients and carers, as well as of the clinical practitioners.

Additionally, AI systems can facilitate communication for individuals requiring translation services, ensuring that language barriers do not impede the delivery of high-quality care. Medical interpretation and translation enabled by natural language processing (NLP) solutions could alleviate language barriers to care in multilingual societies at the planning stage, providing real-time, automated and interactive communication to promote care equity and accessibility. NLP-assisted interpretation enables human connection, eases navigation of challenging discussions such as pregnancy status, enables cultural sensitivity and captures nuances in dialogues that may aid effective planning and ethical attainment of informed consent [42]. The most vulnerable patients, such as those with cognitive impairments, language barriers, cultural differences or other additional needs, are particularly at risk of experiencing breaches in confidentiality and compromised patient safety due to poor translation practices. AI-driven solutions can safeguard these patients by ensuring accurate, timely and confidential communication. For instance, AI can automatically translate medical information into the patient's preferred language, ensuring they fully understand their diagnosis and treatment options. This not only promotes patient safety but also empowers patients to make informed decisions about their care [43]. Moreover, AI could identify and flag any specific requirements needed for vulnerable patients, such as those with mobility issues or modifications to clinical interaction due to sensory preferences or requirements. By integrating this information into the planning and delivery of care, healthcare providers can ensure that patients receive the appropriate support and resources, thereby enhancing their overall care experience.

In recent years healthcare applications have emerged aiming to collect and analyse biometric data and encourage patient collaboration in their own healthcare journey. Healthcare applications in the future are likely to be consolidated into one patient-fronted application, or electronic health

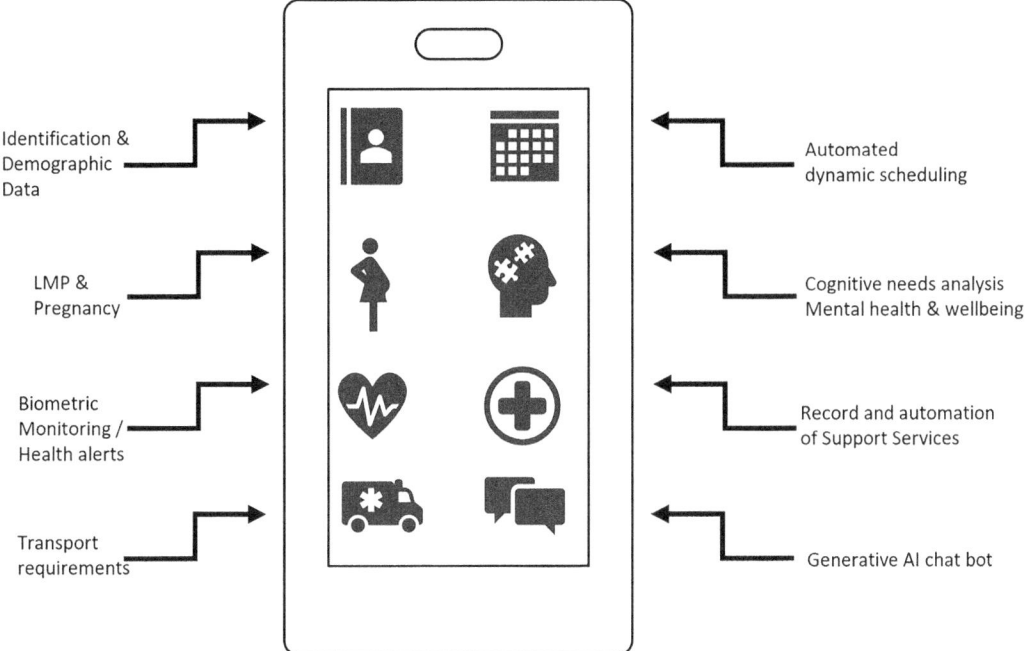

Fig. 5.7 Illustration of an AI-led healthcare portal for personalisation and engagement as a mobile application design. Monitoring and recording of biometric data may facilitate health alerts and personalisation in terms of transport requirements, scheduling and holistic needs analysis. A generative AI chat bot trained in cognitive-behavioural therapies and talking therapies may offer on-demand mental health and well-being support, or answer patient queries regarding diagnostic examinations to help alleviate anxiety

portal, enabling a 'one-stop-shop' for healthcare personalisation (Fig. 5.7).

The capability of AI to assimilate and automate decision-making from patient-specific data permits individualisation. However, on a wider scale, the monitoring of physiological metrics and the deconvolution of complex risk factors, due to advances in population big data analysis, should better enable predictive and preventative care. Indeed, the use of AI in assimilation and processing of multiple health care data from different sources may allow more precise care. This is known as multi-omics, where quantitative data is gathered from multiple data sources, including but not limited to histopathology, genomics and radiographic images ('radiomics') as well as other clinical data. These data are processed to arrive at an outcome, such as diagnosis, prognosis or patient pathway recommendation [44]. Furthermore, in preventative medicine, genomic screening programmes where anatomical, functional and molecular biomarkers for disease can

be used to personalise disease prediction and may be used to support the instigation of pre-emptive diagnostic tests in the future. For more information on big date integration into another modality (radiotherapy), refer to Chap. 11.

5.3.2 Workflow Management and Optimisation

Artificial and automated computing technologies not only benefit the patient as an individual but can have broader applications in wider operational planning, for instance in capacity management and waiting list prioritisation (see Case Study 5.1). Enhancement of diagnostic reproducibility is possible by minimising operator-dependent discrepancies and mechanisation of repetitive tasks, therefore potentially minimising the risk of human error [45, 46]. There is an opportunity for AI optimisation of human resources through shift and workload management based on skill mix, cultural differences and personal preferences, leading to improved work-life balance, which may positively impact recruitment and retention in the workforce.

Some aspects of AI-enabled person-centred care and operational efficiency savings are inevitably automated, but the radiographer is required to quality check data input and validate the AI output. However, it is imperative that radiographers do not become digitally complacent by over-relying on AI tools. Consequently, clinical decision-making is likely to remain radiographer-led, with AI assistive technologies employed as a supporting tool.

Case Study 5.1: Patients Checks & Planning—GE Clinical Command Centre

The clinical challenge: The complex, multi-step patient journey has conventionally been fraught with bottlenecks that are challenging to identify and alleviate.

The AI-enabled solution: The GE Clinical Command Centre is a customisable data analysis software used to improve patient flow and optimise hospital processes [47].

Benefits: Utilisation of AI software may optimise accessibility and efficiency as well as streamline patient flow by digitising the individual patient journey and adopting targeted process improvement software to enable real-time actionable informatics, capacity analytics and workflow prioritisation. For example, imaging referrals for the same patient scheduled on alternate dates may be identified and consolidated, minimising the risk of non-attendance, confusion and inconvenience to the patient in terms of costs, transportation and time. Visualisation and consolidation of information support standardisation of processes across integrated care boards. Data modelling predicts and pre-empts areas of risk such as breaches, patient deterioration, and capacity issues [48]. Discrete event

simulation modelling permits safe evaluation of targeted performance improvement projects, utilising a digital patient population representative of the community, therefore permitting evaluation and adjustments of a service-improvement before implementation.

Diagnostic radiographers are key stakeholders in every patient pathway and are therefore instrumental in leading on a technology assisted culture of collaborative decision-making. The GE Clinical Command Centre supports this vision by narrowing the communication gap between the imaging department, referrers and hospital wards.

Challenges: This, and other functionalities, can be tailored to the bespoke requirements of the service. However, there are barriers to the implementation of such systems, including limitations in infrastructure and integration compatibility, radiographer personal and psychological barriers to technology adoption and a lack of education and training [49].

5.3.3 Image Data Acquisition

When considering image, or data optimisation, AI implementation offers numerous opportunities to enhance patient care and reduce the cognitive burden on radiographers. Currently, radiographers are tasked with selecting and verifying protocols and projections based on patient presentation, individual characteristics and clinical questions. Traditional machine learning (ML) has been shown to assist in the automation of some tasks; however, the advent of deep learning (DL), a subset of ML, has increased the scope and capability of AI to accomplish more complex tasks [50].

In image acquisition, automation may assist with the standardisation of practice, promoting consistency across clinical centres. Variations in operational tasks like patient positioning or exposure factor selection may also highlight suboptimal practice and may, therefore, be utilised as a learning tool for technique improvement [3, 8, 51]. Figure 5.2 outlines some AI-enabled products by Philips Healthcare used to standardise image acquisition in projectional chest radiography. Consistency in image production is crucial both for the patient experience and for the optimal usefulness of the image data beyond individual patient care, such as in research or construction of datasets for further AI training. Case Study 5.2 below describes the use of AI in the optimisation of imaging data acquisition in projectional imaging through AI-enabled noise suppression and scatter correction.

The implementation of technical parameter suggestion and the automation of acquisition could impact various aspects of the image acquisition process. For instance, exposure parameters such as kVp (kilovolt peak), mAs (milliampere-seconds), focal spot size, target and filter material options can be predetermined based on patient demographics and examination requirements to optimise data quality, image quality and dose. Currently, parameters for 'average patients' often require manual adjustments for individual cases, and the lack of standardisation in exposure factor optimisation contributes to the 'dose creep' phenomenon. DL analysis of biometric data could ultimately allow for individualised exposure and dose optimisation in a way that is reproducible and evidence based. Most large manufacturers have created platforms that consider individual patient body habitus. Siemens Healthineers has developed a system which integrates a 3D camera in the examination room, which, along with an AI-based thorax detection algorithm, can calculate collimation and imaging parameters without the patient getting undressed [45] (Fig. 5.8).

Selecting, calibrating and activating the most appropriate detector for each examination and projection will reduce risks and errors. Complementary visual and auditory indications of the active detector can help reduce human error-based clinical incidents, such as exposures occurring when the image receptor is inactive or misaligned. Automatic alignment and centring of the central ray to the image receptor at the opti-

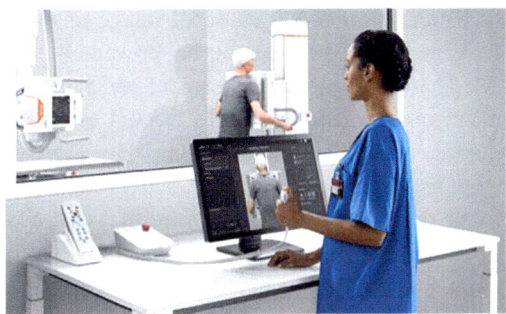

Fig. 5.8 A commercially developed AI-based thorax detection algorithm, which can calculate collimation and imaging parameters without the patient getting undressed [10–12]. (Image courtesy of Siemens Healthineers – LUMINOS Q.namix T)

mal source-to-detector distance (SDD) and in the correct orientation for the examination and projection could increase accuracy and reduce errors. Auto-tracking functionalities could further simplify image acquisition in remote environments by indicating the SDD to the operator. Future developments may include recognising body morphology to ensure accurate alignment of the patient, active detector and X-ray tube [52].

Automatic registration of detector size and collimation to the predicted size and shape of the desired anatomical region helps eliminate unnecessary irradiation and scatter generation, thereby improving image quality and reducing dose [53]. Mechanised selection and positioning of the most appropriate anti-scatter grid for each examination and projection, such as using an anti-scatter grid focused at 180 cm in the wall stand for an erect postero-anterior chest projection, result in physical noise reduction and an improved contrast-to-noise ratio (CNR) [54].

Scatter correction software enhances image quality by modelling the noise within the image and subtracting it, mimicking the effect of a physical grid [55]. This allows for a lower mAs to be used compared to a conventional grid, reducing patient dose. Additionally, it improves workflow by eliminating the need for manual handling of grids, reducing the risk of misalignment and artifacts, and enhancing efficiency by streamlining the imaging process, particularly in bedside or remote environments.

Patient motion is a cause of image unsharpness and one that cannot be prevented with AI. Therefore, patient assessment and radiographer communication is still essential to reduce motion artefacts from occurring. However, AI systems can detect if there is patient motion prior to, or during, acquisition, alerting the radiographer to this. It may also evaluate the extent of motion blur during acquisition and make a recommendation as to the diagnostic quality of the image and the need for repeated acquisition [56, 57]. This may reduce the need for patient recalls or repeat imaging if blurring is only identified during reporting, such as in mammography. Cost savings in terms of time and resources may be achieved and patient recalls for repeat diagnostic examinations could be mitigated.

Not only could AI-enabled acquisition promote a safety culture, but operator inclusion may be further supported via technology-enabled accessibility design features which are intuitive, flexible and customisable. For example, acquisition interfaces that support voice and command recognition to automate physical tasks could widen access to the profession. By enabling representation and rendering complex cognitive and physically demanding tasks obsolete at the acquisition stage, more time may be available for the radiographer to balance person-centred care and diagnostic throughput to meet service demand. That said, care should be taken to ensure that the automation of repetitive tasks does not mean that the potential increased patient throughput results in diminished care and unrealistic expectations on current staffing [58]. Central to this responsibility is the role of the radiographer in communicating AI-driven semi-automated processes to the patient when obtaining informed consent. Herein lies the true value of the human in the loop, in establishing a patient-practitioner relationship to demystify the human-machine interface for patients. There is therefore an onus placed on the radiographer to be able to understand and communicate the role and basic function of the technology used to both patients and other healthcare professionals, as applicable in each patient journey [59].

The advantages of automated image acquisition depend on correct protocol selection, as the automation is determined by the examination protocol selection. Although protocol selection may itself be automatic, the radiographer should ensure appropriate selection of all automated acquisition variables. Vigilance and careful oversight of AI-automated and augmented image acquisition could become an essential responsibility of the radiographer to ensure that optimal diagnostic image quality at minimal radiation dose is achieved [60]. As image acquisition is synonymous with data acquisition, errors at any aspect of the image acquisition stage result in inaccuracies in input data and ultimately suboptimal data processing and image display [61].

It is also important to recognise that any changes made by the radiographer that modify or deviate from the automated processes may be recorded and used to further train the AI system, if this is permitted and desirable. It is therefore essential that any changes are made with clear reasoning and justification of the adaptation and with appropriate governance in place.

Case Study 5.2: Noise Suppression & Scatter Correction AI-Enabled Algorithms
Clinical challenge: When X-ray photons are incident with an object, they interact with matter. Some X-ray photons are transmitted, some are absorbed, and some X-ray photons are scattered. Scattered photons may be detected at the image receptor. These photons do not contribute to useful information on the resultant image, instead, causing 'noise', which leads to contrast degradation and a reduction in image quality. X-ray scatter appears as a 'grey fog' of signal superimposed over anatomical structures resulting in a reduced contrast-to-noise ratio (CNR). High CNR is a key quantitative quality metric in projectional radiography modalities such as mammography and digital radiography. Conventionally, noise is reduced and CNR

(continued)

improved by preventing scattered photons from reaching the image receptor using an anti-scatter grid [62, 63]. The detected signal therefore contains a higher proportion of X-ray photons that have been transmitted and attenuated by anatomical structures of different thickness and density, therefore contributing useful information on the resultant images, resulting in reduced 'noise' and improved contrast resolution. In the context of mobile radiography, a stationary grid may be required for examinations of large anatomical regions. If an anti-scatter grid is stationary during the exposure, for example, during mobile radiography, there is risk of gridline artefact appearing as regularly distributed periodic signal loss on the radiographic image.

AI-enabled solution: Ease of workflow is achieved, and gridline artefacts are avoided through the replacement of the conventional anti-scatter grid with noise suppression AI algorithms in digital imaging systems [55]. Rather than removing scattered photons from the primary beam, noise reduction AI algorithms use software-based correction to estimate noise signal due to scattered photons and correct for scatter radiation effects during image processing, achieving comparable image quality [64]. Carestream's 'Smart Noise Cancellation' software uses convolutional neural networks (a deep learning system and type of 'computer vision') to predict the level of noise present on any image based on prior 'learning' from large image datasets with known noise levels. The system then subtracts the noise it has predicted from the image, leaving the useful image data for interpretation [65]. It is important to remember that in practice, X-ray scatter still contributes to signal in the image histogram. Scatter reduction AI-enabled calculations correct for image deterioration by mimicking the function of a physical anti-scatter grid via scatter estimation and grid effect determination, leading to contrast improvement.

Benefits: Noise reduction processing leads to improvement in image quality by identifying and reducing the component of unstructured noise in the detected signal. Scatter estimation and correction methods include threshold-based 'time-of-flight' scatter rejection, which relies on the additional time taken for scattered photons to reach the detector from the source, and although not 'true AI', uses complex mathematical models to allow removal of non-useful photons and improves overall image quality [62].

Challenge: This method may not always effectively differentiate between scattered photons and diagnostic photons; therefore, further computational methods are required. Iterative deconvolution of the measured point-spread function at each pixel during acquisition allows the magnitude and shape of the scatter contribution to be estimated, permitting improved mitigation of scatter on radiographic images. In practice, the benefits of improved granularity and edge enhancement capabilities of the software can be exploited in conjunction with the physical scatter removal benefits afforded by its integration with anti-scatter hardware.

Computational models estimate scatter distribution and subtract it from the acquired radiographic image and are a viable alternative to anti-scatter grids, particularly during mobile radiography examinations. Benefits include dose reduction potential, improved contrast resolution and workflow efficiency. Radiographers should be mindful of the risk of software overcorrection and validity across diverse patient populations and clinical examinations and be aware of a gap in evidence-based guidelines for the use of scatter correction algorithms [66]. Future developments may include machine learning mod-

(continued)

els trained on large datasets to predict and correct scatter more accurately, with AI-driven noise suppression demonstrating potential in the preservation of diagnostic signal by more effectively differentiating scatter [66].

5.3.4 Image Data Processing

As stated previously, there is some disconnect between image quality and exposure factors, and image processing is an important factor in determining resultant image quality. Image processing can manipulate data that is on the threshold of acceptability and convert it into a diagnostically acceptable image.

Although this data manipulation can reduce the need for repeated imaging, there is a risk that poor-quality data can be converted into seemingly acceptable images, or that inappropriate processing may be applied, causing the data to be displayed sub-optimally. There is no 'right' processing; it is dependent on many factors, with consideration of technical and clinical task-based requirements to guide the most appropriate design and selection [67].

On occasion, images are considered 'poor' due to the processing rather than the acquisition, and it is important to consider this before repeating the examination. By analysing and converting the 'raw' data, AI processes can ensure that appropriate, reproducible processing is undertaken, indicating where images are of poor quality, and adapt processing to ensure optimisation

[56]. AI can also be utilised to undertake continuous improvements and ensure these improvements are implemented without interruption of workflow.

5.3.4.1 Image Pre-processing

Histograms are a way of demonstrating the range and frequency of pixel values within an image and are an essential part of automated image processing and optimisation (Fig. 5.9).

Histograms are a frequency analysis of pixel values and have no spatial information about the image. The images below will have the same histogram, as there are the same number of grey and white pixels (Fig. 5.10).

Whereas postprocessing can mask poor image acquisition, histogram analysis can identify issues with image acquisition and data quality, which AI processes can learn from and adapt image acquisition parameters to optimise the data (Fig. 5.11). Automatic rescaling is where the raw histogram is processed to optimise the image based on the signal received. This means that the image quality is independent of the exposure, but only if the signal is within the dynamic range of the system. This is automatically achieved by comparing the data to an expected histogram based on the selected protocol. Values of interest (VOIs) from the raw data histogram are selected to be displayed in the final image, ensuring an optimised display of the required anatomy in terms of contrast resolution.

Bit depths accessible in modern digital radiography systems mean that even small differences in inherent contrast can be detected, and AI can adapt to different areas within the matrix and

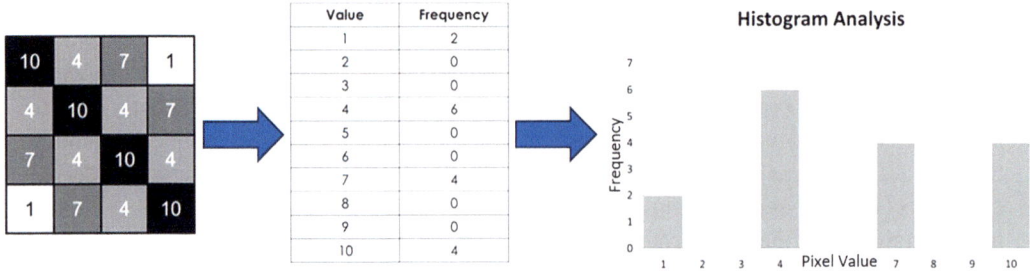

Fig. 5.9 An example of how a histogram is created—a frequency analysis of the pixel values as a bar chart

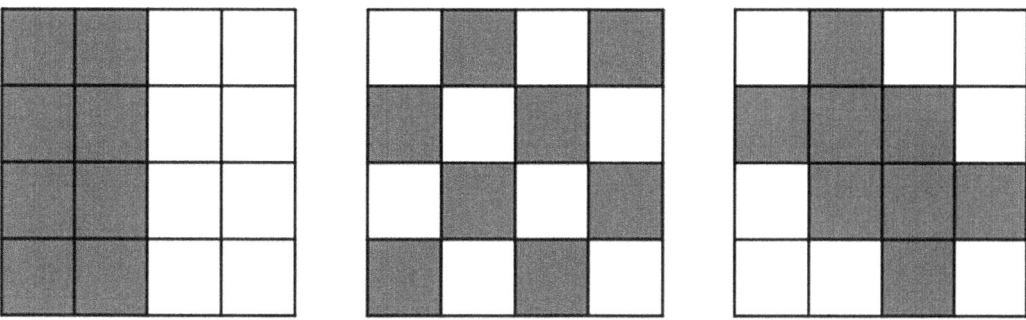

Fig. 5.10 Example of images with the same histogram—histograms have no spatial information

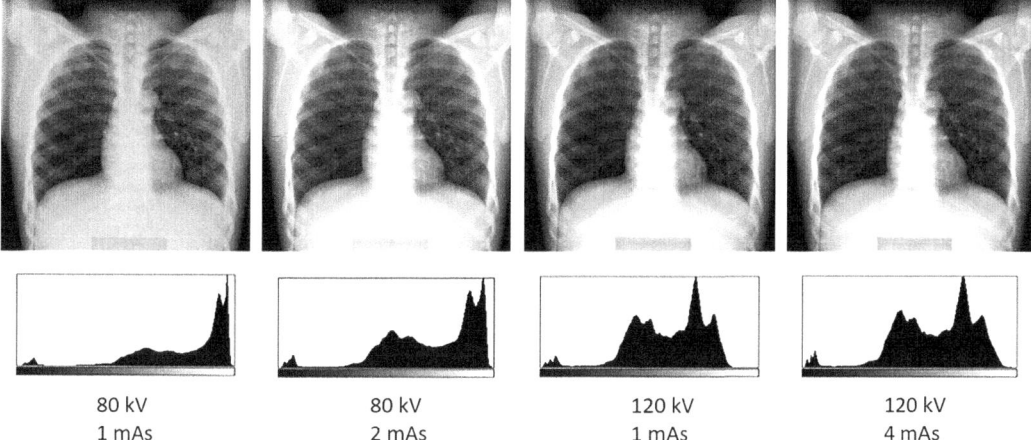

| 80 kV | 80 kV | 120 kV | 120 kV |
| 1 mAs | 2 mAs | 1 mAs | 4 mAs |

Fig. 5.11 Histograms of phantom images taken at different exposure factors on a 16-bit imaging system

optimise them based on the signal received. For example, chest radiographs and mammograms have wide latitudes, with clinically relevant information across the histogram due to the wide differences of tissues within the field of view. Multiscale processing can analyse both spatial and contrast data in multiple ranges across the histogram to ensure non-linear contrast enhancement of all signals of interest within the image automatically.

Windowing is then used to display the appropriate grey levels within the image and adapt the contrast of the image. Although this can be adapted in real time, the optimal window settings are chosen based on the histogram and protocol selection (Fig. 5.12).

As mentioned, noise is non-useful data that obscures the diagnostic signal [68]. Noise reduction has always been an important part of digital image processing, as, although contrast and brightness are controlled through windowing and are no longer limited by latitude and bit depth, noise is still limiting in terms of image quality. Traditionally noise data could not be separated from true anatomical data, and so noise reduction techniques would impact on the whole image, often decreasing spatial or contrast resolution. As explored in Case Study 5.2, advanced noise reduction techniques utilise AI processes by identifying and segmenting true data from noise and supressing noise without impacting on spatial or contrast resolution (Fig. 5.13). It is worth noting that noise preference is subjective and often utilised in diagnostic tasks, so AI systems can adapt how much noise suppression there is within the processed image, dependent on the observer preferences.

Spatial resolution is another important factor when considering pre-processing and image

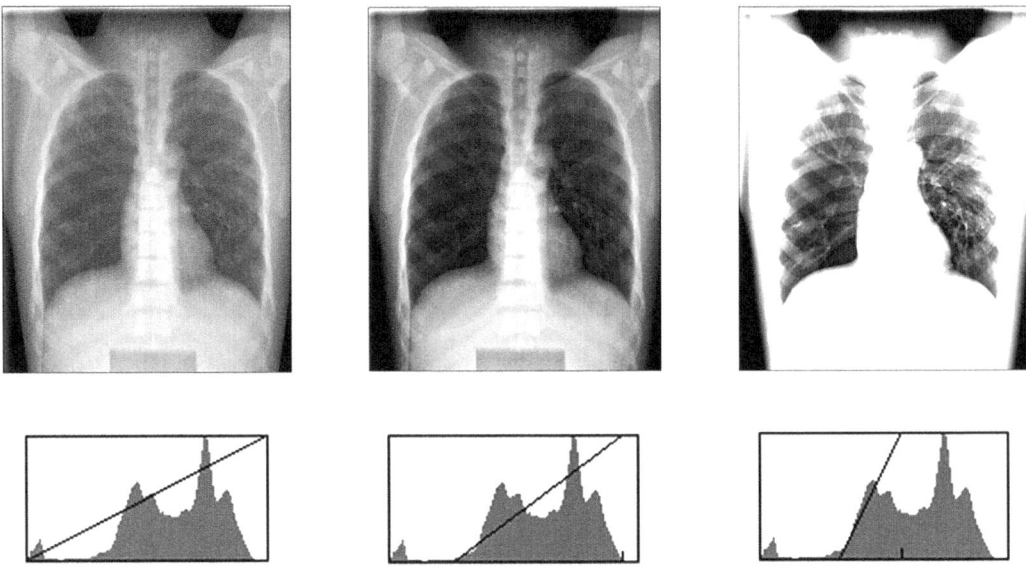

Fig. 5.12 Windowing changes the contrast in the image, whilst the histogram data remains the same

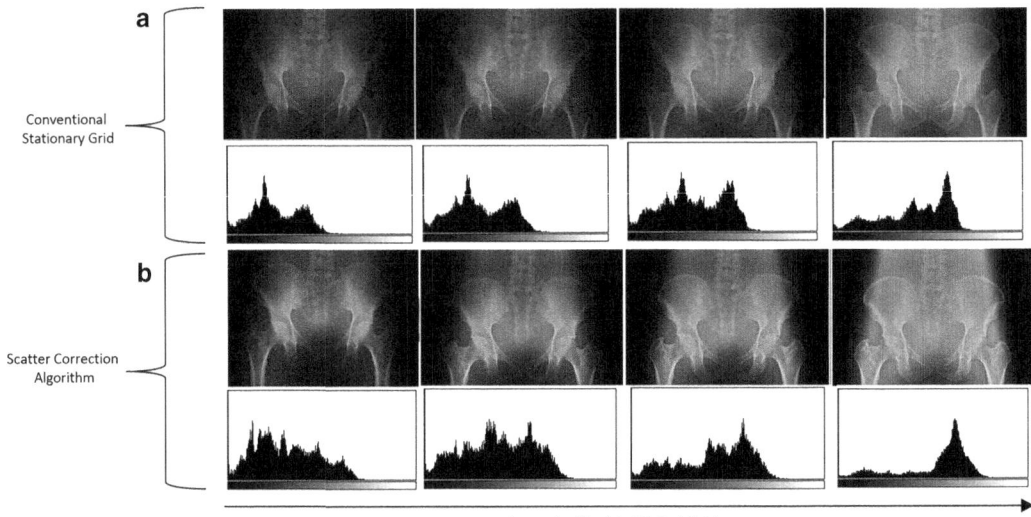

Increasing Simulated Patient Thickness

Fig. 5.13 Illustrative example of AP Pelvis phantom images and associated histograms acquired with (**a**) conventional stationary grid and (**b**) noise reduction AI algorithm. Scatter suppression is comparable to physical removal of scatter by grid devices for standard thickness and distribution of soft tissue. As soft tissue thickness increases, noise reduction algorithms may underperform. It is important to note that on implementation of noise reduction algorithms scatter photons are still detected as evident in the image histograms, which may hinder exposure field recognition and therefore histogram optimisation

quality and may limit the capability of the system to resolve small objects in the image. The smaller the pixel size and the larger the matrix size, the better the spatial resolution of the resultant image; however, traditionally, the smaller the pixels, the less photon quanta available for each pixel, leading to a reduced signal-to-noise ratio (SNR). Previously, this impacted the resultant image quality; however, with AI image processing techniques and increasing bit depths, images can be processed based on the signal received, utilising all signals to ensure optimisation of the data. This means that images can demonstrate significantly higher spatial resolution without impacting on signal or contrast within the image.

5.3.4.2 Image Post-processing

Having considered the functionality of computer-assisted data pre-processing, we must now explore the impact of data post-processing software on image display to guide effective engagement with these tools [69]. Digital annotations permit radiographers to convey examination-specific information which may aid interpretation. However, this functionality has prompted a shift in digital radiography practice from the use of radiopaque anatomical side markers in the primary radiation field to the post-acquisition application of digital anatomical side markers [70, 71]. Furthermore, digital 'cropping' of radiographs post-exposure has become routine to best emulate 'a textbook image' [72]. Such examples of the inappropriate utilisation of digital imaging technologies illustrate the phenomenon of 'digital complacency', where over-reliance on post-processing tools compromises diagnostic quality and patient safety and may lead to an eventual deskilling of the workforce. Although post processing digital side marker functionality is useful in circumstances where patient condition or examination complexity may render radiopaque anatomical side marker placement impossible, it is responsible and preferred practice for the radiographer to situate a physical anatomical side marker within the primary beam. This may avoid potential errors and is, therefore, a recommendation of professional bodies [73].

Post-acquisition autocropping to the region of interest involves identification of pixel intensities attributed to radiographic anatomy and subsequent automatic rescaling of the field of view to the region of interest. Autocropping maximises the anatomical region demonstrated through full-screen visualisation. Field-of-view optimisation via autocropping processing is dependent on collimation accuracy.

Clinical question-dependent presets are a valuable tool for diagnostic radiographers and clinicians such as in the characterisation of foreign bodies or chest line positioning. Evaluation of the position of common lines and tubes such as central venous catheters, nasogastric (NG) and endotracheal tubes (ETT) (see AI-enabled solution described in Fig. 5.3) using enhanced image highlight processing facilitates earlier identification of poor positioning and mitigation of complications [74].

By limiting anatomical detail and applying additional edge enhancement, visualisation of lines and tubes is readily achieved (Fig. 5.3). Deep convolutional neural network (DCNN)-based algorithms perform well in the localisation of common lines and tubes but rely on accurate ground-truth labelling at the point of training and may not be robust in the identification of uncommon devices, which may be under-represented in training datasets [75]. Confounding patient and image characteristics such as excessive noise, rotation, lordosis, or kyphosis must also be considered, as demonstrated in Case Study 5.3.

5.3.5 Data Analysis, Image Evaluation, and Reporting

The post-processing functionalities described facilitate image quality assessment, interpretation, and clinical decision-making. Adjustments to window level and window width can enhance the visualisation of subtle details, while magnification of anatomical regions allows for detailed inspection of pixel values.

Prior to exploring AI-enabled solutions for image evaluation, it is imperative to consider the human-AI interface at this critical juncture of the imaging chain. The 'Explanation User Interface' (EUI) is the component of an AI system designed to provide users with the understandable and interpretable details of the AI outputs. They typically comprise textual reports, heat 'salience' colour maps, or region-of-interest annotations, thereby augmenting image data visualisation and diagnostic accuracy (Fig. 5.14).

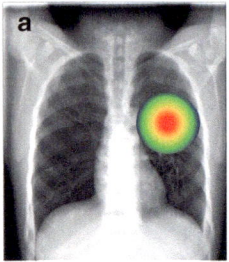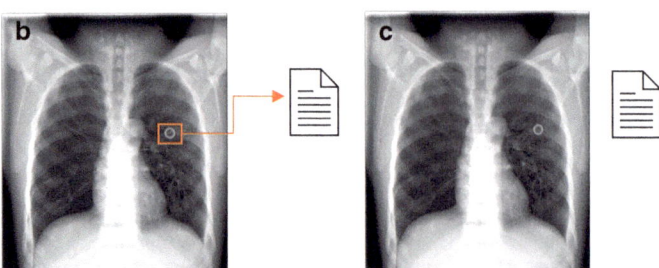

Fig. 5.14 Simplified example of variation in computer-aided detection (CAD) explanation user interface (EUI). Examples of EUIs include (**a**) a salience or 'heat map' to spatially locate suspicious image features for the user (**b**) a region-of-interest indicator to spatially locate suspicious image features with a textual report to explain findings or (**c**) a textual report to explain findings only with no AI-generated image overlay

User preferences of observers regarding interface design and visual presentation remain inadequately understood. A discordance between EUI types and reader preferences may hinder technology adoption and observer performance. This misalignment may exacerbate cognitive load and reduce any potential improvements. It is recommended that radiographers engage in research to evaluate user preferences and performance and collaborate with designers to optimise interface design.

The section of a human-incompatible EUI can result in a lack of trust in the system and bring about a state of under- or misuse of the system [76]. Conversely, the EUI may cause the user to excessively question their professional decision-making, resulting in the user relying on the feedback of the system over their own cognition. This is known as Automation Bias [77]. The user of the system should be aware of the benefits and fallibility of any AI system to reach a responsible relationship, where the user exhibits appropriate 'decision hygiene' [78, 79]. This will come about through user education, involvement in user-centric design and critical awareness of any system frailties, perhaps through case-based failure analysis.

AI systems have demonstrated robust capabilities in the identification and categorisation of image features on radiographs, with their efficacy well-documented. Case Study 5.4 demonstrates an AI-enabled nodule detection tool for lung cancer screening with high diagnostic accuracy, and Case Study 5.5 explores an AI-enabled tool for the diagnosis of COVID19. AI-powered stratification of normal vs. abnormal chest X-rays has been trialled in the United Kingdom, reporting accurate classification and potential for workload reduction [80]. Further studies are required to determine the long-term impact, as there is a risk of observers losing key competencies, like their ability to recognise "normality" in images, and over-dependency on AI systems.

AI-facilitated fatigue alerts may promote image reporter wellbeing by alleviating cognitive fatigue associated with the demanding tasks [81]. Accessibility for readers is further supported via speech recognition and predictive reports based on auto-fill features. The former capability serves to increase reporting throughput, and the latter standardises semantics and classification of image appearances [82]. Natural Language Processing (NLP) and, more recently, Large Language Models (LLM) have the potential to tailor the communication of diagnostic output to the intended audience, rendering them accessible to non-specialist clinicians, patients, and carers [83]. These functionalities may be integrated into existing Picture Arching and Communication Systems (PACS) architecture, enabling seamless communication of diagnostic data [84].

Case Study 5.3: Data Analysis, Image Evaluation and Reporting AI in Spinal Curvature Assessment

Clinical challenge: Spinal curvature disorders such as kyphosis, lordosis, and scoliosis are significant health concerns that require precise assessment and monitoring. Traditional methods of evaluating these conditions involve manual measurements of various spinal parameters, which can be labour-intensive and subject to variability among different observers.

AI enabled solutions: Recent advancements in AI and DL have shown promise in automating these assessments, improving accuracy, and reducing the workload on healthcare professionals. AI, particularly supervised DL models, has emerged as a powerful tool in spinal imaging [85, 86]. These models can be trained to identify or segment specific landmarks on anteroposterior (AP) and lateral spine radiographs, automatically connecting them to calculate spinal parameters. Advanced models can now detect up to 78 landmarks and 18 spinopelvic parameters in whole spine lateral radiographs, demonstrating excellent agreement with human measurements [87].

Benefits: In AP radiographs, automated systems have shown remarkable accuracy in measuring Cobb angles, with lower mean errors compared to human intra- and interobserver measurements ($2°–6.32°$ vs. $±9.6°/±11.8°$). This high level of precision makes AI a valuable tool for scoliosis screening in children, with sensitivity and specificity rates of 95.7% and 88.1%, respectively [88]. Additionally, AI can be used to monitor the progression of spinal curvature in postoperative patients, providing consistent and reliable data [86–88]. The integration of AI in spinal imaging represents a significant advancement in the field of orthopaedics. By automating the measurement of spinal parameters, AI not only enhances accuracy but also reduces the burden on healthcare professionals. As technology continues to evolve, the potential for AI in improving patient outcomes and streamlining clinical workflows will only grow.

Case Study 5.4: Data Analysis, Image Evaluation and Reporting AI for Lung Cancer Screening

Clinical challenge: Lung cancer is the leading cause of cancer-related deaths worldwide [89]. Survival outcomes are strongly linked to early diagnosis [90] Chest X-ray (CXR) are a common and accessible imaging modality used to investigate a wide range of symptoms, for which cancer is a differential diagnosis and can be missed [91] Radiology departments suffer from an increasing shortfall of radiologists combined with higher workloads [92, 93] delaying optimal patient management and time to treatment.

AI-enabled solutions: qXR AI software developed by Qure.ai for CXR is a deep learning-based (convolutional neural network) computer-aided detection software device trained on 9 million datasets to triage, detect and segment 30 findings in a CXR (Fig. 5.15).

Benefits: qXR will triage the radiological worklist for reporting prioritisation and display a 'secondary capture' in PACS demonstrating AI-segmented findings within seconds. This enhances workload efficiency [94], improves sensitivity and specificity [95, 96] reduces missed findings [97] and shortens the time to diagnosis, ultimately leading to better prognosis and treatment outcomes for patients.

qXR detects findings such as nodules, mediastinal widening, masses, hilar enlargement, and cavities—features consistent with lung cancer. This prioritisation allows clinicians to review and report these

(continued)

Urgent Suspicious Cancer (USC) cases first, referring patients for a CT scan ideally the same day, therefore shortening the patient pathway [98].

qXR demonstrates prioritisation initiates a lung cancer AI-accelerated patient pathway to ensure patients are diagnosed and treated early. Prior to AI adoption, the median reporting time for chest X-rays (CXR) was 98 hours. Following the implementation of qXR, prioritised USC cases achieved a reporting time of less than 2 hours, representing a 98% reduction (abstract presented, RSNA 2024) [99].

Patients have reported positive experiences from the AI-enhanced lung cancer pathway, benefiting from reduced waiting times for results, lower anxiety, minimised disease progression, and improved overall outcomes. One patient diagnosed and treated for stage 2 lung cancer commented: "Having the AI enhancement at the beginning of the process is life-saving, really. Who knows how it might have turned out without this AI" [100, 101].

Challenges: As AI publications and evidence highlighting the value grow, its integration into clinical pathways relies on healthcare professionals understanding its purpose, strengths, and limitations, including the risk of false positives or negatives. Healthcare professionals within clinical settings require not only education but also nurturing behavioural changes to support its adoption and effective use.

Case Study 5.5: Data Analysis, Image Evaluation and Reporting—Covid-19 Detection from Chest Radiographs Using Convolutional Neural Networks (CNNs)

Clinical challenge: Application of computer-aided diagnosis accelerated in part due to the pressures associated with the COVID-19 pandemic. AI-based image interpretation was found to reduce interpretation delivery times and enhance diagnostic accuracy by differentiating COVID-19 from pneumonia [102]. Consequently, the application of AI in the identification and categorisation of pulmonary disease in chest radiographs is well-established [103]. Consequently, there has been a surge in applications in this area, facilitated by high-quality curated and benchmarked datasets and ease of scalability of deep learning architecture [104].

AI enabled solution: Machine learning (ML), deep learning (DL), and convolutional neural networks (CNN) emulate and may even surpass the processing, interpretation, and extraction tasks capable of human cognitive ability. Detection capability includes stratification of patient risk via predictive analytics, identification, and differentiation of suspicious regions and a reduction in false positives, thereby improving diagnostic specificity. CNNs interrogate pixel data and demonstrate human-level capability in pathology detection by extracting features from complex image data [83].

Benefits: AI detection in medical imaging has been transformative as exemplified by the plethora of deep learning products entering the market with no signs of abating.

Challenges: Despite this, we must acknowledge and address a crucial limitation of deep learning systems: they are not impervious to bias. Lack of representation and access are the main causes of bias in DL model training data sets [105]. Deployment of bias systems risks widening health inequalities based on sex, gender, race, sexual orientation and socioeconomic status [106]. To mitigate bias, balance of demographic group representation should be considered, and medical imaging data sets should report demographic variables as standard. A viable solution to achieve standardisation of medical imaging demo-

(continued)

graphic labelling is to utilise DICOM headers with diagnostic radiographer oversight to verify metadata. There is future scope for AI training sets representative of the locality, ethnicity, and gender to further individualise diagnostic accuracy. Care should be taken to ensure such initiatives do not widen health inequalities prevalent in the transgender and non-binary community. Continuous quality assurance measures and fine-tuning of the models to the patient population should be considered to ensure responsible AI use in this area.

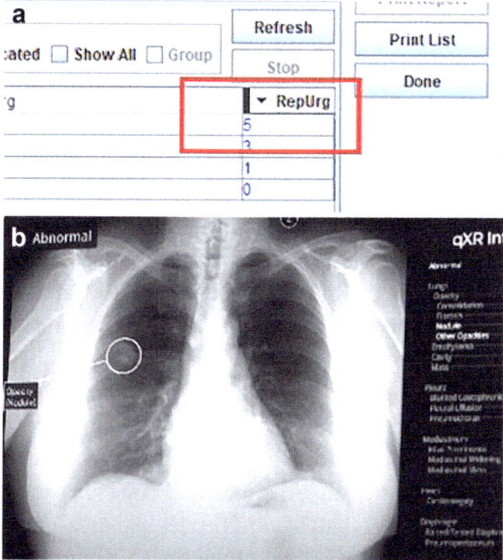

Fig. 5.15 (**a**) qXR Triage on radiologist report urgency column presents as high priority level 5. (**b**) A 60-year-old female, referred by her GP, was diagnosed early with stage 2 lung cancer through AI qXR prioritisation after a suspected nodule was detected on her chest X-ray. Time from X-ray to surgery was 7 weeks

5.3.6 Data Quality & Quality Assurance

With AI, quality control tests can be remotely monitored to make sure that equipment is working optimally in terms of data quality and dose. Data can be constantly checked and measured against baselines and other equipment, finding and forecasting any problems that can be fixed, often remotely. Audits can automatically be performed, on any timescale, on any data, and analysed to improve services. However, it is also important to recognise that the AI systems themselves also need to have quality assurance processes and to ensure that they meet local regulatory requirements [107].

One aspect of machine and deep learning AI algorithms is that they adapt and perform best when they are continuously learning and adapting from the data. However, this may clash with regulatory standards, where approvals depend on the equipment/system presented at the time [108]. To mitigate this, many countries have recognised healthcare AI under the 'medical device' category and have introduced frameworks to enable updates within the AI system whilst ensuring the changes are implemented in a controlled manner and continue to benefit the patient whilst mitigating and limiting risk [107]. More about AI governance and implementation challenges of AI can be found in Chap. 4.

It is essential to understand that all automated processes will be based on the quality of the data provided. Many of these processes will use data that is not necessarily radiographer facing, i.e., DICOM header data. It is therefore imperative that radiographers ensure that all data is accurate and representative if it is to be of the quality required for AI use (e.g. for training, internal or external testing). For example, processing algorithms are often based on acquisition menu, and images can be reprocessed using a different acquisition menu due to personal or local preferences of image presentation. Although this may appear a subtle difference, it could lead to the DICOM data being incorrect. In this example it would be essential to change the processing algorithms within the pipeline to enable different image presentation, rather than applying a mislabelled processing algorithm. Any incorrect data within the DICOM header or any part of the patient journey will mean the quality of the data has been reduced and may risk the data being unusable [109].

In addition to data being of good enough quality for use in AI, it is also essential that data is representative of populations and local demographics. AI methods that are designed and evaluated for specific populations may not work well for different patient groups and may exacerbate existing health disparities [110]. Radiographers are responsible for the quality of the data being generated and for understanding there is more data being created than an image of the patient, and that data quality and curation will become even more relevant to their role in the future. To ensure radiographers are empowered to fulfil these new roles and responsibilities, it is essential that they work in collaboration with the wider teams and external stakeholders, such as academics, vendors and professional bodies, beyond silos [111, 112]. Radiographers need to be consulted and involved in AI developments due to their extensive experience in the patient-facing aspects of medical imaging and background in technology. This places them in a prime position for identification of areas for development beyond disease detection and suggests impactful opportunities for implementation and optimisation. In a study determining the enablers and barriers to the successful implementation of AI into the clinical radiology department, Strohm et al. (2020) [113] found that the engagement of an 'AI champion' was critical to the optimal deployment of clinical AI systems, a position which may be ideally suited to the radiography profession. More about the future roles of radiographers and the changes AI will bring in radiography is discussed in Chap. 15.

Case Study 5.6: Data Quality & Quality Assurance—Volpara AI-Facilitated Feedback and Audit for Mammography

Clinical challenge: Positioning in mammography is essential for optimised image quality and radiation dose. The positioning of the breast impacts on the ability to apply effective compression [114], which in turn determines the effectiveness of the AECs, which control the choice of target, filter, kV and mAs. Therefore, appropriate positioning is essential in mammographic imaging, and poor positioning decreases sensitivity and specificity [115] and can have an impact on the number of patient recalls due to technical factors [116, 117].

Image evaluation of mammograms includes criteria based on accurate positioning of the breast; however, it has been evidenced that this process is subjective [118].

AI-enabled solution: Volpara TruPGMI is an automatic positioning and compression evaluation tool that provides users with feedback on every image they have acquired for both craniocaudal (CC) and medial lateral oblique (MLO) views. This enables longitudinal audit of performance of all data, whereas when undertaken manually, only small sample sizes can be used. The software evaluates the images using the UK PGMI standard [119], and the adapted PGMI criteria from Australia, New Zealand, Norway, and the American College of Radiology. It provides a measure of quality of patient positioning through percentages of images that fall within the PGMI classification (Perfect, Good, Moderate, Inadequate). The software also derives the compression pressure applied by using the recorded compression force from the DICOM header and measuring the contact area of the breast, comparing it to a target compression pressure.

Benefits: The data can then be used by the individual as feedback to identify areas for personal development, with embedded educational resources through the software. Managers can use the software to identify team needs and overall performance across teams and multiple sites.

Evidence has shown improvement in positioning and compression, with related reduction in technical recalls [120]. The largest study to date, with a dataset of over 48,000 exams conducted by 42 mammog-

(continued)

raphers over nine clinics, found that there were significant improvements in breast positioning (6%) and compression quality (8%) with an associated reduction in technical repeats and recalls of 78% [121].

As previously stated, not only should radiographers gain an understanding of the clinical use of AI in radiography, but they should also be involved in all aspects of research, development and implementation to ensure any developments meet the needs of the workforce, patient and profession. There is a risk that if radiographers are not involved in or engaged with AI developments, this can lead to digital complacency, reduced competencies, and accountability for erroneous use of AI equipment. Additionally, this could lead to a reduction in job satisfaction and professional identity due to lack of involvement in this fast-changing AI landscape as part of digital transformation of clinical services. Considering this challenge, we propose some quality criteria for AI integration in the clinical service of projectional radiography to equip an AI-proficient workforce (Table 5.1).

5.3.7 Future Applications of AI in Projectional Radiography and Beyond

Investigation of the impact of user interface on the clinician and patient is a relatively new area of research in radiography. This is despite principles of psychology suggesting that the interface design can impact the decisions made by the user and their future relationship with the technology [122]. Appropriate use of AI requires a balance of appropriate trust in the technology and critical awareness of personal preferences and biases, both based on previous experience with technology and more generally.

However, studies have found that a significant limitation in any interface design research is the disparity between user preference and quantifiable impact, based on actual user behaviour. A study in radiology by Rainey et al., 2024 [123] investigated the impact of different simple user interfaces (binary feedback i.e., pathology/ no pathology and heatmap output as a means of 'explainability'). The study found that the users indicated preference for the binary form of AI feedback, but statistical analysis showed instead that their trust in the AI system was more strongly related to the agreement of the AI with the heatmap explainability. This indicates that user preferences for AI to offer simple, binary form of pathology identification do not always align with what seems to most impact their trust in AI, which in this case it was the level of agreement with the visual form of AI feedback. Furthermore, a study by the same group of researchers found that when accuracy, decision switching and automation bias were considered, radiographers were more often confused by the heatmap and that, in general, the heatmap decreased diagnostic accuracy. Accuracy improved following presentation of the binary feedback. This is particularly paradoxical again, as the users indicated a preference for the heatmap form of AI feedback. Furthermore, this study found that inexperienced users were more susceptible to 'automation bias'—a tendency to trust the recommendation of technology over one's own judgement. Other studies in cardiology involving cardiologists' and cardiology residents' interaction with AI for electrocardiogram (ECG) interpretation found the same phenomenon: that inexperienced users were particularly susceptible to automation bias, and that experienced users were less likely to utilise the system, preferring their own judgement [124]. Whilst this level of critique is useful, and, indeed, a critical approach to technology use should be promoted, experienced users' reticence to engage with technology may become an issue. Algorithmic aversion can be broadly defined as a reluctance of a user to fully utilise or rely on the judgement of technology [125]. This can result in the reluctant user potentially missing out on some of the benefits resulting from utilisation of the AI system. As patients become increasingly aware of and involved in their healthcare journey, clinicians should be able to justify each decision made. This will include the use, or indeed, exclu-

Table 5.1 Proposed quality considerations throughout the patient journey to ensure optimal AI integration in projectional radiography examinations

Stage of patient journey	Questions to consider in ensuring optimal AI integration in projectional radiography examinations
Scheduling and workflow management Throughput and resource optimisation through AI analysis of past data and dynamic alerts to make every contact count.	Has the examination been justified or authorised as appropriate? Is the examination associated with the correct patient? Are the patient's name, age, birthdate and patient identification number accurate? Is demographic data that may feed into big data and ML training such as gender and ethnicity accurate? Has pregnancy status been determined inclusively and respectfully where applicable? Has the system alerted you to any additional requested examinations that you could perform? Have predetermined person-centred support mechanisms such as transport or translation services been implemented effectively? Check with patient, evaluate efficacy and feedback to system.
Procedure selection AI-supported procedure selection, reducing radiation exposure	Has automated vetting and authorisation of referral occurred within acceptability criteria as expected? Is recommended protocol standardised and gold standard? Has correlation of clinical history to appropriate examination occurred accurately? Has data from previous examinations fed into procedure optimisation? On interacting with patient, is the predetermined protocol the most appropriate for the individual's condition and capability? Are any modifications required? Has protocol and preliminary parameter selection been optimised effectively? Evaluate and feedback to system. Promote AI transparency by explaining AI-supported procedure selection to patient
Image acquisition Automated optimisation of technical parameters to improve diagnostic quality	*Pre-exposure* Have you communicated AI-driven semi-automated processes to the patient when obtaining informed consent? Has automation of exposure parameter selection, focal spot selection, filter and target material selection and image acquisition device selection occurred as expected? Are any modifications required? Is the patient positioned accurately, and have you placed correct anatomical side marker within the primary beam if required? Have you explained the procedure and when/why equipment motion, lights or sounds will occur? Have you provided accessible instruction utilising NLP interpretation and visual/aural indicators as appropriate? Has automatic positioning, automatic alignment, automatic collimation, grid selection and predetermined automatic exposure control configuration been optimised? Are any modifications required? Has the correct procedural processing and data display algorithm been determined? *Post-exposure* Was the procedural processing and data display algorithm acceptable? Has contrast and spatial resolution been optimised to maximise visibility of detail? If the projection is suboptimal, does an alternate procedural algorithm improve contrast resolution, ensuring that the alternate algorithm is labelled appropriately? Has effective histogram construction, exposure field recognition, and automatic rescaling to LUTs occurred as expected for the range of signals present? Does windowing allow the values-of-interest to be further demonstrated? Have noise reduction, motion reduction and stitching algorithms performed as expected where applicable? Does the contrast mask align with the edges of the exposure field? Has autocropping maximised the field of view and are collimated borders present on all four sides of the projection as applicable? Is the exposure indicator/deviation indicator within acceptable parameters for the system? Evaluate and feed back into system.

Stage of patient journey	Questions to consider in ensuring optimal AI integration in projectional radiography examinations
Image reporting and Interpretation AI-assisted detection, differentiation and categorisation of image features to support diagnosis and clinical decision-making	Has your reporting worklist been screened and categorised? Has this occurred as expected? Has AI-powered image enhancement occurred, and have any image quality metrics been produced for consideration? Has computer-aided detection identified abnormalities? Does the image appearance correlate to clinical history and risk stratification? Is further augmentation required? Has categorisation and classification of features occurred as expected? Are classifications accurate? Does EUI type meet your personal preference? Does EUI facilitate or impede the image interpretation task? Evaluate and give feedback to system. Has quantitative analysis or precise measurements of anatomical structures and pathologies occurred? If not, should AI-driven quantitative analysis be implemented to aid decision-making? Has the system analysed your performance and offered feedback identifying structural features in which there is scope to hone your diagnostic skills? Consider exploiting AI-powered virtual simulators to meet your training needs.
Reporting & Communication AI-generated and augmented reporting with accessible communication	Has automation of report generation occurred as expected? Validate and give feedback to the system. Does the report meet the standardisation criteria of your facility? Is there scope to apply NLP to improve report accessibility as applicable? How does disease progression map to analytics generated from similar historical cases? Does predictive modelling recommend actionable insight for further diagnostics and treatment? Is expedition of treatment or monitoring required? Has scheduling of all required follow-up and monitoring scans been automated as expected, encompassing a holistic approach to the provision of continuity of care?

The list is not exhaustive but is intended as an enabling and empowering tool for radiographers to engage with AI safely and effectively in promoting people-centred care

sion of the use of AI and advanced technologies in their care. A recent, yet unpublished, study by Busch and colleagues and large group of international contributors (the COMFORT consortium) found that out of 13806 patients from 74 hospitals, 57.6% ($n = 7775$) of respondents had positive attitudes towards AI in healthcare but expressed a desire for the retention of physician-led care. This indicates that the public desire is that AI and advanced technologies form part of their care, but human oversight is a requirement [126]. However, the study also found that the perceptions of AI varied with participants' demographic data. Both findings place the onus on the clinician to justify both the inclusion and exclusion of the use of technology in the patient's care, and these decisions must be made with cognisance of the preferences of each individual patient and scenario.

Other advanced technologies for patient-facing tasks, such as chatbots and large language models (LLMs), are increasingly being developed and tested. A recent study by Can et al. 2024, evaluated a number of LLMs for use in the simplification of interventional radiology reports for patients [127]. In this study, a number of currently available LLMs were assessed for acceptability under a number of headings, such as completeness of the report, accuracy and the ability of the model to present information as a human would, termed 'naturalness'. Some notable errors in the reports generated by LLMs were noted, and these exemplified concerning inaccuracies, or oversimplifications, which may have an impact on patient decision-making and expectations of interventional procedures. This was particularly the case with 'open-source' models, which the public has free access to. Despite the models exhibiting potential for this task, the experienced radiologists assessing the output recommended that further work was required to ensure that the information the patient is accessing is fit for purpose and that conversations around clinical deployment and use of this technology should be carefully considered. There is a paucity of research undertaken in this area within the projectional radiography field; however, the findings from this study may be extrapolated to be relevant to all radiology reports which patients and clinicians may have access to.

Johri et al. (2025) evaluated a framework to determine the conversational abilities of LLMs for use in patient history taking for clinicians [128]. This framework is proposed to be useful to evaluate the acceptability, usefulness and reliability of any LLM proposed for use in the clinical setting. The paper provides a number of recommendations for the use of LLMs for clinical history taking and LLM-facilitated information synthesis and diagnosis; however, these recommendations can apply to many clinical applications and can be extrapolated to situations where patient triage for imaging may be appropriate, for instance in symptomatic mammography or projection radiography in minor trauma. The authors suggest that LLMs may be useful, but further development is needed regarding the type of input data to avoid error which, as supported by Can et al., requires scrutiny before deployment and adequate human input to minimise unintended consequences for the patient.

There is further work required to allow for appropriate AI integration for improving and streamlining workflows. Part of that involves creating platforms that can support a holistic, unified approach where all AI products from different modalities can be embedded and used from a single docking station. A new vendor called deepc.ai proposes a unified product for all AI solutions, called deepcOS [129]. Figure 5.16 illustrates how deepcOS enables secure, scalable and interoperable deployment of AI in healthcare settings. DeepcOS connects seamlessly with any Health Information Technology (HIT) system, including PACS, RIS and EHR platforms. It can be integrated into diverse IT environments without requiring system-specific customisations. Health data from various health systems is ingested and processed regardless of volume or modality. This supports scalability across institutions of all si es. Before any processing or transmission from the edge

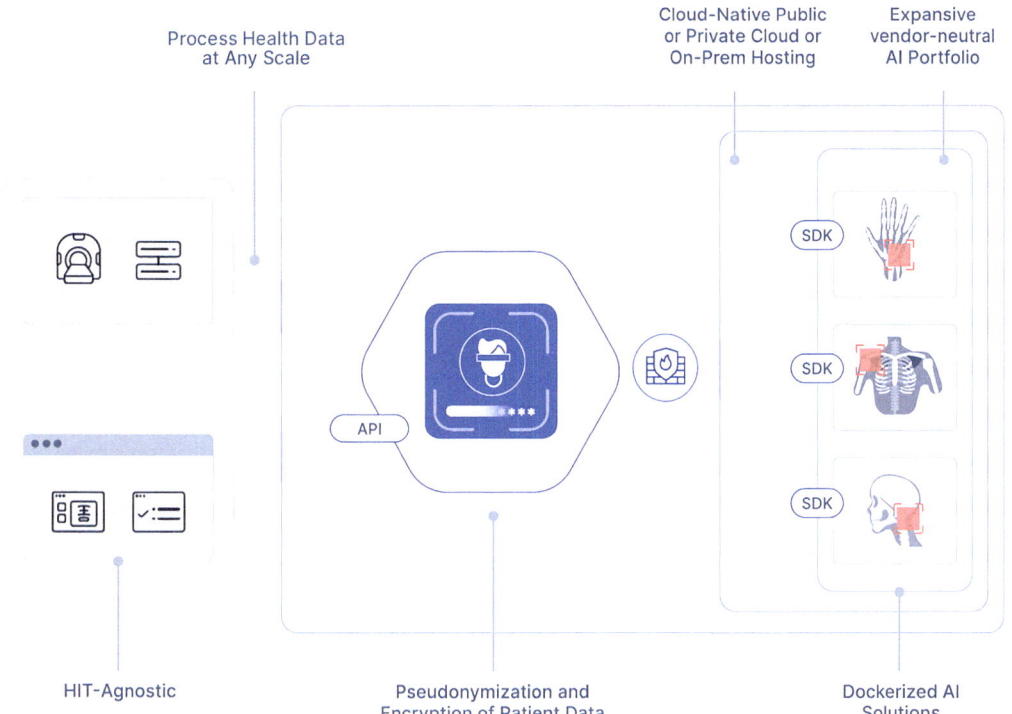

Fig. 5.16 This diagram shows how deepcOS connects with any hospital IT system (HIT-agnostic) through its APIs, securely processes health data at scale, and routes it through a pseudonymisation and encryption layer. AI models are deployed via containerised SDKs and hosted securely and flexibly (cloud, hybrid, or on-prem). A broad, vendor-neutral AI portfolio supports diverse clinical use cases. Abbreviations: *HIT* Health Information Technology, *API* Application Programming Interface, *SDK* Software Development Kit

server, patient data is pseudonymised and encrypted. This ensures compliance with data protection regulations. More on that can be found in Chap. 4. The technology can be deployed flexibly—via public cloud, private cloud or on-premises—depending on the institution's infrastructure and data residency requirements. AI can also support a wide range of models from different vendors, all interoperable through a unified interface, and allows users to integrate their own home-grown AI models [84].

5.3.8   Conclusions

In summary, current and potential applications of AI throughout the patient journey in projectional radiography were explored. Patient, practitioner, and service needs can be predicted, analysed and implemented at the planning stage. Opportunities for dose reduction and image optimisation are available at the acquisition and processing stage. AI-augmented image interpretation and disease detection improve diagnostic accuracy, and accessible NLP/LLM-generated reports may render diagnostic output more meaningful. AI-enabled education, feedback and audits support diagnostic radiographer upskilling and service improvement to ensure appropriate reliance on technology and that AI-human interaction is not only seamless but also continues to work towards patient benefit [130]. The role of other newer technologies like generative AI remains to be seen; currently the lack of regulatory clearance and the resultant hallucinations and lack of adequate testing prevent widespread clinical use in medical imaging [131, 132].

AI offers both threats and opportunities to the diagnostic radiography workforce [133]. As discussed above, it has shown excellent results for patient benefit when used for dynamic image quality assessment and optimisation during image acquisition, for postprocessing image enhancement and for certain cases of augmented image interpretation to facilitate reading time reduction and improved accuracy. Many applications will not be achievable without radiographers leading the way in technology adoption, research, and multidisciplinary collaboration. The profession is known for embracing technology, and as such, we are optimistic that the age of AI will too be embraced.

References

1. Adams SJ, Henderson RDE, Yi X, Babyn P. Artificial Intelligence solutions for analysis of X-ray images. Can Assoc Radiol J. 2021;72(1):60–72. https://doi.org/10.1177/0846537120941671.
2. General Electric. Critical care suite [internet]. 2020. Available at: https://www.gehealthcare.co.uk/-/media/a4846ce0e993461484eb0b71cc16ac47.pdf?rev=-1. Accessed 24 Mar 2025.
3. Poggenborg J, Yaroshenko A, Wieberneit N, Harder T, Gossmann A. Impact of AI-based real time image quality feedback for chest radiographs in the clinical routine. 2021; medrxiv. https://doi.org/10.1101/2021.06.10.21258326.
4. General Electric. Quality care suite 2.0 [internet] 2025. Available at: https://www.gehealthcare.com/products/radiography/quality-care-suite. Accessed 24 Mar 2025.
5. Potočnik J, Foley S, Thomas E. Current and potential applications of artificial intelligence in medical imaging practice: a narrative review. J Med Imaging Radiat Sci. 2023;54(2):376–85. https://doi.org/10.1016/j.jmir.2023.03.033.
6. Toepfer K, Barski L, Vogelsang L, Sehnert W. Denoising in digital radiographic images using a deep convolutional neural network. Carestream. 2020. Accessed 24 Mar 2025.
7. Jin Y, Ben-Jiang X, Wei ZK, Li Y. Chest X-ray image denoising method based on deep convolution neural network. IET Image Process. 2019;13(11):1970–8. https://doi.org/10.1049/iet-ipr.2019.0241.
8. Nousiainen K, Mäkelä T, Piilonen A, Peltonen JI. Automating chest radiograph imaging quality control. Phys Med. 2021;83:138–45. https://doi.org/10.1016/j.ejmp.2021.03.014.
9. Sun H, Wang W, He F, Wang D, Liu X, Xu S, et al. An AI-based image quality control framework for knee radiographs. J Digit Imaging. 2023;36(5):2278–89. https://doi.org/10.1007/s10278-023-00853-6.
10. Siemens Healthineers. YSIO X.pree with myExam companion: a leap forward in intelligent X-ray imaging. 2025. Available at: https://www.siemens-healthineers.com/en-uk/radiography/digital-X-ray/ysio-xpree. Accessed 24 Mar 2025.
11. Siemens Healthineers. Auto thorax collimation. 2025. Available at: https://www.siemens-healthineers.com/fr-lu/infrastructure-it/artificial-intelligence/ai-campaign/auto-thorax-collimation. Accessed 24 Mar 2025.
12. Siemens Healthineers. Siemens Healthineers uses artificial intelligence to take X-ray diagnostics to a new level. 2025. Available at: https://www.siemens-healthineers.com/press/releases/ysioxpree-ai-chest.html. Accessed 24 Mar 2025.
13. Lee HW, Jin KN, Oh S, Kang SY, Lee SM, Jeong IB, et al. Artificial Intelligence solution for chest radiographs in respiratory outpatient clinics: multicenter prospective randomized clinical trial. Ann Am Thorac Soc. 2023;20(5):660–7. https://doi.org/10.1513/AnnalsATS.202206-481OC.
14. Becker J, Decker JA, Römmele C, Kahn M, Messmann H, Wehler M, et al. Artificial Intelligence-based detection of pneumonia in chest radiographs. Diagnostics (Basel). 2022;12(6):1465. https://doi.org/10.3390/diagnostics12061465.
15. Hillis JM, Bizzo BC, Mercaldo S, Chin JK, Newbury-Chaet I, Digumarthy SR, et al. Evaluation of an artificial intelligence model for detection of pneumothorax and tension pneumothorax in chest radiographs. JAMA Netw Open. 2022;5. https://doi.org/10.1001/jamanetworkopen.2022.47172.
16. Niehoff JH, Kalaitzidis J, Kroeger JR, Schoenbeck D, Borggrefe J, Michael AE. Evaluation of the clinical performance of an AI-based application for the automated analysis of chest X-rays. Sci Rep. 2023;13(1):3680. https://doi.org/10.1038/s41598-023-30521-2.
17. Lauritzen AD, Lillholm M, Lynge E, Nielsen M, Karssemeijer N, Vejborg I. Early indicators of the impact of using AI in mammography screening for breast cancer. Radiology. 2024;311(3):e232479. https://doi.org/10.1148/radiol.232479.
18. Philips. Radiology smart assistant. 2022. Available at: https://www.philips.com/c-dam/b2bhc/master/resource-catalog/landing/radiology-smart-assistant/smart-assistant-product-overview-single-pages-rfa-global-final.pdf. Accessed 25 Mar 2025.
19. van Leeuwen KG, Schalekamp S, Rutten MJCM, van Ginneken b, de Rooij M. Artificial intelligence in radiology: 100 commercially available products and their scientific evidence. Eur Radiol.

2021;2021(31):3797–804. https://doi.org/10.1007/s00330-021-07892-z.

20. Radiology AI register. https://radiology.healthairegister.com/products/?subspeciality=Chest&modality=X-ray&ce_under=All&ce_class=All&fda_class=All&sort_by=last+modified&search=&2&page=3. Accessed 24 Mar 2025.

21. Colquitt J, Jordan M, Court R, Loveman E, Parr J, Ghosh I, et al. Artificial intelligence software for analysing chest X-ray images to identify suspected lung cancer: an evidence synthesis early value assessment. Health Technol Assess. 2024 Aug;28(50):1–75. https://doi.org/10.3310/LKRT4721.

22. Akhter Y, Singh R, Vatsa M. AI-based radiodiagnosis using chest X-rays: a review. Front Big Data. 2023;6:1120989. https://doi.org/10.3389/fdata.2023.1120989.

23. Taylor AG, Mielke C, Mongan J. Automated detection of moderate and large pneumothorax on frontal chest X-rays using deep convolutional neural networks: a retrospective study. PLOS Med. 2018;15(11):e1002697. https://doi.org/10.1371/journal.pmed.1002697.

24. Qin ZZ, Ahmed S, Sarker MS, Paul K, Adel ASS, Naheyan T, et al. Tuberculosis detection from chest X-rays for triaging in a high tuberculosis-burden setting: an evaluation of five artificial intelligence algorithms. Lancet Digit Health. 2021;3(9):e543–54. https://doi.org/10.1016/S2589-7500(21)00116-3.

25. Bougias H, Georgiadou E, Malamateniou C, Stogiannos N. Identifying cardiomegaly in chest X-rays: a cross-sectional study of evaluation and comparison between different transfer learning methods. Acta Radiol. 2021;62(12):1601–9. https://doi.org/10.1177/0284185120973630.

26. Gitto S, Serpi F, Albano D, Risoleo G, Fusco S, Messina C, et al. AI applications in musculoskeletal imaging: a narrative review. Eur Radiol Exp. 2024;8(1):22. https://doi.org/10.1186/s41747-024-00422-8.

27. Zech JR, Santomartino SM, Yi PH. Artificial Intelligence (AI) for fracture diagnosis: an overview of current products and considerations for clinical adoption, from the AJR special series on AI applications. AJR Am J Roentgenol. 2022;219(6):869–78. https://doi.org/10.2214/AJR.22.27873.

28. Zhao H, Ou L, Zhang Z, Zhang L, Liu K, Kuang J. The value of deep learning-based X-ray techniques in detecting and classifying K-L grades of knee osteoarthritis: a systematic review and meta-analysis. Eur Radiol. 2025;35(1):327–40. https://doi.org/10.1007/s00330-024-10928-9.

29. Taylor CR, Monga N, Johnson C, Hawley JR, Patel M. Artificial intelligence applications in breast imaging: current status and future directions. Diagnostics (Basel). 2023;13(12):2041. https://doi.org/10.3390/diagnostics13122041.

30. Lamb LR, Lehman CD, Gastounioti A, Conant EF, Bahl M. Artificial Intelligence (AI) for screening mammography, from the AJR special series on AI applications. Am J Roentgenol. 2022;219(3):369–80. https://doi.org/10.2214/AJR.21.27071.

31. Branco PESC, Franco AHS, de Oliveira AP, Carneiro IMC, de Carvalho LMC, de Souza JIN, et al. Artificial intelligence in mammography: a systematic review of the external validation. Rev Bras Ginecol Obstet. 2024:46–71. https://doi.org/10.61622/rbgo/2024rbgo71.

32. Vosper M, England A, Major V. Graham's principles and applications of radiological physics. 7th ed. Elsevier; 2020.

33. Fauber TL, Johnson J. Essentials of radiographic physics and imaging. 3rd ed. Elsevier; 2019.

34. Hayre CM, Cox WAS, editors. General radiography; principles and practices. 1st ed. CRC Press; 2020.

35. Seeram E. Digital radiography. 1st ed. Springer; 2021.

36. Witkowski K, Okhai R, Neely SR. Public perceptions of artificial intelligence in healthcare: ethical concerns and opportunities for patient-centered care. BMC Med Ethics. 2024:25. https://doi.org/10.1186/s12910-024-01066-4.

37. Sauerbrei A, Kerasidou A, Lucivero F, Hallowell N. The impact of artificial intelligence on the person-centred, doctor-patient relationship: some problems and solutions. BMC Med Inform Decis Mak. 2023;23:73. https://doi.org/10.1186/s12911-023-02162-y.

38. Hardy M, Harvey H. Artificial intelligence in diagnostic imaging: impact on the radiography profession. British Journal of Radiology. 2020;93:1108. https://doi.org/10.1259/bjr.20190840.

39. Andargoli AE, Ulapane N, Nguyen TA, Shuakat N, Zelcer J, Wickramasinghe N. Intelligent decision support systems for dementia care: a scoping review. Artif Intell Med. 2024:150. https://doi.org/10.1016/j.artmed.2024.102815.

40. Wolters MK, Kelly F, Kilgour J. Designing a spoken dialogue interface to an intelligent cognitive assistant for people with dementia. Health Informatics J. 2016;22(4):854–66. https://doi.org/10.1177/1460458215593329.

41. Moy S, Irannejad M, Manning SJ, Farahani M, Ahmed Y, Gao E, Prabhune R, Lorenz S, Mirza R, Klinger C. Patient perspectives on the use of artificial intelligence in health care: a scoping review. J Patient Cent Res Rev. 2024;11(1):51–62. https://doi.org/10.17294/2330-0698.2029.

42. Taylor B, McLean G. Exploring the use of mobile translation applications for culturally and linguistically diverse patients during medical imaging examinations in Australia – a systematic review. J Med Radiat Sci. 2024;71:432–44. https://doi.org/10.1002/jmrs.755.

43. Malamateniou C. Technology-enabled patient care in medical radiation sciences: the two sides of the coin. J Med Radiat Sci. 2024;71(3):326–9. https://doi.org/10.1002/jmrs.807. Epub 2024 Jun 24. PMID: 38923225; PMCID: PMC11569419.

44. Dong, D, Liu S, Liu Z, Mu W, Wang S, Shuo W et al. Radiomics and multiomics research. In: Liu, S. (eds) Artificial intelligence in medical imaging in China. Springer. https://doi.org/10.1007/978-981-99-8441-1_4

45. Rasche A, ten Cate G, Hebecker A. YSIO X.pree: How intelligent imaging ensures an efficient and patient-centered radiography workflow, results of a multicenter product evaluation study, Siemens Healthineers white paper 2024.

46. Alowais SA, Alghamdi SS, Alsuhebany N, Alqahtani T, Alshaya AI, Almohareb SN, et al. Revolutionizing healthcare: the role of artificial intelligence in clinical practice. BMC Med Educ. 2023;23:689. https://doi.org/10.1186/s12909-023-04698-z.

47. GE Health Care Command Center: Who are we? Available at: https://www.gehccommandcenter.com/about-us. Accessed 27 Mar 25.

48. Collins BE. Reducing hospital harm: establishing a command centre to foster situational awareness. Healthc Q. 2022;25(2):75–81. https://doi.org/10.12927/hcq.2022.26885.

49. Borges do Nascimento IJ, Abdulazeem H, Vasanthan LT, Martinez EZ, Zucoloto ML, et al. Barriers and facilitators to utilizing digital health technologies by healthcare professionals. NPJ Digit Med. 2023;6(1):161. https://doi.org/10.1038/s41746-023-00899-4.

50. Aggarwal R, Sounderajah V, Martin G, Ting DSW, Karthikesalingam A, King D, et al. Diagnostic accuracy of deep learning in medical imaging: a systematic review and meta-analysis. NPJ Digit Med. 2021;4(65) https://doi.org/10.1038/s41746-021-00438-z.

51. Sun H, Wang W, He F, Wang D, Liu X, Xu S, et al. An AI-based image quality control framework for knee radiographs. J Digit Imaging. 2023 Oct;36(5):2278–89. https://doi.org/10.1007/s10278-023-00853-6.

52. Damilakis J, Stratakis J. Descriptive overview of AI applications in X-ray imaging and radiotherapy. J Radiol Prot. 2024;44(4) https://doi.org/10.1088/1361-6498/ad9f71.

53. Rasche A, Brader P, Borggrefe J, Seuss H, Carr Z, Hebecker A, et al. Impact of intelligent virtual and AI-based automated collimation functionalities on the efficiency of radiographic acquisitions. Radiography. 2024;30(4):1073–9. https://doi.org/10.1016/j.radi.2024.05.002.

54. Siemens Healthineers uses artificial intelligence to take X-ray diagnostics to a new level. Siemens 2020. Available at: https://www.siemens-healthineers.com/press/releases/ysioxpree-ai-chest.html.

55. Lee H, Lee J. A deep learning-based scatter correction of simulated X-ray images. Electronics. 2019;8(9):944. https://doi.org/10.3390/electronics8090944.

56. Kashyap S, Moradi M, Karargyris A, Wu JT, Morris M, Saboury B et al. Artificial intelligence for point of care radiograph quality assessment. Proc. SPIE 2019, Medical Imaging 2019: Computer-Aided Diagnosis. https://doi.org/10.1117/12.2513092.

57. Dasegowda G, Kalra MK, Abi-Ghanem AS, Arru CD, Bernardo M, Saba L, et al. Suboptimal chest radiography and artificial intelligence: the problem and the solution. Diagnostics. 2023;13(3):412. https://doi.org/10.3390/diagnostics13030412.

58. Lawrence A, Hardie T, Zapantis I, Ohenhen O, Hepworth J. AI in London healthcare: the reality behind the hype, UCL Partners and the Health Foundation report, 2025. Available form https://uclpartners.com/wp-content/uploads/UCLP-AI-in-London-healthcare-03.25-final.pdf. Accessed 31 Mar 2025.

59. Rainey C, O'Regan T, Matthew J, Skelton E, Woznitza N, Chu KY, et al. UK reporting radiographers' perceptions of AI in radiographic image interpretation – current perspectives and future developments. Radiography. 2022;28(4):881–8. https://doi.org/10.1016/j.radi.2022.06.006.

60. Moulds A, Horton T, The Health Foundation. What do technology and AI mean for the future of work in health care? 2023. Available from https://www.health.org.uk/reports-and-analysis/briefings/what-do-technology-and-ai-mean-for-the-future-of-work-in-health-care. Accessed 1 Apr 2025.

61. Najjar R. Redefining radiology: a review of artificial intelligence integration in medical imaging. Diagnostics. 2023;13:2760. https://doi.org/10.3390/diagnostics13172760.

62. Rossignol J, Bélanger G, Fromont MC, Therrien A, Fontaine R, Bérubé-Lauzière Y. Time-of-flight computed tomography – proof of principle. Phys Med Biol. 2024;69(17):175017. https://doi.org/10.1088/1361-6560/ab78bf.

63. Tang H, Tong D, Dong Bao X, Dillenseger J-L. A new stationary gridline artifact suppression method based on the 2D discrete wavelet transform. Med Phys. 2015;42(4):1721–9. https://doi.org/10.1118/1.4914861.

64. Gossye T, Buytaert D, Smeets PV, Morbée L, De Wilde C, Vermeiren K, et al. Evaluation of virtual grid processed clinical chest radiographs. Invest Radiol. 2022;57(9):585–91. https://doi.org/10.1097/rli.0000000000000876.

65. Carestream. Smart noise cancellation: a groundbreaking advance in X-ray image quality. 2023. Available at: https://www.carestream.com/blog/2021/05/11/smart-noise-cancellation-a-groundbreaking-advance-in-X-ray-image-quality/#:~:text=Smart%20Noise%20Cancellation%20is%20the%20first%20step%20in,to%20predict%20a%20noise-field%20from%20an%20input%20image.

66. Sayed M, Knapp KM, Fulford J, Heales C, Alqahtani SJ. The principles and effectiveness of X-ray scatter correction software for diagnostic X-ray imaging: a scoping review. Eur J Radiol. 2023:158. https://doi.org/10.1016/j.ejrad.2022.110600.

67. Seeram E, Seeram D. Image postprocessing in digital radiology—a primer for technologists. J Med Imaging Radiat Sci. 2008;19(1):23–41. https://doi.org/10.1016/j.jmir.2008.01.004.

68. McQuillen-Martensen K. Radiographic image analysis. 5th ed. Philadelphia: Saunders; 2019.

69. Song L, Sun H, Xiao H, Lam SK, Zhan Y, Ren G, Cai J. Artificial intelligence for chest X-ray image enhancement. Radiat Med Prot. 2025;6(1):61–8. https://doi.org/10.1016/j.radmp.2024.12.003.

70. Chung L, Kumar S, Oldfield J, Phillips M, Stratfold M. The use of anatomical side markers in general radiology: a systematic review of the current literature. J Patient Saf. 2022;18:1. https://doi.org/10.1097/PTS.0000000000000716.

71. Titley AG, Cosson P. Radiographer use of anatomical side markers and the latent conditions affecting their use in practice. Radiography. 2014;20(1):42–7. https://doi.org/10.1016/j.radi.2013.10.004.

72. Hayre CM, Blackman S, Eyden A, Carlton K. the use of digital side markers (DSMs) and cropping in digital radiography. J Med Imaging Radiat Sci. 2019;50(2):234–42. https://doi.org/10.1016/j.jmir.2018.11.001.

73. Society and College of Radiographers. Use of anatomical side markers. London: Society and College of Radiographers; 2014.

74. Gambato M, Scotti N, Borsari G, Zambon Bertoja J, Gabrieli JD, De Cassai A, et al. Chest X-ray interpretation: detecting devices and device-related complications. Diagnostics (Basel). 2023;13:4. https://doi.org/10.3390/diagnostics13040599.

75. Tang CHM, Seah JCY, Ahmad HK, Milne MR, Wardman JB, Buchlak QD, et al. Analysis of line and tube detection performance of a chest X-ray deep learning model to evaluate hidden stratification. Diagnostics (Basel). 2023;13(14). https://doi.org/10.3390/diagnostics13142317.

76. Rainey C, O'Regan T, Matthew J, Skelton E, Woznitza N, Chu K-Y, et al. Beauty is in the AI of the beholder: are we ready for the clinical integration of artificial intelligence in radiography? An exploratory analysis of perceived AI knowledge, skills, confidence, and education perspectives of UK radiographers. Front Digit Health. 2021;3(739327):1–19. https://doi.org/10.3389/fdgth.2021.739327.

77. Rainey C, Villikudathil A, McConnell J, Hughes C, Bond RR, McFadden S. An experimental machine learning study investigating the decision-making process of students and qualified radiographers when interpreting radiographic images. PLoS Digital Health. 2023;2(10):1–14. https://doi.org/10.1371/journal.pdig.0000229.

78. Kahneman D, Sibony O, Sunstein CR. Noise: a flaw in human judgment. Hachette; 2021.

79. Rainey C, Bond RR, McConnell J, Gill A, Hughes C, Kumar D, McFadden S. The impact of AI feedback on the accuracy of diagnosis, decision switching and trust in radiography. PLoS One. 2025;20(5):e0322051. https://doi.org/10.1371/journal.pone.0322051.

80. Blake SR, Das N, Tadepalli M, Reddy B, Singh A, Agrawal R, et al. Using artificial intelligence to stratify normal versus abnormal chest X-rays: external validation of a deep learning algorithm at East Kent Hospitals University NHS Foundation Trust. Diagnostics (Basel). 2023;13(22). https://doi.org/10.1016/j.ibmed.2022.100049.

81. Derevianko A, Pizzoli SFM, Pesapane F, Rotili A, Monzani D, Grasso R, et al. The use of artificial intelligence (AI) in the radiology field: what is the state of doctor-patient communication in cancer diagnosis? Cancers (Basel). 2023;15(2). https://doi.org/10.3390/cancers1502047.

82. Najjar R. Redefining radiology: a review of artificial intelligence integration in medical imaging. Diagnostics (Basel). 2023;13(17):2760. https://doi.org/10.3390/diagnostics13172760.

83. Salehi AW, Khan S, Gupta G, Alabduallah BI, Almjally A, Alsolai H, et al. A study of CNN and transfer learning in medical imaging: advantages, challenges, future scope. Sustainability. 2023;15(7):5930. https://doi.org/10.3390/su15075930.

84. Kim B, Romeijn S, van Buchem M, Mehrizi MHR, Grootjans W. A holistic approach to implementing artificial intelligence in radiology. Insights Imaging. 2024;15(1):22. https://doi.org/10.1186/s13244-023-01586-4.

85. Lee S, Jung JY, Mahatthanatrakul A, Kim JS. Artificial intelligence in spinal imaging and patient care: a review of recent advances. Neurospine. 2024;21(2):474–86. https://doi.org/10.14245/ns.2448388.194.

86. Berlin C, Adomeit S, Grover P, Dreischarf M, Halm H, Dürr O, et al. Novel AI-based algorithm for the automated computation of coronal parameters in adolescent idiopathic scoliosis patients: a validation study on 100 preoperative full spine X-rays. Global Spine J. 2023;14(6):1728–37. https://doi.org/10.1177/21925682231154543.

87. Goldman SN, Hui AT, Choi S, Mbamalu EK, Tirabady P, Eleswarapu AS, et al. Applications of artificial intelligence for adolescent idiopathic scoliosis: mapping the evidence. Spine Deform. 2024;12:1545–70. https://doi.org/10.1007/s43390-024-00940-w.

88. Li L, Wong MS. The application of machine learning methods for predicting the progression of adolescent idiopathic scoliosis: a systematic review. Biomed Eng. 2024;23(80). https://doi.org/10.1186/s12938-024-01272-6.

89. World Health Organization. Global cancer burden growing, amidst mounting need for services. 2024. Available at: https://www.who.int/news/item/01-02-2024-global-cancer-burden-

growing%2D%2Damidst-mounting-need-for-services. Accessed 28 Mar 25.

90. Tsai CH, Kung PT, Kuo WY, Tsai WC. Effect of time interval from diagnosis to treatment for non-small cell lung cancer on survival: a national cohort study in Taiwan. BMJ Open. 2020;10(4):e034351. https://doi.org/10.1136/bmjopen-2019-034351.

91. Del Ciello A, Franchi P, Contegiacomo A, Cicchetti G, Bonomo L, Larici AR. Missed lung cancer: when, where, and why? Diagn Interv Radiol. 2017;23(2):118–26. https://doi.org/10.5152/dir.2016.16187.

92. Royal College of Radiologists. Clinical Radiology Workforce Census 2023. Research United Kingdom: Royal College of Radiologists, Clinical Radiology; 2023.

93. Everlight Radiology. Radiology unlocked: the global radiologist report 2025. Research United Kingdom: Everlight Radiology, Medical Leadership Council; 2025.

94. Blake SR, Das N, Tadepalli M, Reddy B, Singh A, Agrawal R, et al. Using artificial intelligence to stratify normal versus abnormal chest X-rays: external validation of a deep learning algorithm at East Kent Hospitals University NHS Foundation Trust. Diagnostics (Basel). 2023;13(22):3408. https://doi.org/10.3390/diagnostics13223408.

95. Robert D, Sathyamurthy S, Singh AK, Matta SA, Tadepalli M, Tanamala S, et al. Effect of artificial intelligence as a second reader on the lung nodule detection and localization accuracy of radiologists and non-radiology physicians in chest radiographs: a multicenter reader study. Acad Radiol. 2025;32(3):1706–17. https://doi.org/10.1016/j.acra.2024.11.003.

96. Mahboub B, Tadepalli M, Raj T, Rajalakshmi S, Hachim M, Usama B, et al. Identifying malignant nodules on chest X-rays: a validation study of radiologist versus artificial intelligence diagnostic accuracy. Adv Biomed Health Sci. 2022;1(3):137–43. https://doi.org/10.4103/abhs.abhs_17_22.

97. Kaviani P, Kalra MK, Digumarthy SR, Gupta RV, Dasegowda G, Jagirdar A, et al. Frequency of missed findings on chest radiographs (CXRs) in an international, multicenter study: application of AI to reduce missed findings. Diagnostics (Basel). 2022;12(10):2382. https://doi.org/10.3390/diagnostics12102382.

98. Duncan SF, McConnachie A, Blackwood J, Stobo DB, Maclay JD, Wu O, et al. Radiograph accelerated detection and identification of cancer in the lung (RADICAL): a mixed methods study to assess the clinical effectiveness and acceptability of Qure.ai artificial intelligence software to prioritise chest X-ray (CXR) interpretation. BMJ Open. 2024;20;14(9) https://doi.org/10.1136/bmjopen-2023-081062.

99. Lowe D. The power of Chest X-ray AI and early lung cancer detection: Prelim results of RADICAL study: Qure.ai Technologies. In RSNA; 2024; Chicago.

https://reg.meeting.rsna.org/flow/rsna/rsna24/MeetingCentralRSNA24/page/session-catalog/session/1724433040362001qfLZ.

100. STV News. Gran's lung cancer detected early using AI-powered X-ray. Patient Report. Glasgow; 2024.

101. Kumar S. The impact of AI in early lung cancer detection. Patient Report. Glasgow: Qure.ai; 2025.

102. Annarumma M, Withey SJ, Bakewell RJ, Pesce E, Goh V, Montana G. Automated triaging of adult chest radiographs with deep artificial neural networks. Radiology. 2019;291(1):196–202. https://doi.org/10.1148/radiol.2018180921.

103. Field EL, Tam W, Moore N, McEntee M. Efficacy of artificial intelligence in the categorisation of paediatric pneumonia on chest radiographs: a systematic review. Children (Basel). 2023;10(3) https://doi.org/10.3390/children10030576.

104. Liu T, Siegel E, Shen D. Deep learning and medical image analysis for COVID-19 diagnosis and prediction. Annu Rev Biomed Eng. 2022;24:179–201. https://doi.org/10.1146/annurev-bioeng-110220-012203.

105. Yi PH, Kim TK, Siegel E, Yahyavi-Firouz-Abadi N. Demographic reporting in publicly available chest radiograph data sets: opportunities for mitigating sex and racial disparities in deep learning models. J Am Coll Radiol. 2022;19(1 Pt B):192–200. https://doi.org/10.1016/j.jacr.2021.08.018.

106. Gianfrancesco MA, Tamang S, Yazdany J, Schmajuk G. Potential biases in machine learning algorithms using electronic health record data. JAMA Intern Med. 2018;178(11):1544–7. https://doi.org/10.1001/jamainternmed.2018.3763.

107. Pianykh OS, Langs G, Dewey M, Enzmann DR, Herold CJ, Schoenberg SO, et al. Continuous learning AI in radiology: implementation principles and early applications. Radiology. 2020;297(1):6–14. https://doi.org/10.1148/radiol.2020200038.

108. Geis JR, Brady AP, Wu CC, Spencer J, Ranschaert E, Jaremko JL, et al. Ethics of artificial intelligence in radiology: summary of the joint European and North American multisociety statement. Radiology. 2019;293(2):436–40. https://doi.org/10.1016/j.jacr.2019.07.028.

109. The Medical Imaging Technology Association. AI And DICOM: MITA; 2023. Available from: https://www.dicomstandard.org/ai. Accessed 19 Mar 25.

110. Abràmoff MD, Tarver ME, Loyo-Berrios N, Trujillo S, Char D, Obermeyer Z, et al. Considerations for addressing bias in artificial intelligence for health equity. NPJ Digit Med. 2023;6(1):170 https://doi.org/10.1038/s41746-023-00913-9.

111. Stogiannos N, Gillan C, Precht H, Reis CSD, Kumar A, O'Regan T, et al. A multidisciplinary team and multiagency approach for AI implementation: a commentary for medical imaging and radiotherapy key stakeholders. J Med Imaging Radiat Sci. 2024;55(4):101717. https://doi.org/10.1016/j.jmir.2024.101717.

112. Malamateniou C, McFadden S, McQuinlan Y, England A, Woznitza N, Goldsworthy S. Artificial intelligence: guidance for clinical imaging and therapeutic radiography workforce professionals, vol. 27. The Society of Radiographers. 2021. Available at: https://www.sor.org/news/information-management-technology/sor-publishes-guidance-on-use-of-ai-in-radiography.

113. Strohm L, Hehakaya C, Ranschaert ER, Boon WPC, Moors EHM. Implementation of artificial intelligence (AI) applications in radiology: hindering and facilitating factors. Eur Radiol. 2020;30:5525–32. https://doi.org/10.1007/s00330-020-06946-y.

114. Serwan E, Matthews D, Davies J, Chau M. Mechanical standardisation of mammographic compression using Volpara software. Radiography. 2021;27(3):789–94. https://doi.org/10.1016/j.radi.2020.12.009.

115. Henderson LM, Benefield T, Marsh MW, Schroeder BF, Durham DD, Yankaskas BC, et al. The influence of mammographic technologists on radiologists' ability to interpret screening mammograms in community practice. Acad Radiol. 2015;22(3):278–89. https://doi.org/10.1016/j.acra.2014.09.013.

116. Huppe AI, Overman KL, Gatewood JB, Hill JD, Miller LC, Inciardi MF. Mammography positioning standards in the digital era: is the status quo acceptable? Am J Roentgenol. 2017;209(6):1419–25. https://doi.org/10.2214/AJR.16.17522.

117. Salkowski LR, Elezaby M, Fowler AM, Burnside E, Woods RW, Strigel RM. Comparison of screening full-field digital mammography and digital breast tomosynthesis technical recalls. J Med Imaging (Bellingham). 2019;6(3):031403. https://doi.org/10.1117/1.JMI.6.3.031403.

118. Alukić E, Homar K, Pavić M, Žibert J, Mekiš N. The impact of subjective image quality evaluation in mammography. Radiography. 2023;29(3):526–32. https://doi.org/10.1016/j.radi.2023.02.025.

119. Guidance for breast screening mammographers; 2020. Available from : https://www.gov.uk/government/publications/breast-screening-quality-assurance-for-mammography-and-radiography/guidance-for-breast-screening-mammographers. Accessed 2 Apr 2025.

120. Gennaro G, Povolo L, Del Genio S, Ciampani L, Fasoli C, Carlevaris P, et al. Using automated software evaluation to improve the performance of breast radiographers in tomosynthesis screening. Eur Radiol. 2023. https://doi.org/10.1007/s00330-023-10457-x.

121. Eby PR, Martis LM, Paluch JT, Pak JJ, Chan AHL. Impact of artificial intelligence–driven quality improvement software on mammography technical repeat and recall rates. Radiol Artif Intell. 2023;5(6):e230038. https://doi.org/10.1148/ryai.230038.

122. Johnson J. Designing with the mind in mind: simple guide to understanding user interface design rules. Elsevier Science & Technology; 2010.

123. Rainey C, Bond R, McConnell J, Hughes C, Kumar D, McFadden S. Reporting radiographers' interaction with Artificial Intelligence—how do different forms of AI feedback impact trust and decision switching? PLOS Digit Health. 2024;3(8) https://doi.org/10.1371/journal.pdig.0000560.

124. Bond RR, Novotny T, Andrsova I, Koc L, Sisakova M, Finlay D, et al. Automation bias in medicine: the influence of automated diagnoses on interpreter accuracy and uncertainty when reading electrocardiograms. J Electrocardiol. 2018;51:S6–S11. https://doi.org/10.1016/j.jelectrocard.2018.08.007.

125. Mahmud H, Islam AKMN, Ahmed SI, Smolander K. What influences algorithmic decision-making? A systematic literature review on algorithm aversion. Technol Forecast Soc Chang. 2022:175. https://doi.org/10.1016/j.techfore.2021.121390.

126. Busch F, Hoffmann L, Xu L, Zhang L, Hu B, García-Juárez I, et al. Multinational attitudes towards AI in healthcare and diagnostics among hospital patients. medRxiv. 2024. https://doi.org/10.1101/2024.09.01.24312016.

127. Can E, Uller W, Vogt K, Doppler MC, Busch F, Bayerl N, et al. Large language models for simplified interventional radiology reports: a comparative analysis. Acad Radiol. 2025;32(2). https://doi.org/10.1016/j.acra.2024.09.041.

128. Johri S, Jeong J, Tran BA, Schlessinger DI, Wongvibulsin S, Barnes LA, et al. An evaluation framework for clinical use of large language models in patient interaction tasks. Nat Med. 2025;31:77–86. https://doi.org/10.1038/s41591-024-03328-5.

129. DeepcOS. 2025. Available from https://www.deepc.ai/. Accessed 2 Apr 2025.

130. Li MD, Little BP. Appropriate reliance on artificial intelligence in radiology education. J Am Coll Radiol. 2023;20(11):1126–30. https://doi.org/10.1016/j.jacr.2023.04.019.

131. Huang J, Neill L, Wittbrodt M, Melnick D, Klug M, Thompson M, et al. Generative artificial intelligence for chest radiograph interpretation in the emergency department. JAMA Netw Open. 2023;6(10). https://doi.org/10.1001/jamanetworkopen.2023.36100.

132. Lang O, Yaya-Stupp D, Traynis I, Cole-Lewis H, Bennett CR, Lyles CR, et al. Using generative AI to investigate medical imagery models and datasets. EBioMedicine. 2024;102:105075. https://doi.org/10.1016/j.ebiom.2024.105075.

133. Harcus J, Ferrari G, Berry E, Cadogan E, McNally CS, Bardwell A, et al. "Making it work in the face of extreme adversity" – exploring perceptions for the future of the imaging and oncology workforce using 'soundbite' interviews. Radiography. 2024;31(1):12–9. https://doi.org/10.1016/j.radi.2024.10.017.

Ciara McNally has a background in chemistry and materials science, having worked as a postgraduate researcher before training as a diagnostic radiographer. In 2021, she joined the University of Bradford as a Clinical Teacher in Diagnostic Radiography. Now a lecturer and undergraduate programme leader, she teaches computing in medical imaging. Ciara is interested in AI's application in projectional radiography, focusing on enhancing image acquisition and data fidelity to improve diagnostics. She is dedicated to educating future radiographers on digital fluency and AI's transformative potential in medical imaging.

Dr Clare Rainey works at University College Cork in the Discipline of Radiography in the School of Medicine. She is an experienced academic and researcher in Artificial Intelligence (AI) in medicine with a particular interest in human–computer interaction and how this impacts decision-making. She has published extensively in a number of well-known journals in the field and delivered at a number of international conferences as an invited speaker. She continues to progress her own research whilst also supervising PhD students in user interface design in radiology and the use of technology in specialist modalities, such as mammography.

Professor Katy Szczepura is an Associate Professor in Medical Imaging Physics and co-research lead for the Digital Skills and Medical Imaging research group. Her research focuses on medical image analysis, optimisation, and developing novel acquisition and analysis techniques to improve health outcomes in clinical applications. Katy is an associate editor for the British Journal of Radiology and President-Elect of the Manchester Medical Society Medical Imaging Section. She has supervised over 15 PhD students and numerous MSc students. Katy also teaches medical physics, technology, digital skills, research, and ethics across a number of radiography-focused undergraduate and postgraduate programmes.

AI in Computed Tomography

6

Benard Ohene-Botwe, Bo Mussmann, and Mark F McEntee

6.1 Introduction

Computed tomography (CT) is one of the most invaluable, reliable, and life-saving technologies in radiography. Since its introduction in the early 1970s, the modality has resulted in improvements in patient care, research activities, and CT education [1, 2]. Concerning emergencies alone, studies have suggested that the increased utilisation of the modality has eliminated the need for many exploratory surgical procedures and emergency surgery from 13% to 5% [3, 4]. Recent advances in CT equipment and accessories have further boosted their demand. Interestingly, many of the current advances have been driven partly by the development of AI tools and algorithms. This chapter provides an overview of some of the AI applications in CT and explains how they are being used to improve practice in medical imaging and enhance health outcomes. This discussion broadly covers the following areas: examination workflow and preparation; positioning; image acquisition, reconstruction, and dose reduction; image processing and analysis; detection of abnormalities/clinical decision support systems; future development; and limitations and challenges. Table 6.1 provides an overview of the key areas discussed in this chapter concerning AI tool integration into CT clinical practice.

on behalf of Association of Healthcare Technology Providers for Imaging, Radiotherapy and Care (AXREM)

B. Ohene-Botwe (✉)
Division of Radiography, City St George's, University of London, London, UK
e-mail: benard.ohene-botwe@citystgeorges.ac.uk

B. Mussmann
Odense University Hospital and University of Southern Denmark, Odense, Denmark
e-mail: Bo.mussmann@rsyd.dk

M. F. McEntee
Medical Imaging and Radiation Therapy, University College Cork, School of Medicine, Cork, Ireland
e-mail: mark.mcentee@ucc.ie

© The Author(s), under exclusive license to Springer Nature Switzerland AG 2026
C. Malamateniou et al. (eds.), *Artificial Intelligence for Radiographers*,
https://doi.org/10.1007/978-3-032-05080-9_6

Table 6.1 Important AI applications in CT covered in this chapter, with some examples

Main topics	Examples of areas covered
Examination workflow and preparation	*Appointments and Workflows*
	Contrast Media Administration
Positioning	*Auto Positioning and Alignment to the Iso-centre*
Image acquisition, reconstruction and dose reduction	*Protocol Recommendations*
	Automatic Tube Voltage and Current Selection
	Scan Range Optimisation
	Needle Tracking
	Image Reconstruction and Low Dose Scanning
	Artefacts Reduction
	Dose Tracking
Image processing and analysis	*Segmentation*
AI-assisted Diagnosis	*Flagging, Triaging and Detection*
Future Development and Emerging Trends	*CT Radiomics and Radiogenomics*
	Photon counting
	Screening
Challenges and Limitations of AI in CT	*Data Availability, Uniformity and Quality*
	Generalisation and Interpretability
	Ethical and Regulatory Considerations
	Integration with Clinical Workflow

6.2 Examination Workflow and Preparation

6.2.1 Appointments and Workflows

CT departments rely on Radiology Information Systems (RIS) to manage patient appointments, seamlessly integrated with Electronic Health Records (EHR) for patient information retrieval [5]. RIS facilitates scheduling with calendar management, conflict detection, and automated reminders [6]. Patients can book appointments online, improving convenience. Moreover, integration with Picture Archiving and Communication Systems (PACS) ensures efficient image storage, retrieval, and access for radiologists [7], thus enhancing department workflow and communication between clinical practitioners. This improved efficiency is clearly reflected in the reduced report turnaround times. For instance, Tadia (7) reported that after the integration of RIS and PACS, turnaround times dropped significantly—from 6.8 days in 2006 to just 2.2 days in 2011. This demonstrates the positive impact of technological advancements in streamlining radiology workflows.

While these technologies have significantly streamlined workflows, AI has the potential to push these improvements further. Advances in AI, particularly through machine learning (ML) algorithms that simulate intelligent human decisions (e.g., diagnosis, subsequent referrals), have made AI a crucial element of modern healthcare [8]. However, most AI studies remain in experimental settings, with full integration into clinical environments still a challenge [1–3]. The main difficulty lies in integrating AI seamlessly into existing clinical workflows without disruption [9]. When successfully integrated, AI platforms could assist clinicians at each step—vetting unnecessary examinations, suggesting optimal referral pathways, reducing diagnostic delays, ensuring patient safety, and optimising workloads, all while reducing costs for healthcare systems [10].

Furthermore, the convergence of cloud computing and increased bandwidth (internet capacity and speed of data transmission over a network) across Europe has made it possible to integrate digital data into decision-making processes in ways that were previously not feasible [11]. Radiology, which has been digital for decades, is now especially well-positioned to make further strides with the support of AI, enabling personalised radiology for patients and assisting radiologists and radiographers in decision-making. This AI support will enhance accuracy and efficiency, ultimately reducing errors, morbidity, and mortality.

Current imaging practices can be wasteful and of low value when they involve unnecessary repetition of investigations, excessive use of contrast media, performing investigations unlikely to affect patient management, conducting scans too frequently, prescribing suboptimal diagnostic tests, scanning with insufficient clinical information, acting on less specific referral queries, or over-investigating for reassurance of clinicians and patients [12]. Malone et al. highlighted that 20–77% of radiological examinations performed were either inappropriate or unjustified [13]. Referral criteria have been shown to reduce unnecessary examinations [14]; however, these are often considered challenging, and clinicians may become overwhelmed by the complexity of such tools [15]. AI platforms, however, promise

to provide clinicians with a single, integrated, intelligent tool to navigate the referral process, personalising decisions for patients while focusing on the potential diagnosis.

In addition, errors are prevalent throughout healthcare, including radiology. For instance, 30% of cancers detected were visible on previous imaging but were initially missed [16]. AI has been shown to reduce errors and improve accuracy [17]. Beyond that, AI-driven workflow enhancements have been introduced to address inefficiencies in CT practice. Several vendors have developed advanced integration tools aimed at streamlining radiology workflows, reducing reporting times and minimising delays, and optimising clinical efficiency. For example, some vendors have collaborated on deep integration solutions to enhance radiology workflows and alleviate workload challenges [18].

Integrating AI into clinical workflows could significantly enhance diagnostic efficiency and accuracy while reducing the costs associated with errors and delays. These costs include not only financial burdens, but also the impact on patient experience and outcomes, and the often-overlooked emotional toll on patients and their families. As AI-driven workflow solutions continue to evolve, their potential to improve patient care while reducing clinician burnout remains a critical area of ongoing research and development.

6.3 Contrast Media Administration

Sufficient contrast enhancement is crucial for the detection of various radiographic manifestations of disease, such as liver lesions, where at least 50 Hounsfield units (HU) of enhancement are desired [19]. Before the contrast medium is injected, it is essential to assess the risk of contrast-associated acute kidney injury (AKI), which is defined as reduced kidney function with an increase in serum creatinine >0.3 mg/dl (or >26.5 μmol/l), or >1.5 times baseline, within 48–72 h of intravascular administration of a contrast agent [20, 21]. Currently, the estimated glomerular filtration rate (eGFR) is the standard method for assessing renal health before contrast administration. However, new predictive ML models, which incorporate additional features such as age, sex, heart rate, repeat contrast exams, and diabetes status, have been developed. In experimental settings, these models have shown superior ability to predict reduced kidney function and the need for 30-day dialysis following contrast-enhanced CT [22].

Moreover, in clinical practice, body weight is traditionally used to calculate the iodine dose for contrast administration. However, the enhancement achieved is influenced by various technical parameters and patient-related factors, such as height and cardiac output [23, 24]. These factors may also affect the radiomic features derived from the scan. Additionally, iodine is a scarce and costly resource and is considered nephrotoxic [25, 26]. Therefore, ensuring the delivery of minimally acceptable enhancement is crucial. In clinical scenarios where numerous parameters affect enhancement, AI-enabled contrast administration could offer significant benefits by improving both efficacy and safety. One factor that may more accurately guide contrast dose than simple body weight is lean body weight, which results in less variability in enhancement [27]. Lean body weight can be determined from previous or current unenhanced scans using automated body segmentation algorithms [28]. Haubold et al. developed models for contrast dose reduction using generative adversarial networks, demonstrating a 50% reduction in dose while preserving image quality and diagnostic performance [29]. Furthermore, more consistent positioning of the locator scan in bolus tracking can reduce operator-induced variability [30]. ML models that incorporate patient-related factors, imaging parameters, and test bolus features have also been explored for predicting insufficient contrast enhancement in coronary CT, suggesting that patient-specific contrast administration may be improved through such algorithms [31].

6.4 Positioning

6.4.1 Auto-Positioning and Alignment to the Iso-Centre

Modern CT scanners offer several dose-reduction features such as image reconstruction techniques, filters, and automated adjustments [32, 33]. Among these, automatic exposure control (AEC) has shown promise in reducing radiation dose [34, 35]. However, AEC's effectiveness heavily depends on precise patient positioning within the scanner [32, 36].

Suboptimal patient positioning is a well-established contributor to increased radiation dose and compromised image quality [32, 37–39]. Achieving optimal positioning remains challenging even with current laser systems [37, 40]. The ALARA principle (As Low As Reasonably Achievable), or the UK equivalent ALARP (As Low As Reasonably Practicable), emphasises minimising radiation exposure while maintaining high-quality diagnostic images [41].

Recent advancements in CT technology have led to the development of automated patient-centring systems that significantly enhance positioning accuracy [34]. Leveraging AI algorithms, these systems can analyse patient anatomy and automatically adjust positioning to optimise image quality while minimising radiation exposure. These systems use deep learning algorithms, 3D detection cameras, and automatic table adjustments to align patients within the scanner by detecting their body contours, yielding very good results. For instance, a study evaluating a deep neural network for patient positioning in CT imaging found a significant reduction in body centreline positioning error with AI-based methods compared to manual positioning [42]. The AI method achieved an error of 0.75 ± 7.73 mm, while manual positioning resulted in 9.35 ± 14.94 mm, reflecting a 92% reduction in positioning error [42].

Despite these promising results, the impact of auto-centring on radiation dose and image quality has not yet been universally accepted. While some studies suggest potential dose reduction due to better alignment [42, 43], others show minimal or size-dependent effects [33, 44]. The effectiveness of these systems in diverse scenarios, such as emergencies, paediatric patients, or patients with atypical body habitus, disabilities, neurodegenerative disorders, or special positioning needs, requires further exploration. Additionally, their reliability, integration with existing protocols, and impact on workflow efficiency need further evaluation.

In a study comparing conventional workflows with automatic contactless positioning for COVID-19 patients, scan preparation time, including patient positioning and any necessary adjustments before starting the CT scan, was significantly reduced [43]. Their findings suggest that improved patient alignment can reduce radiation dose, even without an operator in the room. However, further research is needed to fully understand the impact and acceptability of these systems from the patient's perspective. While medical imaging can be isolating, reducing human interaction may mitigate infection risks, improve dose efficiency, and enhance image quality and reproducibility in clinical scenarios. However, emergency situations and those involving patients with atypical body habitus, pain, learning disabilities, movement disorders, pregnancy, or paediatric care may still benefit from keeping the human in the loop when it comes to patient positioning for patient safety, comfort, and quality of the examination.

Additionally, concerns regarding the reliability of these systems in various settings, their integration with existing CT protocols, and their overall impact on workflow efficiency and patient throughput remain. Options to override these automated tools should be available to ensure the safety and success of the examination in case the AI system fails. These factors are crucial for the wider adoption of auto-centring technologies.

6.5 Image Acquisition, Reconstruction, and Dose Reduction

6.5.1 Protocol Recommendations

AI tools are being developed to provide protocol recommendations during CT scans across multiple anatomical areas and pathologies. AI can be helpful in optimising imaging protocols, improving diagnostic accuracy, reducing unnecessary exposure to radiation, and personalising imaging settings [45]. For example, some of the AI algorithms can analyse CT images to detect subtle anomalies indicative of illnesses such as pulmonary nodules when a patient presents with suspected lung pathology and then refine the CT protocol recommendations depending on the pathology's individual characteristics [46]. Where a nodule is detected, the AI may recommend changes to scan settings such as slice thickness or contrast enhancement to optimise pathology visualisation and enable accurate diagnosis [47].

Some AI solutions do not directly offer personalised protocols; however, they can consider individual patient factors, such as age, body habitus, and medical history, to recommend personalised scanning protocols or sequences that optimise examination time, dose, and image quality [45]. For example, in the case when a patient has a known history of renal impairment, the AI tool may recommend adjusting the amount of contrast agent administered or scan parameters to minimise the impact on renal function while maintaining diagnostic quality. Additionally, the AI could optimise the window width (WW) and window level (WL) settings for better tissue differentiation, ensuring consistent image quality across all views. The tool can also generate reformatted views with predefined WW/WL settings and automatically transfer them to PACS, improving qualitative image comparison. These tools are powered by deep learning algorithms, such as convolutional neural networks (CNNs) and recurrent neural networks (RNNs) [45, 46]. With the growing demand for patient-centred care, the prospects of personalised scan protocols are very promising.

6.5.2 Automatic Tube Voltage and Current Selection

CT scanners have in the past used manual exposure selection methods, often employing fixed mAs and/or kVp systems across the anatomy under examination. However, the radiation dose was not optimised, impacting negatively on patient radiation dose accumulation [48, 49]. Automatic control (AEC) systems such as the Automatic Tube Current Modulation (also called mA modulation) and Tube Voltage (kV) Selection were introduced. While not standalone traditional AI tools, they leverage computational algorithms to dynamically adjust imaging parameters, contributing to dose optimisation and improved image quality [50]. AEC systems in CT benefit from advanced image processing, with CNNs playing a significant role in optimising and enhancing scan images [50].

Unlike a fixed system, vendors incorporate elements of AI-assisted technologies within the AEC systems of modern CT scanners, allowing particularly the mA modulation to adjust the tube current, based on the different attenuation profiles of different parts of the object to achieve a target image quality throughout the scan [51]. By adapting the mAs, doses and scan time vary according to the object's changing thickness, in contrast to fixed mAs systems where smaller and larger body areas receive similar doses, thereby customising doses. The automated kV, however, does not modulate kV during the scan, as this could result in inconsistent Hounsfield Unit (HU) values within the individual patient. Instead, kV is selected automatically based on the scout scan and clinical task and then fixed for the scan, depending on patient size, while also considering mAs and image quality requirements [52].

Vendors have different approaches to setting the image quality reference parameter the modulation must maintain. Quality reference mAs (effective mAs), reference image, noise index, and standard deviation (or image quality level) of pixel values in patient-equivalent water phantom are the image quality reference parameters used by Siemens, Philips, GE, and Toshiba (now Canon), respectively [51]. CT scanners commonly employ three adaptive AEC techniques: angular (attenuation characteristics vary with the patient's anatomy in different angular positions), longitudinal (mA modulation adapts the tube current based on variations in patient thickness along the z-axis, which is the direction of the scan), and combined modulations (tube current adjustments based on both angular and longitudinal variations in anatomy) [53]. Modern scanners are equipped with organ-based tube current modulation, allowing for a reduction in anterior dose, which has the potential to decrease radiation exposure to radiosensitive organs, such as the breasts and eye lens [49, 54].

6.5.3 Scan Range Optimisation

In CT imaging, the scan range, also referred to as the scan coverage, is typically determined by radiographers [55], taking into account the anatomy of interest and pathology under investigation, as stipulated in the referral. The use of an effective scan length along the z-axis in CT imaging is an efficient dose optimisation method without compromising image quality. However, there are challenges in consistently achieving this by radiographers [56]. In a study conducted by Botwe et al. [56], over 70% of the scans exceeded their predefined anatomic boundaries along the z-axis, resulting in additional radiation doses to patients.

AI models are available to optimise the scan range automatically without compromising image quality. They can automatically determine the optimal scan range based on predefined parameters, the referral, and the patient's anatomy, to guide the radiographer in scanning. For example, Demircioğlu et al. [57] used three different network architectures: Cascade R-CNN, VFNet, and YOLOX to develop AI models for the detection and determination of the required scan range. They concluded that fully automated delimitation of the scan range using a deep neural network such as the AI model VFNet enables a decrease of up to 12.6% of radiation exposure to the patient during CT coronary angiography compared to manual examination planning, with the added advantage of reducing the workload of radiographers. A previous study [58] also reported a reduction of 6%, suggesting that this technology is promising in improving CT imaging practices.

6.5.4 Needle Tracking Algorithm for CT Biopsy and Interventional Procedures

Another AI tool in CT that plays a crucial role in patient safety is the automatic needle tracking algorithm for CT percutaneous biopsy and interventional procedures like *CT-guided spinal* injection [59]. For example, while tissue samples can be obtained in various ways, CT is a vital radiological method for acquiring biological tissues for histopathological analysis, essential for diagnosis and timely treatment [60]. The technique involves advancing a needle into the tissues of interest under CT guidance to obtain a sample. Although percutaneous needle aspiration or core biopsy is a minimally invasive procedure considered essential in diagnosing many conditions, it can be time-consuming, and there is always the potential for extra-target injury, especially when CT fluoroscopy is not used [60].

To mitigate errors and minimise the risk of damaging healthy tissues, multiple CT scans are performed during biopsy procedures to map the position of the needle and the target. However, this increased imaging results in a considerable radiation dose burden for patients. Despite these precautions, errors in needle tip tracking can still occur. One of this chapter's authors witnessed an unfortunate incident in which poor needle tracking nearly caused a patient's death due to an unintended puncture of a major vessel during a biopsy procedure. Various interventions have been explored, including the use of mobile devices [61] and infrared cameras [62] to enhance

needle tip identification during biopsy and interventional procedures. However, these methods still have significant limitations [61–63].

Fortunately, modern automatic needle-tracking AI algorithms for CT biopsy and spinal injection procedures now exist, leveraging advanced image analysis and ML techniques to overcome this challenge. In the case of biopsy, the algorithms are designed to track the position of the biopsy needle in real-time during the procedure, providing precise guidance to the clinician for targeting lesions or tissues of interest [30]. The process involves advanced imaging analysis, computer vision, and deep learning architectures, particularly CNNs, continuously analysing CT images in real-time to extract features and register them with a reference model in CT biopsy procedures [30, 59]. This enables spatial localisation of the needle and calculation of its distance and angle from the skin entry point.

The real-time pixel-level feedback, overlaid on live CT images, guides clinicians, and the system adapts to patient movement, potentially incorporating ML for enhanced accuracy ensuring precise, safe, and efficient CT-guided percutaneous biopsy interventions [30]. There are also CT-guided robotic needle biopsy systems in which the AI-powered robot swiftly advances biopsy needles, and this has been successful in lung biopsies, even though this is not very common [64–66]. These tools have impacted patient safety, where a difference of a few millimetres may cause damage to adjacent structures [67]. Figure 6.1 shows images of automatic needle tracking during the planning, needle tracking phase, and the final stage of a biopsy procedure.

6.5.5 Image Reconstruction and Low Dose Scanning

Producing diagnostic CT images of appropriate quality, devoid of noise for the intended task, while reducing radiation dose, is very important. Despite various efforts to optimise radiation doses in CT scans, achieving this remains challenging. One of these ways is through different image reconstruction methods. Iterative recon-

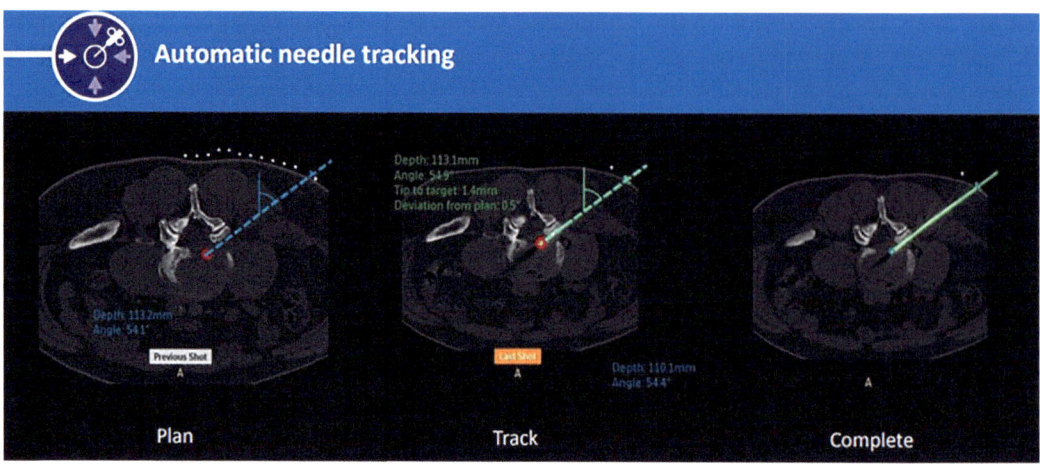

Fig. 6.1 Showing images of automatic needle tracking during the planning phase (plan), the tracking phase (track), and the final stage of the biopsy (Complete). (Source: 'Illustration by courtesy of Koninklijke Philips N.V')

struction refers to techniques that repeatedly refine the image by comparing it to the expected results, reducing noise, and improving image quality. However, the widespread use of iterative reconstruction methods may affect image texture and low-contrast detectability [68], especially when applied at full strength, i.e., without blending with filtered back projection (FBP), a traditional technique that uses mathematical algorithms to create images from raw data.

The resulting images may look unfamiliar to radiologists who perceive images as smooth with little texture, often referred to as '*plastic like*' or '*blotchy*' and therefore, the dose reduction potential of iterative reconstruction comes at a cost to image quality [69]. Changes in scan settings may reduce the dose but can simultaneously increase image noise.

To address this challenge, deep learning-based image reconstruction (DLIR) mechanisms powered by convolutional neural networks (CNN) have been introduced in CT to reduce image noise and enhance image quality by analysing noise profiles within images and subtracting them from the originals [70–73] (Fig. 6.2). The algorithms can work in the projection domain, the image domain, or in a hybrid solution [74]. Application of third-party algorithms working in the image domain results in denoising only, while vendor-specific algorithms with access to raw

data can also improve spatial resolution and edge definition [75].

Before application, the algorithms are trained on numerous images [71], with the specific training approach varying between vendors. Some train the CNN using high-quality filtered back-projection images, while others generate simulated low-dose scans from standard-dose FBP or use phantom images acquired at both high and low doses. In all cases, a noisy image is compared to a low-noise ground truth image [75]. DLIR enables the use of low-dose parameters during data acquisition while still producing low-noise images for intended clinical tasks [71]. Figure 6.3 illustrates a simple example of the denoising AI process, where a low-dose image or sinogram undergoes multiple convolutional operations, with each layer in the network processing a specific feature—such as image texture—ultimately resulting in a denoised image.

CT scans of the abdomen and pelvis account for approximately 50% of the collective CT radiation dose. Deep learning image reconstruction (DLIR) has demonstrated the potential to reduce radiation dose without compromising image quality, contributing to improved patient safety. As a result, DLIR has been applied in numerous clinical examinations. For example, in the detection of low-contrast hepatic metastases, a 50% dose reduction has been achieved while main-

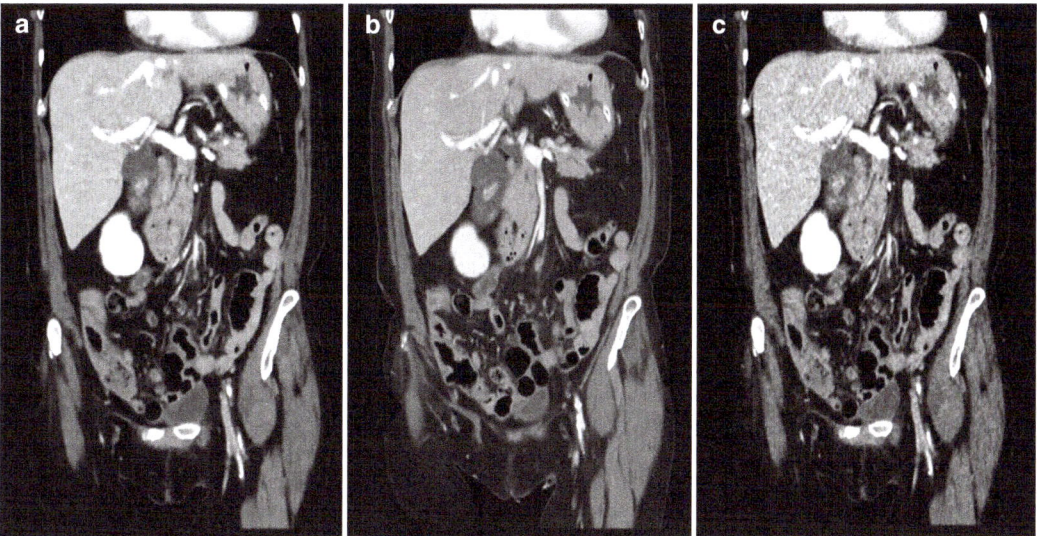

Fig. 6.2 Coronal reformatted 3-mm abdominal CT images of an elderly female patient with a history of a sigmoid resection, presenting with upper abdominal pain for 5 days. (**a**) Standard dose (CTDI$_{vol}$, 6.7 mGy) and medium DLIR strength, noise SD 7.28 HU. (**b**) Low dose (CTDI$_{vol}$, 1.49 mGy) using 50% model-based iterative reconstruction, noise SD 14.28 HU. (**c**) Low dose (CTDI$_{vol}$ (1.49 mGy) and high strength deep learning image reconstruction (DLIR), noise SD 8.95 HU

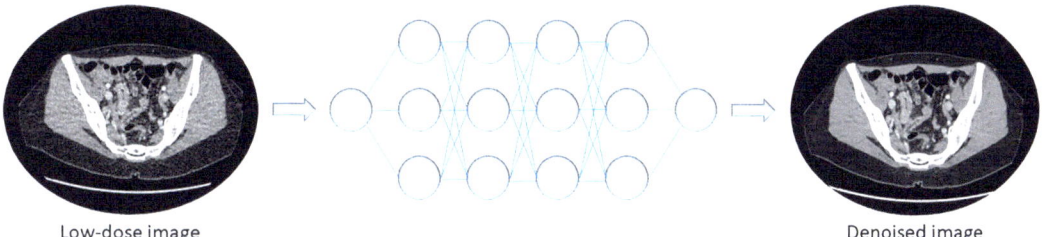

Low-dose image   Denoised image

Fig. 6.3 Deep learning-based denoising can be performed in the image or projection domain. A low-dose image or sinogram undergoes multiple convolutional operations where each layer in the network handles a specific feature, e.g. image texture, resulting in a denoised image

taining image quality comparable to standard-dose filtered back projection (FBP) and standard-dose iterative reconstruction (IR), regardless of tumour size [76]. Notably, despite dose reduction, reader confidence, image quality perception, liver-to-lesion contrast-to-noise ratio (CNR), and lesion conspicuity all showed improvement [76]. Similar benefits have been observed in pancreatic cancer imaging [77, 78]. DLIR has also demonstrated promising results in low-dose chest CT [79, 80] and CT angiography of the lower extremity, where it provided better image quality, reduced noise, sharper delineation of vessel walls, and improved diagnostic accuracy for arterial stenoses [81]. In non-contrast brain CT [82–85], paediatric head CT [86, 87], and CT angiography [88–90], DLIR has been shown to enhance both quantitative and qualitative image quality, as well as the conspicuity of ischemic lesions. However, some disadvantages have been noted, including a slight reduction in the sharpness of fine details and alterations in traditional image metrics such as the noise power spectrum compared to FBP [74]. Additionally,

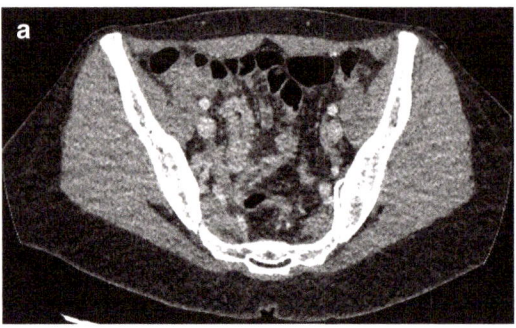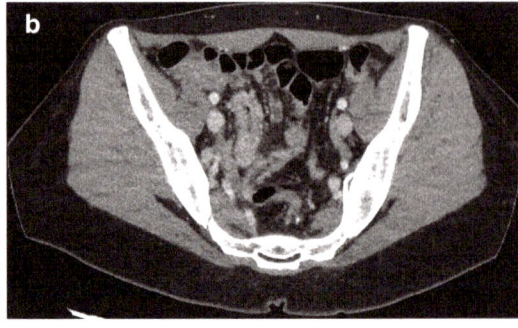

Fig. 6.4 (**a**) Reconstructed with iterative reconstruction. (**b**) Reconstructed with DLIR. A case study of the application of deep learning-based image reconstruction (DLIR).

(Images courtesy of Dr. Anselm Schulz, Department of Radiology and Nuclear Medicine, Oslo University Hospital, Norway)

subtle widespread checkered-line artefacts may occur [91, 92]. A case study of the application of DLIR is presented in Fig. 6.4.

6.5.6 Artefact Reduction

Case Study 1

Use of deep learning-based image reconstruction (DLIR)

Clinical challenge: A 21-year-old female with a history of persistent abdominal pain. Ten months before the examination, she had a negative coloscopy; now presenting with sudden pain in the right lower fossa and was referred for acute abdominal CT with query of appendicitis. Low-dose CT was performed with $CTDI_{vol}$ = 1.3 mGy and reconstruction was done with iterative reconstruction (image 1) and DLIR (image 2).

AI-enabled solution: Use of deep learning-based image reconstruction (DLIR) in abdominal CT

Benefits: Terminal ileitis is apparent in both images, but DLIR demonstrated significantly lower noise levels.

There are many different types of CT artefacts, which originate from different mechanisms, but they can significantly degrade image quality in CT [93]. To overcome some of these problems, CT scanners now use deep learning, CNNs, predictive modelling, and other AI architectures, to detect and correct artefacts during image reconstruction [94, 95]. Despite a reliance on simulated or synthetic data, which may not fully represent real-world CT scans, certain CNNs have been designed to allow for user-controlled reduction in image noise, truncation artefacts, and enhancement of edge sharpness [45].

In the case of metal artefacts, deep learning algorithms, such as CNNs and generative adversarial networks, provide solutions and show promise in overcoming such artefacts and reducing noise [96–99]. However, the difficulty of achieving a balance between removing artefacts while preserving essential tissue information, along with other technical and application challenges, results in the limited generalisation of models and the risks of excessive artefact removal, which may erase essential diagnostic details. Nonetheless, the benefits of a balanced AI-enabled artefact removal are numerous [99, 100]. In particular, these tools may reduce the need for patient repositioning, increasing tube voltage, or using high-energy monoenergetic (monoE) X-ray beams. Monoenergetic beams consist of a single energy level, and when using high-energy X-rays, they help reduce beam hardening artefacts and improve image quality by providing clearer contrast in dense areas, while also mitigating secondary artefacts associated with conventional or projection-based methods [101–104]. This is especially true in the case of sacroiliac joint fusion, where artefacts can be severe [98, 99], as explained further below.

A study by Selles et al. [99] demonstrated the benefit of AI-assisted metal artefact reduction in the image shown in Fig. 6.5, where deep learning-based metal artefact reduction (DL-MAR)-corrected CT images were quantitatively compared with orthopaedic metal artefact reduction (O-MAR)-corrected CT images and uncorrected CT images after sacroiliac joint fusion. They concluded that images corrected with DL-MAR resulted in stronger artifact reduction than images corrected with O-MAR in contralat-

eral bone ($p < 0.001$), ipsilateral gluteus medius ($p = 0.006$), contralateral gluteus medius ($p < 0.001$), ipsilateral iliacus ($p = 0.017$), and contralateral iliacus ($p < 0.001$), while noise was significantly reduced in comparison to images corrected with O-MAR in bone ($p = 0.018$), contralateral bone ($p < 0.001$), contralateral gluteus medius ($p < 0.001$), iliacus ($p < 0.001$), and contralateral iliacus ($p < 0.001$), and also in comparison with uncorrected images.

Motion artefacts, as another example, can also be retrospectively corrected on CT images using deep learning, CNNs, predictive modelling algorithms, and their variants to forecast the expected data of anatomical features while adjusting for motion-related inconsistencies based on gathered data [94, 105, 106]. Moreover, AI-powered systems, such as those used in cardiac CT applications, dynamically track and prospectively adjust for motion during image acquisition [107]. The adaptive nature of AI-driven algorithms allows for real-

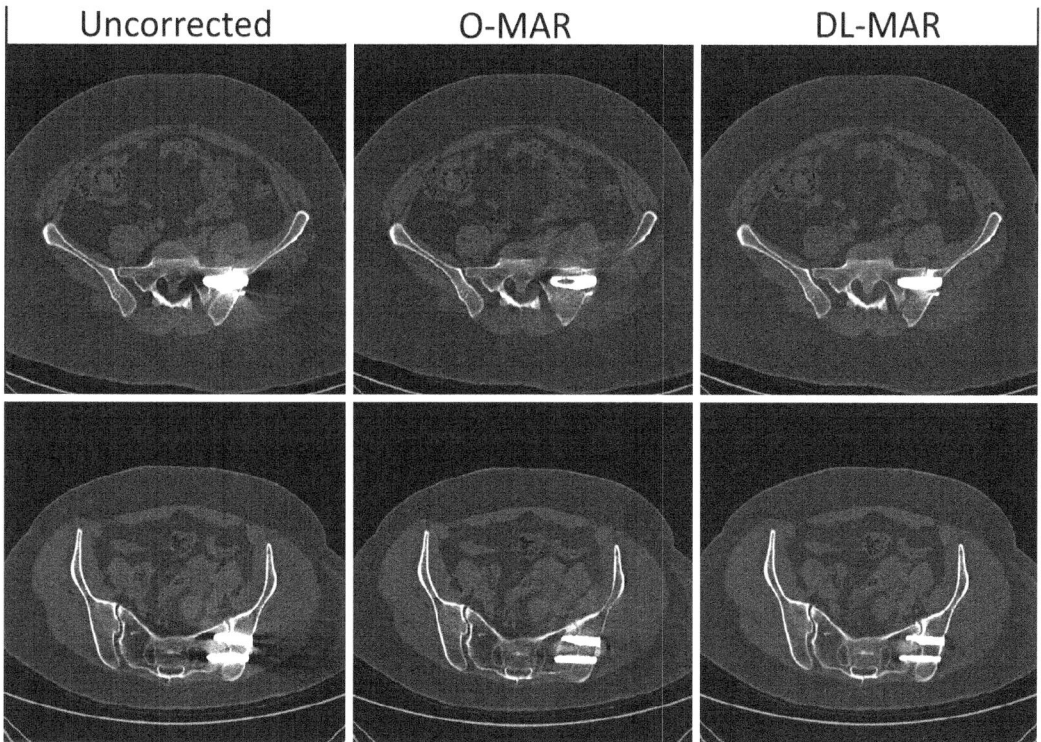

Fig. 6.5 Illustration of the level of artefacts present in CT images, without any metal correction software (uncorrected), with orthopaedic metal artefact reduction (O-MAR)-process and with deep learning-based metal artefact reduction software after sacroiliac (SI) joint fusion [99]

Fig. 6.6 Summarised generic processing steps of AI-enabled motion artefact correction in CT

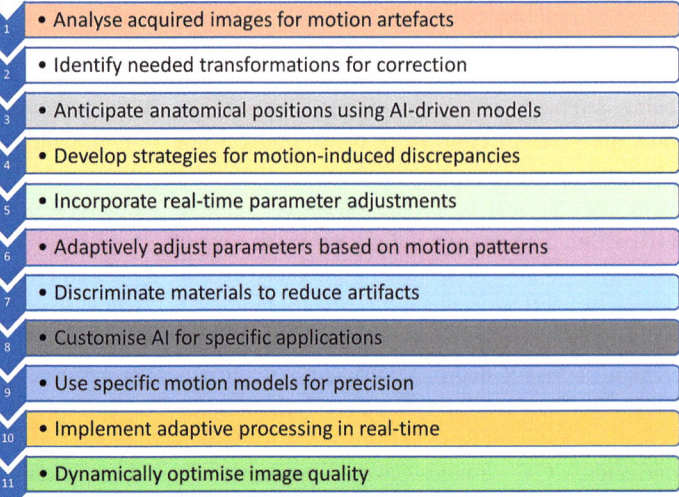

1. • Analyse acquired images for motion artefacts
2. • Identify needed transformations for correction
3. • Anticipate anatomical positions using AI-driven models
4. • Develop strategies for motion-induced discrepancies
5. • Incorporate real-time parameter adjustments
6. • Adaptively adjust parameters based on motion patterns
7. • Discriminate materials to reduce artifacts
8. • Customise AI for specific applications
9. • Use specific motion models for precision
10. • Implement adaptive processing in real-time
11. • Dynamically optimise image quality

time modifications to imaging parameters, optimising image quality despite patient movements [96]. Using vast datasets, AI models generalise motion correction techniques, giving stable solutions across a wide range of clinical circumstances, compensating for motion, and saving a patient from a repeat scan. These clinical circumstances or procedures include cardiac imaging [94], pulmonary angiography [95], Positron Emission Tomography and Computed Tomography (PET-CT) [97], lung CT scans [96], and CT-guided interventions [108], among others. In the case of cardiac CT, for example, deep learning-based motion correction techniques like iterative reconstruction with artefact reduction (iMAR) or deep learning reconstruction (DLR) can examine consecutive CT slices, monitoring the motion of the heart throughout the scan [109]. This enables compensation for blurriness induced by movement, resulting in clearer images of coronary arteries [109].

Of note, different CT vendors present various approaches to how these tools operate on their systems. While some of these AI tools are automated and fully integrated and allow for a zero-click process during the generation of motion-corrected images, others may require radiographers to choose the optimal filtering technique [107]. This means that users must familiarise themselves with the ways of using the software through the operating interfaces provided by different vendors. Additionally, it is

their responsibility to select the right options related to respiratory gating, cardiac gating, or other artefact correction techniques on the scanner or console for the algorithms to work effectively and enable efficient utilisation of the motion reduction tools integrated into the CT scanner. A summary of the generic processing steps of AI-enabled motion artefact correction based on a rapid review of the literature [94, 96, 109] is presented in Fig. 6.6.

6.5.7 Dose Tracking

Optimising Doses with Reference Levels and Monitoring Systems

To address increasing radiation exposure and dose variations [110], Diagnostic Reference Levels (DRLs) have been established and are utilised [111]. Regular audits of delivered doses through DRLs are mandated in Europe to identify high-dose cases and implement reduction strategies [112]. Dose management systems, such as DoseWatch, DoseWise, and Teamplay, have been developed to aid dose auditing and launch and monitor reduction efforts [18, 113–115]. These systems collect, analyse, and report dose data, potentially increasing dose awareness among clinical staff. Although there has been some work on the implementation of such systems, they have not yet been thoroughly studied [116] and there are challenges and opportunities for automated dose monitoring, including the potential for using AI to create alerts and help avoid mistakes and over-radiation of patients.

Automated dose monitoring systems provide real-time feedback to radiographers when radiation exposure exceeds preset limits, triggering red alerts [117]. Their ability to collect, store, and analyse vast amounts of dose data makes them ideal for monitoring purposes. However, integrating these systems into clinical practice poses challenges. The collected data needs careful review, evaluation, and action by CT users, requiring significant changes to workflow and governance. A major challenge in using AI for this purpose is distinguishing true alerts (unjustified high exposures) from false alerts (justifiable high exposures) [116]. Distinguishing unnecessary high exposures from justifiable ones, using dose-tracking devices, is crucial. True alerts may indicate system or protocol errors, while false alerts can be used to refine dose calculations, clean data, and provide operator feedback.

In their 2021 paper, Crowley and colleagues investigate red alerts issued by the DoseWatch software to identify the causes of false alerts and develop mitigation strategies [116]. Additionally, it assessed the effectiveness of a radiographer feedback tool in reducing red alert rates and compared doses triggering red alerts with national benchmarks. They found that '…procedural documentation errors, as well as patient-related factors, are associated with false alerts in DoseWatch…' and '…the implementation of a radiographer feedback tool reduced true alerts…' Thus, in the short term, dose alerts are likely to follow a 'human-in-the-loop approach,' where the system executes the AI model's suggestion only if a qualified human approves it [118, 119]. For an AI system to independently make this determination in the medium to long term, it will need comprehensive data on all aspects of documentation, patient factors, and medical history. The complexity of these factors will need to be addressed in great detail. At present, the system does not have sufficient information, context, or training to interpret the available scanning data, but can be used to create alerts for the clinician's

interpretation and inform proportionate action. These alerts must be useful, or they risk being ignored. Olakotan et al. [120] demonstrate that information may be disregarded unless it adheres to the '5 rights': the right information, person, intervention format, channel, and time.

Predictive Dose Modelling is a potential area where the data is more mature for clinical use. AI models can be trained on historical data to predict the optimal radiation dose for a specific patient and scan type. This personalised approach can help minimise radiation exposure while ensuring sufficient image quality for diagnosis [121].

6.6 Image Processing and Analysis

Segmentation

Interpretation of CT images often requires segmentation to delineate specific anatomical structures or pathological lesions for further analysis [122]. However, the widely used semi-automated methods such as region-growing and threshold-based methods are time-consuming because they often require manual correction of errors and thus are prone to inter-observer variability [123, 124]. Furthermore, lesion edges may be blurred or even embedded in neighbouring tissue of similar attenuation, making manual segmentation challenging. This is often seen in small lung nodules in the hilus area and in iodine contrast-filled vessels adjacent to compact bone structures.

Deep learning (DL) algorithms, such as U-Net, offer automated solutions for CT image segmentation (Fig. 6.7), reducing both image processing and analysis time and variability, and they are applied clinically for many purposes [125, 127]. In cerebral CT, intra-cranial haemorrhage assessment in stroke and head trauma can be performed using DL algorithms [128], and blood vessels may be delineated from non-contrast head CT [129]. In chest CT, nodule segmentation is a crucial part of the classification of nodules into true and false positive findings and can be performed with high DICE similarity coefficients (>92%) [130]. Furthermore, COVID-19-affected lung segments can be visu-

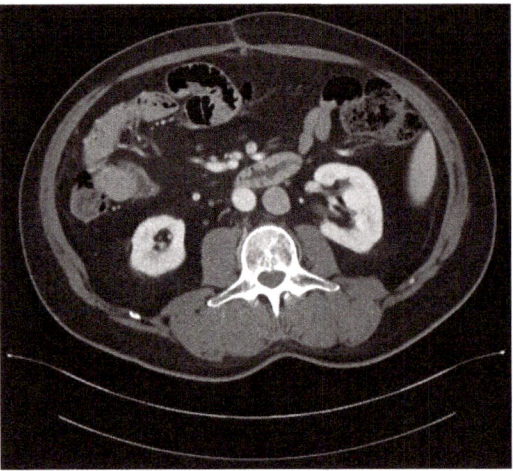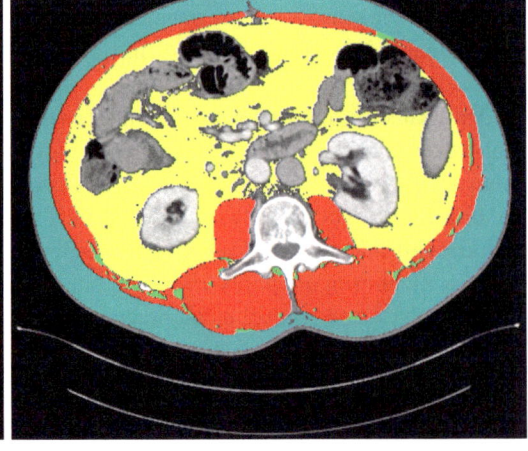

Fig. 6.7 Unsegmented image and AI-assisted segmentation of skeletal muscle (red), visceral adipose tissue (yellow), subcutaneous adipose tissue (green), and intermuscular and intramuscular adipose tissue (green) in abdominal CT. (Adapted from the publication of Alavi et al. [127])

alised, aiding both quantification and diagnosis [122], and lung emphysema can be quantified in chronic obstructive lung disease [126]. In abdominal CT, liver tumours and liver segments can be displayed using DL algorithms [131, 132] and have been suggested as a screening tool for aortic aneurysms [133]. Primary bone tumours and metastases demonstrate broad variation in size and structure and are thus challenging to segment, and though promising, algorithms still need improvement before fully automated methods can be implemented [134]. In maxillo-facial reconstruction, DL-based bone segmentation is crucial in surgical planning as errors may lead to inaccurate implants. Though widely used, there are challenges, especially that the generic DICE similarity coefficient may not always represent clinical relevance within the field [135]. ML and DL are also promising in the segmentation of skeletal muscles, even though the individual shape and similar attenuation of muscles compared with visceral organs may be challenging [136].

As differences in body composition may affect health outcomes, body morphometric analysis using abdominal CT and automated calculation of the cross-sectional area of muscle may contribute to risk stratification [124, 137]. Finally, segmenting organs at risk is widely used in radiation therapy planning, where U-Net is the most used CNN architecture, but others are used, for example, V-Net and Generative Adversarial Networks [138]. Overall, the integration of AI segmentation tools into CT imaging workflow can enhance efficiency by automating repetitive tasks and providing quantitative metrics for image analysis, diagnosis, treatment planning, and assessment.

6.7 AI-Assisted Diagnosis

Several AI applications in radiology have been developed to support reporting radiographers and radiologists in the detection of abnormalities in CT. These tools are primarily utilised in flagging, triaging, detection, diagnosis, and quantitative measurements of abnormalities. These AI algorithms are trained on extensive datasets to recognise patterns associated with abnormalities in medical CT images. They employ ML, deep learning, CNNs, generative adversarial networks (GANs), and other variants of AI, along with image segmentation and pattern recognition techniques, to analyse images and identify regions or patterns indicative of abnormalities [139].

When the AI algorithm detects regions suggestive of abnormalities, it marks or highlights these areas on the medical images for attention. Various approaches are used by different vendors, but all involve a form of notification process that helps automatically identify, alert, classify, and prioritise cases based on the presence of abnormalities, facilitating faster diagnosis and treatment.

In head CT imaging, these tools offer various solutions for clinical decision support, improving detection accuracy across a wide range of clinical findings, including flagging and communicating suspected intracranial haemorrhage [140], detecting occlusions, identifying suspected strokes on CT angiography [141–144], and non-enhanced head CT images [140, 145]. Additionally, AI-driven perfusion maps provide heat maps indicating the probability of hypodensity, outlining infarcted regions to aid acute ischemic stroke assessment [141].

In chest and thoraco-abdominal CT, these tools offer a range of functionalities, including flagging, triaging, detection, classifying, and quantitative measurements of abnormalities such as pulmonary embolism [47, 146, 147], lung lesions or nodules [148, 149], interstitial lung disease, chronic obstructive pulmonary disease (COPD), lung cancer [150], fibrotic conditions [151], aortic dissection [152], and coronary artery disease [153, 154]. They can also detect and prioritise intra-abdominal free gas and rib fractures [155]. Other functionalities include lung cancer screening analysis [156], lung lobe measurements, pneumonia analysis, calcium scoring [149, 157], kidney stone assessment [151], Fractional Flow Reserve CT (FFR-CT), and myocardial perfusion (MP) [158, 159]. They are also a growing area of research on the application of AI in weight-bearing CT WBCT scanners.

Of note with all AI tools is that the accuracy of the results can vary depending on the complexity of the abnormality, hardware and software used, and patient demographics [160]. It may not produce accurate results if the training data is very different from the population the tool is being used on; thus, it is limited to the quality of input CT scans [160]. Moreover, there may be integration challenges with diverse healthcare systems.

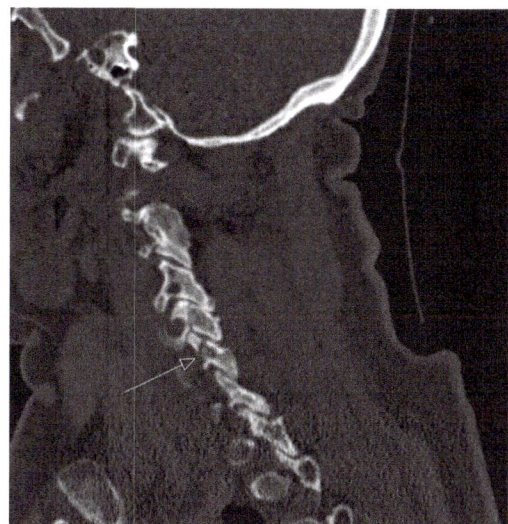

Fig. 6.8 A case study of AI application in fracture detection in CT

Please look more into Chap. 4 about implementation challenges, even if the AI model has been carefully trained and tested.

Figure 6.8 presents a case study of AI application in fracture detection in CT

Case Study 2: AI for Fracture Detection in CT
Clinical challenge: Accurate and timely detection of complex fractures in CT scans is crucial for prompt treatment and care. However, the analysis of trauma CT scans, such as those involving vertebral fractures, can be time-consuming, especially in high-volume settings [161]. Unfortunately, missed fractures may result in prolonged pain, disability, and increased healthcare costs

AI-enabled solution: The use of convolutional neural networks (CNNs) and other AI architecture and image segmentation as well as pattern recognition techniques allow large, trained data processes to flag, triage, and detect different fractures, including occult ones.

Benefits: AI tools are trained to detect specific critical conditions, such as traumatic injuries, acute bleeding, or life-threatening pathologies in CT scans. These

(continued)

tools could assist CT reporting radiographers and radiologists in expediting diagnosis and prioritising critical cases for quick and accurate diagnosis [162]. This can lead to reductions in missed fractures from whole-body CT images and improve workflows and patient care through efficient diagnosis in, for example, polytrauma patients. In a study by Inoue et al. [163], improved sensitivity and precision were observed among orthopaedic surgeons with AI assistance. When assessing fractures, these clinicians displayed variable sensitivities and specificities, both with and without CNN assistance. Without CNN, sensitivity ranged from 58.0% to 85.3%, and specificity from 93.5% to 96.1%. However, with CNN, sensitivity increased to 71.9% to 89.2%, and specificity ranged from 88.5% to 97.6%.

Challenges: The accuracy of the results can vary depending on the complexity of the fracture. It may not produce accurate results if the training data is very different from the population it is being used on (unseen data); thus, it is limited to the quality of input CT scans. This means quality control needs to be put in place before using AI tools for image interpretation purposes. It is important to monitor the AI'S performance over time and track any discrepancies or errors to identify areas for improvement. This further emphasises the importance of maintaining a healthy level of scepticism and not solely relying on AI predictions.

The image here shows an example of a missed fracture by both an attending radiologist and AI emphasising the above point.

Sagittal non-contrast CT view of left-sided C6 facet fracture (annotated with an arrow) in a 66-year-old female patient undetected by both attending radiologist and AI [164]

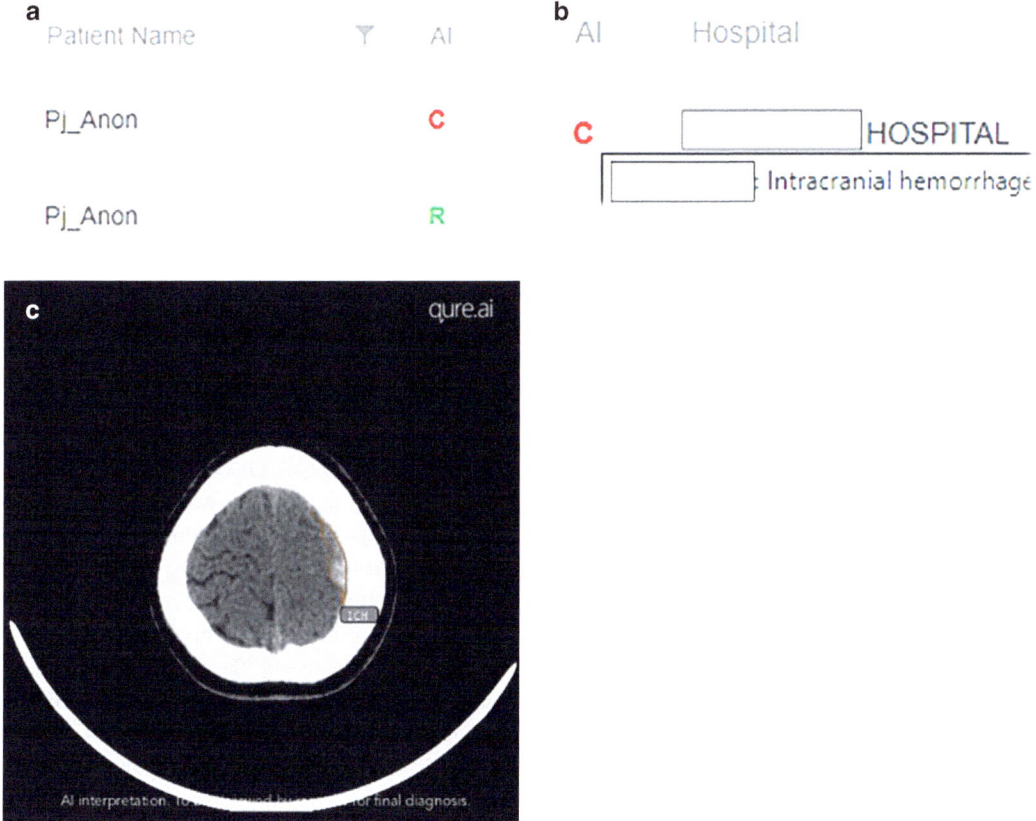

Fig. 6.9 (a–c) A case study of AI application in the rapid detection of a small acute subdural haemorrhage in a CT head scan to support clinical decision making for patient management

Figure 6.9 presents a case study of AI application for the rapid detection of abnormalities in CT head.

Case Study 3: AI for CT Head

Clinical challenge: Computerised tomography (CT) of the head is the most common cross-sectional imaging modality performed in the emergency department (ED) [165]. ED clinicians depend on the non-contrast CT head (NCCTH) report from radiologists to guide their clinical decision [166]. However, radiology services are often unable to provide timely reports, leading to delays in treatment, referral, and discharge decisions [167, 168].

AI-enabled solution: qER AI software developed by qure.Ai for NCCTH is a deep learning-based algorithm using convolutional neural networks (CNNs) techniques, trained on 500,000 NCCTH scans with expert radiologists' annotations as labels to triage, detect, and segment over 10 findings.

Benefits: qER prioritises critical findings such as intracranial haemorrhage, midline shift, mass effect, and fractures by assigning them high priority status on the radiological worklist. Within minutes, qER generates a 'secondary capture' in PACS, visually displaying AI-segmented findings to assist in rapid clinical decision-making.

(continued)

qER has demonstrated diagnostic accuracy with high sensitivity and specificity [169, 171]. When used in conjunction with resident review, qER increases sensitivity from 86% to 95.2% and improves overall diagnostic accuracy to 98.8%, providing valuable support to doctors during out-of-hours shifts and helping to reduce missed findings [170]. Similar improvements have been observed among ED clinicians, with a significant increase in sensitivity for detecting abnormalities, bringing their performance to a level comparable to unaided radiologists [172].

The use of AI triaging in high-volume settings has been shown to reduce turnaround times (TAT) by 6–10 min [173] and to reduce the time to significant intervention for acute stroke suspected patients by approximately 26% [171]. Such tools support faster reporting in environments with high reporting demands. Early diagnosis is particularly beneficial in busy, high-volume departments where resources must be available 24/7 and timely intervention is critical for preventing neurological deterioration and reducing mortality [173].

Challenges: The accuracy of the results can vary depending on the local prevalence and population; thus, a thresholding exercise is undertaken to ensure appropriate balance of sensitivity and specificity as per the use case. It is important to monitor the AI'S performance over time and track any discrepancies to identify areas for improvement.

The CT image is of a 25-year-old male who arrived at ED on a Sunday, after a road traffic accident (RTA), where the qER AI tool detected a small acute subdural Haemorrhage, supporting ED doctors out of hours.

6.8 Future Development and Emerging Trends

6.8.1 Photon-Counting CT Technology

Photon-counting CT technology, known for its superior spatial resolution, dose efficiency, and material decomposition capabilities [174], is a development that has the potential to transform CT imaging. With its detectors' ability to register individual photon interactions, it can detect and classify various energy spectra, providing a detailed material breakdown in scanned areas [174, 175].

The integration of photon-counting CT with deep learning algorithms has the potential to improve image quality by reducing noise, optimising contrast and enhancing workflow efficiency, enabling previously unattainable imaging applications of CT [175]. This fusion allows for more accurate material classification, as well as anatomy and pathology segmentation, thereby supporting lesion detection and the identification of subtle pathological changes—crucial for monitoring conditions like vascular diseases and tumours [175, 176]. Additionally, it facilitates predictive modelling in personalised medicine [177]. A recent study [178] evaluated an AI-based computer-aided detection (CAD) system in photon-counting detector CT (PCD-CT) for pulmonary nodule assessment at different low-dose levels; PCD-CT outperformed energy-integrating detector CT (EID-CT) in subjective image quality with comparable or lower objective image noise. However, attention is needed to address false-positive findings in this maiden research.

6.8.2 CT Radiomics and Radiogenomics

CT radiomics is also rapidly advancing with the integration of AI in imaging. Radiomics involves extracting quantitative imaging features from medical images to characterise tissue properties and their spatial distribution. This method is commonly used to analyse tumour characteristics in CT scans. Radiogenomics, on the other hand, explores the relationships between imaging features and genomic or molecular data [175, 177, 179]. The integration of AI tools such as deep learning algorithms in CT radiomics and radiogenomics helps to automate the extraction and analysis of complex imaging features and reveal new imaging biomarkers [122]. These advancements support personalised medicine and precision oncology and treatment pathways [180].

6.8.3 Screening

Evidence also suggests that as AI tools advance in CT diagnosis and image reporting, screening activities, such as low-dose CT (LDCT) screening for lung cancer, have the potential to expand rapidly in many hospitals [181]. This trend shows promise for a significant reduction in lung cancer morbidity and mortality [182]. Several studies have utilised AI tools, including ML, deep learning, CNNs, Dynamic Bayesian Networks, and others, to develop algorithms capable of identifying specific imaging features from LDCT images related to lung cancer [180, 181, 183, 184]. These algorithms aim to improve the differentiation between benign and cancerous nodules, potentially enhancing cancer screening outcomes [181]. Moreover, efforts are underway to employ AI to identify tissue growth from CT scans [185]. Beyond cancer, novel AI-driven CT of coronary arteries (CTCA) techniques now offer the opportunity for prompt coronary artery screenings [186].

6.9 Challenges and Limitations of AI in CT

AI models in CT have some limitations and challenges. While many have been discussed under various sub-headings above, a few generic ones have been explained below:

(i) *Data Availability, Uniformity, and Quality*

Like the AI tools used in other modalities, CT AI tools are dependent on the quantity, quality, and consistency of input data. This is because unrepresentative, biased, or incomplete data can negatively impact performance and result in inaccurate predictions or biased outcomes that can influence decision-making processes [187].

(ii) *Generalisation and Interpretability*

CT models trained on specific datasets may not generalise successfully to new or unseen data if they were trained on certain datasets. Because patient populations in CT can vary, this can be very problematic. Furthermore, users may find it difficult to trust and accept these AI models due to the lack of transparency surrounding how they make their predictions [188, 189]. More on this can be found in Chap. 4.

(iii) *Ethical and Regulatory Considerations*

Even though there are regulations in place to manage the use of AI tools in CT, and ethical frameworks addressing issues such as data privacy, patient consent, and liability, there are still opportunities for unscrupulous exploitation of data, potentially harming patients or the common good [190]. There is a need for vigilance and oversight by professionals to identify unethical and potentially harmful practices, including but not limited to cybersecurity threats, data breaches, and malicious attacks, associated with AI tools promptly. Chapters 3 and 4 discuss further about ethics and regulation.

(iv) *Integration with Clinical Workflow*

Integrating AI tools seamlessly into existing clinical workflows can be challenging due to a lack of standards for data sharing between digital systems. This is because most radiology practices lack formal frameworks for implementing and governing AI solutions within clinical workflows [191]. Additionally, some AI developers may lack understanding of technologies such as Digital Imaging and Communications in Medicine (DICOM), Picture Archiving and

Communication Systems (PACS), and Vendor Neutral Archives (VNA), leading to offline evaluation of algorithms and creating a gap in a real clinical workflow [192].

ware through the operating interfaces provided by different vendors. They must also be able to make informed choices for the benefit of their patients.

6.10　Chapter Summary

AI tools in CT improve workflows and scan preparation, while also providing precise patient positioning and alignment to ensure consistent and accurate scans. Personalised scanning protocols optimise examination time and image quality, enhancing diagnostic capabilities. AI-driven automated tube voltage and current selection and scan range optimisation ensure efficient and effective imaging without compromising quality. Advanced needle-tracking algorithms improve precision in procedures such as CT biopsies, enhancing patient safety. AI-based image reconstruction reduces noise and artefacts, resulting in clearer and more accurate images with less dose burden. AI-assisted segmentation and diagnosis aid in detecting abnormalities, facilitating timely and accurate diagnosis for improved patient outcomes. Furthermore, there are many areas of AI development in CT, including photon counting, radiomics, radiogenomics, and screening. Challenges remain in data quality, integration with clinical workflows, and ethical considerations, highlighting the need for ongoing research and development in AI implementation in CT.

The integration of AI in CT technology contributes to improving many areas across the CT imaging process and patient journey. Notably, different CT vendors present various approaches to how these tools operate on their systems. While some AI tools are automated, enabling a fully integrated process during the generation of results, others may require the user to choose the optimal technique from a range of different options. Furthermore, many radiation dose alerts serve as warnings, requiring human intervention by the radiographer. This means that while humans remain in the loop for AI-enabled optimisation of scanning, patient experience, and safety, radiographers must familiarise themselves with the optimal and safe use of AI soft-

References

1. IAEA. Radiation protection of patients in the new era of medical imaging [Internet]. 2024 [cited 2024 Dec 20]. Available from: https://www.iaea.org/newscenter/news/radiation-protection-of-patients-in-the-new-era-of-medical-imaging?utm_source=chatgpt.com.
2. World Health Organisation. Strengthening medical imaging [Internet]. 2024 [cited 2024 Feb 29]. Available from: https://www.who.int/activities/strengthening-medical-imaging?utm_source=chatgpt.com.
3. Rud B, Olafsson L, Vejborg TS, Wilhelmsen M, Reitsma JB, Rappeport ED, et al. Diagnostic accuracy of computed tomography for appendicitis in adults. Cochrane Colorectal Cancer Group, editor. Cochrane Database Syst Rev. 2012. [cited 2025 Jan 30]. Available from: https://doi.wiley.com/10.1002/14651858.CD009977
4. Power SP, Moloney F, Twomey M, James K, O'Connor OJ, Maher MM. Computed tomography and patient risk: facts, perceptions and uncertainties. World J Radiol. 2016;8(12):902–15.
5. Ramakrishnan S, Courtney AK, Emick F. Streamlining the workflow at the CT scan area of a healthcare provider. In: IIE annual conference. Proceedings; 2005. p. 1–6.
6. Huang HK. Pacs-based multimedia imaging informatics: basic principles and applications. Wiley; 2019.
7. Vijay Kumar T. Picture archiving and communication systems (PACS): a pre-post comparative analysis. Medico Leg Update. 2021;21(1):1162–7.
8. Cheng JZ, Kim M, Yang X. Editorial: workflow optimisation for radiological imaging. Front Med. 2024;11:1487230.
9. Meng H, Wang TD, Zhuo LY, Hao JW, Sui L-Y, Yang W, et al. Quantitative radiomics analysis of imaging features in adults and children Mycoplasma pneumonia. Front Med. 2024;11:1409477.
10. Lu G, Tian R, Yang W, Liu R, Liu D, Xiang Z, et al. Deep learning radiomics based on multimodal imaging for distinguishing benign and malignant breast tumours. Front Med. 2024;11:1402967.
11. European Commission. Cloud computing. [Internet]. 2024 [cited 2024 Dec 29]. Available from: https://digital-strategy.ec.europa.eu/en/policies/cloud-computing?utm_source=chatgpt.com.
12. Kjelle E, Andersen ER, Krokeide AM, Soril LJJ, Van Bodegom-Vos L, Clement FM, et al. Characterizing and quantifying low-value diagnostic imaging inter-

nationally: a scoping review. BMC Med Imaging. 2022;22(1):73.

13. Malone J, Guleria R, Craven C, Horton P, Järvinen H, Mayo J, et al. Justification of diagnostic medical exposures: some practical issues. Report of an International Atomic Energy Agency Consultation. Br J Radiol. 2012;85(1013):523–38.

14. Del Rosario PM. Referral criteria and clinical decision support: radiological protection aspects for justification. Ann ICRP. 2015;44(1_suppl):276–87.

15. Huber T, Gaskin CM, Krishnaraj A. Early experience with implementation of a commercial decision-support product for imaging order entry. Curr Probl Diagn Radiol. 2016;45(2):133–6.

16. Rawashdeh M, Abdelrahman M, Zaitoun M, McEntee MF, Tapia K, Brennan P. Assessment of Jordanian radiologist performance in the detection of breast cancers. Open J Med Imaging. 2018;08(03):41–53.

17. McKinney SM, Sieniek M, Godbole V, Godwin J, Antropova N, Ashrafian H, et al. International evaluation of an AI system for breast cancer screening. Nature. 2020;577(7788):89–94.

18. GE Healthcare. Addressing radiology workload challenges: GE HealthCare and Sectra plan to leverage deep integration to help enhance clinical efficiency [Internet]. 2023 [cited 2025 Jan 24]. Available from: https://www.gehealthcare.com/about/newsroom/press-releases/addressing-radiology-workload-challenges-ge-healthcare-and-sectra-plan-to-leverage-deep-integration-to-help-enhance-clinical-efficiency?srsltid=AfmBOoryoNURhndlixbLCKBfFJ_lNqfPCU_p6w2NFlIL7YNvtCM.

19. Van Cooten VV, De Jong DJ, Wessels FJ, De Jong PA, Kok M. Liver enhancement on computed tomography is suboptimal in patients with liver steatosis. J Pers Med. 2021;11(12):1255.

20. Mehran R, Dangas GD, Weisbord SD. Contrast-associated acute kidney injury. Ingelfinger JR, editor. N Engl J Med. 2019;380(22):2146–55.

21. Thomsen HS. European Society of Urogenital Radiology (ESUR) guidelines on the safe use of iodinated contrast media. Eur J Radiol. 2006;60(3):307–13.

22. Chen YY, Liu CF, Shen YT, Kuo YT, Ko CC, Chen TY, et al. Development of real-time individualized risk prediction models for contrast associated acute kidney injury and 30-day dialysis after contrast enhanced computed tomography. Eur J Radiol. 2023;167:111034.

23. Bae KT. Intravenous contrast medium administration and scan timing at CT: considerations and approaches. Radiology. 2010;256(1):32–61.

24. Martens B, Hendriks BMF, Wildberger JE, Mihl C. Artificial Intelligence-Based Contrast Medium Optimization. in: De Cecco CN, van Assen M, Leiner T. (eds) artificial intelligence in cardiothoracic imaging. Contemporary medical imaging. Humana, cham. https://doi.org/10.1007/978-3-030-92087-6_16.

25. Gleeson TG, Bulugahapitiya S. Contrast-induced nephropathy. Am J Roentgenol. 2004;183(6):1673–89.

26. Sica GT, Ji H, Ros PR. CT and MR imaging of hepatic metastases. Am J Roentgenol. 2000;174(3):691–8.

27. Ho LM, Nelson RC, DeLong DM. Determining contrast medium dose and rate on basis of lean body weight: does this strategy improve patient-to-patient uniformity of hepatic enhancement during multi-detector row CT? Radiology. 2007;243(2):431–7.

28. de Jong DJ, Veldhuis WB, Wessels FJ, de Vos B, Moeskops P, Kok M. Towards personalised contrast injection: artificial-intelligence-derived body composition and liver enhancement in computed tomography. J Pers Med. 2021;11(3):159.

29. Haubold J, Hosch R, Umutlu L, Wetter A, Haubold P, Radbruch A, et al. Contrast agent dose reduction in computed tomography with deep learning using a conditional generative adversarial network. Eur Radiol. 2021;31(8):6087–95.

30. Li X, Young AS, Raman SS, Lu DS, Lee YH, Tsao TC, et al. Automatic needle tracking using Mask R-CNN for MRI-guided percutaneous interventions. Int J Comput Assist Radiol Surg. 2020;15(10):1673–84.

31. Lopes RR, Van Den Boogert TPW, Lobe NHJ, Verwest TA, Henriques JPS, Marquering HA, et al. Machine learning-based prediction of insufficient contrast enhancement in coronary computed tomography angiography. Eur Radiol. 2022;32(10):7136–45.

32. Kaasalainen T, Palmu K, Lampinen A, Kortesniemi M. Effect of vertical positioning on organ dose, image noise and contrast in pediatric chest CT—phantom study. Pediatr Radiol. 2013;43(6):673–84.

33. Saltybaeva N, Schmidt B, Wimmer A, Flohr T, Alkadhi H. Precise and automatic patient positioning in computed tomography: avatar modeling of the patient surface using a 3-dimensional camera. Investig Radiol. 2018;53(11):641–6.

34. Lell M, Wucherer M, Kachelrieß M. Dosis und Dosisreduktion in der Computertomografie. Radiol Up2date. 2017;17(02):163–78.

35. Schegerer A, Loose R, Heuser LJ, Brix G. Diagnostic reference levels for diagnostic and interventional X-ray procedures in Germany: update and handling. RöFo – Fortschritte Auf Dem Geb Röntgenstrahlen Bildgeb Verfahr. 2019;191(08):739–51.

36. Gudjonsdottir J, Svensson JR, Campling S, Brennan PC, Jonsdottir B. Efficient use of automatic exposure control systems in computed tomography requires correct patient positioning. Acta Radiol. 2009;50(9):1035–41.

37. Al-Hayek Y, Zheng X, Hayre C, Spuur K. The influence of patient positioning on radiation dose in CT imaging: a narrative review. J Med Imaging Radiat Sci. 2022;53(4):737–47.

38. Manava P, Galster M, Ammon J, Singer J, Lell MM, Rieger V. Optimized camera-based patient positioning in CT: impact on radiation exposure. Investig Radiol. 2023;58(2):126–30.

39. Eberhard M, Blüthgen C, Barth BK, Frauenfelder T, Saltybaeva N, Martini K. Vertical off-centering in reduced dose chest-CT: impact on effective dose and image noise values. Acad Radiol. 2020;27(4):508–17.

40. Newman B, Callahan MJ. ALARA (as low as reasonably achievable) CT 2011—executive summary. Pediatr Radiol. 2011;41(S2):453–5.

41. Health and Safety Executive (HSE). Ionising radiations regulations 2017 (IRR 2017) [Internet]. 2017 [cited 2024 Sep 23]. Available from: https://www.hse.gov.uk/pubns/priced/l121.pdf.

42. Salimi Y, Shiri I, Akavanallaf A, Mansouri Z, Arabi H, Zaidi H. Fully automated accurate patient positioning in computed tomography using anterior–posterior localizer images and a deep neural network: a dual-center study. Eur Radiol. 2023;33(5):3243–52.

43. Gang Y, Chen X, Wang H, Li J, Guo Y, Wen B, et al. Accurate and efficient pulmonary CT imaging workflow for COVID-19 patients by the combination of intelligent guided robot and automatic positioning technology. Intell Med. 2021;1(1):3–9.

44. Booij R. The "Knowledgeable" CT scanner optimization by technological advancements [Internet]. 2021. Available from: https://repub.eur.nl/pub/133040/Ronald-Booij-proefschrift-compleet-definitief.pdf.

45. Paudyal R, Shah AD, Akin O, Do RKG, Konar AS, Hatzoglou V, et al. Artificial Intelligence in CT and MR imaging for oncological applications. Cancer. 2023;15(9):2573.

46. Aidoc. Radiologists' Go-To AI Solution [Internet]. 2023 [cited 2023 Jan 2]. Available from: https://www.aidoc.com/solutions/radiology/.

47. Kim Y, Park JY, Hwang EJ, Lee SM, Park CM. Applications of artificial intelligence in the thorax: a narrative review focusing on thoracic radiology. J Thorac Dis. 2021;13(12):6943–62.

48. Bebbington NA, Jørgensen T, Dupont E, Micheelsen MA. Validation of CARE kV automated tube voltage selection for PET-CT: PET quantification and CT radiation dose reduction in phantoms. EJNMMI Phys. 2021;8(1):29.

49. Papadakis AE, Damilakis J. Evaluation of an organ-based tube current modulation tool in pediatric CT examinations. Eur Radiol. 2020;30(10):5728–37.

50. Kalra MK, Rajiah R. CT dose reduction and optimization: a comprehensive guide to CT dose reduction principles. Berlin: Springer; 2018.

51. Merzan D, Nowik P, Poludniowski G, Bujila R. Evaluating the impact of scan settings on automatic tube current modulation in CT using a novel phantom. Br J Radiol. 2017;90(1069):20160308.

52. Mussmann B, Widmann G, Origgi D. Optimisation in automated tube voltage selection. ESR Eurosafe Imaging [Internet]. 2020 [cited 2024 Sep 20]. Available from: https://www.eurosafeimaging.org/wp/wp-content/uploads/2020/02/Automated-tube-voltage.pdf.

53. Van Straten M, Deak P, Shrimpton PC, Kalender WA. The effect of angular and longitudinal tube current modulations on the estimation of organ and effective doses in x-ray computed tomography. Med Phys. 2009;36(11):4881–9.

54. Mussmann BR, Mørup SD, Skov PM, Foley S, Brenøe AS, Eldahl F, et al. Organ-based tube current modulation in chest CT. A comparison of three vendors. Radiography. 2021;27(1):1–7.

55. Demircioğlu A, Bos D, Demircioğlu E, Qaadan S, Glasmachers T, Bruder O, et al. Deep learning–based scan range optimization can reduce radiation exposure in coronary CT angiography. Eur Radiol. 2024;34:411–21.

56. Botwe BO, Schandorf C, Inkoom S, Faanu A. Variability of redundant scan coverages along the Z-axis and dose implications for common computed tomography examinations. J Med Imaging Radiat Sci. 2022;53(1):113–22.

57. Demircioğlu A, Bos D, Demircioğlu E, Qaadan S, Glasmachers T, Bruder O, et al. Deep learning-based scan range optimization can reduce radiation exposure in coronary CT angiography. Eur Radiol. 2024;34(1):411–21.

58. Demircioğlu A, Kim MS, Stein CM, Guberina N, Umutlu L, Nassenstein K. Automatic scan range delimitation in chest CT using deep learning. Radiol Artif Intell. 2021;3(3):e200211.

59. Gulamhussene G, Das A, Spiegel J, Punzet D, Rak M, Hansen C. Needle tip tracking during CT-guided interventions using fuzzy segmentation. In: Deserno TM, Handels H, Maier A, Maier-Hein K, Palm C, Tolxdorff T, editors. Bildverarbeitung für die Medizin 2023 [Internet]. Wiesbaden: Springer Fachmedien Wiesbaden; 2023. p. 285–91. [cited 2025 Jan 30] (Informatik aktuell). Available from: https://link.springer.com/10.1007/978-3-658-41657-7_62.

60. Lehmann S, Frank N. An overview of percutaneous CT-guided lung biopsies. J Radiol Nurs. 2018;37(1):2–8.

61. Xu S, Krishnasamy V, Levy E, Li M, Tse ZTH, Wood BJ. Smartphone-guided needle angle selection during CT-guided procedures. Am J Roentgenol. 2018;210(1):207–13.

62. Shar B, Leis J, Coucher J. Infrared needle mapping to assist biopsy procedures and training. Healthc Technol Lett. 2018;5(2):65–9.

63. Shahriari N, Hekman E, Oudkerk M, Misra S. Design and evaluation of a computed tomography (CT)-compatible needle insertion device using an electromagnetic tracking system and CT images. Int J Comput Assist Radiol Surg. 2015;10(11):1845–52.

64. Liu J, Jiang Y, He R, Cui F, Lin Y, Xu K, et al. Robotic-assisted navigation system for preoperative lung nodule localization: a pilot study. Transl Lung Cancer Res. 2023;12(11):2283–93.

65. Wei L, Jiang S, Yang Z, Zhang G, Ma L. A CT-guided robotic needle puncture method for lung tumours with respiratory motion. Phys Med. 2020;73:48–56.

66. Hiraki T, Kamegawa T, Matsuno T, Komaki T, Sakurai J, Kanazawa S. Zerobot®: a remote-controlled robot for needle insertion in CT-guided

Interventional Radiology Developed at Okayama University [Internet]. Okayama University Medical School; 2018 [cited 2025 Jan 30]. Available from: https://doi.org/10.18926/AMO/56370.

67. Philips. Advancing interventional CT: Precise Intervention [Internet]. 2021 [cited 2014 May 11]. Available from: https://www.philips.co.uk/c-dam/b2bhc/master/resource-catalog/landing/precise-suite/incisive_interventional.download.pdf.

68. Njølstad T, Schulz A, Godt JC, Brøgger HM, Johansen CK, Andersen HK, et al. Improved image quality in abdominal computed tomography reconstructed with a novel deep learning image reconstruction technique—initial clinical experience. Acta Radiol Open. 2021;10(4):20584601211008391.

69. Greffier J, Hamard A, Pereira F, Barrau C, Pasquier H, Beregi JP, et al. Image quality and dose reduction opportunity of deep learning image reconstruction algorithm for CT: a phantom study. Eur Radiol. 2020;30(7):3951–9.

70. Missert AD, Yu L, Leng S, Fletcher JG, McCollough CH. Synthesizing images from multiple kernels using a deep convolutional neural network. Med Phys. 2020;47(2):422–30.

71. McCollough CH, Leng S. Use of artificial intelligence in computed tomography dose optimisation. Ann ICRP. 2020;49(1_suppl):113–25.

72. Chen H, Zhang Y, Zhang W, Liao P, Li K, Zhou J, et al. aLow-dose CT via convolutional neural network. Biomed Opt Express. 2017;8(2):679–94.

73. Chen M, Pu YF, Bai YC. Low-dose CT image denoising using residual convolutional network with fractional TV loss. Neurocomputing. 2021;452:510–20.

74. Koetzier LR, Mastrodicasa D, Szczykutowicz TP, Van Der Werf NR, Wang AS, Sandfort V, et al. Deep learning image reconstruction for CT: technical principles and clinical prospects. Radiology. 2023;306(3):e221257.

75. Brady SL. Implementation of AI image reconstruction in CT—how is it validated and what dose reductions can be achieved. Br J Radiol. 2023;96(1150):20220915.

76. Lyu P, Liu N, Harrawood B, Solomon J, Wang H, Chen Y, et al. Is it possible to use low-dose deep learning reconstruction for the detection of liver metastases on CT routinely? Eur Radiol. 2022;33(3):1629–40.

77. Lyu P, Neely B, Solomon J, Rigiroli F, Ding Y, Schwartz FR, et al. Effect of deep learning image reconstruction in the prediction of resectability of pancreatic cancer: diagnostic performance and reader confidence. Eur J Radiol. 2021;141:109825.

78. Noda Y, Iritani Y, Kawai N, Miyoshi T, Ishihara T, Hyodo F, et al. Deep learning image reconstruction for pancreatic low-dose computed tomography: comparison with hybrid iterative reconstruction. Abdom Radiol. 2021;46(9):4238–44.

79. Jiang JM, Miao L, Liang X, Liu ZH, Zhang L, Li M. The value of deep learning image reconstruction in improving the quality of low-dose chest CT images. Diagnostics. 2022;12(10):2560.

80. Zhao K, Jiang B, Zhang S, Zhang L, Zhang L, Feng Y, et al. Measurement accuracy and repeatability of RECIST-defined pulmonary lesions and lymph nodes in ultra-low-dose CT based on deep learning image reconstruction. Cancer. 2022;14(20):5016.

81. Qu T, Guo Y, Li J, Cao L, Li Y, Chen L, et al. Iterative reconstruction *vs* deep learning image reconstruction: comparison of image quality and diagnostic accuracy of arterial stenosis in low-dose lower extremity CT angiography. Br J Radiol. 2022;95(1140):20220196.

82. Cozzi A, Cè M, De Padova G, Libri D, Caldarelli N, Zucconi F, et al. Deep learning-based versus iterative image reconstruction for unenhanced brain CT: a quantitative comparison of image quality. Tomography. 2023;9(5):1629–37.

83. Okimoto N, Yasaka K, Fujita N, Watanabe Y, Kanzawa J, Abe O. Deep learning reconstruction for improving the visualization of acute brain infarct on computed tomography. Neuroradiology. 2024;66(1):63–71.

84. Oostveen LJ, Meijer FJA, De Lange F, Smit EJ, Pegge SA, Steens SCA, et al. Deep learning–based reconstruction may improve non-contrast cerebral CT imaging compared to other current reconstruction algorithms. Eur Radiol. 2021;31(8):5498–506.

85. Pula M, Kucharczyk E, Zdanowicz A, Guzinski M. Image quality improvement in deep learning image reconstruction of head computed tomography examination. Tomography. 2023;9(4):1485–93.

86. Lee N, Cho HH, Lee SM, You SK. Adaptation of deep learning image reconstruction for pediatric head CT: a focus on the image quality. J Korean Soc Radiol. 2023;84(1):240–52.

87. Sun J, Li H, Wang B, Li J, Li M, Zhou Z, et al. Application of a deep learning image reconstruction (DLIR) algorithm in head CT imaging for children to improve image quality and lesion detection. BMC Med Imaging. 2021;21(1):108.

88. Bernard A, Comby PO, Lemogne B, Haioun K, Ricolfi F, Chevallier O, et al. Deep learning reconstruction versus iterative reconstruction for cardiac CT angiography in a stroke imaging protocol: reduced radiation dose and improved image quality. Quant Imaging Med Surg. 2021;11(1):392–401.

89. Lei L, Zhou Y, Guo X, Wang L, Zhao X, Wang H, et al. The value of a deep learning image reconstruction algorithm in whole-brain computed tomography perfusion in patients with acute ischemic stroke. Quant Imaging Med Surg. 2023;13(12):8173–89.

90. Otgonbaatar C, Ryu JK, Kim S, Seo JW, Shim H, Hwang DH. Improvement of depiction of the intracranial arteries on brain CT angiography using deep learning reconstruction. J Integr Neurosci. 2021;20(4):967–76.

91. Agostini A, Borgheresi A, Granata V, Bruno F, Palumbo P, De Muzio F, et al. Technological

advances in body CT: a primer for beginners. Eur Rev Med Pharmacol Sci. 2022;26(21):7918–37.

92. Nam JG, Hong JH, Kim DS, Oh J, Goo JM. Deep learning reconstruction for contrast-enhanced CT of the upper abdomen: similar image quality with lower radiation dose in direct comparison with iterative reconstruction. Eur Radiol. 2021;31(8):5533–43.

93. Alzain AF, Elhussein N, Fadulelmulla IA, Ahmed AM, Elbashir ME, Elamin BA. Common computed tomography artifact: source and avoidance. Egypt J Radiol Nucl Med. 2021;52(1):151.

94. Lossau T, Nickisch H, Wissel T, Bippus R, Schmitt H, Morlock M, et al. Motion artifact recognition and quantification in coronary CT angiography using convolutional neural networks. Med Image Anal. 2019;52:68–79.

95. Dasegowda G, Bizzo BC, Kaviani P, Karout L, Ebrahimian S, Digumarthy SR, et al. Auto-detection of motion artifacts on CT pulmonary angiograms with a physician-trained AI algorithm. Diagnostics. 2023;13(4):778.

96. Kim D, Choi J, Lee D, Kim H, Jung J, Cho M, et al. Motion correction for routine X-ray lung CT imaging. Sci Rep. 2021;11(1):3695.

97. Arabi H, Zaidi H. Deep learning–based metal artefact reduction in PET/CT imaging. Eur Radiol. 2021;31(8):6384–96.

98. Selles M, Korte JH, Boelhouwers HJ, Nijholt IM, Van Osch JAC, Nijveldt RJ, et al. Metal artifact reduction in computed tomography: is it of benefit in evaluating sacroiliac joint fusion? Eur J Radiol. 2022;148:110159.

99. Selles M, Slotman DJ, Van Osch JAC, Nijholt IM, Wellenberg RHH, Maas M, et al. Is AI the way forward for reducing metal artifacts in CT? Development of a generic deep learning-based method and initial evaluation in patients with sacro-iliac joint implants. Eur J Radiol. 2023;163:110844.

100. Gjesteby L, Yang Q, Xi Y, Claus BEH, Jin Y, De Man B, et al. Deep learning methods for CT image-domain metal artifact reduction. In: Müller B, Wang G, editors. Developments in X-ray tomography XI [Internet]. San Diego: SPIE; 2017. p. 31. [cited 2025 Jan 30]. Available from: https://www.spiedigitallibrary.org/conference-proceedings-of-spie/10391/2274427/Deep-learning-methods-for-CT-image-domain-metal-artifact-reduction/10.1117/12.2274427.full.

101. Wellenberg RHH. Reducing metal artefacts and radiation dose in musculoskeletal CT imaging [Internet] [PhD]. [Faculty of Medicine (AMC-UvA)]: University of Amsterdam; 2018. Available from: https://dare.uva.nl/search?identifier=db9e26c0-499f-4f54-a899-2c425ecb4a37.

102. Bolstad K, Flatabø S, Aadnevik D, Dalehaug I, Vetti N. Metal artifact reduction in CT, a phantom study: subjective and objective evaluation of four commercial metal artifact reduction algorithms when used on three different orthopedic metal implants. Acta Radiol. 2018;59(9):1110–8.

103. Pessis E, Sverzut JM, Campagna R, Guerini H, Feydy A, Drapé JL. Reduction of metal artifact with dual-energy CT: virtual Monospectral imaging with fast Kilovoltage switching and metal artifact reduction software. Semin Musculoskelet Radiol. 2015;19(05):446–55.

104. Andersson KM, Nowik P, Persliden J, Thunberg P, Norrman E. Metal artefact reduction in CT imaging of hip prostheses—an evaluation of commercial techniques provided by four vendors. Br J Radiol. 2015;88(1052):20140473.

105. Ren P, He Y, Zhu Y, Zhang T, Cao J, Wang Z, et al. Motion artefact reduction in coronary CT angiography images with a deep learning method. BMC Med Imaging. 2022;22(1):184.

106. Elss T, Nickisch H, Wissel T, Schmitt H, Vembar M, Morlock MM, et al. Deep-learning-based CT motion artifact recognition in coronary arteries. In: Angelini ED, Landman BA, editors. Medical imaging 2018: image processing. Houston: SPIE; 2018. p. 41. [cited 2025 Jan 30]. Available from: https://www.spiedigitallibrary.org/conference-proceedings-of-spie/10574/2292882/Deep-learning-based-CT-motion-artifact-recognition-in-coronary-arteries/10.1117/12.2292882.full.

107. Gong H, Ahmed Z, Thorne J, Fletcher JG, McCollough CH, Leng S. Improving coronary artery imaging in single source CT with cardiac motion correction using attention and spatial transformer based neural networks. In: Zhao W, Yu L, editors. Medical imaging 2022: physics of medical imaging [Internet]. San Diego: SPIE; 2022. p. 71. [cited 2025 Jan 30] Available from: https://www.spiedigitallibrary.org/conference-proceedings-of-spie/12031/2611794/Improving-coronary-artery-imaging-in-single-source-CT-with-cardiac/10.1117/12.2611794.full.

108. Vernikouskaya I, Bertsche D, Rottbauer W, Rasche V. Deep learning-based framework for motion-compensated image fusion in catheterization procedures. Comput Med Imaging Graph. 2022;98:102069.

109. Shuai T, Zhong S, Zhang G, Wang Z, Zhang Y, Li Z. Deep learning–based motion correction in projection domain for coronary computed tomography angiography: a clinical evaluation. J Comput Assist Tomogr. 2023;47(6):898–905.

110. Mettler FA, Mahesh M, Bhargavan-Chatfield M, Chambers CE, Elee JG, Frush DP, et al. Patient exposure from radiologic and nuclear medicine procedures in the United States: procedure volume and effective dose for the period 2006–2016. Radiology. 2020;295(2):418–27.

111. Vañó E, Miller DL, Martin CJ, Rehani MM, Kang K, Rosenstein M, et al. ICRP publication 135: diagnostic reference levels in medical imaging. Ann ICRP. 2017;46(1):1–144.

112. European Commission. European Commission. Radiation Protection No 185, European guidelines on diagnostic reference levels for paediatric imaging [Internet]. 2018 [cited 2024 Oct 24]. Available from:

https://www.eurosafeimaging.org/wp/wp-content/uploads/2018/09/rp_185.pdf.

113. NICE. Radiation dose monitoring software for medical imaging with ionising radiation [Internet]. 2017 [cited 2024 Dec 20]. Available from: nice.org.uk/guidance/mib127.

114. Philips. DoseWise Education [Internet]. 2022 [cited 2023 Oct 20]. Available from: https://www.learning-connection.philips.com/en/dosewise-education.

115. Siemens. Teamplay Dose [Internet]. 2024 [cited 2024 Dec 12]. Available from: https://www.siemens-healthineers.com/en-uk/digital-health-solutions/teamplay-performance-management-applications/teamplay-dose-management-excellence.

116. Crowley C, Ekpo EU, Carey BW, Joyce S, Kennedy C, Grey T, et al. Radiation dose tracking in computed tomography: red alerts and feedback. Implementing a radiation dose alert system in CT. Radiography. 2021;27(1):67–74.

117. Parakh A, Euler A, Szucs-Farkas Z, Schindera ST. Transatlantic comparison of CT radiation doses in the era of radiation dose–tracking software. Am J Roentgenol. 2017;209(6):1302–7.

118. Parasuraman R, Sheridan TB, Wickens CD. A model for types and levels of human interaction with automation. IEEE Trans Syst Man Cybern – Part Syst Hum. 2000;30(3):286–97.

119. Parasuraman R. Designing automation for human use: empirical studies and quantitative models. Ergonomics. 2000;43(7):931–51.

120. Olakotan OO, Yusof MM. Evaluating the alert appropriateness of clinical decision support systems in supporting clinical workflow. J Biomed Inform. 2020;106:103453.

121. Ng CKC. Artificial intelligence for radiation dose optimization in pediatric radiology: a systematic review. Children. 2022;9(7):1044.

122. Shi F, Wang J, Shi J, Wu Z, Wang Q, Tang Z, et al. Review of artificial intelligence techniques in imaging data acquisition, segmentation, and diagnosis for COVID-19. IEEE Rev Biomed Eng. 2021;14:4–15.

123. Moghbel M, Mashohor S, Mahmud R, Saripan MIB. Review of liver segmentation and computer assisted detection/diagnosis methods in computed tomography. Artif Intell Rev. 2018;50(4):497–537.

124. Lee H, Troschel FM, Tajmir S, Fuchs G, Mario J, Fintelmann FJ, et al. Pixel-level deep segmentation: artificial intelligence quantifies muscle on computed tomography for body morphometric analysis. J Digit Imaging. 2017;30(4):487–98.

125. Bonaldi L, Pretto A, Pirri C, Uccheddu F, Fontanella CG, Stecco C. Deep learning-based medical images segmentation of musculoskeletal anatomical structures: a survey of bottlenecks and strategies. Bioengineering. 2023;10(2):137.

126. Fischer AM, Varga-Szemes A, Martin SS, Sperl JI, Sahbaee P, Neumann D, et al. Artificial intelligence-based fully automated per Lobe segmentation and emphysema-quantification based on chest computed tomography compared with global initiative for chronic obstructive lung disease severity of smokers. J Thorac Imaging. 2020;35(Supplement 1):S28–34.

127. Alavi DH, Sakinis T, Henriksen HB, Beichmann B, Fløtten A, Blomhoff R, et al. Body composition assessment by artificial intelligence from routine computed tomography scans in colorectal cancer: introducing BodySegAI. JCSM Clin Rep. 2022;7(3):55–64.

128. MacIntosh BJ, Liu Q, Schellhorn T, Beyer MK, Groote IR, Morberg PC, et al. Radiological features of brain hemorrhage through automated segmentation from computed tomography in stroke and traumatic brain injury. Front Neurol. 2023;14:1244672.

129. Klimont M, Oronowicz-Jaśkowiak A, Flieger M, Rzeszutek J, Juszkat R, Jończyk-Potoczna K. Deep learning for cerebral angiography segmentation from non-contrast computed tomography. Su Y, editor. PLoS One. 2020;15(7):e0237092.

130. De Margerie-Mellon C, Chassagnon G. Artificial intelligence: a critical review of applications for lung nodule and lung cancer. Diagn Interv Imaging. 2023;104(1):11–7.

131. Lakshmipriya B, Pottakkat B, Ramkumar G. Deep learning techniques in liver tumour diagnosis using CT and MR imaging – a systematic review. Artif Intell Med. 2023;141:102557.

132. Spinella G, Fantazzini A, Finotello A, Vincenzi E, Boschetti GA, Brutti F, et al. Artificial intelligence application to screen abdominal aortic aneurysm using computed tomography angiography. J Digit Imaging. 2023;36(5):2125–37.

133. Artzner C, Bongers MN, Kärgel R, Faby S, Hefferman G, Herrmann J, et al. Assessing the accuracy of an artificial intelligence-based segmentation algorithm for the thoracic aorta in computed tomography applications. Diagnostics. 2022;12(8):1790.

134. Paranavithana IR, Stirling D, Ros M, Field M. Systematic review of tumor segmentation strategies for bone metastases. Cancer. 2023;15(6):1750.

135. Minnema J, Ernst A, Van Eijnatten M, Pauwels R, Forouzanfar T, Batenburg KJ, et al. A review on the application of deep learning for CT reconstruction, bone segmentation and surgical planning in oral and maxillofacial surgery. Dentomaxillofacial Radiol. 2022;51(7):20210437.

136. Kamiya N. Muscle segmentation for orthopedic interventions. In: Zheng G, Tian W, Zhuang X, editors. Intelligent orthopaedics: artificial intelligence and smart image-guided technology for orthopaedics. Singapore: Springer Singapore; 2018. p. 81–91.

137. Bousson V, Benoist N, Guetat P, Attané G, Salvat C, Perronne L. Application of artificial intelligence to imaging interpretations in the musculoskeletal area: where are we? Where are we going? Joint Bone Spine. 2023;90(1):105493.

138. Samarasinghe G, Jameson M, Vinod S, Field M, Dowling J, Sowmya A, et al. Deep learning for segmentation in radiation therapy planning: a review. J Med Imaging Radiat Oncol. 2021;65(5):578–95.

139. Topff L, Ranschaert ER, Bartels-Rutten A, Negoita A, Menezes R, Beets-Tan RGH, et al. Artificial intelligence tool for detection and worklist prioritization reduces time to diagnosis of incidental pulmonary embolism at CT. Radiol Cardiothorac Imaging. 2023;5(2):e220163.

140. Seyam M, Weikert T, Sauter A, Brehm A, Psychogios MN, Blackham KA. Utilization of artificial intelligence–based intracranial hemorrhage detection on emergent noncontrast CT images in clinical workflow. Radiol Artif Intell. 2022;4(2):e210168.

141. Ayobi A. Validation of a deep learning AI-based software for automated ASPECTS assessment. 2023; 1660 words.

142. Hillal A, Sultani G, Ramgren B, Norrving B, Wassélius J, Ullberg T. Accuracy of automated intracerebral hemorrhage volume measurement on non-contrast computed tomography: a Swedish Stroke Register cohort study. Neuroradiology. 2023;65(3):479–88.

143. Kunst M, Gupta R, Coombs LP, Delfino JG, Khan A, Berglar I, et al. Real-world performance of large vessel occlusion artificial intelligence–based computer-aided triage and notification algorithms—what the stroke team needs to know. J Am Coll Radiol. 2024;21(2):329–40.

144. Rava RA, Peterson BA, Seymour SE, Snyder KV, Mokin M, Waqas M, et al. Validation of an artificial intelligence-driven large vessel occlusion detection algorithm for acute ischemic stroke patients. Neuroradiol J. 2021;34(5):408–17.

145. Buchlak QD, Tang CHM, Seah JCY, Johnson A, Holt X, Bottrell GM, et al. Effects of a comprehensive brain computed tomography deep learning model on radiologist detection accuracy. Eur Radiol. 2023;34(2):810–22.

146. Vallée A, Quint R, Laure Brun A, Mellot F, Grenier PA. A deep learning-based algorithm improves radiology residents' diagnoses of acute pulmonary embolism on CT pulmonary angiograms. Eur J Radiol. 2024;171:111324.

147. Rothenberg SA, Savage CH, Abou Elkassem A, Singh S, Abozeed M, Hamki O, et al. Prospective evaluation of AI triage of pulmonary emboli on CT pulmonary angiograms. Radiology. 2023;309(1):e230702.

148. Hempel HL, Engbersen MP, Wakkie J, Van Kelckhoven BJ, De Monyé W. Higher agreement between readers with deep learning CAD software for reporting pulmonary nodules on CT. Eur J Radiol Open. 2022;9:100435.

149. Grenier PA, Ayobi A, Quenet S, Tassy M, Marx M, Chow DS, et al. Deep learning-based algorithm for automatic detection of pulmonary embolism in chest CT angiograms. Diagnostics. 2023;13(7):1324.

150. Röhrich S, Heidinger BH, Prayer F, Weber M, Krenn M, Zhang R, et al. Impact of a content-based image retrieval system on the interpretation of chest CTs of patients with diffuse parenchymal lung disease. Eur Radiol. 2022;33(1):360–7.

151. Cui HW, Devlies W, Ravenscroft S, Heers H, Freidin AJ, Cleveland RO, et al. CT texture analysis of *ex vivo* renal stones predicts ease of fragmentation with shockwave lithotripsy. J Endourol. 2017;31(7):694–700.

152. Mastrodicasa D, Codari M, Bäumler K, Sandfort V, Shen J, Mistelbauer G, et al. Artificial intelligence applications in aortic dissection imaging. Semin Roentgenol. 2022;57(4):357–63.

153. Muscogiuri G, Chiesa M, Trotta M, Gatti M, Palmisano V, Dell'Aversana S, et al. Performance of a deep learning algorithm for the evaluation of CAD-RADS classification with CCTA. Atherosclerosis. 2020;294:25–32.

154. Paul JF, Rohnean A, Giroussens H, Pressat-Laffouilhere T, Wong T. Evaluation of a deep learning model on coronary CT angiography for automatic stenosis detection. Diagn Interv Imaging. 2022;103(6):316–23.

155. Winkel DJ, Heye T, Weikert TJ, Boll DT, Stieltjes B. Evaluation of an AI-based detection software for acute findings in abdominal computed tomography scans: toward an automated work list prioritization of routine CT examinations. Investig Radiol. 2019;54(1):55–9.

156. Van Leeuwen KG, Becks MJ, Grob D, De Lange F, Rutten JHE, Schalekamp S, et al. AI-support for the detection of intracranial large vessel occlusions: one-year prospective evaluation. Heliyon. 2023;9(8):e19065.

157. Bercean BA, Birhala A, Ardelean PG, Barbulescu I, Benta MM, Rasadean CD, et al. Evidence of a cognitive bias in the quantification of COVID-19 with CT: an artificial intelligence randomised clinical trial. Sci Rep. 2023;13(1):4887.

158. Tesche C, Gray HN. Machine learning and deep neural networks applications in coronary flow assessment: the case of computed tomography fractional flow reserve. J Thorac Imaging. 2020;35(Supplement 1):S66–71.

159. Van Hamersvelt RW, Zreik M, Voskuil M, Viergever MA, Išgum I, Leiner T. Deep learning analysis of left ventricular myocardium in CT angiographic intermediate-degree coronary stenosis improves the diagnostic accuracy for identification of functionally significant stenosis. Eur Radiol. 2019;29(5):2350–9.

160. Santos MK, Ferreira Júnior JR, Wada DT, Tenório APM, Nogueira-Barbosa MH, Marques PMDA. Artificial intelligence, machine learning, computer-aided diagnosis, and radiomics: advances in imaging towards to precision medicine. Radiol Bras. 2019;52(6):387–96.

161. Muehlematter UJ, Mannil M, Becker AS, Vokinger KN, Finkenstaedt T, Osterhoff G, et al. Vertebral body insufficiency fractures: detection of vertebrae at risk on standard CT images using texture analysis and machine learning. Eur Radiol. 2019;29(5):2207–17.

162. Dankelman LHM, Schilstra S, IJpma FFA, Doornberg JN, Colaris JW, Verhofstad MHJ, et al. Artificial intelligence fracture recognition on computed tomography: review of literature and recommendations. Eur J Trauma Emerg Surg. 2023;49(2):681–91.

163. Inoue T, Maki S, Furuya T, Mikami Y, Mizutani M, Takada I, et al. Automated fracture screening using an object detection algorithm on whole-body trauma computed tomography. Sci Rep. 2022;12(1):16549.

164. Van Den Wittenboer GJ, Van Der Kolk BYM, Nijholt IM, Langius-Wiffen E, Van Dijk RA, Van Hasselt BAAM, et al. Diagnostic accuracy of an artificial intelligence algorithm versus radiologists for fracture detection on cervical spine CT. Eur Radiol. 2024;34(8):5041–8.

165. Heit JJ, Iv M, Wintermark M. Imaging of intracranial hemorrhage. J Stroke. 2017;19(1):11–27. https://doi.org/10.5853/jos.2016.00563.

166. Arhami Dolatabadi A, Baratloo A, Rouhipour A, Abdalvand A, Hatamabadi H, Forouzanfar M, Shojaee M, Hashemi B. Interpretation of computed tomography of the head: emergency physicians versus radiologists. Trauma Mon. 2013;18(2):86–9. https://doi.org/10.5812/traumamon.12023.

167. Richards M. Diagnostics: recovery and renewal report of the independent review of diagnostic services for NHS England. Review. NHS England; 2020.

168. Chong ST, Robinson JD, Davis MA, Bruno MA, Roberge EA, Reddy S, Pyatt RS Jr, Friedberg EB. Emergency radiology: current challenges and preparing for continued growth. J Am Coll Radiol. 2019;16(10):1447–55. https://doi.org/10.1016/j.jacr.2019.03.009.

169. Hillal A, Sultani G, Ramgren B, Norrving B, Wassélius J, Ullberg T. Accuracy of automated intracerebral hemorrhage volume measurement on non-contrast computed tomography: a Swedish Stroke Register cohort study. Neuroradiology. 2023;65(3):479–88. https://doi.org/10.1007/s00234-022-03075-9.

170. Mabit L, Herpe G, Poitiers/FR. Real life performance of a commercially available AI for post-traumatic intracranial haemorrhage detection on CT-scans: a supportive tool. ECR; 2025; Vienna. https://connect.myesr.org/course/emergency-radiology-new-technologies-and-workload-challenges/.

171. Chiramal JA, Johnson J, Webster J, Nag DR, Robert D, Ghosh T, Golla S, Pawar S, Krishnan P, Drain PK, Mooney SJ. Artificial intelligence-based automated CT brain interpretation to accelerate treatment for acute stroke in rural India: an interrupted time series study. PLOS Glob Public Health. 2024;4(7):e0003351. https://doi.org/10.1371/journal.pgph.0003351.

172. Novak A. Can ED clinicians use AI to reliably interpret CT Head scans? Results from the AI-REACT multireader multicase study. Royal College of Emergency Medicine; 2024; https://rcem.ac.uk/wp-content/uploads/2024/10/Annual-Scientific-Conference-2024-Virtual-Programme-8-10-October-V17.pdf.

173. Morais J. Improving stroke patient pathway, with AI assisted diagnosis. Case Report. USA: vRad, Radiology; 2023.

174. Nakamura Y, Higaki T, Kondo S, Kawashita I, Takahashi I, Awai K. An introduction to photon-counting detector CT (PCD CT) for radiologists. Jpn J Radiol. 2022. [cited 2025 Jan 30]; Available from: https://link.springer.com/10.1007/s11604-022-01350-6.

175. Mese I, Altintas Taslicay C, Sivrioglu AK. Synergizing photon-counting CT with deep learning: potential enhancements in medical imaging. Acta Radiol. 2024;65(2):159–66.

176. Van Timmeren JE, Cester D, Tanadini-Lang S, Alkadhi H, Baessler B. Radiomics in medical imaging—"how-to" guide and critical reflection. Insights Imaging. 2020;11(1):91.

177. Johnson KB, Wei W, Weeraratne D, Frisse ME, Misulis K, Rhee K, et al. Precision medicine, AI, and the future of personalized health care. Clin Transl Sci. 2021;14(1):86–93.

178. Jungblut L, Blüthgen C, Polacin M, Messerli M, Schmidt B, Euler A, et al. First performance evaluation of an artificial intelligence-based computer-aided detection system for pulmonary nodule evaluation in dual-source photon-counting detector CT at different low-dose levels. Investig Radiol. 2022;57(2):108–14.

179. Beig N, Bera K, Tiwari P. Introduction to radiomics and radiogenomics in neuro-oncology: implications and challenges. Neuro-Oncol Adv. 2020;2(Supplement_4):iv3–v14.

180. Liu Z, Duan T, Zhang Y, Weng S, Xu H, Ren Y, et al. Radiogenomics: a key component of precision cancer medicine. Br J Cancer. 2023;129(5):741–53.

181. Espinoza JL, Dong LT. Artificial intelligence tools for refining lung cancer screening. J Clin Med. 2020;9(12):3860.

182. Becker N, Motsch E, Trotter A, Heussel CP, Dienemann H, Schnabel PA, et al. Lung cancer mortality reduction by LDCT screening—results from the randomized German LUSI trial. Int J Cancer. 2020;146(6):1503–13.

183. Cellina M, Cacioppa LM, Cè M, Chiarpenello V, Costa M, Vincenzo Z, et al. Artificial intelligence in lung cancer screening: the future is now. Cancer. 2023;15(17):4344.

184. Shah AA, Malik HAM, Muhammad A, Alourani A, Butt ZA. Deep learning ensemble 2D CNN approach towards the detection of lung cancer. Sci Rep. 2023;13(1):2987.

185. NHS Egland. Using AI to identify tissue growth from CT scans [Internet]. 2024 [cited 2025

Jan 20]. Available from: https://transform. england.nhs.uk/ai-lab/explore-all-resources/ develop-ai/using-ai-to-identify-tissue-growth-from-ct-scans/https://transform.england.nhs. uk/ai-lab/explore-all-resources/develop-ai/ using-ai-to-identify-tissue-growth-from-ct-scans/.

186. Baeßler B, Götz M, Antoniades C, Heidenreich JF, Leiner T, Beer M. Artificial intelligence in coronary computed tomography angiography: demands and solutions from a clinical perspective. Front Cardiovasc Med. 2023;10:1120361.

187. Aldoseri A, Al-Khalifa KN, Hamouda AM. Re-thinking data strategy and integration for artificial intelligence: concepts, opportunities, and challenges. Appl Sci. 2023;13(12):7082.

188. Abgrall G, Holder AL, Chelly Dagdia Z, Zeitouni K, Monnet X. Should AI models be explainable to clinicians? Crit Care (Lond Engl). 2024;28(1):301.

189. Cheong BC. Transparency and accountability in AI systems: safeguarding wellbeing in the age of algorithmic decision-making. Front Hum Dyn. 2024;6:1421273.

190. Geis JR, Brady AP, Wu CC, Spencer J, Ranschaert E, Jaremko JL, et al. Ethics of artificial intelligence in radiology: summary of the joint European and north American multisociety statement. Radiology. 2019;293(2):436–40.

191. Kotter E, Ranschaert E. Challenges and solutions for introducing artificial intelligence (AI) in daily clinical workflow. Eur Radiol. 2021;31(1):5–7.

192. Blezek DJ, Olson-Williams L, Missert A, Korfiatis P. AI integration in the clinical workflow. J Digit Imaging. 2021;34(6):1435–46.

Dr. Benard Ohene-Botwe is the Programme Director of Postgraduate Radiography (CT/MRI) at City St George's, University of London. His research focuses on artificial intelligence, medical imaging safety and clinical education. He is also an Editorial Board member of the *Journal of Medical Imaging and Radiation Sciences* (JMIRS) and a member (Lead for CT and Quantitative Research) of the CRRAG research group at City St George's, University of London. Additionally, he is a mentor for the Formal Radiography Research Mentoring (FoRRM) scheme of the College of Radiographers in the UK.

Dr. Bo Mussmann is head of Research and Associate Professor at the Department of Radiology, Odense University Hospital, and the Department of Clinical Research, University of Southern Denmark. He also holds the position of associate professor at the Faculty of Health Sciences, Department of Radiography, Oslo Metropolitan University in Norway. His research primarily focuses on computed tomography and professional issues within radiographic practice. Earlier in his career, Dr. Mussmann gained extensive clinical experience in computed tomography, interventional radiography, and general radiography. He is currently serving as an Editorial Fellow for the *Radiography* journal (2023–2025).

Professor Mark F McEntee is a full professor and chair of Medical Imaging and Radiation Therapy at University College Cork. He is vice head for Teaching and Learning in the College of Medicine and Health and Chair of the School of Medicine Athena Swan Team. He is also an honorary professor of Radiography at the University of Sydney and South Denmark, deputy editor of the *Journal of Medical Imaging and Radiation Science*, past president of the Irish Institute of Radiography, executive board member of the European Federation of Radiographer Societies (RFRS), vice president of the EFRS 2024–26, and president of EFRS 2026–28.

AI in Magnetic Resonance Imaging

7

Nikolaos Stogiannos, Stephanos Leandrou, and Charalampos Bougias

7.1 Introduction

The tremendous increase which has been noted in the clinical applications of AI tools in medical imaging has also started impacting the field of MRI. AI-based solutions in MRI are now capable of assisting MRI radiographers in their scanning, such as protocol optimisation [1], automated slice prescription [2], and patient positioning [3]. In addition, DL-based image reconstruction techniques are now available from all major MR vendors, and this has resulted in improved image quality, faster scan times, and increased diagnostic accuracy [4–6]. The future of AI-powered MRI may be both promising and challenging; to reach its full potential, all key stakeholders should engage in explainable AI (XAI) approaches to build trust and mitigate the 'black box' effect [7]. This chapter provides an overview of the fundamental AI-based MRI techniques and their beneficial impact in MRI acquisition, image reconstruction, and image analysis, as well as some key concerns regarding AI ethics and challenges in the adoption of AI in clinical MRI practice.

7.2 AI Techniques in MRI Image Acquisition

7.2.1 Image Quality Enhancement

Nowadays, most MRI vendors have already developed AI techniques which aim to enhance image quality in a prospective way. This can be achieved by DL-based image reconstruction models applied directly on the raw data in the k-space, while also preserving any data acquired without DL methods [8]. Another application of AI in this field is the use of convolutional neural networks (CNNs) to interpolate the fully sampled centre of k-space to estimate the unsampled k-space lines, a technique called robust artificial-neural-networks for k-space interpolation (RAKI) [9]. A similar example is DL used to benefit from the properties of half-Fourier acquisition single-shot MRI sequences to enhance image quality. The combination of a DL-based approach for image reconstruction of these sequences resulted in better mage quality and enhanced contrast, which has allowed better detection of challenging pathologies, such as liver lesions [10].

on behalf of Association of Healthcare Technology Providers for Imaging, Radiotherapy and Care (AXREM)

N. Stogiannos (✉)
City St George's, University of London, Northampton Square, London, UK
e-mail: nikos.stogiannos@citystgeorges.ac.uk

S. Leandrou
European University Cyprus, Nicosia, Cyprus
e-mail: s.leandrou@euc.ac.cy

C. Bougias
University Hospital of Ioannina, Ioannina, Greece

© The Author(s), under exclusive license to Springer Nature Switzerland AG 2026
C. Malamateniou et al. (eds.), *Artificial Intelligence for Radiographers*,
https://doi.org/10.1007/978-3-032-05080-9_7

7.2.2 Accelerated Imaging

Many efforts have been made during the last years to reduce image acquisition times in MRI, since the duration of MRI scans can be challenging for the patients, result in prematurely terminated examinations, or reduce image quality [11]. The most important innovations around MRI scan times were the development of parallel imaging (PI) techniques and the simultaneous multi-slice acquisition [12]. PI achieves shortened scan times by reducing the number of acquired cartesian k-space lines and relies on spatial information acquired from an array of receiver coils, while multi-slice acquisition uses certain radiofrequency pulses to simultaneously excite several slices within a slice stack [13]. However, both these methods may produce certain artefacts due to misregistration of data and other reasons [14]. Novel approaches, based on DL techniques, have achieved excellent results in this field, since this task is performed in a data-driven way, being able to achieve reduced scan times and state-of-the-art image reconstruction at the same time [15]. AI-assisted compressed sensing (ACS) techniques have been already applied to optimise musculoskeletal MRI protocols (Fig. 7.1), with 3D ACS sequences demonstrating a significant reduction in MRI acquisition times (over 50%) compared to the conventional 2D PI protocol, while also preserving image quality [16].

ACS proved to be superior compared to PI in other anatomical areas too, such as in the head and neck regions, where it achieved statistically significant reductions in scan times (e.g. 40.08 s vs 60.21 s, $p < 0.001$), enabling to improve the MRI experience of cancer patients [18]. The combination of PI, compressed sensing (CS) and DL using an adaptive CNN to integrate and enhance the conventional CS algorithm has achieved a reduction of 47% in scan times without compromising image quality [19].

Finally, another field where AI can assist with MRI acquisition times is automated slice prescription, which can lead to faster protocols, reducing the need for slice parameter optimisation [2]. Selection and optimisation of MRI protocols is a complex process, requiring deep knowledge of the underlying physical principles of MRI. The application of machine learning (ML)-based, domain-specific languages has showed promising results in facilitating the process of selecting optimal MRI sequences and protocols, which can assist radiographers based on clinical needs and scenarios, and also reduce the time needed for a scan [1]. It does not, though, take away the unique and extensive expertise required by radiographers to modify scan parameters, patient or slice positioning, and whole protocols on a patient-by-patient basis to offer truly personalised care for different patient populations (e.g. a patient with claustrophobia, low back pain, unusual anatomy, inability to understand instructions for different reasons, or tremor in extremities) or different clinical scenarios than those the AI was trained on. Table 7.1 summarises the different AI-enabled products and their commercial names that have been produced by major medical equipment vendors for AI-powered enhanced image acquisition.

7.2.3 Acoustic Noise Reduction

The acoustic noise generated by MRI scanners can be overwhelming for many patients undergoing these examinations [20]. Although there are currently no specific AI techniques to reduce the acoustic noise exhibited during the scans, some preliminary approaches have been proposed, using CNNs to achieve a 10–15 dB noise reduction [21]. In addition, there are some AI-based approaches that have been used in conjunction with zero-echo time (ZTE) MRI. These are simply presented here, since they have not been primarily used to reduce the acoustic noise, but mainly were developed to capture signal from short-T2 tissues. ZTE employs non-selective excitation and 3D radial k-space encoding, and it uses a gradient amplitude that remains constant throughout the examination. ZTE images are

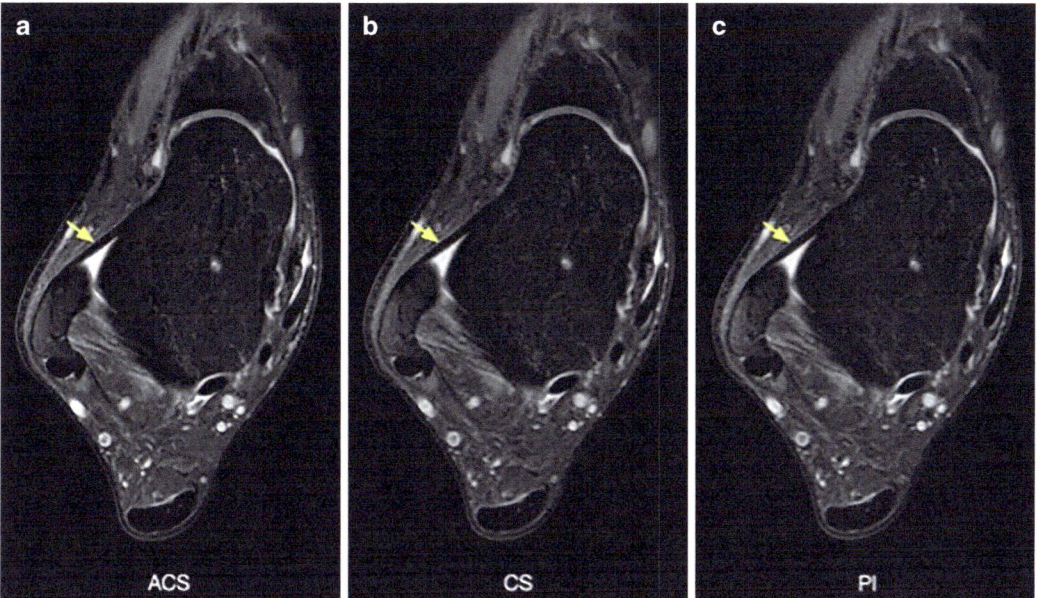

Fig. 7.1 Axial PD-weighted images of the ankle with fat saturation. Example of the performance of ACS technique on MR images of the ankle, compared to conventional CS and PI [17]. Note the quality of the images for the anterior talofibular ligament (yellow arrows) when using ACS, CS, and PI

often used in musculoskeletal images and look very similar to CT scans in terms of the bony features present and tissue contrast. Additional sequence advantages include silent scanning, but also rapid imaging times, and artefact resistance [22, 23].

7.2.4 Automated Patient Positioning

Optimal patient positioning is vital in MRI examinations, and this will result in a better image quality (due to optimal signal-to-noise ratio), enhanced patient safety, and improved patient comfort during the scan. Most major MRI vendors have now introduced AI-based techniques to assist MRI radiographers in patient positioning.

This can be achieved by automatically detecting certain anatomical landmarks on the patient positioned on the scanner table, using a database of optimal positioning guidance for different anatomical areas and then positioning the anatomical area of interest in the isocentre of the magnet with a single push of a button [24]. Also, automated coil selection based on patient anatomy using an AI-based landmarking tool has been developed to help streamline the process and adjust protocols based on patient anatomy [25]. AI-assisted guidance on patient positioning, coil, and protocol selection can result in reduced variations between different MRI radiographers and similar anatomical coverage between scans, vital for longitudinal examinations and research studies [26].

Table 7.1 Commercial names of AI-powered solutions by vendor

Vendor	Product commercial name	Aim
Siemens Healthineers	myExam Companion	Automated scanning workflows
	myExam 3D Camera	AI-based automated positioning
	AutoSuite	Automated slice coverage, automated bolus detection, automated coil selection
	Deep Resolve	Image noise reduction, reduced scan times, enhanced image sharpness, reduced energy consumption
Philips	SmartSpeed	Increased image resolution, reduced scan times
	MR Smart Workflow	Automated scanning workflows
GE	Sonic DL	Reduced scan times, reduced motion artefacts
	AIR Recon DL	Enhanced image sharpness, reduced image noise, increased SNR
	AIR x	Automated slice prescription
Canon Medical Systems	AiCE	Higher SNR, reduced image noise
	PIQE	Automated matrix increase, enhanced image sharpness
United Imaging Healthcare	DeepRecon	Increased image sharpness, higher SNR
	uAIFI ACS	Reduced scan times
	uAIFI QScan	Reduced acoustic noise
	uAIFI EasyScan	Automated scanning workflows

7.3 AI Techniques in MRI Image Reconstruction

7.3.1 Artefact Correction and Denoising

One of the major drawbacks of MRI is the presence of different types of artefacts, arising from the nature and physics of this modality, and often altering image quality, minimising diagnostic accuracy, and sometimes even leading to misdiagnosis. AI tools have now been developed to retrospectively remove some types of artefacts and denoise MRI images. AI-based image filtering, especially when combined with interpolation, has proved superior to the conventional filtering methods, with statistically significant ($p < 0.05$) but varying results for all sequence weightings [27]. AI-assisted denoising applications combine iterative reconstruction with statistical methods of identifying noise distribution on the images that were acquired with suboptimal parameters, and this can lead to image denoising and subsequently improve the signal-to-noise-ratio (SNR) [28]. DL-based algorithms are now effectively used to improve image quality and remove noise from MRI images, and these have been superior even in challenging cases in the abdomen, such as in prostate imaging without the use of endorectal coils [29]. CNNs are useful tools in image denoising, as they use convolution and non-linear operations to learn a hierarchy of features. To optimise the performance of deep CNNs, a residual learning approach has been employed to connect low-level features to high-level representations [30]. A recent application of an improved U-type CNN, based on U-Net, has achieved very promising results in image denoising by introducing the separation attention residual module in the U-Net CNN [31]. Thermal noise, arising from the patient being scanned and the electronic components in the receiver chain, is also another important source of image noise in MRI. U-type CNNs have been effectively employed to denoise images even without the use of ground-truth noise-free images (Fig. 7.2). This was achieved by employing Stein's unbiased risk estimator (SURE) to estimate the true mean square error [32]. This creates the advantage of model training without requiring noise-free images.

7.3.2 Parallel Imaging Reconstruction

As noted, PI refers to the acquisition of fewer k-space data, so this under-sampled data can

| Input | SURE | Noise2Void | Residual |

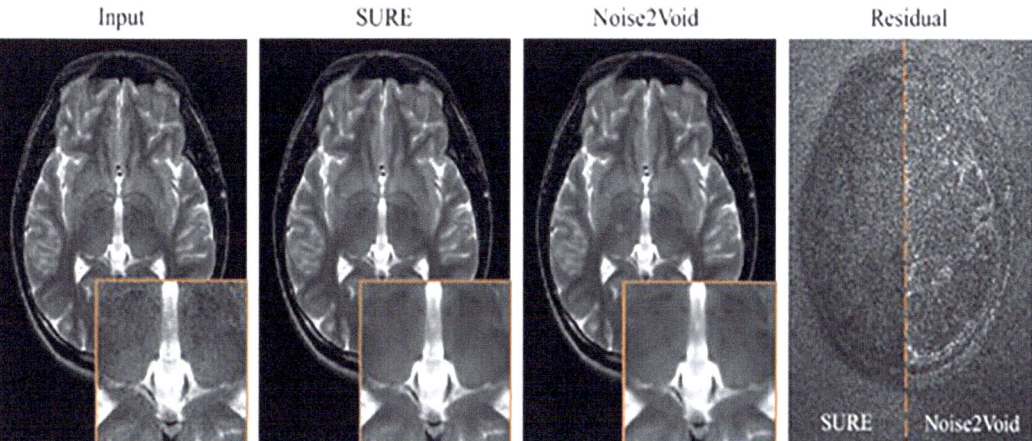

Fig. 7.2 T2-weighted image of the brain on the transverse plane demonstrating self-supervised denoising without the use of ground-truth images. SURE provides superior image sharpness and clarity, compared to the reference method. The residual image shows the difference between the input and denoised images [32]

accelerate MRI scans. The main PI techniques used in MRI are generalised auto-calibrated partially parallel acquisition (GRAPPA) and sensitivity encoding (SENSE), which were not originally AI-enabled [33]. GRAPPA operates in the k-space domain, while SENSE in the image domain. ML-based approaches to further improve PI gains in MRI include either using specific auto-calibrated lines to train neural networks for interpolation or using training databases [34]. A non-linear version of GRAPPA has been developed and integrated into a CNN. This is called GrappaNet and it has shown high performance (peak signal to noise ratio [PSNR] = 40.74; structural similarity loss function [SSIM] = 0.957) in image reconstruction, thus considered as one of the best performing methods [35]. As mentioned above, RAKI is also an effective example of employing robust networks for k-space interpolation [9]. Deep neural networks are now effectively used to further accelerate MRI sequences that already use PI acceleration, and this has proved superior both in terms of SNR/CNR and scan time [36]. In addition, PI has been also combined with the architecture of generative adversarial networks (GAN). GANs consist of a generator and a discriminator, where the generator is used to learn from the dataset and the discriminator to distinguish the generated images from the original. Such approach has been supe-rior to other DL-based methods for MR image reconstruction in terms of reducing aliasing artefacts and restoring tissue structures, and it has been tested in different anatomical areas and datasets [37].

7.3.3 Compressed Sensing

Compressed sensing (CS) is another technique developed to accelerate MRI acquisition by reconstructing incomplete k-space data. However, CS does not require to collect complementary data, unlike PI reconstruction [38]. Many efforts have been made to integrate AI techniques into CS. AI-assisted CS methods have been successfully applied to further improve image quality and decrease scan time in MR sequences that already use PI techniques. This has shown superior outcomes, even in cases of uncooperative patients with involuntary head motion (Case Study 7.1) [39]. Another approach to AI-assisted reconstruction is the use of networks that operate first in the k-space domain, then in the image domain, and then they repeat in a hybrid fashion. KIKI-net (named after its operation in k-space, image, k-space, and image sequentially) has shown promising results in reconstruction, but it failed in removing artefacts [40]. Another novel technique used to further improve image reconstruction is automated transform by manifold approximation (AUTOMAP). The AUTOMAP neural network can learn from the raw MR data using the forward-encoding model [41]. This

approach can achieve real-time reconstruction of radial data and it can be used in MR-guided radiotherapy to adapt to anatomical changes.

Case Study 7.1

Case: A patient with involuntary head motion, suspicious of brain disease, underwent a brain MRI to establish diagnosis.

Clinical challenge: Motion-induced arte-facts significantly decreased image quality.

AI-enabled solution: An AI-enabled com-pressed sensing fluid attenuation inversion recovery (FLAIR) sequence was acquired to reduce artefacts and scan time.

Benefits: ACS FLAIR facilitated detection of a hyperintense lesion in the right lateral paraventricular area (image b; white arrow) and another lesion in the posterior corner of the left lateral ventricle (image b; white arrow-head). The subacute infarction was also con-firmed on the diffusion-weighted images (image c; white arrow). These lesions were not obvious on the conventional FLAIR images (image a) [39].

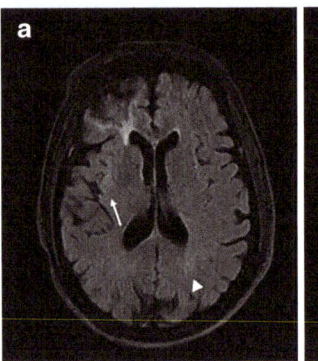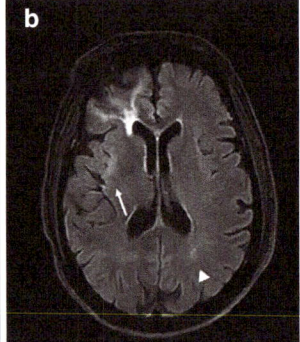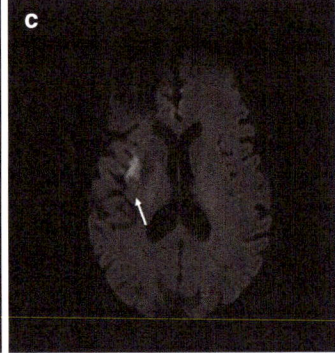

7.3.4   Super-Resolution Reconstruction

Another great achievement of AI in the field of MRI is super-resolution [42]. Super-resolution refers to the task of creating high-resolution images from low-resolution images, and this can be applied either to raw or reconstructed data [43]. These replace the originally used zero-fill strategy to increase the matrix size, and thus the sharpness of the images results in the so-called super-resolution reconstructions. A 3D DL-based CNN has been used to learn residual-based trans-formations between high-resolution thin images and low-resolution thick images [44]. Prospective

DL-based super-resolution has been also used to enhance image quality in conjunction with newly developed quantitative Double-echo steady-state pulse sequences (qDESS) for musculoskeletal MRI applications [45]. Segmentation of super-resolved images has been superior to that of interpolated images in MRI, and recent methods of AI-based super-resolution also include some interpretability-orientated aspects, such as self-attention methods [46]. Unified DL-based super-resolution frameworks have been also introduced, offering the advantage of standardised datasets, stronger feature extraction, learning from a large number of data, and achievement of a more stable and improved reconstruction [47].

7.4   AI Techniques in MRI Image Segmentation

7.4.1   Tissue, Organ, and Lesion Segmentation

Tissue Segmentation AI techniques in tissue segmentation help distinguish different types of tissues within MRI scans. For instance, AI can differentiate between grey matter, white matter, and cerebrospinal fluid in brain MRI images [48]. This segmentation is an essential task and aids in the precise analysis of tissue characteristics, assisting in diagnosing conditions like tumours, lesions, or degenerative diseases. Segmentation in medical imaging involves dividing an image into distinct areas for studying anatomy, pinpointing specific regions of interest (ROIs), or gauging tissue volume.

Organ Segmentation AI helps segment and outline organs within MRI images, enabling accurate volumetric measurements and providing insights into organ health. Organ segmentation in medical images is also necessary for many clinical applications such as computer-aided diagnosis (CAD) and radiation therapy. Brain and vessels are two of the most commonly used areas for organ segmentation. Brain segmentation involves dividing a brain MRI scan into distinct regions or structures to analyse and understand brain anatomy, pathology, and function. This segmentation is crucial for various applications, such as studying normal brain development and growth, diagnosing neurological disorders, treatment planning, and monitoring disease progression [49]. With regards to vessel segmentation, in MRI angiography, AI assists in segmenting blood vessels, especially in patients with different cerebrovascular diseases. Automated vessel segmentation can assist in the identification and delineation of complex network of blood vessels, understanding blood flow patterns within the body, aiding in the diagnosis of vascular diseases, planning surgeries, and monitoring pharmacological and other treatments. Further than clinical practice, it can speed up the diagnosis of complex vessel pathologies and potentially help pinpoint

in the future important biomarkers for preventing cerebrovascular events [50].

Lesion Segmentation Lesion segmentation is perhaps the most refined function, as AI contributes to identifying and characterising abnormalities like tumours, cysts, or infarcts. AI algorithms are trained to recognise these irregularities within MRI scans by differentiating them from healthy tissues. Usually, these slight changes in texture cannot be identified with the naked eye by radiologists. Therefore, AI may assist in precisely locating, quantifying, and monitoring the progression or regression of such lesions. Furthermore, after segmentation, valuable quantitative measurements (e.g. radiomics, see Chap. 2 for further details) are calculated on the segmented ROI, providing valuable information essential for the assessment of pathologies [51]. An example is using semi-automated segmentation with dedicated tools for breast lesions in multiparametric breast MRI [52] (Fig. 7.3).

AI can achieve these segmentations through various methods like:

ML Algorithms Until 2015, ML was the dominant strategy in the field of medical image segmentation. These algorithms learn patterns from annotated medical images to classify and segment different structures [53].

DL Techniques Compared to ML-based methods, DL has the advantage of being able to automatically extract features [54]. Advanced neural network architectures, such as U-Net [55], are tailored for image segmentation tasks. These advanced CNNs have outstanding feature extraction and expression capabilities in image segmentation, and they can handle large numbers of features and complex structures and produce high-precision segmentations [56].

Semantic Segmentation In this technique, AI models perform pixel-level classification, labelling each pixel value (0, 1, … .255) on an image to a specific class (e.g. tissue type, blood vessel, lesion) [57].

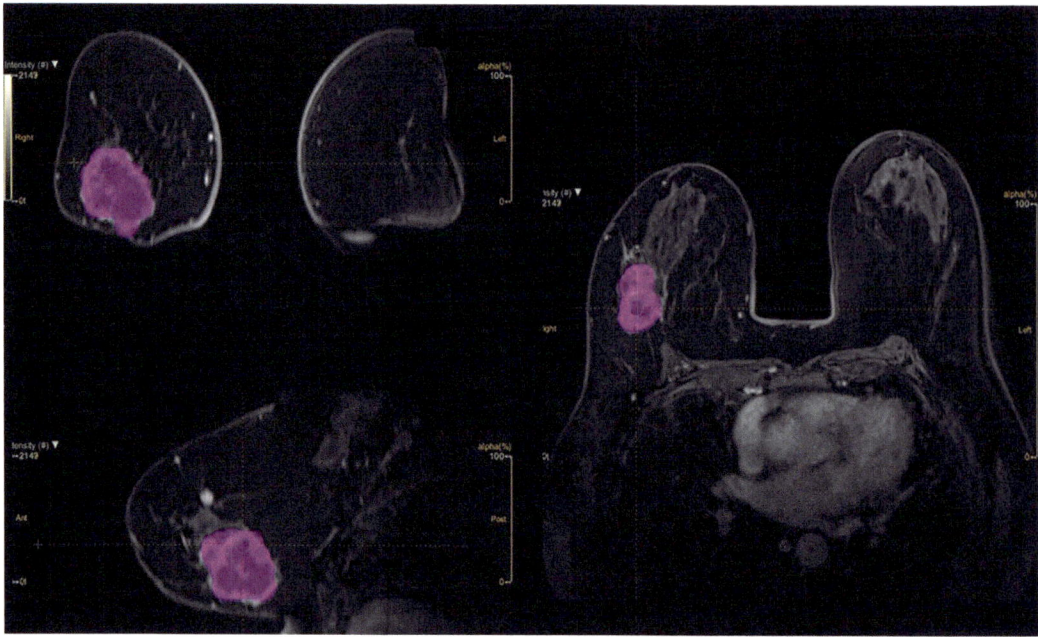

Fig. 7.3 Female patient (54 years old) with invasive ductal carcinoma of the right breast. Segmentation of this breast lesion in breast MRI was initially employed to extract radiomic features for the differentiation between malignant and benign lesions [52]

Probabilistic Models These models estimate the probability of a voxel belonging to a particular structure, providing a more nuanced segmentation output [58, 59].

Numerous software packages have been developed based on these segmentation methods for automated brain tissue analysis. They typically encompass skull stripping, correcting intensity irregularities, and automated segmentation of grey matter, white matter, and cerebrospinal fluid. FreeSurfer [60], an open-source suite (Massachusetts General Hospital, Boston, MA), stands out for its Bayesian-based approach in automatically segmenting brain MRI scans. Research by Morey et al. [61] has favoured FreeSurfer over older methods [62] when comparing automated methods to manual tracing for hippocampus segmentation. FreeSurfer has also

been successfully used in the segmentation of ROIs in radiomics studies on Alsheimer's disease, using skull striping and normalisation of signal intensities with the N3 algorithm [63]. Another notable software, Statistical Parameter Mapping, freely available and utilising MATLAB, specialises in segmentation, normalisation, registration, and volume measurements, among other image analysis tasks [64].

Overall, AI-driven segmentation in MRI can significantly boost the speed and consistency of identifying and delineating tissues and lesions, assisting healthcare professionals in making more informed diagnoses and treatment decisions.

7.4.2   Mapping

Mapping refers to a technique used in MRI to quantify the relaxation times (T1, T2, T2*) of all pixels within an image, which results in parametric maps not affected by scan-specific parameters and inter-observer variability [65]. Mapping has been widely used in certain anatomical areas and examinations, such as multiparametric MRI of the prostate or cardiac MRI (CMR). DL-based applications using CNNs have been employed to create cancer estimation maps of the prostate gland in MRI to predict the extent of clinically significant disease [66]. In CMR, parametric mapping of myocardial tissue properties is vital to detect any intracellular and/or extracellular changes related to certain cardiac pathologies. Different AI-based approaches have been implemented in CMR mapping, such as U-Net CNNs, and have shown similar accuracy with this of human experts [67]. Similarly, neural networks have been applied to automatically assess femoral cartilage degradation in MRI scans of the knee [68].

7.5   Clinical Applications of AI in MRI

With the advancements in computational technology, AI is increasingly used to improve image interpretation and analysis in medical imaging. Within the following sections, we discuss the role of AI in disease classification, treatment response assessment, prognostic prediction, radiomics, and radiogenomics.

7.5.1   Disease Classification

Valuable Feature Extraction AI algorithms can be trained to automatically analyse and extract complex features from MRI images that may be difficult for the humans to detect. These features could include texture patterns, shape characteristics, or intensity distributions within the images [69]. This can further lead to increased diagnostic accuracy and patient outcomes (Case Study 7.2) [70].

Case Study 7.2

Case: A 67-year-old patient with chronic hepatitis B underwent abdominal MRI.

Clinical challenge: Diagnosis of liver cirrhosis is often difficult to establish with certainty due to subtle changes in images.

AI-enabled solution: A combined CNN model was developed, in which data from serum biomarkers were integrated.

Benefits: T1-weighted in- and opposed-phase images (A, B), T2-weighted image (C), pre-contrast T1-weighted image (D), and portal venous phase images (E, F) did not reveal any indications of liver cirrhosis. However, activation maps overlaid on T2-weighted images (G) and pre-contrast T1-weighted images (H) showed abnormalities in liver parenchyma, and this led to a cirrhosis diagnosis [70].

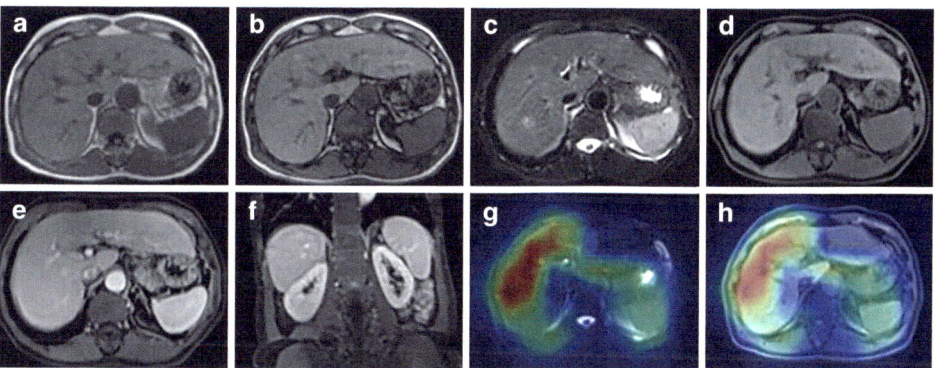

Segmentation, Analysis, and Diagnosis Trained AI algorithms can automatically segment and label structures in MRI images to pinpoint specific ROIs, such as regions of abnormality. Then, AI analyses unseen MRI data and classifies them into different disease categories or determines the likelihood of a particular condition. For instance, in neuroimaging, AI models might classify MRIs into categories like Alzheimer's disease [71], multiple sclerosis [72], or other neurological conditions [73], based on identified patterns within the images.

Enhancing Efficiency and Accuracy One major advantage of using AI in medical image analysis is its efficiency in analysing large amounts of data quickly and accurately [74]. It helps radiologists and other clinicians by providing additional insights, reducing interpretation time, and potentially detecting subtle abnormalities that might be missed during standard observation.

Personalised Medicine Personalised treatment planning involves tailoring medical treatment according to the patients [75]. AI could assist in the identification of patient-specific features in MR imaging, the discovery of new imaging biomarkers associated with diseases and help inform customised treatments [76].

7.5.2 Monitoring Response to Treatment

Another area in which AI is becoming increasingly valuable is assessing treatment response [77]. AI algorithms help in quantifying changes observed in MRI images before and after treatment. They analyse subtle variations in tissue characteristics, such as size, volume, texture, or enhancement patterns, to assess how a particular treatment impacts the targeted area [78]. Furthermore, through AI, accurate delineation of tumour boundaries could be automatically performed and assess their size or volume over time. This assists in tracking tumour growth, shrinkage, or stability, providing critical information on treatment efficacy [79]. This, in turn, can result in accurate quantification of tumour burden, while it also helps mitigate the challenges with inter-reader variability (Fig. 7.4).

7.5.3 Prognostic Prediction

The integration of AI in treatment models allows predictive modelling by analysing the patients' response patterns in comparison to large datasets (big data). AI algorithms can extract intricate features from MRI images that might be indicative of disease progression or prognosis [81]. These

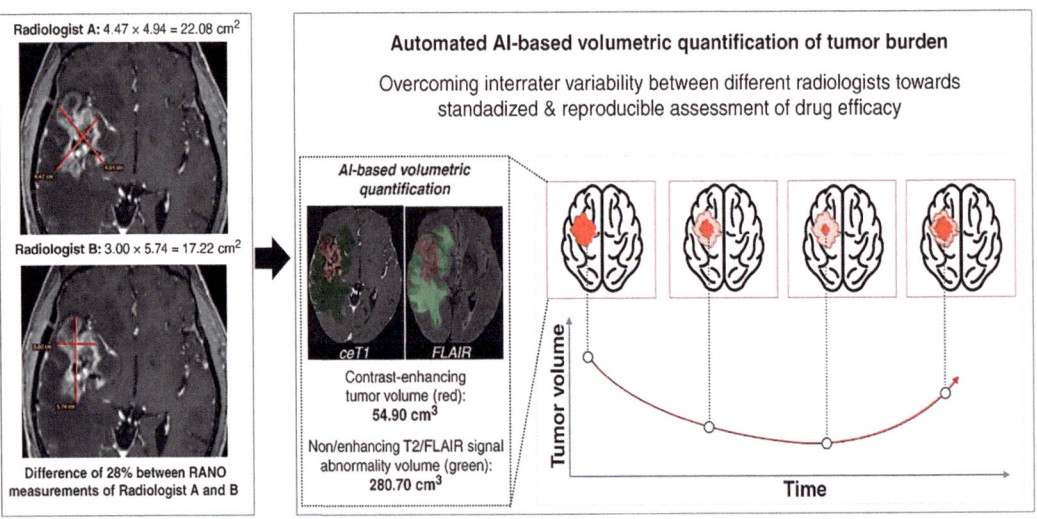

Fig. 7.4 AI-based quantification of brain tumour burden [80]

algorithms will be trained using established MR imaging biomarkers combined with clinical history or longitudinal monitoring data to offer patient prognoses. As a result, clinicians will be assisted in making informed decisions about treatment adjustments, continuation, or interruption, based on objective MRI-based evidence. This will also assist risk stratification for each patient [82]. AI models could link quantitative measures from MR images and associated patient data to identify risk factors that may lead to certain medical conditions.

7.5.4 Radiomics and Radiogenomics

Radiomics and radiogenomics are advanced techniques that harness the power of data extraction and use advanced quantitative analysis from medical images to provide insights into tissue characteristics, treatment response, and patient outcomes [83]. The integration of AI in disease classification analysis has the potential to revolutionise medical imaging, aiding in earlier and more accurate diagnoses, personalised treatment plans, and improved patient outcomes. An example of the radiomic analysis pipeline is given below (Fig. 7.5). More details about radiomic analysis can be found in Chap. 2.

The integration of radiomics with genomic data (radiogenomics) aims to understand how genetic variations (genotypes) manifest as specific imaging traits (phenotypes). Radiogenomics focuses on correlating imaging features with underlying genomic characteristics of tumours. Radiogenomics can identify imaging-based biomarkers associated with specific genetic mutations or gene expression patterns, therefore understanding a tumour's biology even without biopsy (often called 'virtual biopsy', used in breast imaging) [85, 86]. This offers a more holistic view of patient medical history and can inform future treatment.

7.6 Challenges and Limitations of AI in MRI

As AI continues to revolutionise various fields, its integration into medical imaging, particularly MRI, has emerged as a promising area of advancement. AI holds the potential to enhance diagnostic accuracy, streamline workflows, optimise imaging protocols, and personalise treatment plans [87]. However, the successful implementation of AI in MRI presents unique challenges that require careful consideration.

7.6.1 Data Availability, Uniformity, and Quality

AI models are heavily reliant on large datasets for algorithm training and validation. However, obtaining high-quality, annotated MRI data remains a significant challenge. Data used for AI development, training, and validation should be large enough to allow optimal algorithm training, have minimal noise, and be complete and consistent [88]. MRI scans are complex and can be affected by various factors, such as individual anatomy, scan parameters, and technical inconsistencies. Acquiring a sufficiently robust, diverse, representative, and large dataset to train AI models can be very challenging [89], particularly for specific pathologies or rare diseases.

7.6.2 Bias, Generalisability, and Interpretability

The potential for data bias presents an important challenge in AI-assisted MRI analysis. Bias can arise from various sources, including the composition of the training data, inherent biases in the data collection process, and human-generated annotations. If not addressed, data bias can lead to inaccurate or discriminatory results, poten-

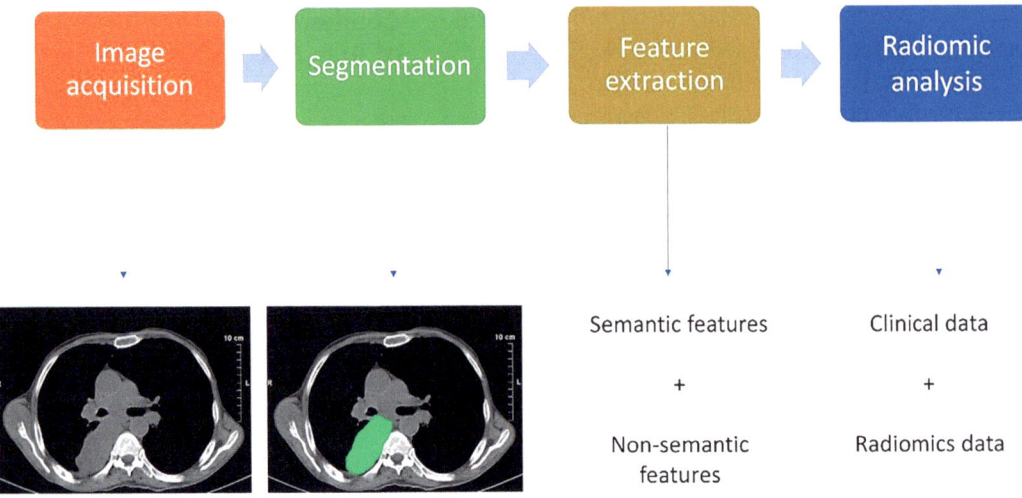

Fig. 7.5 Radiomic analysis pipeline [84]. Semantic features refer to qualitative features introduced by human vision, which cannot be described with mathematical procedures; non-semantic features are mathematically extracted quantitative features

tially harming patient care [90]. Ensuring data diversity and implementing robust bias mitigation techniques are essential to prevent these issues. One of the key aspects of AI models is their ability to make decisions based on complex patterns and interactions in the data. However, this opacity ingrained in AI models can hinder understanding and trust in the AI's reasoning process. Explainability techniques are crucial for enabling clinicians to comprehend how the AI reached its conclusions, facilitating informed decision-making and enhancing transparency [91, 92].

7.6.3 Ethical and Regulatory Considerations

The integration of AI into clinical practice raises important regulatory and ethical considerations. As AI algorithms are increasingly used for decision-making in healthcare, it is crucial to establish clear guidelines for their development, validation, and deployment. Ensuring patient privacy, data security, and informed consent are paramount to ethical and responsible AI implementation [93]. Freedom, dignity, and accountability should be central to AI implementation

[94]. More about AI ethics and regulation can be found in Chaps. 3 and 4, respectively.

7.6.4 Implementation into Clinical Workflows

To overcome the above challenges and effectively implement AI into MRI clinical workflows, several strategies can be employed. Clear regulatory guidance should be developed to assist medical imaging professionals in AI implementation and standardisation of procedures [87]. In addition, it is vital to ensure adequate training and education of all professionals involved in the AI ecosystem [95]. MRI protocols, image acquisition parameters, and data formats can vary significantly across institutions and regions. This lack of standardisation poses challenges for AI models trained on one dataset to generalise effectively to other settings. Establishing standardised practices and data management protocols are essential for ensuring the interoperability and scalability of AI-driven MRI solutions. Also, collaboration between medical imaging professionals from different professional backgrounds and industry could enable the development of large, diverse, and carefully annotated MRI datasets

[96]. AI models should be continuously evaluated and refined, based on real-world clinical experience, ensuring their accuracy, efficiency, and relevance in patient care [97]. Rigorous techniques should be employed for the identification and mitigation of data and algorithmic bias. Interoperability of AI solutions should be explored to allow seamless integration of AI into clinical practice across different clinical settings and hardware. More about implementation challenges and enablers for AI in medical imaging can be found in Chap. 4.

7.7 Future Directions and Emerging Trends

7.7.1 Multimodal Integration

One of the most important parts of clinical practice in healthcare is the management and integration of a diverse set of data formats, such as tabular data, imaging data, electronic health records, in vitro tests, blood tests, etc. AI models are already being used to leverage multiple data modalities, and this can also have applications in medical imaging [98]. Multimodal AI will have the ability to transcend unimodal tasks and broaden machine capabilities to encompass all input modes [99]. An example of multimodal AI framework is demonstrated below (Fig. 7.6), as it has been suggested by Soenksen et al. [98].

To achieve multimodal integration of AI in MRI, all anatomical structures must be aligned across images, and this is referred as registration of images. Segmentation of MRI images and fusion of multimodal images are also vital for further evaluation [100]. Recent studies have suggested DL-based techniques for fusion segmentation of aortas between CT and MRI in CMR examinations. Other novel applications of multimodal AI include simultaneous segmentation of multi-source images in a common space using multivariate mixture models [101], application of CNNs to align CT with MR images [102], or ML-based techniques to fuse MRI images with electronic health data, mental state examination scores, laboratory tests, cognitive tests and many more [103].

7.7.2 Federated Learning and Data Privacy

Federated Learning (FL) is a novel strategy employed to protect the users' data during procedures related to AI algorithm training. FL allows multiple developers to jointly train AI models without having to transfer data outside the clinical setting, thus preserving the privacy of data owners [104]. According to the global shared model, in FL all participating organisations operate under a central server, and each organisation maintains access to its model locally [104]. AI-based solutions have been tested to further enhance FL approaches in MRI. DL can be used in conjunction with FL, and this includes federated semantic segmentation using deep neural networks. This results in protection of patient data, improved training processes, and cross-site platforms to facilitate image reconstruction from data acquired at different scanners and organisations [105]. The challenge of not having fully labelled data across different clinical settings can be addressed using semi-supervised FL associated with pseudo-labelling of unlabelled data based on these with labels [106].

7.7.3 Explainable AI in MRI

Explainable AI (XAI) refers to the strategies and tools developed to mitigate the 'black box' narrative and lack of transparency in the way that AI algorithms make decisions. XAI is a move to improve transparency of AI models, facilitate seamless interactions between humans and AI tools, and enhance the reliability of the decisions made by AI models [7]. The techniques developed to apply XAI in MRI can be divided into model-specific and model-agnostic techniques. Model-specific techniques are those that can be only applied to specific AI models, while model-agnostic techniques are independent of DL models. The most widely used model-specific explanation methods are (a) class activation mapping, (b) gradient-weighted class activation mapping, (c) layer-wise relevance propagation, and (d) guided backpropagation [107]. A widely

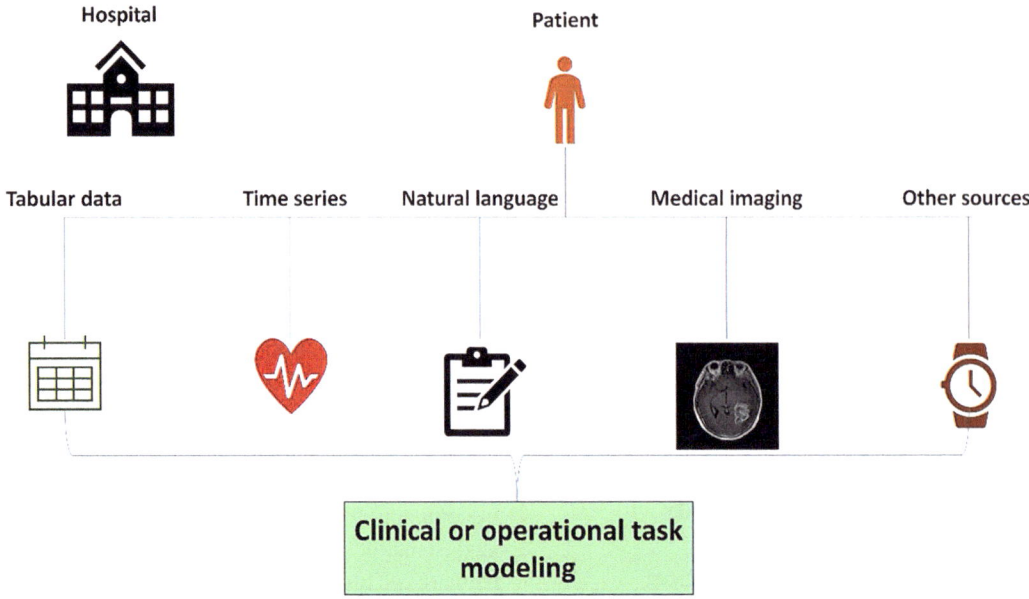

Fig. 7.6 Suggested pipeline for multimodal AI in healthcare. This requires the combination of different data formats, such as tabular data, medical imaging data, etc.

used method to enhance explainability in medical imaging is by employing heat maps, which are generated by gradient-weighted class activation mapping [108]. On the contrary, Shapley additive explanations (SHAP), local interpretable model-agnostic explanations (LIME), and prediction difference analysis are at the frontline of model-agnostic methods [109]. SHAP is a method derived from game theory and it allows the interpretability of the AI model. An example of a SHAP beeswarm summary plot is depicted below (Fig. 7.7), showing the contribution of each extracted feature to the model. High SHAP values refer to features that had a significant contribution to the model, and similarly positive values refer to features that had a positive impact on prediction [52].

XAI is essential to continue the development, training, and deployment of AI tools in MRI and build trust between developers and service users. Future approaches to XAI should opt to directly engage with the users' needs [92]. Chapters 2 and 4 discuss explainable AI from a methods and an implementation perspective, respectively.

7.8   Chapter Summary

The advancements and applications of AI in MRI can be seen in AI-assisted image reconstruction which is already widely used to accelerate MR imaging and enhance image quality. AI solutions can assist in creating an AI-powered seamless workflow in MRI, mainly employing automated patient positioning, slice prescription, scan time reduction, and streamlining of scan acquisition and image post-processing. AI tools can assist in disease classification, monitoring of treatment response, and prognosis. AI adoption into MRI clinical practice should address ethical and legal considerations, data availability and quality issues, and seamless integration into clinical workflows. XAI and federated learning can enhance trust in AI, ensure data privacy, and offer explainability to professionals and patients, to accelerate AI implementation for real patient benefit.

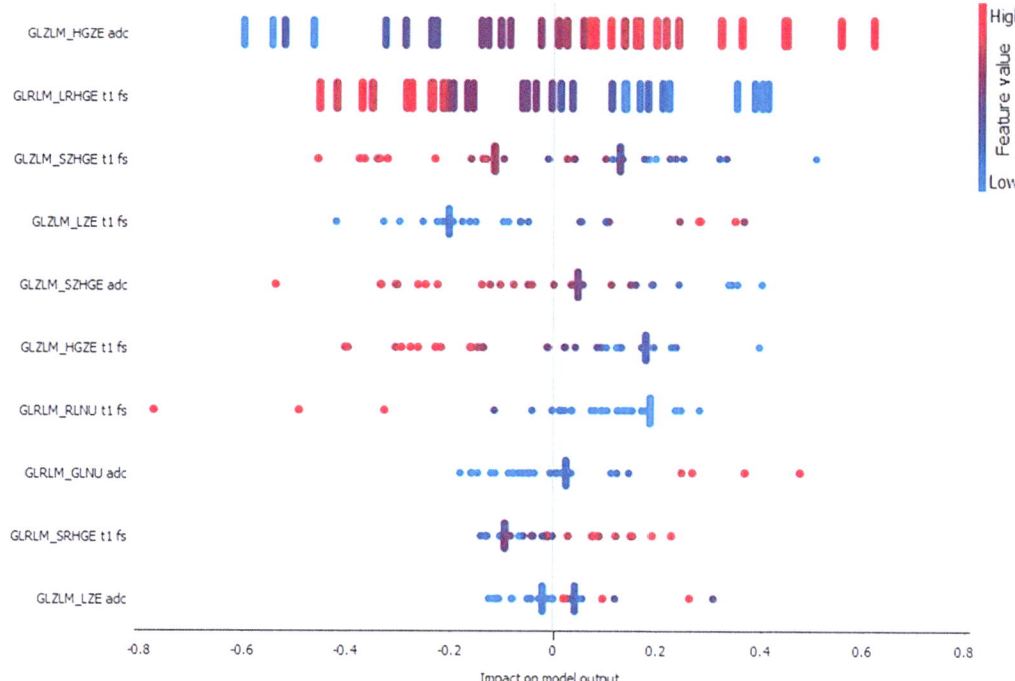

Fig. 7.7 Example of a SHAP beeswarm summary plot. This demonstrates how each of the features impacts the model's output. High values of features appear with red colour, and low value variables appear with blue colour. The colour distribution along the x axis reveals the relationship between each variable and its SHAP values

References

1. Hoinkiss DC, Huber J, Plump C, Lüth C, Drechsler R, Günther M. AI-driven and automated MRI sequence optimisation in scanner-independent MRI sequences formulated by a domain-specific language. Front Neuroimaging. 2023;2:1090054. https://doi.org/10.3389/fnimg.2023.1090054.
2. Morales MA, Manning WJ, Nesafat R. Present and future innovations in AI and cardiac MRI. Radiology. 2024;310(1):e231269. https://doi.org/10.1148/radiol.231269.
3. Sparnon E, How AI. Can help streamline the patient experience. Biomed Instrum Technol. 2022;56(4):139–41. https://doi.org/10.2345/0899-8205-56.4.139.
4. Estler A, Serweck L, Brunnée M, Estler B, Richter V, Örgel A, Bürkle E, Becker H, Hurth H, Stahl S, Konrad EM, Kelbsch C, Ernemann U, Hauser TK, Gohla G. Deep learning-accelerated image reconstruction in MRI of the orbit to shorten acquisition time and enhance image quality. J Neuroimaging. 2024;34(2):232–40. https://doi.org/10.1111/jon.13187.
5. Jurka M, Macova I, Wagnerova M, Capoun O, Jakubicek R, Ourednicek P, et al. Deep-learning-based reconstruction of T2-weighted magnetic resonance imaging of the prostate accelerated by compressed sensing provides improved image quality at half the acquisition time. Quant Imaging Med Surg. 2024;14(5):3534–43. https://doi.org/10.21037/qims-23-1488.
6. Allen TJ, Hense Bancroft LC, Unal O, Estkowski LD, Cashen TA, Korosec F, et al. Evaluation of a deep learning reconstruction for high-quality T2-weighted breast magnetic resonance imaging. Tomography. 2023;9(5):1949–64. https://doi.org/10.3390/tomography9050152.
7. Qian J, Li H, Wang J, He L. Recent advances in explainable artificial intelligence for magnetic resonance imaging. Diagnostics (Basel). 2023;13(9):1571. https://doi.org/10.3390/diagnostics13091571.
8. Serunian M, Pucciarelli F, Caruso D, Polici M, Masci B, Guido G, et al. Artificial intelligence based image quality enhancement in liver MRI: a quantitative and qualitative evaluation. Radiol Med. 2022;127(10):1098–105. https://doi.org/10.1007/s11547-022-01539-9.
9. Akçakaya M, Moeller S, Weingärtner S, Uğurbil K. Scan-specific robust artificial-neural-networks for k-space interpolation (RAKI) reconstruction: database-free deep learning for fast imaging.

Magn Reson Med. 2019;81(1):439–53. https://doi.org/10.1002/mrm.27420.

10. Wary P, Hossu G, Ambarki K, Nickel D, Arberet A, Oster J, et al. Deep learning HASTE sequence compared with T2-weighted BLADE sequence for liver MRI at 3 Tesla: a qualitative and quantitative prospective study. Eur Radiol. 2023;33(10):6817–27. https://doi.org/10.1007/s00330-023-09693-y.

11. Ostek MA, Brunnquell CL, Hoff MN, Boulter DJ, Mossa-Basha M, Beauchamp LH, et al. Practical considerations for radiologists in implementing a patient-friendly MRI experience. Top Magn Reson Imaging. 2020;29(4):181–6. https://doi.org/10.1097/rmr.0000000000000247.

12. Barth M, Breuer F, Koopmans PJ, Norris DG, Poser BA. Simultaneous multislice (SMS) imaging techniques. Magn Reson Med. 2016;75(1):63–81. https://doi.org/10.1002/mrm.25897.

13. Lin DJ, Walter SS, Frits J. Artificial intelligence-driven ultra-fast superresolution MRI: 10-fold accelerated musculoskeletal turbo spin echo MRI within reach. Investg Radiol. 2023;58(1):28–42. https://doi.org/10.1097/rli.0000000000000928.

14. Noël P, Bammer R, Reinhold C, Haider MA. Parallel imaging artifacts in body magnetic resonance imaging. Can Assoc Radiol J. 2009;60(2):91–8. https://doi.org/10.1016/j.carj.2009.02.036.

15. Shimron E, Perlman O. AI in MRI: computational frameworks for a faster, optimised, and automated imaging workflow. Bioengineering (Basel). 2023;10(4):492. https://doi.org/10.3390%2Fbioengineering10040492

16. Ni M, He M, Yang Y, Wen X, Shao Y, Gao L, et al. Application research of AI-assisted compressed sensing technology in MRI scanning of the knee joint: 3D-MRI perspective. Eur Radiol. 2023;34(5):3046–58. https://doi.org/10.1007/s00330-023-10368-x.

17. Shao Q, Xu J, Yang YX, Yu D, Shao Y, Wang Q, et al. AI-assisted accelerated MRI of the ankle: clinical practice assessment. Eur Radiol Exp. 2023;7:62. https://doi.org/10.1186/s41747-023-00374-5.

18. Liu H, Deng D, Seng W, Huang Y, Sheng C, Li X, et al. AI-assisted compressed sensing and parallel imaging sequences for MRI of patients with nasopharyngeal carcinoma: comparison of their capabilities in terms of examination time and image quality. Eur Radiol. 2023;33(11):7686–96. https://doi.org/10.1007/s00330-023-09742-6.

19. Foreman SC, Neumann J, Han J, Harrasser N, Weiss K, Peeters JM, et al. Deep learning–based acceleration of compressed Sense MR imaging of the ankle. Eur Radiol. 2022;32:8376–85. https://doi.org/10.1007/s00330-022-08919-9.

20. Stogiannos N. Reducing patient's psychological stress. A guide for MR technologists. HJR. 2019;4(1):26–30. https://doi.org/10.36162/hjr.v4i1.256.

21. Almeer MH. MRI acoustic noise cancellation using CNN. J Eng Res. 2022. https://doi.org/10.36909/jer.17661.

22. Wiesinger F, Ho ML. Zero-TE MRI: principles and applications in the head and neck. Br J Radiol. 2022;95(1136):20220059. https://doi.org/10.1259/bjr.20220059.

23. Aydıngös Ü, Yıldız AE, Ergen FB. Zero Echo time musculoskeletal MRI: technique, optimisation, applications, and pitfalls. Radiographics. 2022;42(5):1398–414. https://doi.org/10.1148/rg.220029.

24. Philips Magnetic Resonance. SmartWorkflow Solutions: patient-centred productivity. https://www.philips.com/c-dam/b2bhc/master/resource-catalog/landing/smartworkflow/philips_mr_smartworkflow_brochur.pdf.

25. GE HealthCare. AIR Touch. Intelligent coil selection that automatically knows the best coil-element configuration for every patient. https://www.gehealthcare.com/products/magnetic-resonance-imaging/mr-workflow-solutions.

26. Potočnik J, Foley S, Thomas E. Current and potential applications of artificial intelligence in medical imaging practice: a narrative review. J Med Imaging Radiat Sci. 2023;54(2):376–85. https://doi.org/10.1016/j.jmir.2023.03.033.

27. Xu X, Peng WL, Shang JG, Liu KL, Hu SX, Seng LM, et al. The application value of artificial intelligence-based filtering and interpolated image reconstruction algorithm in abdominal magnetic resonance image Denoising. Sichuan Da Xue Xue Bao Yi Xue Ban. 2021;52(2):293–9. https://doi.org/10.12182/20210360104.

28. Kanemaru N, Takao H, Amemiya S, Abe O. The effect of a post-scan processing denoising system on image quality and morphometric analysis. J Neuroradiol. 2022;49(2):205–12. https://doi.org/10.1016/j.neurad.2021.11.007.

29. Wang X, Ma J, Bhosale P, Ibarra Rovira JJ, Qayyum A, Sun J, et al. Novel deep learning-based noise reduction technique for prostate magnetic resonance imaging. Abdom Radiol (NY). 2021;46(7):3378–86. https://doi.org/10.1007/s00261-021-02964-6.

30. Shao S, Cahill DG, Li S, Xiao F, Blu T, Griffith JF, et al. Denoising of three-dimensional fast spin echo magnetic resonance images of knee joints using spatial-variant noise-relevant residual learning of convolution neural network. Comput Biol Med. 2022;151(Pt A):106295. https://doi.org/10.1016/j.compbiomed.2022.106295.

31. Liu H, Ren L, Fan B, Wang W, Hu X, Shang X. Artificial intelligence algorithm-based MRI in the diagnosis of complications after renal transplantation. Contrast Media Mol Imaging. 2022;2022:8930584. https://doi.org/10.1155/2022/8930584.

32. Pfaff L, Hossbach J, Preuhs E, Wagner F, Arroyo Camejo S, Kannengiesser S, et al. Self-supervised

MRI denoising: leveraging Stein's unbiased risk estimator and spatially resolved noise maps. Sci Rep. 2023;13:22629. https://doi.org/10.1038/s41598-023-49023-2.

33. Pruessmann KP, Weiger M, Scheidegger MB, Boesiger P. SENSE: sensitivity encoding for fast MRI. Magn Reson Med. 1999;42(5):952–62.

34. Knoll F, Hammernik K, Shang C, Moeller S, Pock T, Sodickson DK, et al. Deep-learning methods for parallel magnetic resonance imaging reconstruction: a survey of the current approaches, trends, and issues. IEEE Signal Process Mag. 2020;37(1):128–40. https://doi.org/10.1109/msp.2019.2950640.

35. Pal A, Rathi Y. A review and experimental evaluation of deep learning methods for MRI reconstruction. J Mach Learn Biomed Imaging. 2022;1:001.

36. Lee J, Jung M, Park J, Kim S, Im Y, Lee N, et al. Highly accelerated knee magnetic resonance imaging using deep neural network (DNN)–based reconstruction: prospective, multi-reader, multi-vendor study. Sci Rep. 2023;13:17264. https://doi.org/10.1038/s41598-023-44248-7.

37. Lv J, Wang C, Yang G. PIC-GAN: a parallel imaging coupled generative adversarial network for accelerated multi-channel MRI reconstruction. Diagnostics (Basel). 2021;11(1):61. https://doi.org/10.3390/diagnostics11010061.

38. Jaspan ON, Fleysher R, Lipton ML. Compressed sensing MRI: a review of the clinical literature. Br J Radiol. 2015;88(1056):20150487. https://doi.org/10.1259/bjr.20150487.

39. Liu K, Xi B, Sun H, Wang J, Chen C, Wen X, et al. The clinical feasibility of artificial intelligence-assisted compressed sensing single-shot fluid-attenuated inversion recovery (ACS-SS-FLAIR) for evaluation of uncooperative patients with brain diseases: comparison with the conventional T2-FLAIR with parallel imaging. Acta Radiol. 2023;64(5):1943–9. https://doi.org/10.1177/02841851221139125.

40. Noordman CR, Yakar D, Bosma J, Simonis FFJ, Huisman H. Complexities of deep learning-based undersampled MR image reconstruction. Eur Radiol Exp. 2023;7:58. https://doi.org/10.1186/s41747-023-00372-7.

41. Waddington DEJ, Hindley N, Koonjoo N, Chiu C, Reynolds T, Liu PSY, et al. Real-time radial reconstruction with domain transform manifold learning for MRI-guided radiotherapy. Med Phys. 2023;50(4):1962–74. https://doi.org/10.1002/mp.16224.

42. Yang J, Wright J, Huang TS, Ma Y. Image super-resolution via sparse representation. IEEE Trans Image Process. 2010;19(11):2861–73. https://doi.org/10.1109/TIP.2010.2050625.

43. Nguyen X, Ostek M, Nelakurti DD, Brunnquell CL, Mossa-Basha M, Haynor DR, et al. Applying artificial intelligence to mitigate effects of patient motion or other complicating factors on image quality. Top Magn Reson Imaging. 2020;29(4):175–80. https://doi.org/10.1097/RMR.0000000000000249.

44. Chaudhari AS, Fang S, Kogan F, Wood J, Stevens KJ, Gibbons EK, et al. Super-resolution musculoskeletal MRI using deep learning. Magn Reson Med. 2018;80(5):2139–54. https://doi.org/10.1002/mrm.27178.

45. Chaudhari AS, Grissom MJ, Fang S, Sveinsson B, Lee JH, Gold GE, et al. Diagnostic accuracy of quantitative multicontrast 5-minute knee MRI using prospective artificial intelligence image quality enhancement. AJR Am J Roentgenol. 2021;216(6):1614–25. https://doi.org/10.2214/ajr.20.24172.

46. Li BM, Castorina LV, Valdés Hernándes MDC, Clancy U, Wiseman SJ, Sakka E, et al. Deep attention super-resolution of brain magnetic resonance images acquired under clinical protocols. Front Comput Neurosci. 2022;16:887633. https://doi.org/10.3389/fncom.2022.887633.

47. Liu H, Liu J, Li J, Pan JS, Yu X. DL-MRI: a unified framework of deep learning-based MRI super resolution. J Healthc Eng. 2021;2021:5594649. https://doi.org/10.1155/2021/5594649.

48. Weiss DA, Saluja R, Xie L, Gee JC, Sugrue LP, Pradhan A, et al. Automated multiclass tissue segmentation of clinical brain MRIs with lesions. Neuroimage Clin. 2021;31:102769. https://doi.org/10.1016/j.nicl.2021.102769.

49. Despotović I, Goossens B, Philips W. MRI segmentation of the human brain: challenges, methods, and applications. Comput Math Methods Med. 2015;2015:450341. https://doi.org/10.1155/2015/450341.

50. Hilbert A, Madai VI, Akay EM, Aydin OU, Behland J, Sobesky J, et al. BRAVE-NET: fully automated arterial brain vessel segmentation in patients with cerebrovascular disease. Front Artif Intell. 2020;3:552258. https://doi.org/10.3389/frai.2020.552258.

51. Kim H, Kang SW, Kim J-H, Nagar H, Sabuncu M, Margolis D, et al. The role of AI in prostate MRI quality and interpretation: opportunities and challenges. Eur J Radiol. 2023;165:110887. https://doi.org/10.1016/j.ejrad.2023.110887.

52. Stogiannos N, Bougias H, Georgiadou E, Leandrou S, Papavasileiou P. Analysis of radiomic features derived from post-contrast T1-weighted images and apparent diffusion coefficient (ADC) maps for breast lesion evaluation: a retrospective study. Radiography (Lond). 2023;29(2):355–61. https://doi.org/10.1016/j.radi.2023.01.019.

53. de Bruijne M. Machine learning approaches in medical image analysis: from detection to diagnosis. Med Image Anal. 2016;33:94–7. https://doi.org/10.1016/j.media.2016.06.032.

54. LeCun Y, Bengio Y, Hinton G. Deep learning. Nature. 2015;521:436–44. https://doi.org/10.1038/nature14539.

55. Ronneberger O, Fischer P, Brox T. U-net: convolutional networks for biomedical image segmentation. In: Navab N, Hornegger J, Wells WM, Frangi AF,

editors. Medical Image Computing and Computer-Assisted Intervention—MICCAI 2015. October 5–9, 2015; Munich, Germany, vol. 2015. Cham: Springer International Publishing; 2015. p. 234241.

56. Minaee S, Boykov Y, Porikli F, Plasa A, Kehtarnavas N, Tersopoulos D. Image segmentation using deep learning: a survey. IEEE Trans Pattern Anal Mach Intell. 2022;44(7):3523–42. https://doi.org/10.1109/tpami.2021.3059968.

57. Hao S, Shou Y, Guo Y. A brief survey on semantic segmentation with deep learning. Neurocomputing. 2020;406:302–21. https://doi.org/10.1016/j.neucom.2019.11.118.

58. Wang T, Yang J, Ji S, Sun Q. Probabilistic diffusion for interactive image segmentation. IEEE Trans Image Process. 2019;28(1):330–42. https://doi.org/10.1109/tip.2018.2867941.

59. Qiu L, Ren H. U-RSNet: an unsupervised probabilistic model for joint registration and segmentation. Neurocomputing. 2021;450:264–74. https://doi.org/10.1016/j.neucom.2021.04.042.

60. Fischl B, van der Kouwe A, Destrieux C, Halgren E, Ségonne F, Salat DH, et al. Automatically parcellating the human cerebral cortex. Cereb Cortex. 2004;14(1):11–22. https://doi.org/10.1093/cercor/bhg087.

61. Morey RA, Petty CM, Xu Y, Hayes JP, Wagner HR 2nd, Lewis DV, et al. A comparison of automated segmentation and manual tracing for quantifying hippocampal and amygdala volumes. NeuroImage. 2009;45(3):855–66. https://doi.org/10.1016/j.neuroimage.2008.12.033.

62. Smith SM, Jenkinson M, Woolrich MW, Beckmann CF, Behrens TE, Johansen-Berg H, et al. Advances in functional and structural MR image analysis and implementation as FSL. NeuroImage. 2004;23(Suppl 1):S208–19. https://doi.org/10.1016/j.neuroimage.2004.07.051.

63. Leandrou S, Lamnisos D, Bougias H, Stogiannos N, Georgiadou E, Achilleos KG, et al. A cross-sectional study of explainable machine learning in Alzheimer's disease: diagnostic classification using MR radiomic features. Front Aging Neurosci. 2023;15:1149871. https://doi.org/10.3389/fnagi.2023.1149871.

64. The MathWorks. Statistical parametric mapping. Available at: https://uk.mathworks.com/matlab-central/fileexchange/68729-statistical-parametric-mapping. Accessed 15 Jan 2025.

65. Ogier AC, Bustin A, Cochet H, Schwitter J, van Heeswijk RB. The road toward reproducibility of parametric mapping of the heart: a technical review. Front Cardiovasc Med. 2022;9:876475. https://doi.org/10.3389/fcvm.2022.876475.

66. Priester A, Fan RE, Shubert J, Rusu M, Vesal S, Shao W, et al. Prediction and mapping of intraprostatic tumor extent with artificial intelligence. Eur Urol Open Sci. 2023;54:20–7. https://doi.org/10.1016/j.euros.2023.05.018.

67. Kalapos A, Ssabó L, Dohy S, Kiss M, Merkely B, Gyires-Tóth B, et al. Automated T1 and T2 mapping

segmentation on cardiovascular magnetic resonance imaging using deep learning. Front Cardiovasc Med. 2023;10:1147581. https://doi.org/10.3389/fcvm.2023.1147581.

68. Thomas KA, Krsemiński D, Kidsiński Ł, Paul R, Rubin EB, Halilaj E, et al. Open source software for automatic subregional assessment of knee cartilage degradation using quantitative T2 Relaxometry and deep learning. Cartilage. 2021;13(1_suppl):747S–56S. https://doi.org/10.1177/19476035211042406.

69. Tang X. The role of artificial intelligence in medical imaging research. BJR Open. 2020;2(1):20190031. https://doi.org/10.1259/bjro.20190031.

70. Sheng T, Shu Y, Chen Y, Mai S, Xu L, Jiang H, et al. Fully automated MRI-based convolutional neural network for noninvasive diagnosis of cirrhosis. Insights Imaging. 2024;15(1):298. https://doi.org/10.1186/s13244-024-01872-9.

71. Rathore S, Habes M, Iftikhar MA, Shacklett A, Davatsikos C. A review on neuroimaging-based classification studies and associated feature extraction methods for Alzheimer's disease and its prodromal stages. NeuroImage. 2017;155:530–48. https://doi.org/10.1016/j.neuroimage.2017.03.057.

72. Khattap MG, Abd Elasis M, Hassan HGEMA, Elgarayhi A, Sallah M. AI-based model for automatic identification of multiple sclerosis based on enhanced sea-horse optimiser and MRI scans. Sci Rep. 2024;14(1):12104. https://doi.org/10.1038/s41598-024-61876-9.

73. Shang S, Li G, Xu Y, Tang X. Application of artificial intelligence in the MRI classification task of human brain neurological and psychiatric diseases: a scoping review. Diagnostics (Basel). 2021;11(8):1402. https://doi.org/10.3390/diagnostics11081402.

74. Oren O, Gersh BJ, Bhatt DL. Artificial intelligence in medical imaging: switching from radiographic pathological data to clinically meaningful endpoints. Lancet Digit Health. 2020;2(9):e486–8. https://doi.org/10.1016/S2589-7500(20)30160-6.

75. Mathur S, Sutton J. Personalised medicine could transform healthcare. Biomed Rep. 2017;7(1):3–5. https://doi.org/10.3892/br.2017.922.

76. Khalifa M, Albadawy M. AI in diagnostic imaging: Revolutionising accuracy and efficiency. Comput Methods Programs Biomed Update. 2024;5:100146. https://doi.org/10.1016/j.cmpbup.2024.100146.

77. Hsieh C, Laguna A, Ikeda I, Maxwell AWP, Chapiro J, Nadolski G, et al. Using machine learning to predict response to image-guided therapies for hepatocellular carcinoma. Radiology. 2023;309(2):e222891. https://doi.org/10.1148/radiol.222891.

78. Ke J, Jin C, Tang J, Cao H, He S, Ding P, et al. A longitudinal MRI-based artificial intelligence system to predict pathological complete response after neoadjuvant therapy in rectal cancer: a multicenter validation study. Dis Colon Rectum. 2023;66(12):e1195–206. https://doi.org/10.1097/dcr.0000000000002931.

79. Arita Y, Kwee TC, Akin O, Shigeta K, Paudyal R, Roest C, et al. Multiparametric MRI and artificial intelligence in predicting and monitoring treatment response in bladder cancer. Insights Imaging. 2025;16(1):7. https://doi.org/10.1186/s13244-024-01884-5.

80. Vollmuth P, Foltyn M, Huang RY, Galldiks N, Petersen J, Isensee F, et al. Artificial intelligence (AI)-based decision support improves reproducibility of tumor response assessment in neuro-oncology: an international multi-reader study. Neuro-Oncology. 2023;25(3):533–43. https://doi.org/10.1093/neuonc/noac189.

81. Qi X. Artificial intelligence-assisted magnetic resonance imaging technology in the differential diagnosis and prognosis prediction of endometrial cancer. Sci Rep. 2024;14(1):26878. https://doi.org/10.1038/s41598-024-78081-3.

82. Tovar DR, Rosenthal MH, Maitra A, Koay EJ. Potential of artificial intelligence in the risk stratification for and early detection of pancreatic cancer. Artif Intell Surg. 2023;3(1):14–26. https://doi.org/10.20517/ais.2022.38.

83. Bodalal S, Trebeschi S, Nguyen-Kim TDL, Schats W, Beets-Tan R. Radiogenomics: bridging imaging and genomics. Abdom Radiol (NY). 2019;44(6):1960–84. https://doi.org/10.1007/s00261-019-02028-w.

84. Georgiadou E, Bougias H, Leandrou S, Stogiannos N. Radiomics for Alzheimer's disease: fundamental principles and clinical applications. In: Vlamos P, editor. GeNeDis 2022: computational biology and bioinformatics. Switzerland: Springer Nature; 2023. p. 297–310.

85. Shui L, Ren H, Yang X, Li J, Chen S, Yi C, et al. The era of radiogenomics in precision medicine: an emerging approach to support diagnosis, treatment decisions, and prognostication in oncology. Front Oncol. 2021;10:570465. https://doi.org/10.3389/fonc.2020.570465.

86. Barros V, Tlusty T, Barkan E, Hexter E, Gruen D, Guindy M, et al. Virtual biopsy by using artificial intelligence-based multimodal modeling of binational mammography data. Radiology. 2023;306(3):e220027. https://doi.org/10.1148/radiol.220027.

87. Stogiannos N, Malik R, Kumar A, Barnes A, Pogose M, Harvey H, et al. Black box no more: a scoping review of AI governance frameworks to guide procurement and adoption of AI in medical imaging and radiotherapy in the UK. Br J Radiol. 2023;96(1152):20221157. https://doi.org/10.1259/bjr.20221157.

88. Shah RM, Gautam R. Overcoming diagnostic challenges of artificial intelligence in pathology and radiology: innovative solutions and strategies. Indian J Med Sci. 2023;75:107–13. https://doi.org/10.25259/IJMS_98_2023.

89. Sourlos N, Vliegenthart R, Santinha J, Klontzas ME, Cuocolo R, Huisman M, et al. Recommendations for the creation of benchmark datasets for reproducible artificial intelligence in radiology. Insights Imaging. 2024;15(1):24. https://doi.org/10.1186/s13244-024-01833-2.

90. Najjar R. Redefining radiology: a review of artificial intelligence integration in medical imaging. Diagnostics (Basel). 2023;13(17):2760. https://doi.org/10.3390/diagnostics13172760.

91. Ueda D, Kakinuma T, Fujita S, Kamagata K, Fushimi Y, Ito R, et al. Fairness of artificial intelligence in healthcare: review and recommendations. Jpn J Radiol. 2024;42(1):3–15. https://doi.org/10.1007/s11604-023-01474-3.

92. Champendal M, Müller H, Prior JO, Dos Reis CS. A scoping review of interpretability and explainability concerning artificial intelligence methods in medical imaging. Eur J Radiol. 2023;169:111159. https://doi.org/10.1016/j.ejrad.2023.111159.

93. Walsh G, Stogiannos N, van de Venter R, Rainey C, Tam W, McFadden S, et al. Responsible AI practice and AI education are central to AI implementation: a rapid review for all medical imaging professionals in Europe. BJR Open. 2023;5(1):20230033. https://doi.org/10.1259/bjro.20230033.

94. Waller J, O'Connor A, Rafaat E, Amireh A, Dempsey J, Martin C, et al. Applications and challenges of artificial intelligence in diagnostic and interventional radiology. Pol J Radiol. 2022;87:e113–7. https://doi.org/10.5114/pjr.2022.113531.

95. Stogiannos N, O'Regan T, Scurr E, Litosseliti L, Pogose M, Harvey H, et al. AI implementation in the UK landscape: knowledge of AI governance, perceived challenges and opportunities, and ways forward for radiographers. Radiography (Lond). 2024;30(2):612–21. https://doi.org/10.1016/j.radi.2024.01.019.

96. Stogiannos N, Gillan C, Precht H, Reis CSD, Kumar A, O'Regan T, et al. A multidisciplinary team and multiagency approach for AI implementation: a commentary for medical imaging and radiotherapy key stakeholders. J Med Imaging Radiat Sci. 2024;55(4):101717. https://doi.org/10.1016/j.jmir.2024.101717.

97. Shelmerdine SC, Togher D, Rickaby S, Dean G. Artificial intelligence (AI) implementation within the National Health Service (NHS): the South West London AI working group experience. Clin Radiol. 2024;79(9):665–72. https://doi.org/10.1016/j.crad.2024.05.018.

98. Soenksen LR, Ma Y, Seng C, Boussioux L, Villalobos Carballo K, Na L, et al. Integrated multimodal artificial intelligence framework for healthcare applications. NPJ Digit Med. 2022;5(1):149. https://doi.org/10.1038/s41746-022-00689-4.

99. Topol EJ. As artificial intelligence goes multimodal, medical applications multiply. Science. 2023;381(6663):adk6139. https://doi.org/10.1126/science.adk6139.

100. Milosevic M, Jin Q, Singh A, Amal S. Applications of AI in multi-modal imaging for cardiovascular

disease. Front Radiol. 2024;3:1294068. https://doi.org/10.3389/fradi.2023.1294068.

101. Shuang X. Multivariate mixture model for myocardial segmentation combining multi-source images. IEEE Trans Pattern Anal Mach Intell. 2019;41(12):2933–46. https://doi.org/10.1109/tpami.2018.2869576.

102. Blendowski M, Bouteldja N, Heinrich MP. Multimodal 3D medical image registration guided by shape encoder-decoder networks. Int J Comput Assist Radiol Surg. 2020;15(2):269–76. https://doi.org/10.1007/s11548-019-02089-8.

103. Mohsen F, Ali H, El Hajj N, Shah S. Artificial intelligence-based methods for fusion of electronic health records and imaging data. Sci Rep. 2022;12(1):17981. https://doi.org/10.1038/s41598-022-22514-4.

104. Rehman MHU, Hugo Lopes Pinaya W, Nachev P, Teo JT, Ourselin S, Cardoso MJ. Federated learning for medical imaging radiology. Br J Radiol. 2023;96(1150):20220890. https://doi.org/10.1259/bjr.20220890.

105. Naeem A, Anees T, Naqvi RA, Loh WK. A comprehensive analysis of recent deep and federated-learning-based methodologies for brain tumor diagnosis. J Pers Med. 2022;12(2):275. https://doi.org/10.3390/jpm12020275.

106. Qiu L, Cheng J, Gao H, Xiong W, Ren H. Federated semi-supervised learning for medical image segmentation via pseudo-label denoising. IEEE J Biomed Health Inform. 2023;27(10):4672–83. https://doi.org/10.1109/jbhi.2023.3274498.

107. Karim MR, Islam T, Shajalal M, Beyan O, Lange C, Coches M, et al. Explainable AI for bioinformatics: methods, tools and applications. Brief Bioinform. 2023;24(5):bbad236. https://doi.org/10.1093/bib/bbad236.

108. Lysdahlgaard S. Utilising heat maps as explainable artificial intelligence for detecting abnormalities on wrist and elbow radiographs. Radiography. 2023;29(6):1132–8. https://doi.org/10.1016/j.radi.2023.09.012.

109. Abgrall G, Holder AL, Chelly Dagdia S, Seitouni K, Monnet X. Should AI models be explainable to clinicians? Crit Care. 2024;28(1):301. https://doi.org/10.1186/s13054-024-05005-y.

Nikolaos Stogiannos is an expert MRI radiographer with over 16 years of clinical experience. In addition, he is deeply involved in research and academic publishing, and he is currently a PhD researcher and Honorary Research Fellow at City St George's, University of London. He is an associate editor for *Journal of Medical Imaging & Radiation Sciences*, as well as for BMC Medical Imaging. Nikos has given many invited talks at major international conferences, and he has a steadily growing publication record. Currently, he works towards safe and successful integration of AI in radiography clinical practice.

Dr Stephanos Leandrou is a radiologic technologist with a Bachelor of Science in Medical Radiologic Technology and a Master of Science in Diagnostic Imaging from the University of Oxford, where he also gained clinical experience in magnetic resonance imaging (MRI). He holds a PhD in Biomedical from City, University of London, with research focused on quantitative texture analysis of MRI images in the assessment of Alzheimer's disease. His main areas of interest include diagnostic radiology with emphasis on MRI, medical image analysis, and the development of computer-aided diagnosis (CAD) systems to support clinical decision-making and improve patient outcomes. Since 2013, Dr. Leandrou has been a faculty member at European University Cyprus.

Charalampos Bougias earned his degree as a Radiographer from the Department of Radiologic Technologists at the National Technological Institution of Athens (University of West Attica), Greece, in 1998. In 2018, he obtained a Master of Science diploma in Advanced Ultrasonic Functional Imaging and Research for the Prevention and Diagnosis of Vascular Diseases from the University of Thessaly, Greece. He currently serves as a radiographer in the Department of Molecular Imaging at the University Hospital of Ioannina, Greece. Since 2017, he has been a member of the MRI Experts Committee of the European Federation of Radiographer Societies (EFRS) and is the co-chair of the MRI Safety Working Group. In 2023, he became a member of the ESMRMB-EFRS MRI Radiographers Working Group. Mr Bougias is a co-author of 5 book chapters and has published over 30 scientific papers in peer-reviewed international journals. He has delivered more than 40 lectures at international congresses and educational courses. His primary research interests include medical image processing, artificial intelligence in radiology, molecular imaging, and advanced MRI applications for neurology and body imaging. Since 2022, he has been a visiting lecturer at the University of West Attica in the Department of Biomedical Sciences. He currently works as an MRI application specialist and consultant.

AI in Interventional Radiology and Cardiology

8

Christopher Steelman

8.1 Introduction to Interventional Radiology and Cardiology Imaging Environments

Fluoroscopy serves as the cornerstone of angiographic imaging, enabling real-time, dynamic visualisation of vascular structures. The cardiac imaging environment exemplifies the critical principles of fluoroscopy, offering a comprehensive model that informs best practices across a range of fluoroscopic procedures. Precision, adaptability, and radiation safety are paramount in this setting, where operators must balance image quality with patient and staff protection. By exploring the cardiac imaging environment, this section highlights core imaging techniques, radiation safety protocols, and workflow considerations that are transferable to other fluoroscopic applications. This approach provides a holistic understanding of fluoroscopy's role in both diagnostic and interventional procedures.

Recent technological advancements, particularly the integration of artificial intelligence (AI), have significantly enhanced the effectiveness and safety of fluoroscopic imaging. AI encompasses a

on behalf of Association of Healthcare Technology Providers for Imaging, Radiotherapy and Care (AXREM)

C. Steelman (✉)
Cath Lab International, LLC, New Orleans, Louisanna, USA

range of computational methods designed to perform tasks typically requiring human intelligence. Machine learning (ML), a subset of AI, utilises algorithms that learn from and make predictions based on large datasets. In cardiovascular imaging, these technologies are applied to modalities such as echocardiography, computed tomography (CT), magnetic resonance imaging (MRI), and nuclear imaging, facilitating improved image interpretation and automation of repetitive tasks [1]. The incorporation of AI into fluoroscopic workflows enhances diagnostic accuracy, reduces reliance on human interpretation, and accelerates clinical decision-making, ultimately improving procedural efficiency.

The integration of AI has also transformed the broader fields of interventional cardiology and interventional radiology. While interventional cardiology focuses on heart-related conditions such as coronary artery disease (CAD) and heart valve disorders through procedures like angioplasty, stent placement, and cardiac catheterisation, interventional radiology addresses a wider range of conditions, including cancer, vascular diseases, and musculoskeletal issues [2]. Procedures like embolisation, thrombolysis, and ablation rely on fluoroscopy for guidance, and both fields increasingly depend on AI-driven solutions to improve care quality, safety, and efficiency.

One of the most transformative impacts of AI is seen in angiography, a vital imaging tool in cardiovascular care. Traditional two-dimensional imaging posed challenges in precision and depth perception, often requiring expert interpretation. However, AI-driven tools, such as convolutional neural networks (CNNs), process large datasets to provide enhanced image analysis and real-time guidance during procedures [3, 4]. These advancements have improved the accuracy of CAD diagnosis and streamlined clinical workflows, ensuring faster and more precise interventions. By reducing reliance on manual interpretation, AI supports real-time decision-making, enabling more efficient patient care.

Radiation safety, a critical issue in interventional procedures, has also improved with the adoption of AI-based dose optimisation systems. These systems monitor and adjust radiation parameters in real time, reducing cumulative exposure for both patients and healthcare professionals [5]. For interventional teams who perform multiple procedures daily, AI's ability to predict and mitigate radiation exposure represents a vital advancement in procedural safety. This development addresses a long-standing challenge in fluoroscopy, where operators, often radiographers, face significant occupational exposure to ionising radiation.

AI's influence extends beyond imaging and radiation safety into procedural automation and robotics. AI-powered robotic systems enhance procedural precision, reduce human error, and improve operator ergonomics. By enabling precise, controlled manipulation of devices, AI-guided robotics reduce operator fatigue and minimise the risk of manual errors [6]. The potential for remote-guided procedures further expands the impact of robotics in interventional practice. Through teleoperated interventions, experienced interventional cardiologists can guide procedures remotely, increasing access to specialised care in underserved regions. This convergence of AI, robotics, and fluoroscopy introduces a paradigm shift in how interventional procedures are performed and accessed.

AI's role in physiological assessments, such as fractional flow reserve (FFR) and intracoronary imaging, further illustrates its transformative potential [7]. FFR measurements and intracoronary imaging are essential for evaluat-

ing the functional significance of coronary lesions. AI-enabled tools analyse patient-specific data in real time, allowing personalised, data-driven treatment decisions. This precision reduces the need for invasive testing and supports more tailored treatment strategies, promoting a shift towards precision medicine.

Beyond AI, emerging computational advancements such as computational simulations (CS) and extended reality (XR) are revolutionising procedural planning, training, and education. CS employs mathematical models to simulate cardiovascular interventions, generating patient-specific data that guides treatment strategy, stent placement, and device selection. By providing a virtual representation of a patient's cardiovascular system, CS enables clinicians to anticipate and plan for procedural challenges, reducing uncertainty and enhancing pre-procedure planning.

Extended reality (XR) technologies, which include virtual reality (VR), augmented reality (AR), and mixed reality (MR), offer immersive training environments where healthcare professionals can hone technical skills in a risk-free, controlled setting. These tools enable medical device developers and healthcare providers to visualise and practice complex interventions before engaging in live procedures. For interventional cardiologists, XR provides a 3D, interactive view of vascular structures, enhancing spatial awareness and improving procedural planning. Despite these challenges, the combined potential of AI, CS, and XR is undeniable. By enhancing procedural safety, accuracy, and access to expert care, these technologies are transforming interventional cardiology and radiology. The continued evolution of AI-driven decision support systems, robotic-assisted interventions, and immersive training platforms signals a future in which healthcare delivery is faster, safer, and more accessible to patients worldwide. Through the thoughtful integration of these innovations, interventional procedures are poised for a new era of precision medicine and data-driven care.

The teams in both the cardiac catheterisation laboratory and the interventional radiology suite are multidisciplinary and must function in a highly coordinated manner to ensure the safety, efficacy, and efficiency of clinical care. These teams typically include physicians—such as interventional cardiologists, interventional radiologists, and other specialists—as well as radiographers, cardiovascular technologists, nurses, and other support staff. Radiographers and cardiovascular technologists play essential roles in both diagnostic and interventional procedures across cardiac and non-cardiac vascular systems. Their contributions are grounded in technical expertise, radiologic proficiency, clinical awareness, and strong communication skills. In both the cath lab and IR settings, these professionals must adapt to rapidly changing clinical demands and apply a broad range of techniques in high-pressure environments. These team members are also integral to emergency response and are often part of the on-call roster, providing critical support for urgent, life-saving interventions around the clock [8, 9]. In this Chapter, the term operator refers to various members of the interventional team. The specific responsibilities associated with this role may differ across professional groups and international contexts, depending on local policy, credentialing frameworks, and scope of practice.

8.2 Angiography

The use of fluoroscopy has been a pivotal tool in interventional cardiology, and novel technology has introduced several new techniques to overcome the limitations of two-dimensional (2D) fluoroscopy imaging. Assistant robots controlled by humans and cardiovascular imaging modalities are employed in catheterisation laboratories and hybrid theaters [10, 11].

Imaging has become an essential diagnostic tool in clinical decision-making in cardiovascular diseases and stroke. Invasive coronary angiography is the gold standard for diagnosing coronary artery disease (CAD) [12–14], despite challenges posed by patient-specific anatomy and image quality [13]. Visual estimation of coronary stenosis severity from angiograms remains the most common, guideline-supported approach to evaluate angiographic narrowing of the coronary artery

lumen [15]. However, expertise in image interpretation takes years to acquire, and experts are often overburdened with tasks such as image processing, segmentation, quantitation, and interpretation. Moreover, expertise in image interpretation is scarce, exacerbating inequities in access to high-quality patient care in under-resourced areas, between lower and higher income populations, and between low- and rich-resource countries [16]. In clinical practice and also for quality control purposes in research settings, screening coronary angiogram visually to distinguish cases with normal or mild stenosis from those with higher stenosis severity is a time-consuming process even for experienced readers [12]. The limitations of visual estimation for coronary stenosis severity are well described, and include intra- and inter-observer variability, operator bias and poor reproducibility. Variability in visual stenosis assessment ranges from 7.6% to 22.5% [17]. The difference in mean diameter stenosis between quantitative coronary angiography and visual estimation varies from 10% to 20% and is dependent on stenosis severity [15]. Visual assessment of stenosis can overestimate the severity of stenosis in over a quarter of cases [18] and may contribute to inappropriate coronary artery bypass surgery in 17% of patients and stent usage in at least 10% of patients [17].

There is an increasing interest in AI- and ML-based tools for vascular imaging as they help resolve numerous of the above challenges in the field. Establishing a consistent and reliable approach for interpreting angiograms and evaluating coronary stenosis would be highly valuable for clinical practice. Deep learning (DL) technology, a more advanced version of machine learning (see Chap. 2), can be used in the interpretation of diagnostic angiography. Artificial intelligence techniques, such as DL and computer vision, can be utilised for the purposes of image quantification (e.g. angiography quantify lesion, intravascular imaging assisted diagnosis) and the results thus far have been promising.

Several studies have demonstrated that AI can quantify angiographic lesions with similar accuracy to human experts [19]. DL models have been developed to identify lesion morphology, stenosis, calcification, thrombosis, total occlusion, and dissection from coronary angiography and they demonstrated good accuracy (98.4%) and sensitivity (85.2%) [20]. In the future, it may serve as a more powerful tool to standardise screening and risk stratification of patients with CAD.

8.3   Artificial Intelligence Dose Reduction

While the use of X-rays for visualisation of coronary arteries and catheters has resulted in many positive technological achievements and significant treatment benefits, it also has major disadvantages due to the long-term adverse effects of radiation exposure [21]. Use of ionising radiation during cardiac catheterisation interventions adversely impacts both the patients and medical staff. Radiation exposure can result in long-term health effects, including skin and eye damage, and may cause certain forms of cancer by interacting with and altering cellular DNA [22].

Radiation exposure in interventional cardiology and radiology poses significant risks to both patients and healthcare personnel. Interventional cardiology procedures, such as coronary angiography and percutaneous coronary interventions, involve substantial use of ionising radiation. These procedures account for approximately 12% of all radiological examinations, contributing to nearly 50% of the total radiation dose received in medical settings. For instance, the radiation exposure from a coronary angiography examination can be equivalent to that of 300 chest X-rays, while more complex interventions can result in exposures ranging from 1000 to several thousand chest X-rays [23, 24].

8.3.1   Health Risks to Personnel

Interventional cardiologists are at higher risk for developing various cancers due to prolonged exposure to radiation including brain tumors, particularly on the left side of the head, as well as thyroid cancers and other malignancies [25, 26]. There is also a documented increase in the inci-

dence of cataracts, particularly posterior subcapsular cataracts, among this professional group, particularly those who do not utilise protective eyewear [25, 27]. There is emerging evidence suggesting that radiation exposure may contribute to macrovascular and microvascular abnormalities, although the occupational significance of these findings is still being evaluated [25, 26].

8.3.2   Risks to Patients

Patients undergoing interventional procedures are also at risk from radiation exposure. The potential adverse effects include skin reactions [24, 27] and long-term cancer risk [24, 28].

In the pursuit of advancing transcatheter therapies, it is essential to address the harmful physical effects that can result from cumulative radiation exposure among catheter lab personnel. This issue is becoming increasingly significant due to the rising complexity of interventional procedures and the growth of structural cardiology interventions in modern interventional practice. AI offers promising, long-term solutions to radiation protection challenges, helping to create a safer and more efficient working environment in interventional cardiology and radiology departments within hospitals and other healthcare facilities.

Staff education and training in minimising radiation exposure remains essential for safe radiation practices in the catheterisation lab. However, with the emergence of AI technology, new innovations offer great potential to enhance fluoroscopic procedures and reduce radiation exposure for healthcare workers.

8.3.3   Dynamic Coronary Roadmap

Static vascular roadmaps, like Digital Subtraction Angiography (DSA), are commonly used in peripheral interventions where there is minimal blood vessel movement. In comparison to fluoroscopic dose rates, cine dose rates are 9–13 times higher, while DSA dose rates are 22–30 times greater—more than twice the cine dose rates during various interventional radiology procedures [29]. However, in coronary interventions, vessel movement prevents the use of static roadmaps, requiring navigation through visual comparison to a displayed angiographic image and the use of additional contrast injections for verification during wire passage, ballooning, and stent placement. Deep learning has been introduced to aid in percutaneous coronary intervention (PCI) navigation, increasing procedural efficiency and ease [30]. One notable application is the dynamic coronary roadmap (DCR) developed by Philips Healthcare [31], which provides a motion-compensated, real-time view of coronary arteries (see Fig. 8.1). This system overlays a highlighted coronary angiogram onto a live 2D fluoroscopic image, creating a dynamic, coloured roadmap that adjusts automatically, offering continuous visual feedback on wire and catheter positioning. Clinical studies have shown that DCR reduces the total iodine contrast volume per PCI procedure by an average of 28.8% and lowers the number of contrast-enhanced cineangiograms per procedure by approximately 26.3%

[32]. These technologies clearly have the potential to improve both procedural efficiency and patient outcomes [33].

8.3.4 Fluoroshield

The Fluoroshield system also utilises an AI-enabled approach towards radiation exposure reduction. In a study conducted by Bang et al. [34], on using AI to reduce radiation dose in fluoroscopy, it was discovered that Fluoroshield [35], a type of fluoroscopy system has AI technology embedded in it for the purposes of radiation protection. Unlike the conventional technology, Fluoroshield uses ultrafast collimation to reduce radiation exposure during examinations [34]. The system automatically tracks the region of interest (ROI) in real time, controls a rapid lead shutter for collimating the X-ray beam to the ROI, and blends the imaged ROI with the entire field of view that is updated at a lower frame rate to present, at all times, a full image to the operator (see also Fig. 8.2) [36].

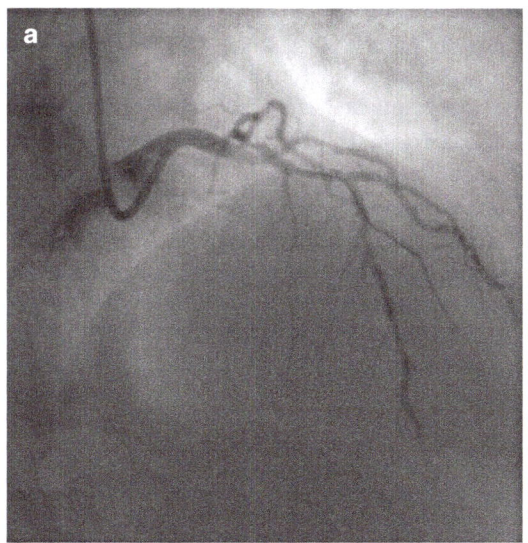
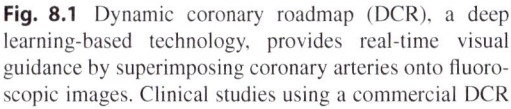
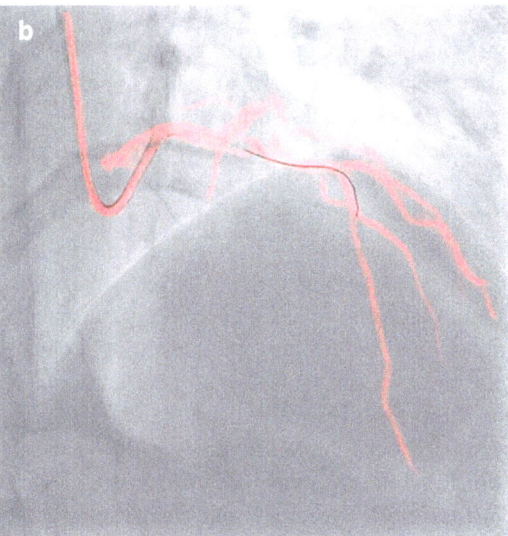

Fig. 8.1 Dynamic coronary roadmap (DCR), a deep learning-based technology, provides real-time visual guidance by superimposing coronary arteries onto fluoroscopic images. Clinical studies using a commercial DCR system (Philips Healthcare) have demonstrated a significant reduction in contrast volume and fluoroscopy time [31, 32]

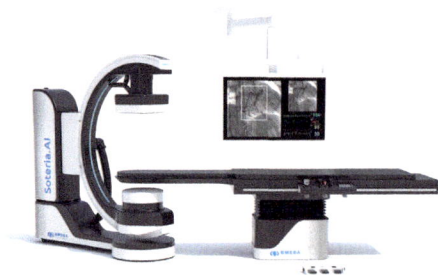

Fig. 8.2 Fluoroshield™ utilises AI-driven automation to detect the interventionalist's region of interest (ROI) in real time, dynamically adjusting collimation to optimise visualisation while minimising radiation exposure [34–36]

8.4 Robotics

Robotic-assisted percutaneous coronary intervention (R-PCI) is a transformative advancement in interventional cardiology, addressing major occupational hazards like radiation exposure and orthopedic strain. Traditional percutaneous coronary intervention (T-PCI) exposes operators to continuous fluoroscopic radiation, increasing the risk of DNA damage, cancer, and orthopedic injuries from prolonged use of heavy lead aprons. Approximately 49% of interventional cardiologists report at least one orthopedic injury [37–42]. R-PCI mitigates these risks by allowing operators to control procedures from a radiation-shielded cockpit, significantly reducing exposure and eliminating the need for lead aprons [40, 41].

R-PCI systems enable interventionalists to remotely control guidewires, catheters, and devices via joystick or touchscreen interfaces. Early platforms relied on basic axial and rotational controls, limiting the ability to replicate complex manual maneuvers, like wiring side branches [36]. However, the CorPath GRX system introduced the AI-driven TechnIQ software, which replicates essential manual techniques, such as "spin," "wiggle," and "rotate-on-retract" manoeuvres [37, 43]. Operators can now execute complex navigations using pre-programmed controls on wires (0.014″ or 0.018″) within the system's active wire drive, enabling more precise navigation through challenging coronary anatomy [43].

R-PCI provides substantial benefits for both patient and operator radiation safety. Traditional PCI exposes operators to continuous radiation, but R-PCI reduces this exposure significantly. The R-EVOLUTION study demonstrated that, compared to T-PCI, R-PCI lowered patient air kerma (AK) from 1110 mGy to 884 mGy ($p = 0.002$) and dose-area product (DAP) from 5746 cGycm^2 to 4734 cGycm^2 both of which were statistically significant ($p = 0.003$) [44, 45]. These reductions are achieved through optimised table height, shielding, and real-time dose adjustments guided by the ALARA (as low as reasonably achievable) principle. Ergonomically, R-PCI eliminates the need for lead aprons, reducing chronic musculoskeletal injuries like neck, back, and joint pain injuries reported by nearly half of interventional cardiologists [40–42].

The R-EVOLUTION study further confirmed that R-PCI is both safe and effective, with a technical success rate of 95% and a clinical success rate of 100%, with no major complications reported within 30 days [45, 46]. Advances in precision control allow R-PCI to address complex lesions, such as chronic total occlusions (CTOs) and side-branch access, which were challenging for earlier robotic platforms. One notable limitation of R-PCI is its longer procedural time. R-PCI requires 37 min, compared to 27 min for T-PCI ($P < 0.0005$), due to the need to load devices into the robotic system [44]. Efforts to reduce this time include faster cassette loading mechanisms and automated device recognition, which are expected to close the time gap in future iterations of robotic platforms.

AI and machine learning (ML) are revolutionising R-PCI through procedural automation. Current systems rely on human input for critical tasks like wire navigation, but AI aims to reduce this dependency. Emerging computer vision and image analysis tools allow AI to detect lesion morphology, guide catheter positioning, and predict optimal procedural strategies [41]. Additionally, AI-enabled predictive analytics could analyse past procedures to support real-time decision-making, such as optimal device selection and lesion access strategies. These capabilities will reduce procedural variability and enhance operator efficiency [12, 41].

A major frontier for R-PCI is remote-operated intervention, where interventional cardiologists control robotic systems from distant locations. Supported by 5G infrastructure, remote R-PCI could democratise access to expert care, especially in underserved regions (see Fig. 8.3) [36]. By enabling operators to guide interventions remotely, hospitals could increase procedural efficacy, and efficiency while reducing the need for specialist travel. This concept aligns with the growing field of telehealth and teleintervention, which utilises telecommunications to expand access to healthcare services [36, 41].

Despite its advantages, R-PCI has limitations. Current robotic systems cannot interpret anatomical variability or patient-specific complexities without human oversight. However, advancements in AI, deep learning, and image recognition are expected to bridge this gap. Future systems may feature automated lesion recognition and pattern recognition algorithms to support autonomous decision-making [41]. Additionally, as discussed above, procedural time for R-PCI remains longer than T-PCI, driven by the manual step of loading devices into the robotic system. Innovations like automatic wire recognition and automated guidewire exchange aim to address this challenge (see Case Study 8.1). As coronary artery disease prevalence rises, robotic platforms are poised to become essential in catheterisation laboratories, driving safer, more precise, and more efficient interventional procedures [40].

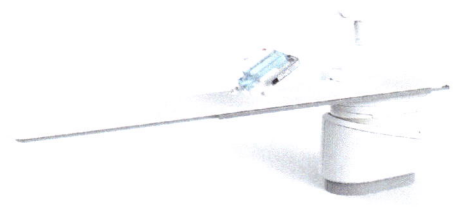

Fig. 8.3 Robocath, a robotic system for treating cardiovascular diseases, successfully performed the first remote robotic coronary angioplasty from 1700 miles (2800 km) away. Conducted entirely over a 5G connection, this milestone paves the way for future long-distance endovascular procedures

Robotic-assisted PCI (R-PCI) represents a pivotal advancement in interventional cardiology. By significantly reducing radiation exposure, improving ergonomics, and enhancing procedural precision, R-PCI addresses long-standing challenges in operator safety and procedural efficiency. Innovations like TechnIQ, AI-guided automation, and remote intervention further highlight R-PCI's transformative potential. While current robotic platforms face challenges related to procedural time and operator oversight, future iterations are expected to overcome these hurdles through AI integration and automation enhancements. With the global burden of coronary artery disease on the rise, R-PCI is positioned as a critical component in the future of interventional cardiology, offering safer, faster, and more accessible care [40, 41, 44, 45].

Case Study 8.1: Comparison of AI-enabled Robotic Percutaneous Coronary Intervention (R-PCI) with Traditional Percutaneous Coronary Intervention (T-PCI) [47]

Clinical Challenge

The adoption of robotic percutaneous coronary intervention (R-PCI) is increasing as an alternative to traditional percutaneous coronary intervention (T-PCI). While previous studies have demonstrated reduced radiation exposure for operators during R-PCI, evidence of patient benefit has been limited. Patel et al. conducted a propensity score-matched analysis of a large cohort to evaluate the comparative outcomes of R-PCI and T-PCI [47]. The study aimed to assess differences in key clinical and procedural metrics, including radiation exposure, fluoroscopy time, contrast usage, and total procedure duration.

AI-enabled solution

This retrospective study included 996 patients who underwent PCI at the Apex Heart Institute, India, from December 2017

(continued)

to March 2019. Of these, 310 (31.1%) patients underwent AI -enabled R-PCI using the Corindus CorePath GRX system, while 686 (68.9%) underwent T-PCI. Propensity score matching (caliper = 0.05) was used to create a cohort of 280 R-PCI and 280 T-PCI patients with comparable baseline characteristics. Data on air kerma (AK), dose-area product (DAP), fluoroscopy time, contrast volume, and total procedural time were collected. Key procedural and angiographic characteristics, such as SYNTAX score and lesion complexity, were also recorded. Statistical analysis was conducted using Mann-Whitney U tests for continuous variables and Pearson's χ^2 tests for categorical data.

Benefits and challenges

The study revealed significant differences in key procedural outcomes between R-PCI and T-PCI.

- *Radiation exposure*: R-PCI demonstrated significantly lower patient exposure to radiation, with median AK of 884 mGy compared to 1110 mGy for T-PCI ($P = 0.002$). Similarly, DAP was lower in R-PCI (4734 cGycm^2) compared to T-PCI (5746 cGycm^2, $P = 0.003$).
- *Fluoroscopy time*: There was no significant difference in fluoroscopy time between R-PCI (5.48 min) and T-PCI (5.51 min, $P = 0.936$).
- *Contrast utilisation*: R-PCI and T-PCI showed comparable median contrast volumes (140 mL vs. 130 mL, $P = 0.905$).
- *Procedure time*: R-PCI had a longer procedure time (37 min) compared to T-PCI (27 min, $P < 0.0005$).
- *Implications*

The results highlight the advantages of R-PCI, particularly in reducing patient radiation exposure. Reduced AK and DAP suggest that R-PCI aligns with the 'as low as reasonably achievable' (ALARA) principle for radiation safety. These findings support the use of robotics to enhance patient safety during PCI. Moreover, comparable fluoroscopy time and contrast usage indicate that R-PCI does not increase patient burden for these metrics. The increased procedure time for R-PCI reflects the setup and preparation required for robotic systems but may be offset by improved operator ergonomics and safety.

Conclusion

R-PCI significantly reduces patient radiation exposure compared to T-PCI, while maintaining comparable fluoroscopy time and contrast utilisation. Although procedure time is longer for R-PCI, the reduction in radiation exposure represents a significant benefit for patients. These findings support the growing role of robotics in coronary interventions, with potential for further efficiency improvements as operators gain experience with robotic systems.

8.5 Augmented and Virtual Reality (Combined with AI)

8.5.1 Integration of AI with Augmented and Virtual Reality

The use of fluoroscopically guided cardiology procedures has significantly improved patient outcomes but has simultaneously increased healthcare professionals' exposure to occupational radiation, resulting in health risks. This underscores the necessity for effective radiation safety training. Traditional training methods, which rely on passive learning, fail to replicate the dynamic environment of a catheterisation laboratory. Augmented and Virtual Reality presents a promising alternative, offering immersive, interactive training experiences without actual radiation exposure. The integration of AI with AR/VR creates advanced imaging solutions where pre-procedural 3D data can be fused with real-time fluoroscopic images. This fusion provides interventional care teams with critical feedback during procedures, enhancing accuracy and further reducing the need for additional imaging that would increase radiation exposure [48]. VR is also being utilised for training purposes, allowing medical professionals to practice procedures in a simulated environment without exposing patients or themselves to radiation. Studies indicate that VR training can lead to a significant reduction in radiation exposure compared to traditional training methods [49].

While large language models (LLMs) have demonstrated remarkable capabilities, small language models (SLMs) offer distinct advantages in educational VR for fluoroscopy and angiography imaging. Due to their focused training, operational efficiency, and ability to deliver contextually relevant content, SLMs are better suited for domain-specific applications without requiring extensive computational resources [50].

Virtual reality (VR) plays a significant role in enhancing training and education for healthcare professionals in the cath lab. By providing immersive, interactive training experiences that replicate real-world scenarios, VR allows practitioners to practice procedural techniques and radiation safety measures without the risks associated with live procedures. This approach promotes active learning and immediate feedback, which are essential for mastering complex procedural skills and learn safely from mistakes or act on feedback. Furthermore, VR enables the simulation of various clinical scenarios commonly encountered in the cath lab. Practitioners can refine their technical skills and decision-making abilities in a controlled, risk-free environment. Research indicates that VR training improves

healthcare professionals' understanding of radiation safety principles, leading to a measurable reduction in radiation exposure among cath lab staff.

In addition to its role in training, VR integrates seamlessly with other emerging technologies such as artificial intelligence (AI) and augmented reality (AR). During procedures, AR can overlay imaging data onto the patient's anatomy to enhance visualisation, while VR facilitates collaborative planning and education among medical teams [51]. This synergy between VR, AI, and AR is transforming procedural workflows, promoting efficiency, and supporting better patient outcomes. VR also contributes to improving patient experience in the transcatheter lab. Patients can visualise their anatomy and procedure in 3D, allowing for a clearer understanding of their treatment plan. This approach reduces anxiety, fosters patient engagement, and encourages compliance with recommended care plans.

The combination of AI, AR, and VR technologies in fluoroscopy represents a promising advancement in reducing radiation exposure. By enhancing visualisation, improving procedural accuracy, and minimising unnecessary imaging, these technologies not only protect patient health but also safeguard healthcare providers from the risks associated with ionising radiation. As these technologies continue to evolve, their application in clinical settings is expected to expand further, leading to safer medical practices overall.

8.6   AI-Enhanced Imaging and Physiological Assessment Technologies

Intracoronary imaging and physiological assessment technologies are well-established diagnostic tools that supplement traditional coronary angiography. Physiological assessment technology is a critical tool for guiding revascularisation decisions. It assesses the severity of coronary artery stenosis to determine if it is significant enough to cause ischemia, which would necessitate interventions such as angioplasty or coronary artery bypass grafting. Similarly, intracoronary imaging is essential in interventional cardiology. These imaging technologies provide detailed views of arterial pathology, aiding in precise device placement and overall management of coronary artery disease. The integration of AI into these technologies improves preprocedural planning, intra-procedure guidance, and post-procedure analysis. Such advancements enhance the precision and effectiveness of treatments, significantly improving patient care.

8.7   Intracoronary Imaging

Coronary angiography has long been the standard for coronary imaging, but it has limitations in assessing vessel wall anatomy and guiding percutaneous coronary intervention (PCI).

Intracoronary imaging overcomes many of the limitations of angiography, which utilises X-ray technology to produce a two-dimensional lumenogram of a three-dimensional structure. Intravascular ultrasound (IVUS) utilises a catheter equipped with an ultrasound probe, which is inserted into the coronary arteries to emit sound waves, producing cross-sectional images of the arterial walls.

Optical coherence tomography (OCT) employs a catheter that uses light waves to generate high-resolution images of the coronary artery's inner layers, offering superior detail compared to IVUS [52].

Intravascular imaging technology, such as IVUS/OCT, can be used to accurately diagnose angiographic lesions, characterise plaque morphology, and identify microvascular dysfunction. Intravascular imaging guidance improves outcomes by adequately informing clinicians of true vessel size, landing zones to guide stent length selection, plaque morphology to guide debulking strategies, identify PCI complications (edge dissection, stent malapposition) and mechanisms of stent failure (stent thrombosis/under expansion/fracture, neointimal hyperplasia, neoatherosclerosis [53]. Clinical studies and meta-analyses have demonstrated that both OCT and IVUS improve PCI results, reducing mortality, major adverse cardiovascular events, and the length of the hospitalisation [54–56].

It is now well established that intracoronary imaging in PCI can improve clinical outcome measures compared with angiography-guided procedures [57, 58]. Despite its crucial role, and recommendation in societal guidelines, the global adoption of preintervention IVUS, the real-world usage of IVUS guidance remains low [59, 60]. In a recent survey, the most common reasons for reluctance to use intravascular imaging include high cost, uncertainty whether it provides additional clinical benefit, and concerns about receiving adequate training [61]. Perceived barriers to utilisation include familiarity with, and ability to interpret imaging, concerns over added procedure time and contrast load, alongside a lack of actionable outcome data [62]. One possible reason is the lack of physician education leading to misinterpretation of IVUS images [63]. AI-based tools can automate analysis and the interpretation of OCT and IVUS to improve cardiovascular diagnosis and treatment [64].

8.7.1   AI-Enhanced Intravascular Ultrasound

Since its introduction in the 1980s, intravascular ultrasound (IVUS) has significantly contributed to the quantitative analysis of coronary artery stenotic lesions and the advancement of percutaneous coronary interventions (PCIs). Despite its crucial role, however, the global adoption of preintervention IVUS, as explained above, is limited due to the procedural complexities that require added time and substantial expertise necessary for optimal image interpretation. The advent of artificial intelligence (AI) may overcome challenges in the IVUS interpretation process through innovative techniques for image processing, feature extraction, plaque identification, and automated quantitation [65].

AI programs can automatically recognise and delineate vascular structures in IVUS images of coronary arteries with complex lesions. Several studies showed that machine learning could be implemented in IVUS imaging [19, 52, 66]. There is a growing list of literature showing high level of agreement between deep learning-based models and manual expert analysis for IVUS interpretation during PCI [67]. Scientists from Emory University have demonstrated an ML algorithm for segmenting IVUS images. After training, it showed excellent agreement with an expert analyst in automatically calculating the lumen area and plaque burden [68]. Similarly, Yang et al. introduced IVUS-Net, a fully convolution network (FCN) architecture model that classifies IVUS segmentation of lumen, vessel, and stent areas. Their results matched the accuracy of manual segmentation by human experts and performed well even in challenging conditions such as bifurcations, shadows, and side branches [69].

DeepIVUS, a convolutional neural network, could potentially be used to segment and classify the phenotype of each IVUS image (e.g. normal, fibrotic, fibroatheroma, calcified, or stented) [70]. This model can be improved to identify various plaque subtypes (lipidic, fibrofatty, fibrous) or calcified plaque with a certain degree arc of calcium. With sufficient training, the model could potentially recommend interventional strategies based on plaque characteristics and severity of calcification (e.g. angioplasty alone, shockwave lithotripsy, orbital atherectomy, or rotational atherectomy) [19, 71]. Shinohara et al. applied a U-Net model for IVUS image interpretation to classify vessels that may require treatment or special devices with high accuracy [67]. ML algorithms have been used for automatic calculation of vascular luminal area and the plaque burden on intravascular ultrasound images [72].

Artificial intelligence (AI) has the potential to significantly enhance intravascular ultrasound (IVUS) guidance for stenting by improving performance and accuracy. This automated DL-based IVUS segmentation of lumen, vessel, and stent area showed an excellent agreement with manual segmentation by experts, supporting the feasibility of artificial intelligence-assisted IVUS assessment in patients undergoing coronary stent implantation [73]. Another study assessed the accuracy of machine learning-enabled automatic

segmentation of coronary artery vessel and lumen dimensions and balloon sizing. The IVUS segmentation of lumen, vessel, and stent areas by machine learning was strongly and positively correlated with those obtained in manually labelled expert analysis. More than 90% of images selected an appropriate balloon size by using both vessel and lumen diameters [74]. Additionally, AI programs are able to automatically recognise and delineate vascular structures in IVUS images of coronary arteries with complex lesions. and can classify vessels that are likely to require treatment or special devices with a high accuracy [67]. Min et al. developed a deep learning model, based on a convolutional neural network architecture, which predicts postprocedural stent area and expansion with an impressive accuracy of 94% [75]. This data-driven approach may assist clinicians in making treatment decisions to avoid incomplete stent expansion as a preventable cause of stent failure.

Postintervention, ML-guided IVUS could identify edge dissections and minimal stent area (MSA), ultimately predicting the risk of in-stent restenosis. Based on the results of these prior studies, ML/DL-assisted IVUS interpretation is one of the most promising areas in interventional cardiology. IVUS could potentially preemptively identify physiologically significant lesions [76] or as demonstrated in preliminary data, the U-Net model can also automate the generation of measurements like minimal lumen area and lesion length, and identify postintervention issues such as edge dissections and minimal stent area, aiding in predicting the risk of in-stent restenosis [67].

Further research has linked IVUS characteristics with significant physiological measurements, suggesting a reduced need for intraprocedural measurements. Lee et al. utilised IVUS-based supervised machine learning algorithms to identify lesions with fractional flow reserve below 0.80 [76]. AI technology has the potential to eliminate the need for vascular physiology assessments using Fractional Flow Reserve (FFR) and instantaneous wave-free ratio (iFR).

Case Study 8.2: Predicting Plaque Vulnerability Using Intravascular Ultrasound, Optical Coherence Tomography, and Machine Learning [71]
Clinical challenge

Predicting coronary plaque vulnerability is critical for preventing myocardial infarction and stroke. Plaque rupture, particularly in thin-cap fibroatheromas (TCFAs), poses a significant risk. Traditional imaging like intravascular ultrasound (IVUS) offers limited resolution (150–200 μm) for detecting thin caps (<65 μm), while optical coherence tomography (OCT) provides superior resolution (~10 μm) but limited penetration. Combining IVUS and OCT allows for more accurate assessments of plaque morphology and stress conditions. In this study, Guo et al. leveraged IVUS + OCT-based fluid–structure interaction (FSI) models and machine learning methods to predict changes in plaque vulnerability indices: Lipid Percentage Index (LPI), Cap Thickness Index (CTI), and Morphological Plaque Vulnerability Index (MPVI) [71].

AI enabled solution

The study analysed two coronary arteries from one patient with stable angina. Baseline and 10-month follow-up IVUS, OCT, and angiography data were collected. 3D FSI models were created to calculate stress and strain distributions in the plaques. From 45 paired slices, 13 key morphological and biomechanical factors were extracted to quantify changes in LPI, CTI, and MPVI. Four machine learning models—support vector machine (SVM), random forest (RF), discriminant analysis (DA), and ensemble learning (EL)—were applied to predict changes in these indices using fivefold cross-validation. More about these models can be found in Chap. 2.

Benefits and challenges

The use of combined morphological and biomechanical predictors resulted in more accurate predictions of plaque vulnerability indices than single-factor predictors.

- *Lipid Percentage Index (ΔLPI)*: SVM achieved the highest area under the curve (AUC) of 0.963 using lipid percentage, wall shear stress, and plaque stress/strain.
- *Cap Thickness Index (ΔCTI)*: DA produced the best AUC (0.836) using minimum cap thickness, mean cap thickness, and cap stress/strain as predictors.
- *Morphological Plaque Vulnerability Index (ΔMPVI)*: RF attained the best AUC (0.847) using minimum cap thickness, plaque area, and critical stress as predictors.

Single-factor predictors, such as wall thickness and minimum cap thickness, produced lower AUCs, confirming that multifactor predictors improve prediction accuracy. Each machine learning model excelled for specific indices: SVM for ΔLPI, DA for ΔCTI, and RF for ΔMPVI.

Implications

This study demonstrates the power of integrating IVUS and OCT imaging with FSI modelling and ML techniques to enhance the prediction of plaque vulnerability. The multi-factor approach improves the ability to predict future changes in LPI, CTI, and MPVI, providing insights that could support early detection and timely intervention for high-risk plaques. By incorporating machine learning, cardiovascular risk assessment could become more precise, ultimately improving clinical decision-making in the management of coronary artery disease.

(continued)

Conclusion

The combination of IVUS, OCT, FSI modelling, and machine learning enables accurate prediction of changes in plaque vulnerability indices. Combinational-factor predictors outperform single-factor predictors, offering a powerful approach for assessing cardiovascular risk. This innovative approach highlights the potential for data-driven predictive modelling in cardiovascular research and patient care.

8.7.2   AI-Enhanced Optical Coherence Tomography

Optical coherence tomography (OCT) is also a catheter-based intravascular imaging modality used in cardiology to provide high-resolution, cross-sectional views of coronary arteries. OCT provides high-resolution, detailed imaging of atherosclerotic plaque, allowing for precise identification of different tissue compositions. This information is crucial for tailoring lesion preparation to the specific plaque characteristics and for selecting the most appropriate therapeutic approach during OCT-guided interventions. However, plaque characterisation is currently challenging, time-consuming, difficult to systematise, based on subjective interpretation of the operators and largely dependent on their expertise, thus posing problems for reproducibility.

An AI-based model [77] has been developed and validated for automatic plaque characterisation on OCT. This substantially improved the objectivity and reproducibility of OCT quantification. The AI model allows for detailed plaque characterisation and identification of inflammatory markers, offering promising opportunities for future research on plaque progression monitoring and risk stratification. This model could enhance OCT-guided PCI by customising interventions based on plaque composition and using the internal elastic lamina as a guide for stent sizing. By reducing subjectivity in image interpretation and aiding in the quantification of plaque composition, the model has significant potential for both research applications and OCT-guided PCI procedures. Another project utilised a convolutional neural network to delineate arterial wall areas and characterise various plaque components, including calcium, lipid, fibrous, and mixed tissues [78]. A comparative study was conducted to evaluate AI-driven assessments of calcification detected through OCT against visual assessments, in order to determine the need for lesion modification before stenting. The study concluded that the accuracy of AI evaluations was comparable to that of human assessments [19].

8.8   Vascular Physiology

Coronary angiography, while an essential imaging tool, primarily gives a two-dimensional view of the coronary arteries and shows the anatomical narrowing (stenosis) of these vessels. However, angiography cannot always reliably predict the physiological impact of stenosis on blood flow, particularly for intermediate lesions (40–70% stenosis). Visual estimation alone may not accurately reflect whether a narrowing is causing significant ischemia or whether it requires intervention, such as stenting or bypass surgery.

Vascular physiology assessment, such as fractional flow reserve (FFR) and instantaneous wave-free ratio (iFR), goes beyond anatomical visualisation by measuring the actual impact of a stenosis on coronary blood flow. By incorporating these physiological assessments, we can better understand whether a stenosis is functionally significant and likely to cause ischemia. This allows for more tailored decision-making, ensuring that only patients with ischemia-causing lesions receive revascularisation, while patients with non-significant lesions can avoid unnecessary procedures. In essence, vascular physiology provides a more complete picture of coronary artery disease, helping to guide appropriate clinical interventions based on the actual physiological burden rather than purely anatomical appearances.

Fractional flow reserve (FFR) and instantaneous wave-free ratio (iFR) are two of the most commonly used physiological methods of assessing lesion significance. FFR is defined as the ratio of maximal blood flow in a region distal to a lesion compared with the normal maximal blood flow of an artery. The iFR, an index of lesion severity, is the instantaneous wave-free ratio (in diastole) of coronary pressure distal to the coronary lesion (Pd) to the aortic pressure (Pa). The potential advantage of iFR, which is a resting physiological index, is that it obviates the use of adenosine because it does not require a state of maximal hyperemia [15].

According to the current international guidelines, fractional flow reserve (FFR), represents the gold standard in guiding the decision to proceed or not with coronary revascularisation [15, 79–81]. Over the past two decades, the use of invasive intracoronary measurement of fractional flow reserve, (FFR) to evaluate the physiological significance of coronary lesions and to guide revascularisation strategy has been shown to improve clinical outcomes [82–84] and is recommended in both the European Society of Cardiology and American College of Cardiology guidelines [15, 79].

8.8.1 Fractional Flow Reserve

FFR, involves inserting a specialised pressure wire into the coronary artery and comparing the blood pressure before and after the stenosis while the patient is given a medication to induce maximal blood flow. An FFR value of 0.80 or less indicates that the stenosis is likely causing a significant obstruction to blood flow, justifying intervention such as stenting or bypass surgery. As the most frequently used pressure-derived index for assessing stenosis severity, FFR is indispensable in guiding coronary revascularisation decisions. Its use in the catheterisation laboratory accurately identifies which lesions should be stented, thereby improving outcomes in most elective clinical and angiographic conditions [85–88]. The results of coronary physiological assessment have been shown to change the treatment strategy in more than 40% of cases and save inappropriate stent implantations and bypass surgeries with a significant reduction in healthcare costs [89].

Despite the well-established evidence of FFR-guided revascularisation therapy, its utilisation is still low with significant variation in adoption level between different countries ranging from less than 1% to close to 20% [90–92]. FFR remains underutilised for a number of potential reasons, including the additional time needed to measure pressure wire–derived FFR, technical challenges and the small risk associated with manoeuvering a pressure wire down a coronary artery, the added time to assess multiple vessels, issues with drift in the pressure wire reading, and the time, expense, and associated side effects with some hyperemic agents necessary to measure FFR. Other cited reasons for the lack of adoption of FFR are discordance between the clinician's interpretation of the angiogram and physiological tracings and the perceived lack of reproducibility of the measurements. Inherent physiological variability and lack of standardisation in performing these measurements account for some of the negative perceptions of physiology, but the interpretation of pressure tracings is also subject to technical errors, pressure drift, or waveform artifacts [93]. It has been demonstrated that suboptimal FFR measurements occur in almost one-third of tracings [74]. Furthermore, more detailed physiological measurements using pressure pull back curves performed to define lesion-level hemodynamic significance in diffuse or tandem lesions are even more complex and vulnerable to errors and biases [94]. In the last few years, non-invasive techniques for measuring FFR, by employing computational flow dynamics (CFD) calculations from specific coronary angiograms have been developed aiming to address the limitations of invasive techniques.

8.8.2 Coronary Angiography-Based Fractional Flow Reserve

Several groups have devised techniques to calculate FFR from invasive angiography without the need to insert a pressure wire or induce hyperemia, thereby eliminating the key obstacles to its broader use. These software systems generate a 3D model of the coronary anatomy from cineangiography and utilise a flow dynamics model to determine an FFR value [90]. Angiography-derived FFR therefore has the potential to extend the benefits of physiological coronary lesion assessment to considerably more patients [95]. In the catheterisation laboratory, computational fluid dynamics has enabled the creation of wire-free algorithms that utilise computer vision and 3D reconstruction to identify functionally significant coronary stenoses [45]. Fractional Flow Reserve measured from the coronary angiogram alone has a high sensitivity, specificity, and accuracy compared with pressure wire-derived FFR [92]. In addition, a recent study found that AI-based FFR was as accurate as wire-based FFR in predicting hemodynamically significant lesions [90].

Growing evidence suggests good diagnostic performance of angiography-based FFR measurements, both in chronic and acute coronary syndromes, as well as in specific lesion subsets, such as long and calcified lesions, left main coronary stenosis, and bifurcations. In a multi-centre retrospective study, research has shown that AI-FFR calculated by an AI-based, angio-derived FFR method, demonstrated excellent diagnostic performance against invasive FFR [96]. More recently, promising results on the superiority of angiography-based FFR as compared to angiography-guided PCI have been published [96]. Furthermore, AI-FFR calculation was fast and showed high reproducibility with minimal requirement from the interventional cardiologist, allowing for potential easy integration into catheterisation laboratories [97].

Several companies have developed systems to derive fractional flow reserve (FFR) values from coronary angiography performed in catheterisation labs, improving the assessment of coronary artery disease. CathWorks offers the FFRangio System (Fig. 8.4), which delivers real-time FFR values from routine 2D angiograms, enabling interventional cardiologists to evaluate the entire coronary tree. This system uses advanced algo-

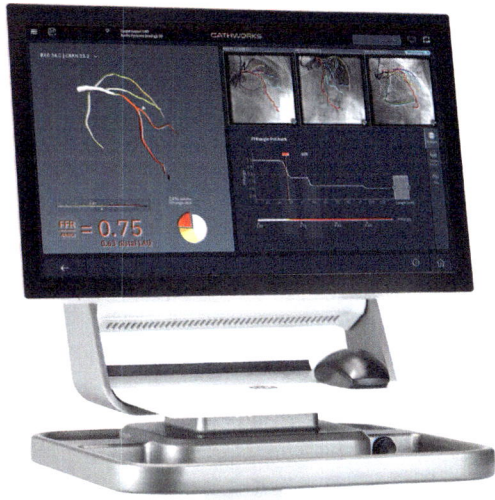

Fig. 8.4 The CathWorks FFRangio® System utilises advanced AI-based computational modelling to derive fractional flow reserve (FFR) values non-invasively from standard angiography images

rithms and artificial intelligence to analyse blood flow resistance in both normal and diseased vessels, providing results in about 4 min without requiring invasive pressure wires or drug stimulation [98]. Medis offers Medis QFR, a software solution that evaluates angiography-derived physiological data to assess coronary lesions. It uses deep learning to enhance measurement precision and reduce variability, making it a reliable option for assessing the severity of coronary artery disease [99]. Siemens Healthineers offers various FFR measurement solutions through its Angio-FFR Solutions suite, including catheter-based and image-derived methods that aim to improve decision-making regarding the hemodynamic significance of coronary stenoses [100].

Coronary Angiography-Based Fractional Flow Reserve has the potential to eventually replace wire-based FFR measurement and substantially increase physiological coronary lesion assessment in the catheterisation laboratory, thereby leading to improved patient outcomes [92]

8.9 Applications of AI in Clinical Decision Support

AI is being increasingly incorporated into clinical decision support systems (CDSS) within interventional cardiology, improving decision-making and enhancing patient outcomes. These systems are being developed with autonomous computing capabilities, utilising self-learning machine learning algorithms, deep learning, and pattern recognition techniques to emulate human cognitive processes [101].

Clinical decision support systems hold great promise for enhancing patient safety and aiding in making prognostic and diagnostic predictions during interventional cardiology procedures. While the widespread adoption of fully automated or semi-autonomous interventions remains distant, the implementation of decision-making algorithms to assist operators and aid in procedure planning could become a reality in the coming years [45].

Utilising the vast amounts of cardiovascular imaging data allows for data-driven phenotypic differentiation by enabling the identification of subtle patterns and variations in vascular structures and functions that might not be visible through traditional analysis. With advanced computational tools like AI and machine learning, large-scale imaging datasets can be analysed to uncover distinct phenotypic subgroups based on variations in heart size, wall thickness, blood flow patterns, and other anatomical or functional traits. These phenotypic distinctions are crucial for better understanding the progression of cardiovascular diseases, identifying high-risk patients, and tailoring treatments to specific patient subgroups. This has particular relevance in the field of interventional cardiology and transcatheter therapies for enabling individualised, person-centered treatment [44]. Algorithms integrating ML and cardiovascular imaging can help generate patient-specific risk scores, which can yield diagnostic significance in procedural planning [45]. Furthermore, ML may play a paramount role in automating cardiovascular imaging workflow for referral of patients to cardiac catheterisation laboratory by facilitating faster reading, interpretation and diagnosis [45, 102]. More about person-centered care with the help of AI, ML and DL techniques is touched upon in Chap. 12.

AI-assisted precision percutaneous intervention is a highly promising field in interventional cardiology, offering opportunities to enhance lesion preparation, achieve complete revascularisation, and ensure lasting results. AI can be applied to optimise PCI strategy selection through anatomical and functional assessments, or to provide guidance for complex PCI procedures using data derived from training sets containing millions of angiographic images.

For instance, AI could analyse lesion features like angulation and tortuosity observed in diagnostic angiography to aid in guidewire selection or suggest various atherectomy techniques for calcified lesions, drawing on knowledge from multiple experts and data from Clinical Outcomes Research (CORE) laboratories and clinical trials. [19] Computational modelling and AI, have the potential to improve transcatheter mitral and aortic valves intervention planning, selection, and outcome prediction [103].

8.10 Future Directions

To improve radiation safety in cardiac catheterisation labs, future research should prioritise enhancing safety protocols and conducting thorough assessments of radiation effects on specific organs. Key research areas include developing advanced protocols using artificial intelligence for real-time monitoring, personalising radiation doses based on individual patient characteristics, and evaluating new technologies for dose reduction. Additionally, collecting comprehensive data on operators, including their experience, the volume of procedures performed, and the types of procedures – such as chronic total occlusions (CTOs), bifurcations, structural interventions, and electrophysiological procedures like pacemaker insertions – will enhance the understanding of operator-related human factors that impact both performance and safety [104].

In-depth studies on organ-specific radiation impacts, long-term follow-up of healthcare professionals, and patient-focused approaches are critical, and the integration of AI can play a pivotal role in these areas. AI can enhance multicentre collaborations by streamlining data collection and analysis, enabling real-time monitoring, and identifying patterns in radiation exposure across various centres. Additionally, AI can support the development of personalised radiation safety protocols, adapting dose levels based on individual patient characteristics and procedural complexities. The use of AI in quality improvement strategies can further optimise radiation safety practices, while ensuring ethical research practices remain a priority. Addressing these research priorities, with the help of AI, could significantly advance radiation safety in cardiac catheterisation labs, creating a safer, more efficient environment for both patients and healthcare staff.

In the future, AI-powered simulations will play a pivotal role in training interventional cardiologists, radiographers and the wider teams offering a safe and controlled environment for practicing complex procedures and refining their expertise. These simulations will enable cardiologists to perform intricate interventions in a risk-free setting, underscoring AI's contribution to advancing medical education and enhancing proficiency in cardiac interventions. It will also help radiographers in the optimal, more efficient and safer use of equipment in this environment. The incorporation of AI into immersive technologies will be key in transforming cardiology by simplifying the analysis of complex 3D medical data and improving education and clinical practice for all professionals through personalised, interactive, and efficient solutions [105]. Moreover, innovative approaches will integrate AI with immersive technologies like mixed reality or virtual reality for conducting remote multidisciplinary heart team meetings. AI will facilitate these remote consultations and diagnostics, overcoming geographical barriers and making advanced interventional cardiology care and expert consultations accessible from a distance.

The combination of AI with these cutting-edge technologies will be transformative, significantly enhancing healthcare delivery by connecting interdisciplinary teams across various locations, ultimately expanding the scope and quality of cardiac care. Table 8.1 summarises the potential roles of AI in enhancing interventional cardiology.

8.11 Chapter Summary

Artificial Intelligence (AI) is revolutionising interventional cardiology and radiology, transforming patient care, operator safety, and procedural efficiency. By integrating machine learning, computer vision, and robotics, AI-driven advancements enhance procedural precision, reduce radiation exposure, and support the standardisation of complex interventions. From optical coherence tomography (OCT) to intravascular ultrasound (IVUS), AI automates image interpretation, facilitating accurate diagnosis and real-time decision-making. Fractional flow reserve (FFR) and angiography-based physiological assessments further streamline clinical workflows, enabling personalised treatment strategies with minimal invasiveness. Robotics and remote-controlled interventions not only protect operators from radiation but also allow for remote guidance, expanding access to expert care. Meanwhile, immersive technologies like virtual and augmented reality transform training and education, offering a risk-free environment for skill development. Future directions include AI-enhanced simulations, augmented clinical decision support, and personalised procedural planning. As the prevalence of cardiovascular disease continues to rise, the integration of AI will play a pivotal role in enhancing procedural efficiency, patient safety, and equitable access to advanced cardiovascular care. Collectively, these innovations position AI as a driving force in the future of interventional cardiology and radiology, setting new standards for precision, safety, and global accessibility in cardiovascular healthcare.

Table 8.1 Summary of AI potential in interventional cardiology [19]

Conditions/situations	AI potentials
Cath lab workflow	ML could learn simple pattern in the cath lab and generate automated recommendations (driving the tables, checking ACT, warning for radiation safety)
Spontaneous coronary artery dissection (SCAD)	DL could predict SCAD recurrence based on angiographic and IVUS characteristics.
CTO	ML could learn pattern how to tackle CTO from experts and generate recommendation for approaching CTO lesions
SYNTAX	DL could predict outcomes that are more granular than SYNTAX score. For example, predicting outcomes between PCI and CABG in patients with or without diabetes
IVUS measurement	DL could learn from millions of IVUS images and data regarding adverse outcomes in order to generate an optimal MLA cut-off. In addition, AI could generate an MSA recommendation
Contrast utilisation	DL could potentially be used for contrast recommendation in high-risk patients [coronary artery dissection (CAD) with chronic kidney disease (CKD)]
Cardiogenic shock	ML classification and management of cardiogenic shock or mixed shock. For example, it has been shown that cardiogenic shock can be classified into three phenotypes using ML
Complication assessment	DL combined fluoroscopic and ultrasound imaging to generate recommendations for precise femoral site access to avoid RP bleed, pseudoaneurysm, and hematoma
Physiologic measurements	ML could help with physiologic measurements (FFR, iFR, RFR) to precisely characterise lesion (e.g. location and length). A combination of clinical and imaging
A combination of clinical and imaging	A combination of clinical and imaging variables could better predict outcomes using DL. For example, incorporating variables such as hemoglobin A1C, atherosclerotic cardiovascular disease (ASCVD) score, and a h/o PAD with bifurcation LM, ML could learn from million patients' outcome and generate Optimal recommendation.
Low contrast angiography	ML could identify dissection or perforation from low-contrast angiography

References

1. Glielmo P, Fusco S, Gitto S, et al. Artificial intelligence in interventional radiology: state of the art. Eur Radiol Exp. 2024;8:62. https://doi.org/10.1186/s41747-024-00452-2.
2. Subhan S, Malik J, Haq AU, Qadeer MS, Zaidi SMJ, Orooj F, Zaman H, Mehmoodi A, Majeedi U. Role of artificial Intelligence and machine learning in interventional cardiology. Curr Probl Cardiol. 2023;48(7):101698.
3. Kim Y, Roh JH, Kweon J, Kwon H, Chae J, Park K, Lee JH, Jeong JO, Kang DY, Lee PH, Ahn JM, Kang SJ, Park DW, Lee SW, Lee CW, Park SW, Park SJ, Kim YH. Artificial intelligence-based quantitative coronary angiography of major vessels using deep-learning. Int J Cardiol. 2024;405:131945.
4. Samant S, Panagopoulos AN, Wu W, Zhao S, Chatzizisis YS. Artificial intelligence in coronary artery interventions: preprocedural planning and procedural assistance. J Soc Cardiovasc Angiogr Interv. 2025;4(3Part B):102519.
5. Bang JY, Hough M, Hawes RH, Varadarajulu S. Use of artificial intelligence to reduce radiation exposure at fluoroscopy-guided endoscopic procedures. Am J Gastroenterol. 2020;115(4):555–61.
6. Zhang J, Fang J, Xu Y, Si G. How AI and Robotics will advance interventional radiology: narrative review and future perspectives. Diagnostics. 2024;14:1393.
7. Farhad A, Reza R, Azamossadat H, Ali G, Arash R, Mehrad A, Zahra K. Artificial intelligence in estimating fractional flow reserve: a systematic literature review of techniques. BMC Cardiovasc Disord. 2023;23(1):407.
8. University Hospitals Coventry and Warwickshire. Radiographers in interventional radiology [Internet]. 2025. Available from https://www.uhcw.nhs.uk/interventional-radiology/radiographers-in-interventional-radiology/. Accessed 31 March 2025.
9. RadiologyInfo.org. Professions in interventional radiology [Internet]. 2024. Available from https://www.radiologyinfo.org/en/info/professions-interventional-radiology. Accessed 31 March 2025.

10. Wegermann ZK, Swaminathan RV, Rao SV. Cath Lab Robotics: paradigm change in interventional cardiology? Curr Cardiol Rep [Internet]. 2019 Aug 31 [cited 2024 Sep 15];21(10):119. Available from: https://doi.org/10.1007/s11886-019-1218-5.

11. Wang N, Zhou JJ, Phan S, Yan TD, Phan K. Robot-assisted hybrid coronary revascularisation: systematic review. Heart Lung Circ [Internet]. 2015 Dec 1 [cited 2024 Sep 15];24(12):1171–9. Available from: https://www.sciencedirect.com/science/article/pii/S1443950615012561.

12. Cong C, Kato Y, Vasconcellos HDD, Ostovaneh MR, Lima JAC, Ambale-Venkatesh B. Deep learning-based end-to-end automated stenosis classification and localisation on catheter coronary angiography. Front Cardiovasc Med [Internet]. 2023 Feb 7 [cited 2024 Jul 20];10:944135. Available from: https://www.ncbi.nlm.nih.gov/pmc/articles/PMC9941145/.

13. Danilov VV, Klyshnikov KY, Gerget OM, Kutikhin AG, Ganyukov VI, Frangi AF, et al. Real-time coronary artery stenosis detection based on modern neural networks. Sci Rep [Internet]. 2021 Apr 7 [cited 2024 Jul 20];11(1):7582. Available from: https://www.nature.com/articles/s41598-021-87174-2.

14. Wu W, Zhang J, Xie H, Zhao Y, Zhang S, Gu L. Automatic detection of coronary artery stenosis by convolutional neural network with temporal constraint. Comput Biol Med [Internet]. 2020 Mar 1 [cited 2024 Jul 20];118:103657. Available from: https://www.sciencedirect.com/science/article/pii/S0010482520300512.

15. Lawton JS, Tamis-Holland JE, Bangalore S, Bates ER, Beckie TM, Bischoff JM, et al. 2021 ACC/AHA/SCAI guideline for coronary artery revascularisation: a report of the American College of Cardiology/American Heart Association Joint Committee on Clinical Practice Guidelines. Circulation [Internet]. 2022 Jan 18 [cited 2024 Jul 20];145(3):e18–114. Available from: https://www.ahajournals.org/doi/10.1161/CIR.0000000000001038.

16. Armoundas AA, Narayan SM, Arnett DK, Spector-Bagdady K, Bennett DA, Celi LA, et al. Use of artificial intelligence in improving outcomes in heart disease: a statement from the American Heart Association. Circulation [Internet]. 2024 Apr 2 [cited 2024 Aug 13];149(14):e1028–50. Available from: https://www.ahajournals.org/doi/10.1161/CIR.0000000000001201.

17. Avram R, Olgin JE, Ahmed Z, Verreault-Julien L, Wan A, Barrios J, et al. CathAI: fully automated coronary angiography interpretation and stenosis estimation. npj Digit Med [Internet]. 2023 Aug 11 [cited 2024 Jul 20];6(1):1–12. Available from: https://www.nature.com/articles/s41746-023-00880-1.

18. Nallamothu BK, Spertus JA, Lansky AJ, Cohen DJ, Jones PG, Kureshi F, et al. Comparison of clinical interpretation with visual assessment and quantitative coronary angiography in patients undergoing percutaneous coronary intervention in contemporary practice: the assessing angiography (A2) proj-

ect. Circulation [Internet]. 2013 Apr 30 [cited 2024 Jul 20];127(17):1793–800. Available from: https://www.ncbi.nlm.nih.gov/pmc/articles/PMC3908681/.

19. Krittanawong C, Kaplin S, Sharma SK. Chapter 6 - artificial intelligence on interventional cardiology. In: Krittanawong C, editor. Artificial intelligence in clinical practice [Internet]. Academic; 2024 [cited 2024 Jul 19]. p. 51–63. Available from: https://www.sciencedirect.com/science/article/pii/B9780443156885000401.

20. Du T, Xie L, Zhang H, Liu X, Wang X, Chen D, et al. Training and validation of a deep learning architecture for the automatic analysis of coronary angiography [Internet]. [cited 2024 Jul 20]. Available from: https://eurointervention.pcronline.com/article/automatic-and-multimodal-analysis-for-coronary-angiography-training-and-validation-of-a-deep-learning-architecture.

21. Bruining N. Robotics in interventional cardiology: a new era of safe and efficient procedures [Internet]. [cited 2024 Aug 17]. Available from: https://eurointervention.pcronline.com/article/robotics-in-interventional-cardiology-a-new-era-of-safe-and-efficient-procedures.

22. Elmaraezy A, Morra ME, Mohammed AT, Al-Habbaa A, Elgebaly A, Ghazy AA, et al. Risk of cataract among interventional cardiologists and catheterisation lab staff: a systematic review and meta-analysis. Catheter Cardiovasc Interv [Internet]. 2017 Jul 1 [cited 2024 Aug 17];90(1):1–9. Available from: https://onlinelibrary.wiley.com/doi/10.1002/ccd.27114.

23. Mohammadi M, Danaee L, Alisadeh E. Reduction of radiation risk to interventional cardiologists and patients during angiography and coronary angioplasty. J Tehran Heart Cent [Internet]. 2017 Jul [cited 2024 Sep 14];12(3):101–6. Available from: https://www.ncbi.nlm.nih.gov/pmc/articles/PMC5643866/.

24. Andreassi MG. Radiation risks and interventional cardiology: the value of radiation reduction exposure. J Cardiovasc Dev Dis [Internet]. 2023 Mar [cited 2024 Sep 14];10(3):121. Available from: https://www.mdpi.com/2308-3425/10/3/121.

25. American College of Cardiology [Internet]. [cited 2024 Sep 14]. Radiation safety for the interventional cardiologist—a practical approach to protecting ourselves from the dangers of ionising radiation. Available from: https://www.acc.org/latest-in-cardiology/articles/2015/12/31/10/12/; http://www.acc.org/latest-in-cardiology/articles/2015/12/31/10/12/radiation-safety-for-the-interventional-cardiologist.

26. McNamara DA, Chopra R, Decker JM, McNamara MW, Van Oosterhout SM, Berkompas DC, et al. Comparison of radiation exposure among interventional echocardiographers, interventional cardiologists, and sonographers during percutaneous structural heart interventions. JAMA Network Open [Internet]. 2022 Jul 7 [cited 2024 Sep

14];5(7):e2220597. Available from: https://doi.org/10.1001/jamanetworkopen.2022.20597.

27. Radiation protection of staff during interventional cardiology [Internet]. IAEA; 2017 [cited 2024 Sep 14]. Available from: https://www.iaea.org/resources/rpop/health-professionals/interventional-procedures/interventional-cardiology/staff.

28. Tamirisa KP, Alasnag M, Calvert P, Islam S, Bhardwaj A, Pakanati K, et al. Radiation exposure, training, and safety in cardiology. JACC Adv [Internet]. 2024 Apr [cited 2024 Sep 14];3(4):100863. Available from: https://www.jacc.org/doi/10.1016/j.jacadv.2024.100863.

29. Takeda K, Hayashi T, Sakiyama K, Hasegawa R, Watanabe Y, Tajima O, et al. Multicenter evaluation of cine angiography and digital subtraction angiography dose rate for various angiography programs: comparison with fluoroscopic dose rate. Nihon Hoshasen Gijutsu Gakkai Zasshi. 2021;77(7):718–25.

30. Chu M, Wu P, Li G, Yang W, Gutiérrez-Chico JL, Tu S. Advances in diagnosis, therapy, and prognosis of coronary artery disease powered by deep learning algorithms. JACC Asia [Internet] 2023 Feb [cited 2024 Jul 19];3(1):1–14. Available from: https://www.jacc.org/doi/10.1016/j.jacasi.2022.12.005.

31. Philips [Internet]. [cited 2024 Aug 9]. Philips - dynamic coronary roadmap. Available from: https://www.philips.com/healthcare/product/HCDCR01/dynamic-coronary-roadmap-see-clearly-guide-confidently.

32. Hennessey B, Danenberg H, Vroey FD, Kirtane AJ, Parikh M, Karmpaliotis D, et al. Dynamic Coronary Roadmap versus standard angiography for percutaneous coronary intervention: the randomised, multicentre DCR4Contrast trial [Internet]. [cited 2024 Jul 19]. Available from: https://eurointervention.pcronline.com/article/dynamic-coronary-roadmap-versus-standard-angiography-for-percutaneous-coronary-intervention-the-randomised-multicentre-dcr4contrast-trial.

33. Beyar R, Davies J, Cook C, Dudek D, Cummins P, Bruining N. Robotics, imaging, and artificial intelligence in the catheterisation laboratory [Internet]. [cited 2024 Jul 19]. Available from: https://eurointervention.pcronline.com/article/robotics-imaging-and-artificial-intelligence-in-the-catheterisation-laboratory.

34. Bang JY, Hough M, Hawes RH, Varadarajulu S. Use of artificial intelligence to reduce radiation exposure at fluoroscopy-guided endoscopic procedures. Am J Gastroenterol [Internet]. 2020 Apr [cited 2024 Jul 19];115(4):555–61. Available from: https://journals.lww.com/10.14309/ajg.0000000000000565.

35. Omega Medical Imaging [Internet]. [cited 2024 Aug 9]. Soteria.AI. Available from: https://www.omega-medicalimaging.com/soteria-ai/.

36. Nir G, Machan LS, Donnellan F, Brounstein ABM, Singh K, Wait DG, et al. Automatic detection and tracking of the region of interest during fluoroscopy-guided procedures for radiation exposure reduction. 2021 Feb 1 [cited 2024 Jul 19];11598:1159828. Available from: https://ui.adsabs.harvard.edu/abs/2021SPIE11598E..28N.

37. Durand E, Sabatier R, Smits PC, Verheye S, Pereira B, Fajadet J. Evaluation of the R-One robotic system for percutaneous coronary intervention: the R-EVOLUTION study [Internet]. [cited 2024 Aug 17]. Available from: https://eurointervention.pcronline.com/article/evaluation-of-the-r-one-robotic-system-for-percutaneous-coronary-intervention-the-r-evolution-study.

38. Andreassi MG, Piccaluga E, Guagliumi G, Del Greco M, Gaita F, Picano E. Occupational health risks in cardiac catheterisation laboratory workers. Circ Cardiovasc Interv. 2016;9(4):e003273.

39. Klein LW, Miller DL, Balter S, Laskey W, Naito N, Haines D, et al. Occupational health hazards in the interventional laboratory: time for a safer environment. Catheter Cardiovasc Interv [Internet]. 2018 Jan 4 [cited 2024 Aug 18]; Available from: https://onlinelibrary.wiley.com/doi/10.1002/ccd.21772.

40. Gupta R, Malik AH, Chan JSK, Lawrence H, Mehta A, Venkata VS, et al. Robotic assisted versus manual percutaneous coronary intervention: systematic review and meta-analysis. Cardiol Rev [Internet]. 2024 Feb [cited 2024 Aug 17];32(1):24. Available from: https://journals.lww.com/cardiologyinreview/abstract/2024/01000/robotic_assisted_versus_manual_percutaneous.5.aspx.

41. Patel TM, Shah SC, Soni YY, Radadiya RC, Patel GA, Tiwari PO, et al. Comparison of robotic percutaneous coronary intervention with traditional percutaneous coronary intervention. Circ Cardiovasc Interv[Internet]. 2020 May [cited 2024 Aug 17];13(5):e008888. Available from: https://www.ahajournals.org/doi/10.1161/CIRCINTERVENTIONS.119.008888.

42. Bujak M, Liszka R, Gasior P, Kidoń J, Gasior M, Dudek D, et al. TCT-749 the R-one robotic system for percutaneous coronary intervention: insights from the Robo-SIL registry. J Am Coll Cardiol [Internet]. 2024 Oct 29 [cited 2024 Dec 15];84(18_Supplement):B298–9. Available from: https://www.jacc.org/doi/10.1016/j.jacc.2024.09.894.

43. Seetharam K, Shrestha S, Sengupta PP. Cardiovascular imaging and intervention through the lens of artificial intelligence. Interv Cardiol [Internet]. 2021 Oct 20 [cited 2024 Aug 16];16:e31. Available from: https://www.ncbi.nlm.nih.gov/pmc/articles/PMC8559149/.

44. Sardar P, Abbott JD, Kundu A, Aronow HD, Granada JF, Giri J. Impact of artificial intelligence on interventional cardiology. JACC Cardiovasc Interv [Internet]. 2019 Jul 22 [cited 2024 Jul 19];12(14):1293–303. Available from: https://www.jacc.org/doi/full/10.1016/j.jcin.2019.04.048.

45. Khokhar A, Zelias A, Zlahoda-Huzior A, Chandra K, Ruggiero R, Toselli M, et al. Advancements in

robotic PCI technology: time to tackle the complex lesions! AsiaIntervention [Internet]. 2022 Mar [cited 2024 Dec 15];8(1):50–1. Available from: https://www.ncbi.nlm.nih.gov/pmc/articles/PMC8922457/.

46. Khokhar AA, Marrone A, Bermpeis K, Wyffels E, Tamargo M, Fernandez-Avilez F, et al. Latest developments in robotic percutaneous coronary interventions. Interv Cardiol [Internet]. 2023 Dec 6 [cited 2024 Dec 14];18:e30. Available from: https://www.ncbi.nlm.nih.gov/pmc/articles/PMC10782427/.

47. Patel TM, Shah SC, Patel AT, Patel B, Pancholy SB. Learning curve of robotic percutaneous coronary intervention: a single-center experience. J Soc Cardiovasc Angiogr Interv. 2022;1(6):100508.

48. von Ende E, Ryan S, Crain MA, Makary MS. Artificial intelligence, augmented reality, and virtual reality advances and applications in interventional radiology. Diagnostics (Basel) [Internet]. 2023 Feb 27 [cited 2024 Dec 14];13(5):892. Available from: https://www.ncbi.nlm.nih.gov/pmc/articles/PMC10000832/.

49. Rezaei A, Karimi H, Jafari R, Esmaili M, Naseri S. Comparing Virtual Reality and Traditional Training in Radiation Safety Practices Over Three Years Among Cardiologists and Scrub Nurses. JVS-Vascular Insights [Internet]. 2024 Oct 10 [cited 2024 Dec 14];100146. Available from: https://www.sciencedirect.com/science/article/pii/S2949912724000941.

50. Hayes J. Incorporating AI-Driven Conversations in VR Simulations [Internet]. [cited 2024 Dec 14]. Available from: https://blog.virtualmedicalcoaching.com/en/incorporating-ai-driven-conversations-in-vr-simulations.

51. Lastrucci A, Wandael Y, Barra A, Ricci R, Maccioni G, Pirrera A, et al. Exploring augmented reality integration in diagnostic imaging: myth or reality? Diagnostics (Basel) [Internet]. 2024 Jun 23 [cited 2024 Dec 14];14(13):1333. Available from: https://www.ncbi.nlm.nih.gov/pmc/articles/PMC11240696/.

52. Sarwar M, Adedokun S, Narayanan MA. Role of intravascular ultrasound and optical coherence tomography in intracoronary imaging for coronary artery disease: a systematic review. J Geriatr Cardiol [Internet]. 2024 Jan 28 [cited 2024 Jul 21];21(1):104–29. Available from: https://www.ncbi.nlm.nih.gov/pmc/articles/PMC10908578/.

53. Nagaraja V, Kalra A, Puri R. When to use intravascular ultrasound or optical coherence tomography during percutaneous coronary intervention? Cardiovasc Diagn Ther [Internet]. 2020 Oct [cited 2024 Jul 21];10(5):1429–44. Available from: https://www.ncbi.nlm.nih.gov/pmc/articles/PMC7666918/.

54. Buccheri S, Franchina G, Romano S, Puglisi S, Venuti G, D'Arrigo P, et al. Clinical outcomes following intravascular imaging-guided versus coronary angiography–guided percutaneous coronary intervention with stent implantation: a systematic review and Bayesian network meta-analysis of 31 studies and 17,882 patients. JACC Cardiovasc Interv [Internet]. 2017 Dec 26 [cited 2024 Jul 21];10(24):2488–98. Available from: https://www.sciencedirect.com/science/article/pii/S193687981731823X.

55. Baruś P, Modrzewski J, Gumiężna K, Dunaj P, Głód M, Bednarek A, et al. Comparative appraisal of intravascular ultrasound and optical coherence tomography in invasive coronary imaging: 2022 update. J Clin Med [Internet]. 2022 Jan [cited 2024 Jul 19];11(14):4055. Available from: https://www.mdpi.com/2077-0383/11/14/4055.

56. Matsumura M, Mintz GS, Dohi T, Li W, Shang A, Fall K, et al. Accuracy of IVUS-based machine learning segmentation assessment of coronary artery dimensions and balloon sizing. JACC Adv [Internet]. 2023 Sep 1 [cited 2024 Jul 21];2(7):100564. Available from: https://www.sciencedirect.com/science/article/pii/S2772963X2300501X.

57. Hong SJ, Mintz GS, Ahn CM, Kim JS, Kim BK, Ko YG, et al. Effect of intravascular ultrasound–guided drug-eluting stent implantation: 5-year follow-up of the IVUS-XPL randomised trial. JACC Cardiovasc Interv [Internet]. 2020 Jan 13 [cited 2024 Jul 21];13(1):62–71. Available from: https://www.sciencedirect.com/science/article/pii/S1936879819320199.

58. Gao XF, Ge Z, Kong XQ, Kan J, Han L, Lu S, et al. 3-Year outcomes of the ULTIMATE trial comparing intravascular ultrasound versus angiography-guided drug-eluting stent implantation. JACC Cardiovasc Interv [Internet]. 2021 Feb 8 [cited 2024 Jul 21];14(3):247–57. Available from: https://www.sciencedirect.com/science/article/pii/S1936879820320203.

59. Smilowitz NR, Mohananey D, Razzouk L, Weisz G, Slater JN. Impact and trends of intravascular imaging in diagnostic coronary angiography and percutaneous coronary intervention in inpatients in the United States. Catheter Cardiovasc Interv [Internet]. 2018 [cited 2024 Jul 21];92(6):E410–5. Available from: https://onlinelibrary.wiley.com/doi/abs/10.1002/ccd.27673.

60. Mentias A, Sarrazin MV, Saad M, Panaich S, Kapadia S, Horwitz PA, et al. Long-term outcomes of coronary stenting with and without use of intravascular ultrasound. JACC Cardiovasc Interv [Internet]. 2020 Aug 24 [cited 2024 Jul 21];13(16):1880–90. Available from: https://www.ncbi.nlm.nih.gov/pmc/articles/PMC7444477/.

61. Park DY, Vemmou E, An S, Nikolakopoulos I, Regan CJ, Cambi BC, et al. Trends and impact of intravascular ultrasound and optical coherence tomography on percutaneous coronary intervention for myocardial infarction. Int J Cardiol Heart Vasc [Internet]. 2023 Feb 13 [cited 2024 Aug 15];45:101186. Available from: https://www.ncbi.nlm.nih.gov/pmc/articles/PMC9957744/.

62. Buccola J, Meinen J, Spinelli J, Hammerstone M, Rapoza R, West NEJ. Investigating real-world impact of optical coherence tomography workflow-

guided coronary interventions: design and rationale of the LightLab clinical initiative. Catheter Cardiovasc Interv [Internet]. 2023 Jan 20 [cited 2024 Aug 15];100:S1–6. Available from: https://onlinelibrary.wiley.com/doi/10.1002/ccd.30394.

63. Flattery E, Rahim HM, Petrossian G, Shlofmitz E, Gkargkoulas F, Matsumura M, et al. Competency-based assessment of interventional cardiology fellows' abilities in intracoronary physiology and imaging. Circ Cardiovasc Interv [Internet]. 2020 Feb [cited 2024 Jul 21];13(2):e008760. Available from: https://www.ahajournals.org/doi/10.1161/CIRCINTERVENTIONS.119.008760.

64. Samant S, Bakhos JJ, Wu W, Zhao S, Kassab GS, Khan B, et al. Artificial intelligence, computational simulations, and extended reality in cardiovascular interventions. JACC Cardiovasc Interv [Internet]. 2023 Oct 23 [cited 2024 Jul 19];16(20):2479–97. Available from: https://www.jacc.org/doi/10.1016/j.jcin.2023.07.022.

65. Sengupta PP, Bavishi C. Harnessing artificial intelligence for intravascular imaging. JACC Adv [Internet]. 2023 Aug 22 [cited 2024 Jul 21];2(7):100565. Available from: https://www.ncbi.nlm.nih.gov/pmc/articles/PMC11198631/.

66. Hong D, Lee SH, Lee J, Lee H, Shin D, Kim HK, et al. Cost-effectiveness of fractional flow reserve–guided treatment for acute myocardial infarction and multivessel disease: a prespecified analysis of the FRAME-AMI randomised clinical trial. JAMA Network Open [Internet]. 2024 Jan 25 [cited 2024 Jul 22];7(1):e2352427. Available from: https://doi.org/10.1001/jamanetworkopen.2023.52427.

67. Shinohara H, Kodera S, Ninomiya K, Nakamoto M, Katsushika S, Saito A, et al. Automatic detection of vessel structure by deep learning using intravascular ultrasound images of the coronary arteries. PLoS One [Internet]. 2021 Aug 5 [cited 2024 Aug 12];16(8):e0255577. Available from: https://journals.plos.org/plosone/article?id=10.1371/journal.pone.0255577.

68. Molony D, Hosseini H, Samady H. TCT-2 deep IVUS: a machine learning framework for fully automatic IVUS segmentation. J Am Coll Cardiol [Internet]. 2018 Sep 25 [cited 2024 Jul 23];72(13_Supplement):B1–B1. Available from: https://www.jacc.org/doi/full/10.1016/j.jacc.2018.08.1077.

69. Yang J, Tong L, Faraji M, Basu A. IVUS-net: An intravascular ultrasound segmentation network. In: Basu A, Berretti S, editors. Smart multimedia [Internet]. Cham: Springer; 2018 [cited 2024 Aug 18]. p. 367–77. (Lecture Notes in Computer Science; vol. 11010). Available from: http://link.springer.com/10.1007/978-3-030-04375-9_31.

70. Molony D, Samady H. TCT-342 DeepIVUS: a machine learning platform for fully automatic IVUS segmentation and phenotyping. J Am Coll Cardiol [Internet]. 2019 Oct [cited 2024 Aug 15];74(13_Supplement):B339–B339. Available from: https://www.jacc.org/doi/full/10.1016/j.jacc.2019.08.424.

71. Guo X, Maehara A, Matsumura M, Wang L, Zheng J, Samady H, et al. Predicting plaque vulnerability change using intravascular ultrasound + optical coherence tomography image-based fluid–structure interaction models and machine learning methods with patient follow-up data: a feasibility study. Biomed Eng Online [Internet]. 2021 Apr 6 [cited 2024 Aug 15];20(1):34. Available from: https://doi.org/10.1186/s12938-021-00868-6.

72. Zhang J, Han R, Shao G, Lv B, Sun K. Artificial intelligence in cardiovascular atherosclerosis imaging. J Pers Med [Internet]. 2022 Mar 8 [cited 2024 Jul 24];12(3):420. Available from: https://www.ncbi.nlm.nih.gov/pmc/articles/PMC8952318/.

73. Nishi T, Yamashita R, Imura S, Tateishi K, Kitahara H, Kobayashi Y, et al. Deep learning-based intravascular ultrasound segmentation for the assessment of coronary artery disease. International Journal of Cardiology [Internet]. 2021 Jun 15 [cited 2024 Aug 18];333:55–9. Available from: https://www.internationaljournalofcardiology.com/article/S0167-5273(21)00477-0/abstract.

74. Matsumura M, Johnson NP, Fearon WF, Mintz GS, Stone GW, Oldroyd KG, et al. Accuracy of fractional flow reserve measurements in clinical practice: observations from a core laboratory analysis. JACC: Cardiovasc Interv [Internet]. 2017 Jul 24 [cited 2024 Jul 24];10(14):1392–401. Available from: https://www.sciencedirect.com/science/article/pii/S1936879817306465.

75. Min HS, Ryu D, Kang SJ, Lee JG, Yoo JH, Cho H, et al. Prediction of coronary stent underexpansion by Pre-procedural intravascular ultrasound–based deep learning. JACC: Cardiovasc Interv [Internet]. 2021 May 10 [cited 2024 Aug 18];14(9):1021–9. Available from: https://www.jacc.org/doi/10.1016/j.jcin.2021.01.033.

76. Lee JG, Ko J, Hae H, Kang SJ, Kang DY, Lee PH, et al. Intravascular ultrasound-based machine learning for predicting fractional flow reserve in intermediate coronary artery lesions. Atherosclerosis [Internet]. 2020 Jan 1 [cited 2024 Aug 15];292:171–7. Available from: https://www.sciencedirect.com/science/article/pii/S0021915019315527.

77. Chu M, Jia H, Gutiérrez-Chico J, Maehara A, Ali ZA, Zeng X, et al. Artificial intelligence and optical coherence tomography for the automatic characterisation of human atherosclerotic plaques [Internet]. [cited 2024 Jul 21]. Available from: https://eurointervention.pcronline.com/article/automatic-characterisation-of-human-atherosclerotic-plaque-composition-from-intravascular-optical-coherence-tomography-using-artificial-intelligence.

78. Athanasiou LS, Olender ML, de la Torre Hernandez JM, Ben-Assa E, Edelman ER. A deep learning approach to classify atherosclerosis using intracoronary optical coherence tomography. 2019 Mar 1 [cited 2024 Aug 12];10950:109500N.

Available from: https://ui.adsabs.harvard.edu/abs/2019SPIE10950E..0NA.

79. Neumann FJ, Sousa-Uva M, Ahlsson A, Alfonso F, Banning AP, Benedetto U, et al. 2018 ESC/EACTS guidelines on myocardial revascularisation. Eur Heart J [Internet]. 2019 Jan 7 [cited 2024 Jul 23];40(2):87–165. Available from: https://doi.org/10.1093/eurheartj/ehy394.

80. Vergallo R, Lombardi M, Kakuta T, Pawlowski T, Leone AM, Sardella G, et al. Optical coherence tomography measures predicting fractional flow reserve: the OMEF study. J Soc Cardiovasc Angiogr Interv [Internet]. 2024 Apr 1 [cited 2024 Jul 23];3(4). Available from: https://www.jscai.org/article/S2772-9303(23)01513-2/fulltext.

81. Farhad A, Reza R, Azamossadat H, Ali G, Arash R, Mehrad A, et al. Artificial intelligence in estimating fractional flow reserve: a systematic literature review of techniques. BMC Cardiovasc Disord [Internet]. 2023 Aug 18 [cited 2024 Jul 25];23(1):407. Available from: https://bmccardiovascdisord.biomedcentral.com/articles/10.1186/s12872-023-03447-w.

82. Bruyne BD, Pijls NHJ, Kalesan B, Barbato E, Tonino PAL, Piroth Z, et al. Fractional flow reserve–guided PCI versus medical therapy in stable coronary disease. N Engl J Med [Internet]. 2012 Sep 13 [cited 2024 Jul 25];367(11):991–1001. Available from: https://www.nejm.org/doi/full/10.1056/NEJMoa1205361.

83. Pijls NH, van Schaardenburgh P, Manoharan G, Boersma E, Bech JW, van't Veer M, et al. Percutaneous coronary intervention of functionally nonsignificant stenosis. J Am Coll Cardiol [Internet]. 2007 May 29 [cited 2024 Jul 25];49(21):2105–11. Available from: https://www.jacc.org/doi/abs/10.1016/j.jacc.2007.01.087.

84. Tonino PA, De Bruyne B, Pijls NH, Siebert U, Ikeno F, vant Veer M, et al. Fractional flow reserve versus angiography for guiding percutaneous coronary intervention. N Engl J Med [Internet]. 2009 Jan 15 [cited 2024 Jul 25];360(3). Available from: https://pubmed.ncbi.nlm.nih.gov/19144937/.

85. Pijls NHJ, Sels JWEM. Functional measurement of coronary stenosis. J Am Coll Cardiol [Internet]. 2012 Mar 20 [cited 2024 Jul 22];59(12):1045–57. Available from: https://www.jacc.org/doi/abs/10.1016/j.jacc.2011.09.077.

86. Stegehuis VE, Wijntjens GW, Piek JJ, van de Hoef TP. Fractional flow reserve or coronary flow reserve for the assessment of myocardial perfusion. Curr Cardiol Rep [Internet]. 2018 Jul 26 [cited 2024 Jul 22];20(9):77. Available from: https://doi.org/10.1007/s11886-018-1017-4.

87. Park SJ, Ahn JM. Should we be using fractional flow reserve more routinely to select stable coronary patients for percutaneous coronary intervention? Curr Opin Cardiol. 2012;27(6):675–81.

88. De Maria GL, Garcia-Garcia HM, Scarsini R, Hideo-Kajita A, Gonzalo López N, Leone AM, et al. Novel indices of coronary physiology. Circ Cardiovasc Interv [Internet]. 2020 Apr [cited 2024 Jul 22];13(4):e008487. Available from: https://www.ahajournals.org/doi/full/10.1161/CIRCINTERVENTIONS.119.008487.

89. Van Belle E, Rioufol G, Pouillot C, Cuisset T, Bougrini K, Teiger E, et al. Outcome impact of coronary revascularisation strategy reclassification with fractional flow reserve at time of diagnostic angiography. Circulation [Internet]. 2014 Jan 14 [cited 2024 Jul 25];129(2):173–85. Available from: https://www.ahajournals.org/doi/10.1161/CIRCULATIONAHA.113.006646.

90. Roguin A, Abu Dogosh A, Feld Y, Konigstein M, Lerman A, Koifman E. Early feasibility of automated artificial intelligence angiography based fractional flow reserve estimation. Am J Cardiol [Internet]. 2021 Jan 15 [cited 2024 Jul 23];139:8–14. Available from: https://www.sciencedirect.com/science/article/pii/S0002914920310961.

91. Härle T, Zeymer U, Hochadel M, Zahn R, Kerber S, Zrenner B, et al. Real-world use of fractional flow reserve in Germany: results of the prospective ALKK coronary angiography and PCI registry. Clin Res Cardiol [Internet]. 2017 Feb 1 [cited 2024 Jul 23];106(2):140–50. Available from: https://doi.org/10.1007/s00392-016-1034-5.

92. Fearon WF, Achenbach S, Engstrom T, Assali A, Shlofmitz R, Jeremias A, et al. Accuracy of fractional flow reserve derived from coronary angiography. Circulation [Internet]. 2019 Jan 22 [cited 2024 Jul 22];139(4):477–84. Available from: https://www.ahajournals.org/doi/full/10.1161/CIRCULATIONAHA.118.037350.

93. Koo BK, Samady H. Strap in for the artificial intelligence revolution in interventional cardiology. JACC: Cardiovasc Interv [Internet]. 2019 Jul 22 [cited 2024 Jul 23];12(14):1325–7. Available from: https://www.sciencedirect.com/science/article/pii/S1936879819312397.

94. Kim HL, Koo BK, Nam CW, Doh JH, Kim JH, Yang HM, et al. Clinical and physiological outcomes of fractional flow reserve-guided percutaneous coronary intervention in patients with serial Stenoses within one coronary artery. JACC: Cardiovasc Interv [Internet]. 2012 Oct 1 [cited 2024 Jul 24];5(10):1013–8. Available from: https://www.sciencedirect.com/science/article/pii/S1936879812007595.

95. Morris PD, Curzen N, Gunn JP. Angiography-derived fractional flow reserve: more or less physiology? J Am Heart Assoc [Internet]. 2020 Mar 17 [cited 2024 Jul 25];9(6):e015586. Available from: https://www.ahajournals.org/doi/10.1161/JAHA.119.015586.

96. Scoccia A, Tomaniak M, Neleman T, Groenland FTW, Plantes ACZD, Daemen J. Angiography-based fractional flow reserve: state of the art. Curr Cardiol Rep [Internet] 2022 [cited 2024 Jul 25];24(6):667–78. Available from: https://www.ncbi.nlm.nih.gov/pmc/articles/PMC9188492/.

97. Ben-Assa E, Abu Salman A, Cafri C, Roguin A, Hellou E, Koifman E, et al. Performance of a novel artificial intelligence software developed to derive coronary fractional flow reserve values from diagnostic angiograms. Coron Artery Dis [Internet]. 2023 Dec [cited 2024 Jul 25];34(8):533. Available from: https://journals.lww.com/coronary-artery/fulltext/2023/12000/performance_of_a_novel_artificial_intelligence.1.aspx.

98. Cathworks FFRangio [Internet]. CathWorks FFRangio System. [cited 2024 Sep 18]. Available from: https://cath.works/cathworks-ffrangio/.

99. medisimaging [Internet]. [cited 2024 Sep 18]. Medis QFR® - Physiology made simple. Available from: https://medisimaging.com/software-solutions/medis-qfr/.

100. Snapshot [Internet]. [cited 2024 Sep 18]. Available from: https://www.siemens-healthineers.com/en-us/angio/innovations-technologies/ffr.

101. Subhan S, Malik J, ul Haq A, Qadeer MS, Zaidi SMJ, Orooj F, et al. Role of artificial intelligence and machine learning in interventional cardiology. Curr Probl Cardiol [Internet]. 2023 Jul 1 [cited 2024 Jul 23];48(7):101698. Available from: https://www.sciencedirect.com/science/article/pii/S0146280623001159.

102. Narula S, Shameer K, Salem Omar AM, Dudley JT, Sengupta PP. Machine-learning algorithms to automate morphological and functional assessments in 2D echocardiography. J Am Coll Cardiol. 2016;68(21):2287–95.

103. Alharbi Y. Artificial intelligence in cardiology: present state and prospective directions. J Radiat Res Appl Sci [Internet]. 2024 Sep 1 [cited 2024 Aug 14];17(3):101012. Available from: https://www.sciencedirect.com/science/article/pii/S1687850724001961.

104. Ghallab M, Abdelhamid M, Nassar M, Mostafa KS, Salama DH, Elnaggar W, et al. Assessing and improving radiation safety in cardiac catheterisation: a study from Cairo University Hospital. Egypt Heart J [Internet]. 2024 Feb 9 [cited 2024 Aug 12];76(1):17. Available from: https://doi.org/10.1186/s43044-024-00449-7.

105. Rudnicka Z, Pręgowska A, Glądys K, Perkins M, Proniewska K. Advancements in artificial intelligence-driven techniques for interventional cardiology. Cardiol J [Internet]. 2024 [cited 2024 Aug 14];31(2):321–41. Available from: https://journals.viamedica.pl/cardiology_journal/article/view/98650.

Christopher Steelman MS, R.T.(R)(CI) (ARRT), RCIS, FACVP, AACC is the Founder and Principal Consultant of Cath Lab International, LLC, and an educator and thought leader in cardiovascular imaging and intervention. As Founding Director of the Cardiac Specialist Program at Weber State University in Ogden, Utah, he pioneered innovations in advanced cardiovascular education and curriculum design. He has held key leadership roles with numerous professional societies, including chairing the Cardiac and Vascular Interventional Chapter of the American Society of Radiologic Technologists, serving on the Board of Advisors for Cardiovascular Credentialing International, and co-chairing the American College of Cardiology Allied Health Professionals Workgroup. He has addressed audiences in over 20 countries and authored pivotal publications advancing clinical practice worldwide.

AI Applications in Ultrasound Imaging

9

Martin Weber Kusk, Simon Lysdahlgaard, and Malene Roland Vils Pedersen

9.1 Introduction

Ultrasound (US) differs from other imaging modalities in several key parameters. This presents some unique challenges to the implementation of AI.

In planar and volumetric modalities, image data are spatially correlated in a fixed coordinate system determined by scanner or tube/detector geometry. Thus, if the patient is correctly positioned in, for example, MRI, CT or DR, the pixel/voxel signal can be accurately located relative to the modality in two or three dimensions, and using appropriate acquisition and/or reconstruction parameters, the desired image resolution and contrast can be achieved. In US, the coordinate system originates at the transducer. The position is variable and dynamically adjusted by the sonographer during scanning. Furthermore, multiple acquisitions are often performed with various patient positioning, for example, supine and decubitus positions. Acquisition parameters can change 'on the fly', affecting image quality, resolution and penetration [1], requiring constant balancing dependent on the diagnostic task. The achievable tissue contrast is influenced by acoustic scattering, which varies with patient appearance, while the interposition of, for example, air can restrict tissue visualisation. This may involve altering transducer pressure, which, in turn, can lead to a shift in organ positions. The variability is reflected in the archived data, typically as single snapshots or cine loops, the selection of which is down to operator discretion and experience.

Artefacts, such as speckle and signal dropout, can present challenges to image interpretation. Correct organ or lesion quantification is dependent on the anatomical scan planes. Thus, a high degree of variability can present challenges in obtaining training and validation data for AI algorithms. Much of the information available to the operator in terms of visual, dynamic, and tactile information, which enters into the decision process and leads to a diagnosis, is not stored with the pixel data.

There is also a large diversity of ultrasound equipment vendors, making standardisation difficult, especially in quantitative imaging [2]. The low risks associated with the modality means that

on behalf of Association of Healthcare Technology Providers for Imaging, Radiotherapy and Care (AXREM)

M. W. Kusk (✉) · S. Lysdahlgaard
University of Southern Denmark, Department of Regional Health Research, Esbjerg, Denmark

Esbjerg & Grindsted Hospital, University Hospital of Southern Denmark - Department of Radiology & Nuclear Medicine, Esbjerg, Denmark
e-mail: martin.weber.kusk@rsyd.dk;
simon.lysdahlgaard@rsyd.dk

M. R. V. Pedersen
University of Southern Denmark, Esbjerg, Denmark

Sygehus Lillebælt, Vejle Hospital, Department of Radiology, Vejle, Denmark
e-mail: malene.roland.vils.pedersen@rsyd.dk

there are limited legislative safeguards for determining who can operate ultrasound. This, combined with the relatively low price, has led to the increased availability of ultrasound equipment with varying degrees of operator experience and quality control [3].

Given these factors, AI implementation in US has been described as 'driving on an unpaved road' [4]. On the other hand, the very same challenges also offer unique areas of application for AI, some of which will be described in the following, an overview of which is illustrated in Fig. 9.1. We also present two case studies where AI-powered solutions have already proved their value in clinical imaging.

9.2 Acquisition Support and Guidance

As mentioned above, operator experience is crucial in securing reliable and reproducible diagnosis by standardising the anatomical imaging planes as much as possible. While trained physicians and sonographers can achieve consistent results, this may not be the case in resource-poor settings or in clinics where ultrasound is performed by non-experts. Thus, AI has been proposed as a supporting tool for the standardisation of anatomical scan planes.

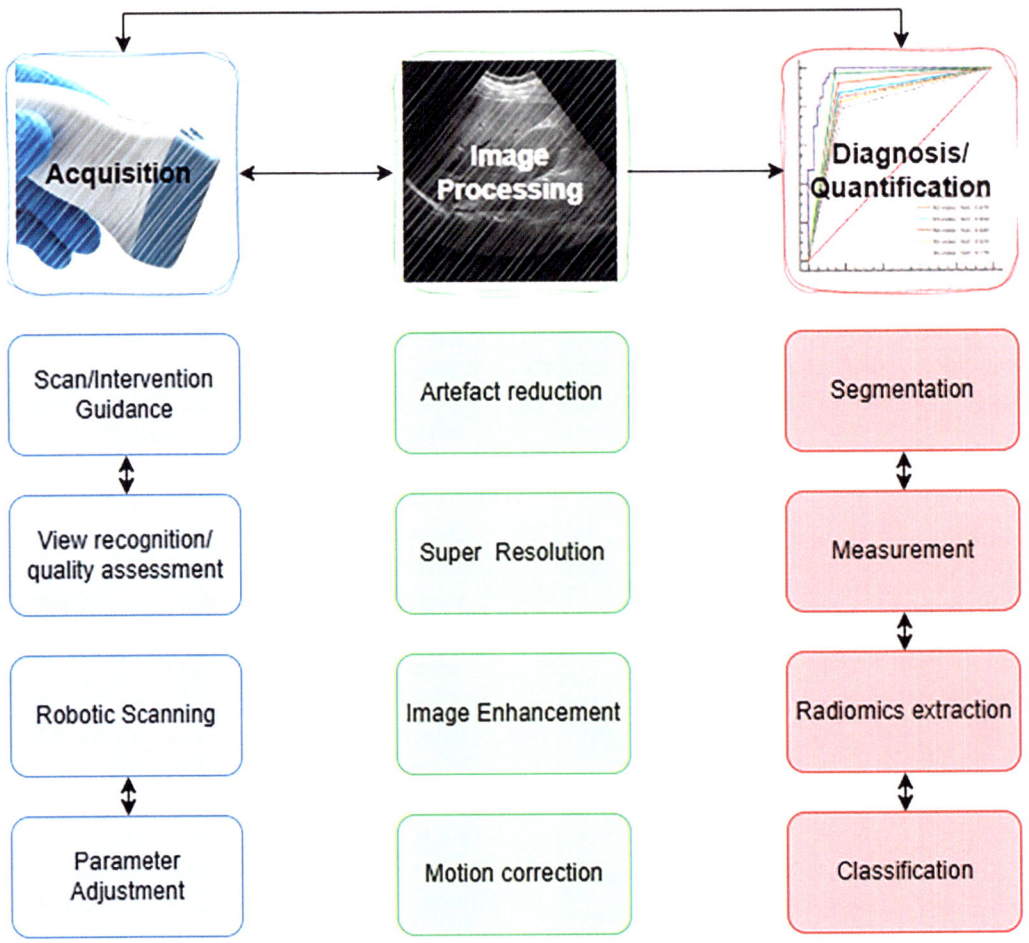

Fig. 9.1 The three main areas of use for AI in ultrasound, with detailed applications for each area. Many applications influence the results of others, which is illustrated with arrows. Image by the authors

Retrospective automated extraction of scan planes from 3D-US images has been demonstrated, for example, for fetal US [5, 6], to allow for reproducible measurements. Other solutions provide cues and quality indicators relating to specific anatomical views and automatically capture images at the optimal positioning. Chiu et al. [7] showed that US novices were able to perform focused assessment with sonography in trauma (FAST) scans with a median image quality score of 5 out of 5, as assessed by three expert sonographers, although AI-guided scans took longer to perform.

Nakayama et al. [8] even demonstrated the use of deep convolutional neural networks (DCNN) to guide disaster victims without access to medical professionals to screen themselves for risk of deep vein thrombosis. They achieved an AUC of 0.89 for the classification for the classification of images as suitable for diagnosis. Nhat et al. [9] demonstrated a real-time AI-assisted ultrasound

solution to allow clinicians to perform lung US in intensive care units.

Finally, in combination with robot technology and 3D cameras, AI has the potential to fully automate acquisition in well-defined, repetitive diagnostic tasks [10]. This technology is termed robotic ultrasound systems (RUSS) [11]. One example that is clinically available today is ARTHUR, where a generic transducer, mounted robot arm, is used to automatically scan 11 joints per hand for detection and monitoring of synovitis in rheumatoid arthritis. The patients simply place their hands on a dedicated plate, and the acquisition can be performed completely operator-free, thus minimising the pressure for experienced sonographers [12]. The technology can even be combined with automated reporting and scoring of disease activity using the standardised EULAR-OMERACT scoring system [13], making for a complete "self-service" US experience (Fig. 9.2).

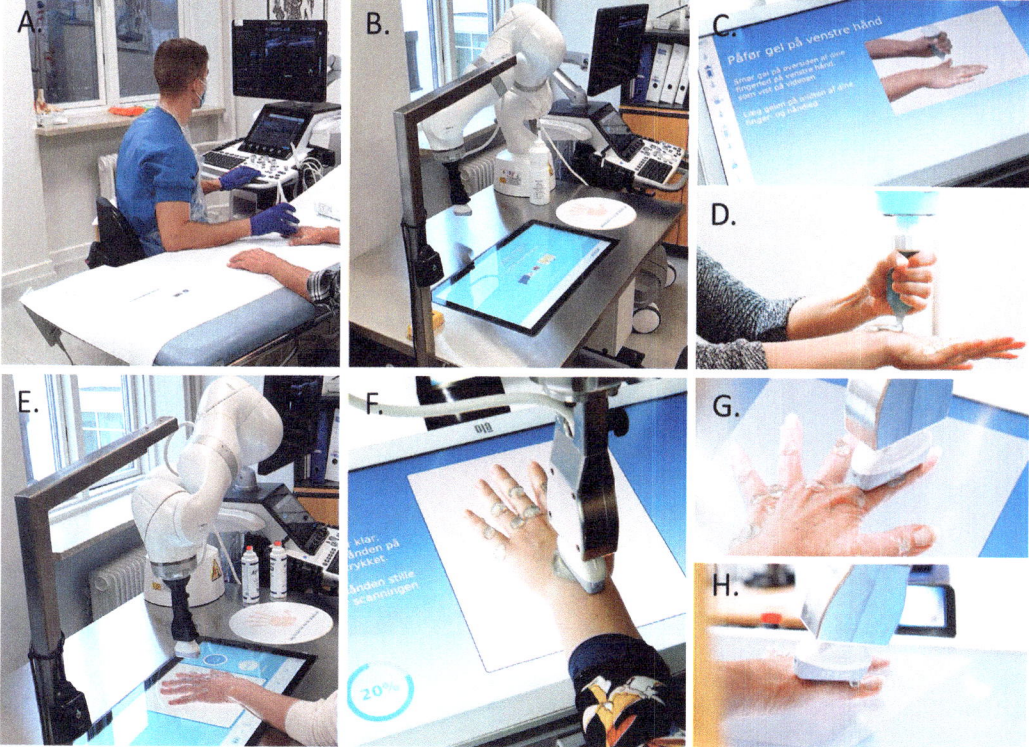

Fig. 9.2 ARTHUR completely automated workflow for scanning and reporting rheumatoid arthritis in fingers and wrist joints. (**a**) Conventional scanning by sonographer. (**b**) The ARTHUR self-service ultrasound station. (**c**) Visual step-by-step patient guidance. (**d**) Patient applies gel on hands and wrist. (**e**) Patient places hand on designated scanning area. (**f**) Scanning of wrist. (**g** & **h**) Patient is instructed to spread fingers, after which these are in turn scanned automatically. The procedure is repeated for both hands. From Frederiksen et al. [12] shared with permission

Algorithms are also being studied for varying degrees of AI-assisted ultrasonically guided interventions. This can be as simple as using AI to detect the needle tip [14, 15], which can be difficult to visualise at a speed of up to 10 frames per second. Palladino et al. [16] developed a robotic system for prostate biopsy (PROST), a new robotic system integrated with DL for prostate biopsies, utilising a CNN named PROST-Net for segmenting the prostate in MRI and US images across different planes and sensor alignments (Fig. 9.3).

9.3 Image Enhancement

AI can be used to enhance ultrasound image quality. Removal of speckle artefacts caused by small-structure wave scattering can help to enhance diagnostic confidence or facilitate more precise quantitative measurements, as depicted in Fig. 9.4, using CNN [17] or recurrent neural network (RNN) [18] networks.

As mentioned previously, image quality depends on the correct adjustment and optimisation of acquisition parameters, which are usually

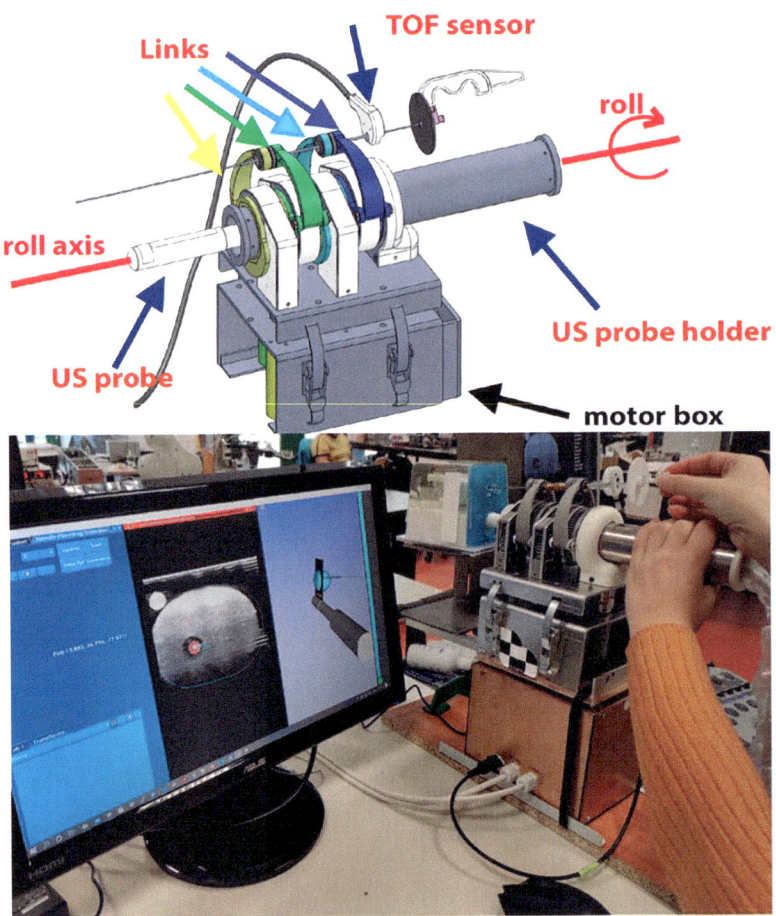

Fig. 9.3 Illustration of autonomous prostate biopsy by real-time DL-enabled fusion of MRI and US images [16]. The probe is actuated to rotate on the sagittal plane (roll). A sensor measures the depth of the needle insertion. Right is the probe robot prepared for a cadaver test

adapted based on the sonographers' individual visual perception. Annangi et al. [19] used RetinaNet, a special neural network, to adjust transmit parameters in trans-thoracic echocardiography (TTE) based on global image quality and found the proposed parameters in accordance with experts in 21 out of 26 cases.

Another example is increasing the spatial resolution beyond the limits imposed by the system's design parameters. This is called super-resolution, where AI algorithms are trained to interpolate pixel information not originally present in the image [20, 21]. At present, this has only been demonstrated retrospectively, as it requires large computational effort. Still, it is not unrealistic to expect that real-time super-resolution may be achieved in the near future. Such technologies may mitigate some of the tradeoffs between resolution and signal quality, as demonstrated by You et al. [22], shown in Fig. 9.5. An interesting application is the proposed use of CycleGANs to harmonise US image quality acquired at different institutions [23]. If successful, this could tackle some of the challenges of data diversity alluded to in the introduction.

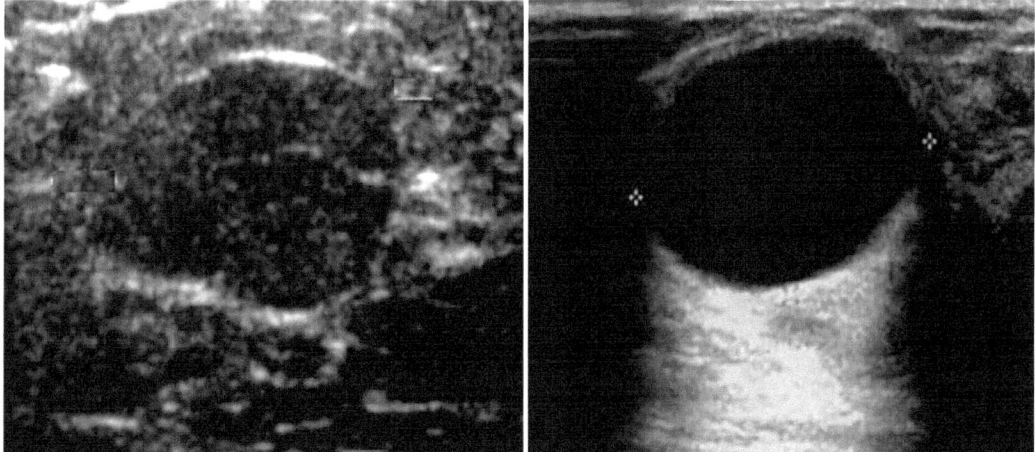

Fig. 9.4 Cystic breast lesion. Left: Original image. Right: After speckle noise suppression by CNN-based algorithm [17] (CC-BY license)

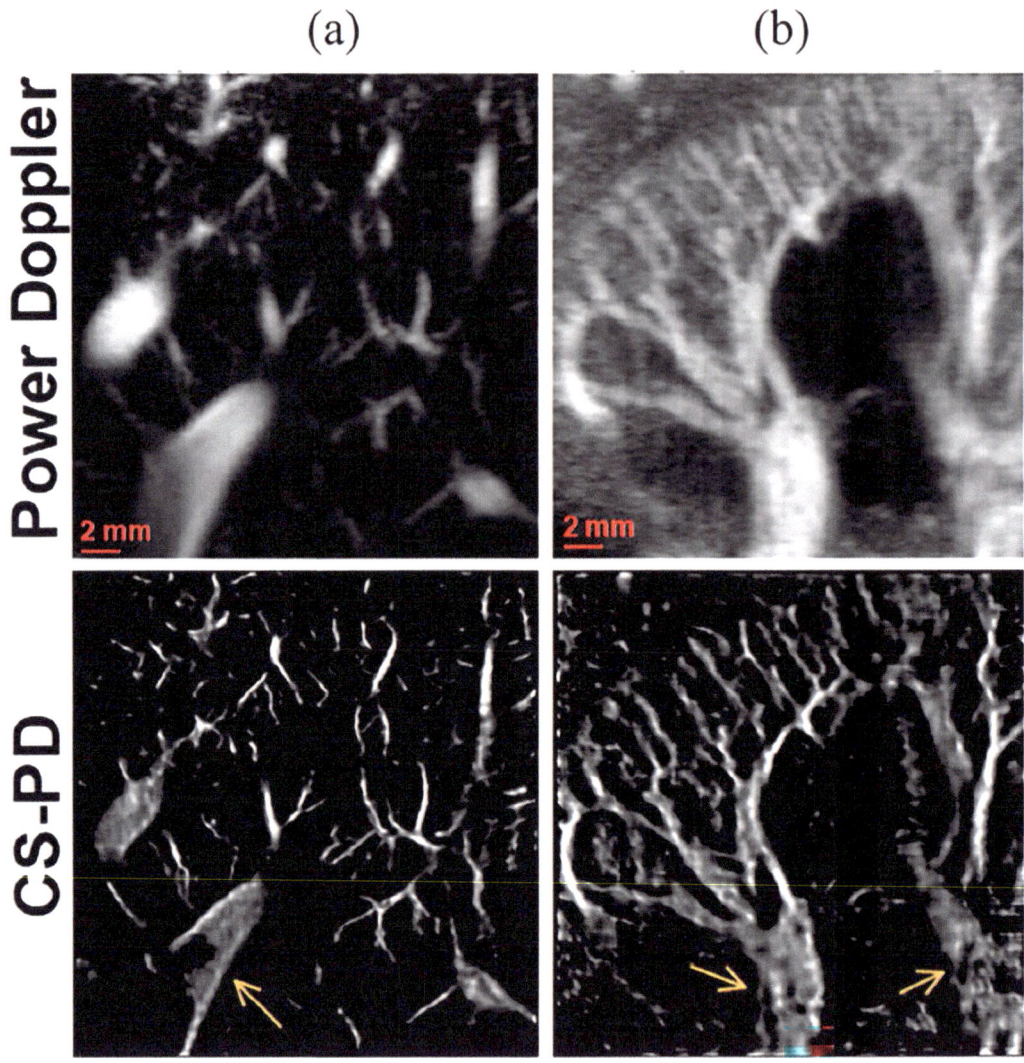

Fig. 9.5 Top row: Power Doppler imaging of a human liver (**a**), kidney (**b**). Bottom row: The same images are processed with contrast-free super-resolution (CS-PD) based on DNN architecture [22]. (License: CC-BY)

9.4 Segmentation, Measurement, Classification and Diagnosis

As in other modalities, the probably most prevalent use in the public mind is the potential of AI to provide 'automatic diagnoses'. Again, the performance of such models is inextricably linked to image quality and the acquisition of correct anatomic views. Thus, there is an overlap in segmentation and classification tasks. The term 'radiomics' (see Chap. 2 for more information on radiomics), in the broadest possible interpretation of pixel statistics, plays a role in such classification but relies on precise delineation of the area/volume of interest, as including non-relevant tissue may produce erroneous results [24]. This delineation, known as segmentation, can be accomplished manually by drawing regions of interest (ROIs) on images.

Needless to say, this can be very time-consuming, especially in US, where the position and size of a tissue of interest may change from frame to frame, requiring review of many images. As shown in Fig. 9.6, lesions present with different shapes dependent on acquisition plane and technique.

It is also highly subjective, as it is based on the segmenters' skill in acquiring images and their experience in discriminating the anatomical tissue signal in the presence of noise and artefacts. Therefore, this task is an ideal candidate for AI enabled automation. It should, however, be noted that as human ground truth segmentations are used for training such algorithms, the model's accuracy is highly dependent on the quality of training data and, as such, cannot be expected to outperform humans.

Chen et al. [25] developed an automatic segmentation algorithm to be able to extract radiomic features separately from renal parenchyma and pelvis to classify diabetic kidney damage (DKD) from US. They found that the area under the curve (AUC) for prediction of DKD was not significantly lower with radiomics features extracted from automated compared to manual segmentations (Fig. 9.7).

Other examples of automated segmentations include carotid plaques [26], ovarian cancer lesions [27] and prostate [28], but they can potentially applied in all anatomies.

Su et al. [29] achieved sensitivities and specificities from 70% to 96% and 67% to 95% in predicting early diabetic nephropathy from radiomic features from US images, classified with KNN, support vector machine (SVM) or linear regression. More information on these and other AI models can be found in Chap. 2. Ahmadi et al. [30] introduced a DL framework for assessing aortic stenosis from 2D echocardiography, achieving high accuracy in detecting and classifying aortic stenosis severity compared to board-certified sonographers and cardiologists. Weng et al. [31] applied a DL algorithm to a new dataset of thyroid nodule US images, finding its diagnostic performance comparable to that of experienced radiologists, with the algorithm's effectiveness not significantly affected by variations in US scanner types. Dadoun et al. [32] trained a DL network to detect, localise and characterise focal liver lesions in US images, achieving a sensitivity of 82% (95% CI: 62–100) and a specificity of 81% (95% CI: 67, 91) compared to three healthcare professionals (one nonexpert and two experts) in a multi-centre study, as shown in Fig. 9.8.

Compared to static image input, Zhao et al. [32] found that dynamic videos improved the classification of benign from malignant breast lesions (with biopsy reference). They outperformed six expert radiologists in the classification task with an AUC of 0.97 (Fig. 9.9). US radiomics features also promise to predict response to neoadjuvant chemotherapy in breast cancers [33, 34]. Such findings may improve the utilisation of US as a radiation-free modality in the diagnosis and follow-up of breast cancer. More about the potential use of radiomics can be found in Chap. 2.

However, many of the included studies suffer from being either single-centre or performed on select US equipment with experienced sonographers. Whether the results can be replicated in clinical practice is unknown. Phantom studies indicate that few features are reproducible across different scanners, acquisition parameters and segmentation localisations [36, 37]. For diagnostic acceptability of US radiomics, it is of utmost importance to reliably identify predictive and reproducible features in diverse patient populations and acquisition conditions.

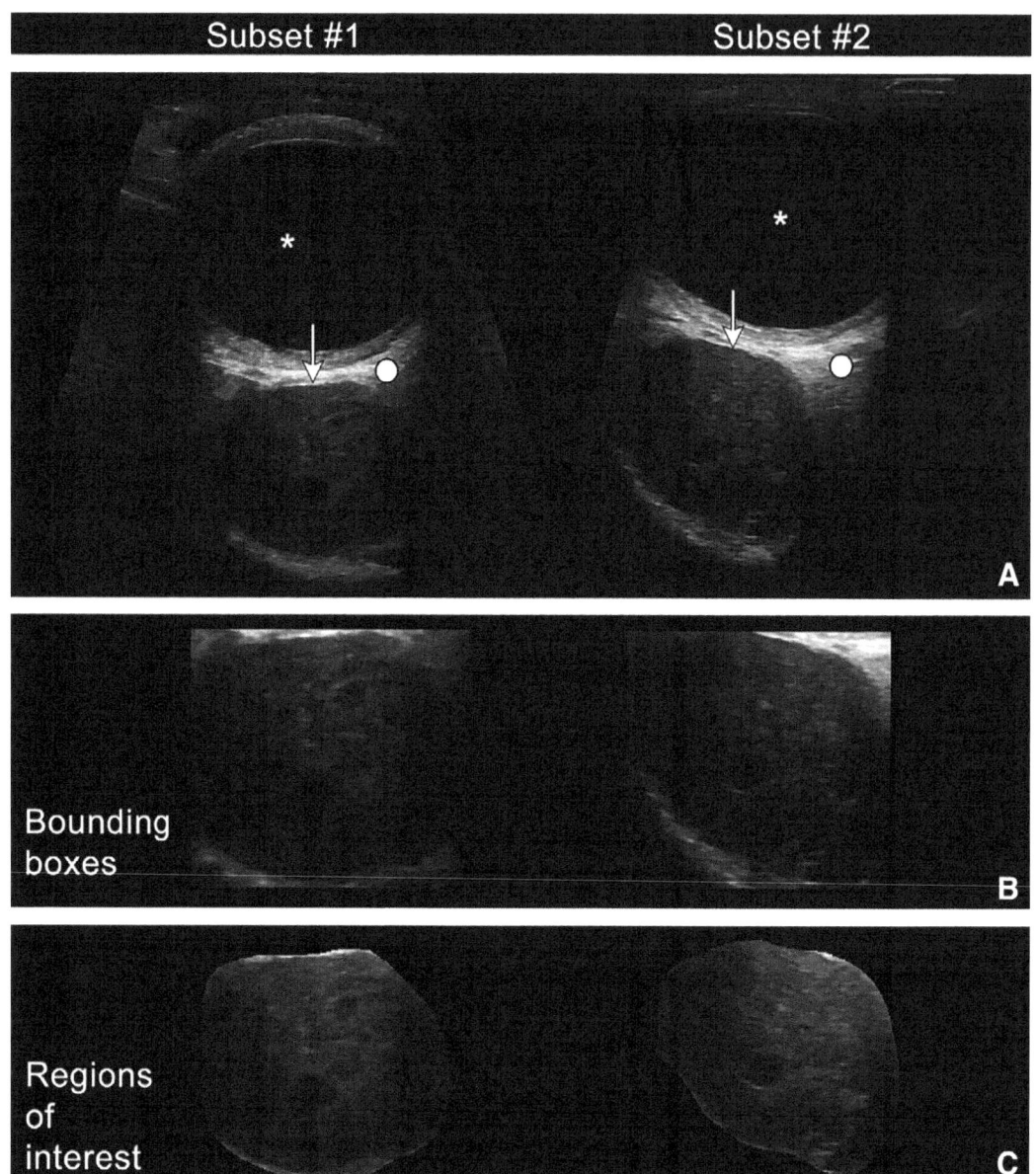

Fig. 9.6 Example of segmentations acquired from two different views of the same orbital lesion (denoted by white arrow). In the bottom row, the ROIs are drawn by a human reader. The challenges in obtaining consistent US segmentations are evident [24] CC-BY license

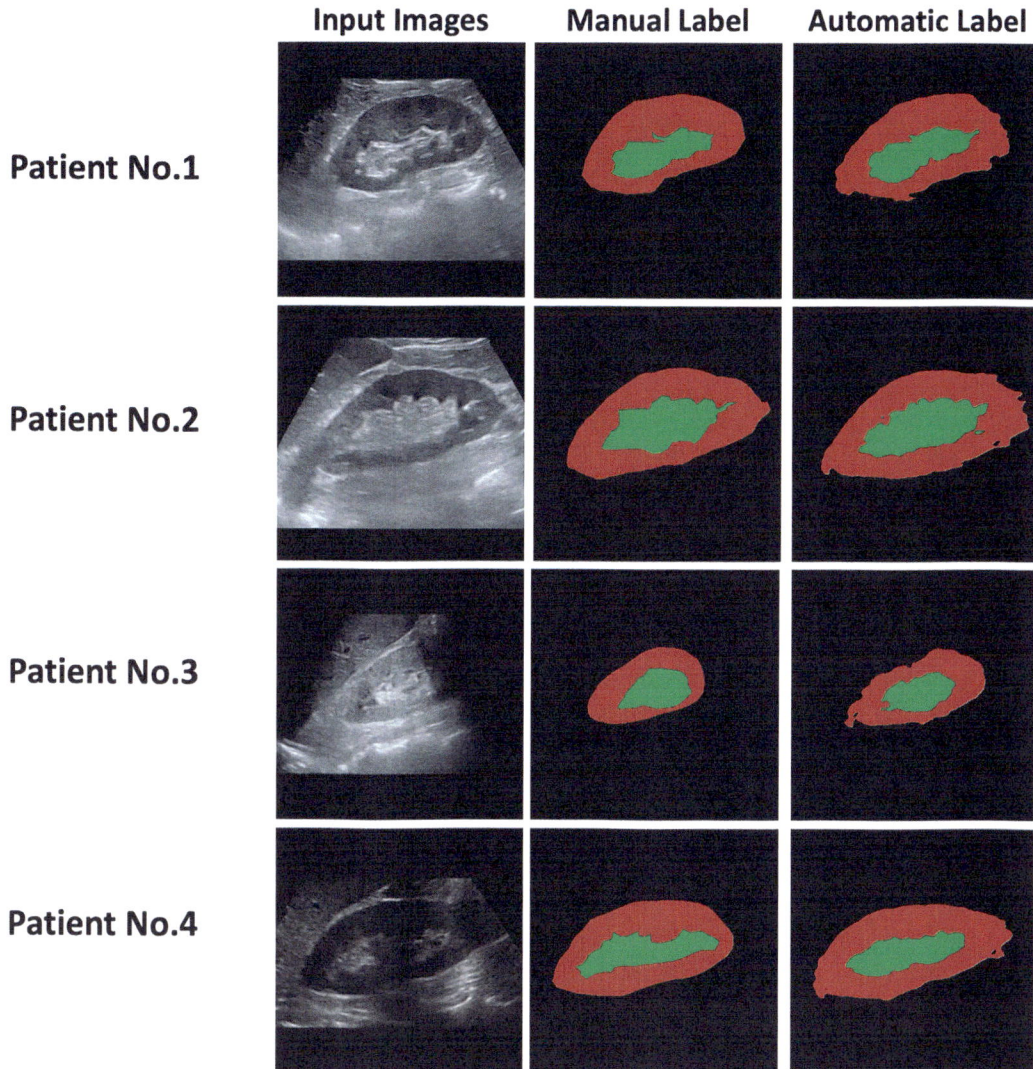

Fig. 9.7 Input images, manual and automated kidney parenchyma (red) and pelvis (green) segmentations from four patients [25]. (Shared with permission)

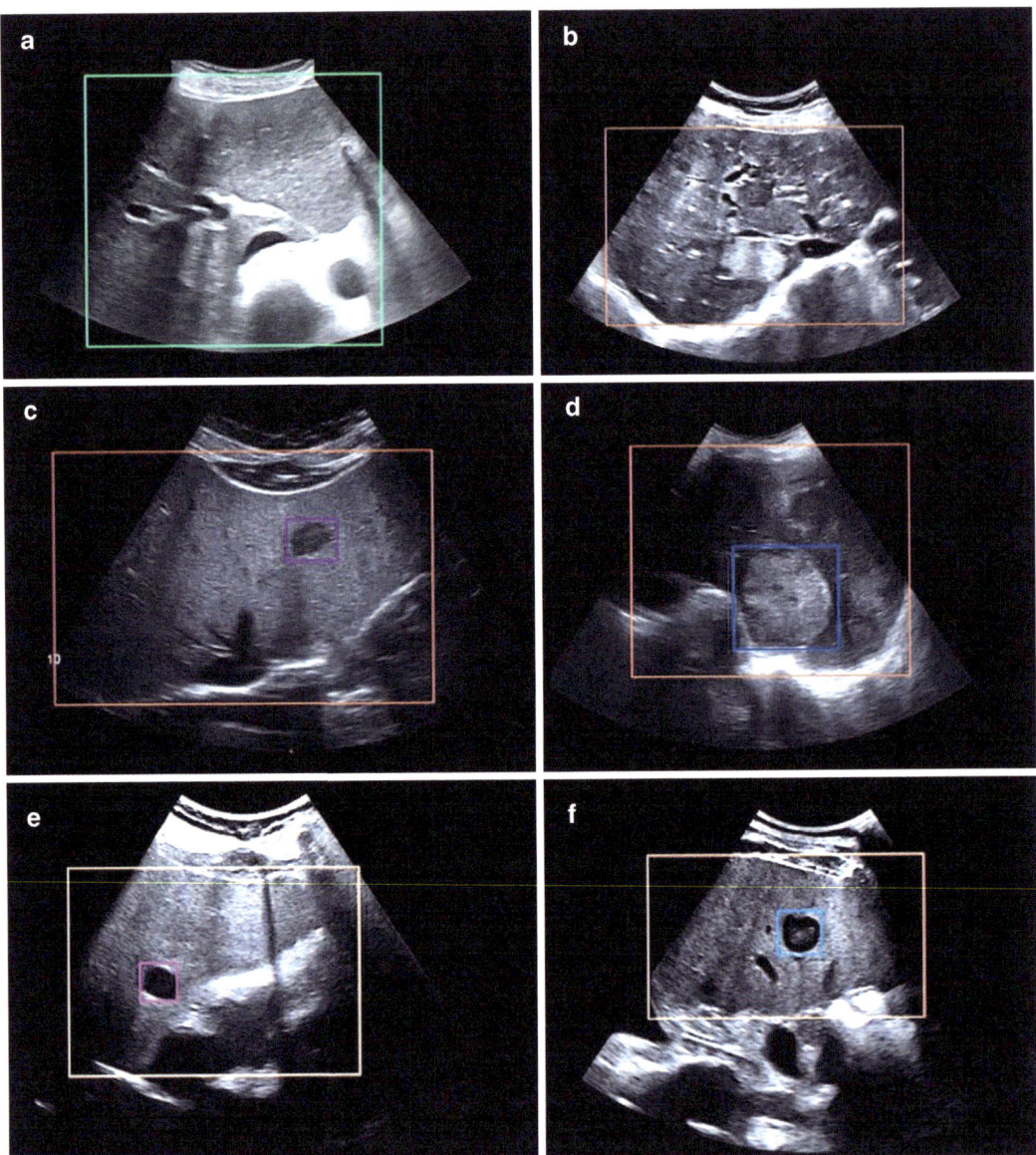

Fig. 9.8 (**a**) A liver without lesions (green box), (**b**) a liver with lesions (orange box), (**c**) a benign lesion (focal nodular hyperplasia [small purple box]), (**d**) a malignant lesion [hepatocellular carcinoma (small blue box)]. (**c**, **d**) In this pairing, the benign and malignant lesions have different textures and sizes. (**e**) A benign lesion [cyst (purple box)] with a circular shape and dark pixel intensities, (**f**) a malignant lesion [metastasis (blue box)] with similar characteristics [32]

Fig. 9.9 Comparison of a deep-learning algorithm (DL-video) and six radiologists (R1–6) in classifying malignant breast lesions from US video clips [35]

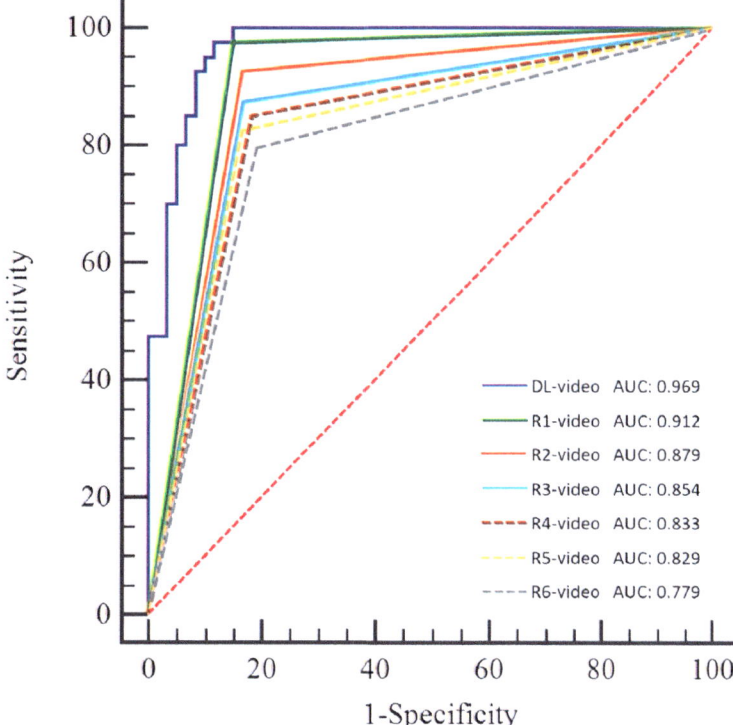

DL-video AUC: 0.969
R1-video AUC: 0.912
R2-video AUC: 0.879
R3-video AUC: 0.854
R4-video AUC: 0.833
R5-video AUC: 0.829
R6-video AUC: 0.779

9.5   Case Studies

9.5.1   Case Study 1: Cardiac Echocardiography

Case Study 9.5.1

Clinical challenge

A common application of ultrasound is for functional evaluation of the heart with TTE. The dynamic nature of ultrasound makes it particularly well suited to visualise and quantify the motion of valves and heart chambers. Besides an overall reader interpretation of pathologies and motion patterns, derived results are quantitative, e.g. vessel diameters, ejection fraction (EF) and global longitudinal strain (GLS). The heart is a small, well-defined, isolated organ, and anatomical acquisition planes are standardised, making segmentation manageable. Quantitative outcome mea-

sures has made it well suited for early studies on AI, and a substantial body of work has already been published in this area.

Incorrect transducer placement relative to the cardiac apex can induce geometric distortions ("foreshortening") and affect EF measurements [38], as the ventricular volumes are estimated from area measurements in two perpendicular planes.

AI-enabled solution

Sabo et al. [39] demonstrated small improvements in apical foreshortening errors caused by incorrect probe position using real-time cueing for expert sonographers (Fig. 9.10). Smistad et al. [40] combined foreshortening detection in multiple planes with fully automatic CNN-based left ventricle segmentation.

One study [41] demonstrated that nurses without prior TTE experience could achieve

(continued)

satisfactory quality for evaluating left and right ventricular sizes, left ventricular function and significant pericardial effusions in 92.5–98.8% of 240 cases. This was achieved using an AI-powered "quality meter" that provided cues to transducer placement and automatically captured systolic/diastolic images when the desired image quality was achieved, as demonstrated in Fig. 9.11.

Automatic derivation of ventricular volumetric measurements can be completely automated [42] using AI. These measurements have been shown to correlate well with measures obtained from expert TTE [43], invasive angiography and cardiac MRI, the latter being considered the reference standard [44]. This was achieved even when the acquisition was performed by clinicians with limited experience [45–47]. Similar results for right ventricular ejection fraction, compared to MRI, were obtained by Otani et al. [48], showing no difference compared to traditional semi-automated methods with user interaction. Heart failure can roughly be classified into types with reduced (HFrEF), mid-range (HFmrEF) and preserved EF (HFpEF) [49]. Obviously, while precise EF measurement, as mentioned above, is important in classifying HFrEF, algorithms have also been demonstrated to detect HFpEF from a single four-chamber TTE video clip [50]. This study was able to demonstrate sensitivity and specificity of 87.8% and 81.9%, respectively (compared to advanced clinical algorithms), while also predicting patients with increased mortality (hazard ratio 1.9) during follow-up (Fig. 9.12). Increased reproducibility is another important contribution of AI in settings where precise longitudinal measurements have precluded the routine use of echocardiography due to concerns over reproducibility, for example, monitoring for chemotherapy-induced cardiotoxicity. One study showed that the use of an artificial neural network (ANN)-based algorithm could reduce test-retest variability, as well as inter-reader variability of global longitudinal strain (GLS) significantly [51].

Benefits and challenges

The above-mentioned solutions has the potential to overcome the issues of reproducibility and observer variability in TTE. This may make the modality more acceptable in serial imaging of quantitative cardiac parameters. Similarly, guided acquisition can make measurements more precise, also when performed by less experienced operators, for example, during night shift. However, evaluating absolute measurement accuracy remains challenging as no in vivo reference standard exists. Measurements must be compared to other imaging modalities, each with their own strengths and weaknesses.

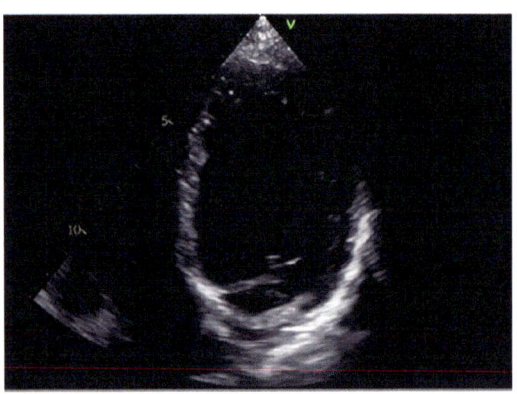 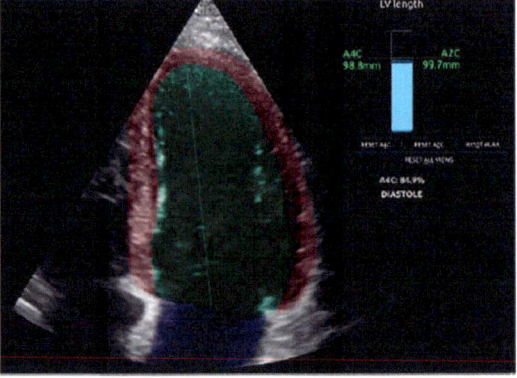

Fig. 9.10 Four-chamber echocardiographic view, with(right) and without(left) positioning guidance [39]

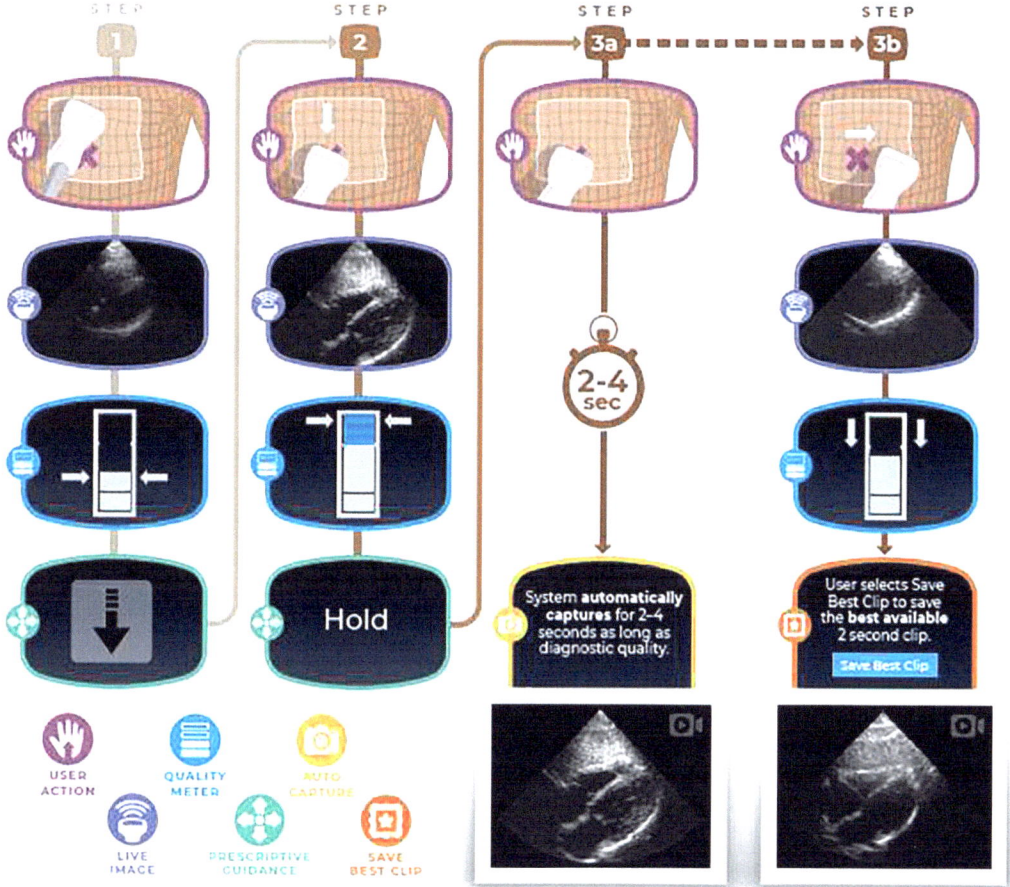

Fig. 9.11 Image describing the working of automatically guidance and recording of TTE, with possibility of manual correction. Adapted from [41] under CC-BY license

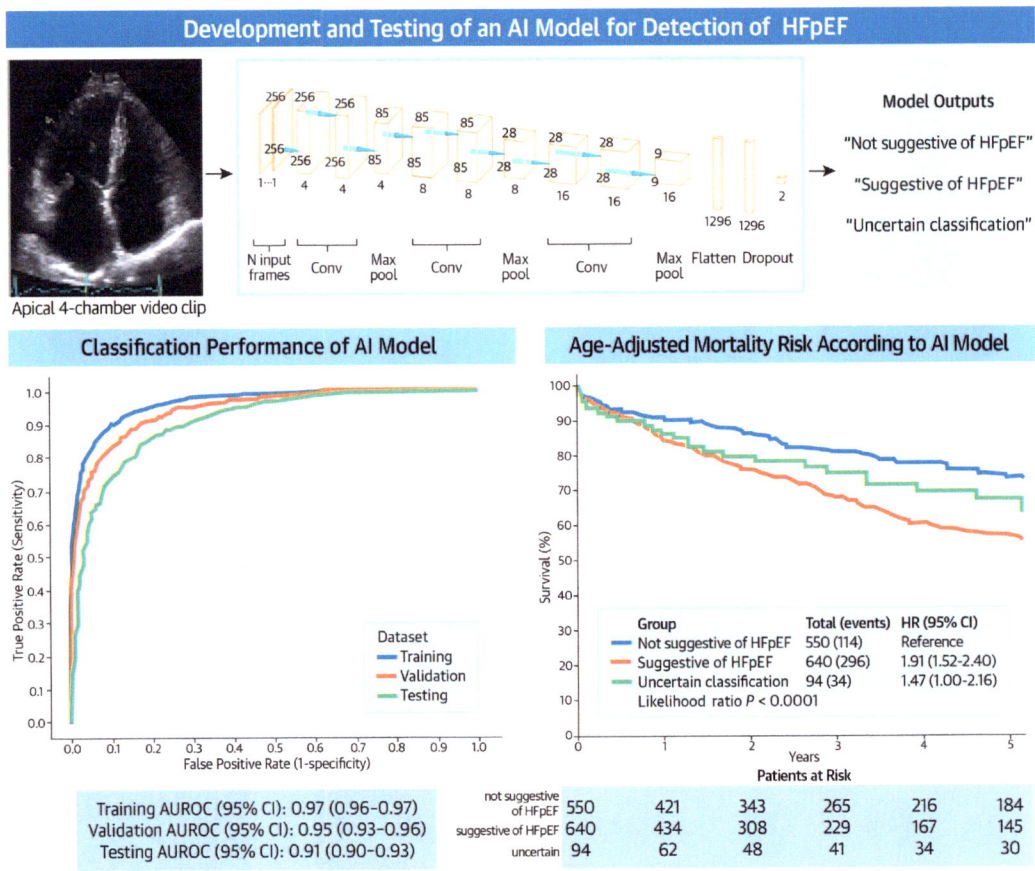

Fig. 9.12 Model and performance of a three-dimensional CNN model for prediction of heart failure with preserved ejection fraction (HFpEF) [50]. *AUROC* area under receiver-operating characteristic curve. (License CC-BY)

9.5.2 Case Study 2: Obstetric Ultrasound

Case Study 9.5.2

Clinical challenge: In pregnancy, ultrasound is a common examination in observing fetal growth and development and diagnosing diseases, facilitating measurements and assessments of fetal anatomy, structures, and organs. At the early stages of pregnancy, the examination is easily subject to involuntary fetal movements. At the same time, in the second and last trimester, structures become occluded, which may cause difficulties for the examination and increase the risk of misdiagnosis. Introducing AI to obstetric US improves diagnostic accuracy and automatic measurements of organs while reducing examination time, improving workflow and maintaining inter-observer agreement variations [52, 53].

AI-enabled solution: Convolutional neural networks (CNNs) is applied to improve ultrasound diagnostics in obstetrics. By employing 3D CNN algorithms, AI can automatically segment key anatomical features, such as the fetus, gestational sac, and placenta, to calculate fetal volume, a task previously challenging due to time constraints and potential operator dependence. This solution enhances diagnostic accuracy and consistency by providing standardised, automated measurements, which are par-

(continued)

ticularly beneficial for complex cases or when visibility is limited in later pregnancy stages. Additionally, AI-based models have been shown to surpass human performance in specific tasks, such as placenta segmentation, with faster execution and higher accuracy, thereby improving workflow and diagnostic reliability.

In another study conducted by Ryou et al. [56], they constructed software for automatic biometry measurements and detection of fetal limbs by segmenting the fetus on 3D-US, as shown in Fig. 9.14.

Another important US scan during the first trimester is the nuchal translucency (NT) thickness scan to detect chromosomal malformations, done by 2D-US. The measurement of the NT, denoting the maximal thickness between the fetal skin and the subcutaneous soft tissue at the cervical spine level, necessitates a standard median sagittal image and demands high accuracy and expertise. The measurement of NT thickness often necessitates multiple

attempts due to small fetal structures, frequent fetal movements, and poor image quality. In a study by Nie et al. [5], the thickness of the fetal NT was determined through a combination of standard median sagittal imaging and deep belief networks, which supplied prior knowledge for identifying the NT structure, where a 3D-US automatic recognition model was created by combining sagittal planes, which achieved a detection accuracy of 88.6%. Figure 9.15 illustrates the semi-automatic segmentation and calculation of the NT in a fetus.

Benefits and challenges: The benefits of AI in obstetric ultrasound include improved diagnostic accuracy, faster examination times, and reduced variability between observers, leading to more reliable assessments. However, challenges remain in ensuring sufficient data quality and diversity for training models and addressing potential resistance to adopting AI-based tools in clinical practice.

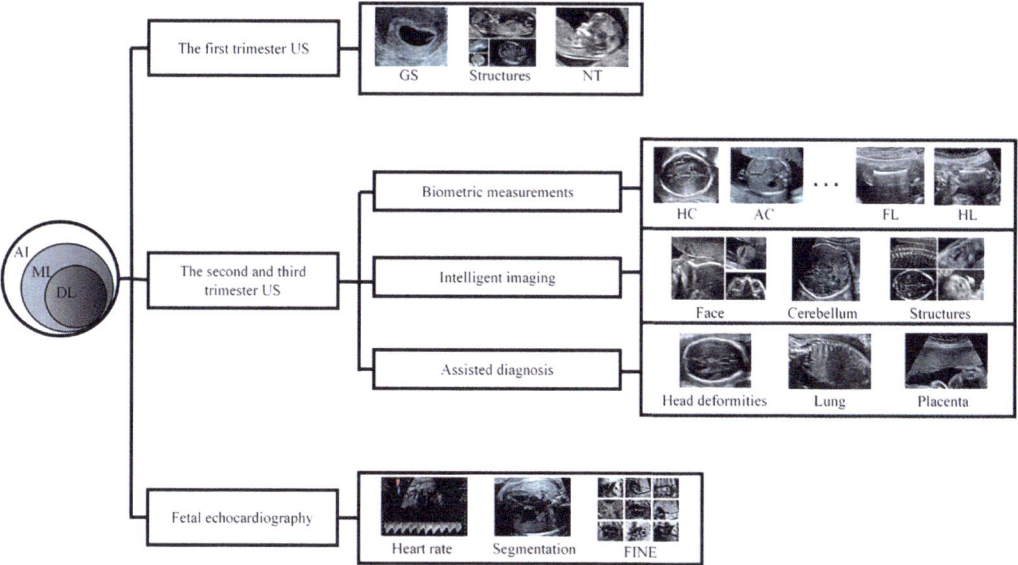

Fig. 9.13 Illustration of (**a**) prenatal ultrasound volume and (**b**) semantic segmentation of fetus, gestational sac and placenta, denoted with green, blue and red color, respectively [54]

Fig. 9.14 Example of fetal body part segmentation [56]. Left: original image. Right: Anatomical labels

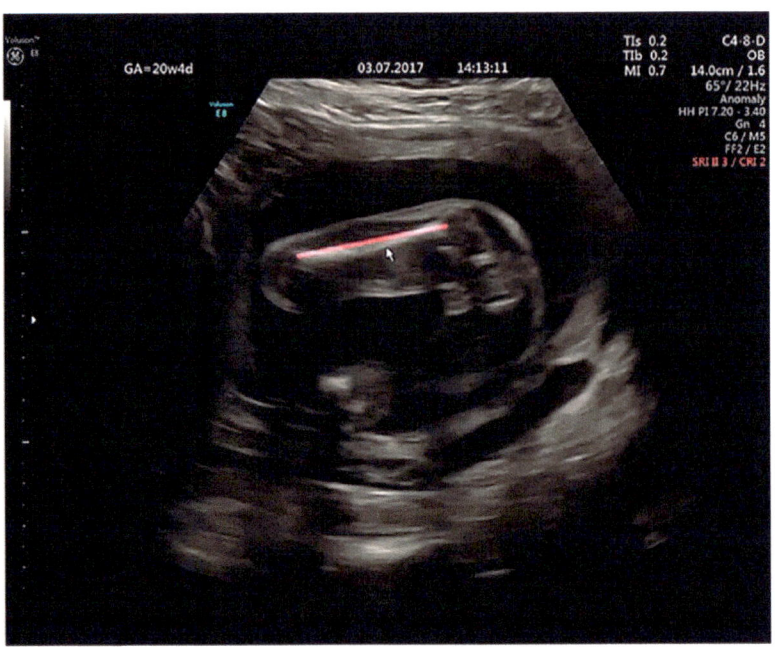

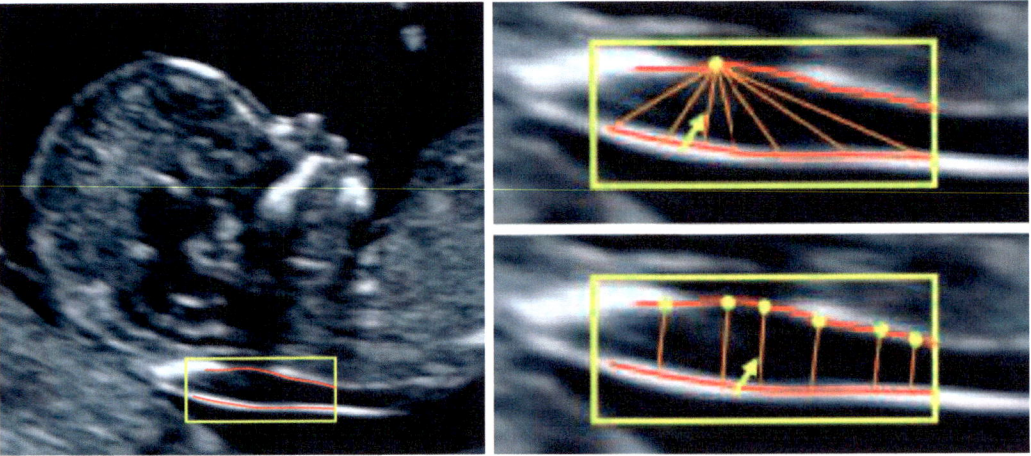

Fig. 9.15 (a) A semi-automated method involves placing an adjustable, yellow-outlined box on a mid-sagittal section of the fetal head and upper thorax to measure nuchal translucency (NT) thickness, where the system automatically draws lines through the nuchal membrane's centre and along the soft tissue edge over the cervical spine. (b) The system determines the NT measurement by calculating and selecting the largest vertical distance between two lines along the nuchal membrane [57]

In pregnancy, ultrasound is a common examination in observing fetal growth and development and diagnosing diseases, facilitating measurements and assessments of fetal anatomy, structures and organs. At the early stages of pregnancy, the examination is easily subject to involuntary fetal movements. At the same time, in the second and last trimester, structures become occluded, which may cause difficulties for the examination and increase the risk of misdiagnosis. Introducing AI to obstetric US improves diagnostic accuracy and automatic measurements of organs while reducing examination time, improving workflow and maintaining inter-observer agreement variations [52, 53].

During the first trimester, US is important in the assessment of fetal growth and development in avoiding pregnancy complications such as premature delivery and low birth weight. 2D-US for measuring the crown-rump length is the routine method of fetal growth assessment. Still, it has been subject to operator dependence and shown no significant difference in the crown-rump length between normal and abnormal fetuses in the first trimester. Volume measurements of the crown-rump length with 3D-US provide more information but are time-consuming, and volume measurements can be underestimated if the 3D examination is insufficient. As shown in Fig. 9.13, a study by Yang et al. [54] used a 3D CNN algorithm to automatically segment multiple anatomical features, including the fetus, gestational sac and placenta, to calculate the fetal volume. Andreasen et al. [55] demonstrated that placenta segmentation could be performed faster with a CNN-based model trained on 7500 labelled images from a Danish screening program and with better accuracy than resident physicians and midwives in all trimesters, with an average intersection over union (IOU) score of 0.78.

9.6 Chapter Summary

The evolution of US technology through the integration of AI underscores a pivotal shift towards more accurate, efficient, and accessible diagnostic imaging. These advancements, illustrated by various studies, highlight AI's role in enhancing image analysis, enabling precise lesion differentiation, and improving disease characterisation with accuracy surpassing traditional methods. Such innovations promise to elevate the standard of care in diagnosing and monitoring diseases like aortic stenosis, thyroid nodules, and liver lesions and aim to democratise healthcare by mitigating the shortage of experienced sonographers. However, for these technologies to be fully embraced in clinical practice, it is crucial that US operators trust AI systems' capabilities and understand that they ultimately retain control over the final diagnostic decisions. Trust must be built through transparent AI system designs with explanations of the system's predictions [58]. This collaborative approach between human expertise and AI precision paves the way for a future where US imaging is more reliable, accessible and patient-centric. More about AI-enabled patient centered care is discussed in Chap. 12.

References

1. Zander D, Hüske S, Hoffmann B, Cui X-W, Dong Y, Lim A, et al. Ultrasound image optimization ("Knobology"): B-mode. Ultrasound Int Open. 2020;06(01):E14–24.
2. Jeon SK, Lee JM. Inter-platform reproducibility of ultrasound-based fat fraction for evaluating hepatic steatosis in nonalcoholic fatty liver disease. Insights Imaging. 2024;15(1):46.
3. Brage K, Pank KTT, Hansen S, Sondergaard LK, McEntee MF, Pedersen MRV. Technical ultrasonic quality assurance in Danish radiology departments. WFUMB Ultrasound Open. 2023;1(1):100005.
4. Kim YH. Artificial intelligence in medical ultrasonography: driving on an unpaved road. Ultrasonography. 2021;40(3):313–7.
5. Nie S, Yu J, Chen P, Wang Y, Zhang JQ. Automatic detection of standard sagittal plane in the first trimester of pregnancy using 3-D ultrasound data. Ultrasound Med Biol. 2017;43(1):286–300.
6. Skelton E, Matthew J, Li Y, Khanal B, Cerrolaza Martinez JJ, Toussaint N, et al. Towards automated extraction of 2D standard fetal head planes from 3D ultrasound acquisitions: a clinical evaluation and quality assessment comparison. Radiography. 2021;27(2):519–26.
7. Chiu I-M, Lin C-HR, Yau F-FF, Cheng F-J, Pan H-Y, Lin X-H, et al. Use of a deep-learning algorithm to guide novices in performing focused assessment with sonography in trauma. JAMA Netw Open. 2023;6(3):e235102.
8. Nakayama Y, Sato M, Okamoto M, Kondo Y, Tamura M, Minagawa Y, et al. Deep learning-based classification of adequate sonographic images for self-diagnosing deep vein thrombosis. PLoS One. 2023;18(3):e0282747.
9. Nhat PTH, Van Hao N, Tho PV, Kerdegari H, Pisani L, Thu LNM, et al. Clinical benefit of AI-assisted lung ultrasound in a resource-limited intensive care unit. Crit Care. 2023;27(1):257.
10. Hidalgo EM, Wright L, Isaksson M, Lambert G, Marwick TH. Current applications of robot-assisted ultrasound examination. JACC Cardiovasc Imaging. 2023;16(2):239–47.
11. Jiang Z, Salcudean SE, Navab N. Robotic ultrasound imaging: state-of-the-art and future perspectives. Med Image Anal. 2023;89:102878.

12. Frederiksen BA, Schousboe M, Terslev L, Iversen N, Lindegaard H, Savarimuthu TR, et al. Ultrasound joint examination by an automated system versus by a rheumatologist: from a patient perspective. Adv Rheumatol. 2022;62(1):30.

13. D'Agostino M-A, Terslev L, Aegerter P, Backhaus M, Balint P, Bruyn GA, et al. Scoring ultrasound synovitis in rheumatoid arthritis: a EULAR-OMERACT ultrasound taskforce. Part 1: definition and development of a standardised, consensus-based scoring system. RMD Open. 2017;3(1):e000428.

14. Pourtaherian A, Ghazvinian Zanjani F, Zinger S, Mihajlovic N, Ng GC, Korsten HHM, et al. Robust and semantic needle detection in 3D ultrasound using orthogonal-plane convolutional neural networks. Int J Comput Assist Radiol Surg. 2018;13(9):1321–33.

15. Amiri Tehrani Zade A, Jalili Aziz M, Majedi H, Mirbagheri A, Ahmadian A. Spatiotemporal analysis of speckle dynamics to track invisible needle in ultrasound sequences using convolutional neural networks: a phantom study. Int J Comput Assist Radiol Surg. 2023;18(8):1373–82.

16. Palladino L, Maris B, Antonelli A, Fiorini P, editors. Autonomy in robotic prostate biopsy through AI-assisted fusion. 2021 20th International Conference on Advanced Robotics (ICAR); 2021-12-06: IEEE.

17. Li X, Wang Y, Zhao Y, Wei Y. Fast speckle noise suppression algorithm in breast ultrasound image using three-dimensional deep learning. Front Physiol. 2022;13:880966.

18. Vimala B, Srinivasan S, Mathivanan S, Muthukumaran V, Babu J, Herencsar N, et al. Image noise removal in ultrasound breast images based on hybrid deep learning technique. Sensors (Basel). 2023;23(3):1167.

19. Annangi P, Ravishankar H, Patil R, Tore B, Aase SA, Steen E, editors. AI assisted feedback system for transmit parameter optimization in Cardiac Ultrasound. 2020 IEEE International Ultrasonics Symposium (IUS); 2020-09-07: IEEE.

20. Cammarasana S, Nicolardi P, Patanè G. Super-resolution of 2D ultrasound images and videos. Med Biol Eng Comput. 2023;61(10):2511–26.

21. Christensen-Jeffries K, Couture O, Dayton PA, Eldar YC, Hynynen K, Kiessling F, et al. Super-resolution ultrasound imaging. Ultrasound Med Biol. 2020;46(4):865–91.

22. You Q, Lowerison M, Shin Y, Chen X, Sekaran N, Dong Z, et al. Contrast-free Super-resolution Power Doppler (CS-PD) based on deep neural networks. IEEE Trans Ultrason Ferroelectr Freq Control. 2023;70:1355–68.

23. Huang L, Zhou Z, Guo Y, Wang Y. A stability-enhanced CycleGAN for effective domain transformation of unpaired ultrasound images. Biomed Signal Process Control. 2022;77:103831.

24. Duron L, Savatovsky J, Fournier L, Lecler A. Can we use radiomics in ultrasound imaging? Impact of preprocessing on feature repeatability. Diagn Interv Imaging. 2021;102(11):659–67.

25. Chen J, Jin P, Song Y, Feng L, Lu J, Chen H, et al. Auto-segmentation ultrasound-based Radiomics technology to stratify patient with diabetic kidney disease: a multi-center retrospective study. Front Oncol. 2022;12:876967.

26. Jain PK, Sharma N, Saba L, Paraskevas KI, Kalra MK, Johri A, et al. Unseen artificial intelligence—deep learning paradigm for segmentation of low atherosclerotic plaque in carotid ultrasound: a multicenter cardiovascular study. Diagnostics. 2021;11(12):2257.

27. Jin J, Zhu H, Zhang J, Ai Y, Zhang J, Teng Y, et al. Multiple U-net-based automatic segmentations and Radiomics feature stability on ultrasound images for patients with ovarian cancer. Front Oncol. 2021;10:614201.

28. Peng T, Wu Y, Zhao J, Wang C, Wang J, Cai J. Ultrasound prostate segmentation using adaptive selection principal curve and smooth mathematical model. J Digit Imaging. 2023;36(3):947–63.

29. Su X, Lin S, Huang Y. Value of radiomics-based two-dimensional ultrasound for diagnosing early diabetic nephropathy. Sci Rep. 2023;13(1):20427.

30. Ahmadi N, Tsang MY, Gu AN, Tsang TSM, Abolmaesumi P. Transformer-based spatio-temporal analysis for classification of aortic stenosis severity from echocardiography cine series. IEEE Trans Med Imaging. 2024;43(1):366–76.

31. Weng J, Wildman-Tobriner B, Buda M, Yang J, Ho LM, Allen BC, et al. Deep learning for classification of thyroid nodules on ultrasound: validation on an independent dataset. Clin Imaging. 2023;99:60–6.

32. Dadoun H, Rousseau A-L, De Kerviler E, Correas J-M, Tissier A-M, Joujou F, et al. Deep learning for the detection, localization, and characterization of focal liver lesions on abdominal US images. Radiol Artif Intell. 2022;4(3):e210110.

33. Yu F, Miao S, Li C, Hang J, Deng J, Ye X, et al. Pretreatment ultrasound-based deep learning radiomics model for the early prediction of pathologic response to neoadjuvant chemotherapy in breast cancer. Eur Radiol. 2023;33(8):5634–44.

34. Gu J, Tong T, He C, Xu M, Yang X, Tian J, et al. Deep learning radiomics of ultrasonography can predict response to neoadjuvant chemotherapy in breast cancer at an early stage of treatment: a prospective study. Eur Radiol. 2022;32(3):2099–109.

35. Zhao G, Kong D, Xu X, Hu S, Li Z, Tian J. Deep learning-based classification of breast lesions using dynamic ultrasound video. Eur J Radiol. 2023;165:110885.

36. Li M-D, Cheng M-Q, Chen L-D, Hu H-T, Zhang J-C, Ruan S-M, et al. Reproducibility of radiomics features from ultrasound images: influence of image acquisition and processing. Eur Radiol. 2022;32(9):5843–51.

37. Soleymani Y, Jahanshahi AR, Pourfarshid A, Khezerloo D. Reproducibility assessment of radiomics features in various ultrasound scan settings and different scanner vendors. J Med Imaging Radiat Sci. 2022;53(4):664–71.

38. Ünlü S, Duchenne J, Mirea O, Pagourelias ED, Bézy S, Cvijic M, et al. Impact of apical fore-shortening on deformation measurements: a report from the EACVI-ASE Strain Standardization Task Force. Eur Heart J Cardiovasc Imaging. 2019;21(3):337–43.

39. Sabo S, Pettersen HN, Smistad E, Pasdeloup D, Stølen SB, Grenne BL, et al. Real-time guiding by deep learning during echocardiography to reduce left ventricular foreshortening and measurement variability. Eur Heart J Imaging Methods Pract. 2023;1(1):qyad012.

40. Smistad E, Ostvik A, Salte IM, Melichova D, Nguyen TM, Haugaa K, et al. Real-time automatic ejection fraction and foreshortening detection using deep learning. IEEE Trans Ultrason Ferroelectr Freq Control. 2020;67(12):2595–604.

41. Narang A, Bae R, Hong H, Thomas Y, Surette S, Cadieu C, et al. Utility of a deep-learning algorithm to guide novices to acquire echocardiograms for limited diagnostic use. JAMA Cardiol. 2021;6(6):624.

42. Li H, Wang Y, Qu M, Cao P, Feng C, Yang J. EchoEFNet: multi-task deep learning network for automatic calculation of left ventricular ejection fraction in 2D echocardiography. Comput Biol Med. 2023;156:106705.

43. Tromp J, Seekings PJ, Hung C-L, Iversen MB, Frost MJ, Ouwerkerk W, et al. Automated interpretation of systolic and diastolic function on the echocardiogram: a multicohort study. The Lancet Digital Health. 2022;4(1):e46–54.

44. Nicol P, Rank A, Lenz T, Schürmann F, Syryca F, Trenkwalder T, et al. Echocardiographic evaluation of left ventricular function using an automated analysis algorithm is feasible for beginners and experts: comparison with invasive and non-invasive methods. J Echocardiogr. 2023;21(2):65–73.

45. Yamaguchi N, Kosaka Y, Haga A, Sata M, Kusunose K. Artificial intelligence-assisted interpretation of systolic function by echocardiogram. Open Heart. 2023;10(2):e002287.

46. Asch FM, Mor-Avi V, Rubenson D, Goldstein S, Saric M, Mikati I, et al. Deep learning–based automated echocardiographic quantification of left ventricular ejection fraction: a point-of-care solution. Circ Cardiovasc Imaging. 2021;14(6):e012293.

47. Baum E, Tandel MD, Ren C, Weng Y, Pascucci M, Kugler J, et al. Acquisition of cardiac point-of-care ultrasound images with deep learning. CHEST Pulmonary. 2023;1(3):100023.

48. Otani K, Nabeshima Y, Kitano T, Takeuchi M. Accuracy of fully automated right ventricular quantification software with 3D echocardiography: direct comparison with cardiac magnetic resonance and semi-automated quantification software. Eur Heart J Cardiovasc Imaging. 2020;21(7):787–95.

49. Bozkurt B, Coats AJ, Tsutsui H, Abdelhamid M, Adamopoulos S, Albert N, et al. Universal definition and classification of heart failure. J Card Fail. 2021;27(4):387–413.

50. Akerman AP, Porumb M, Scott CG, Beqiri A, Chartsias A, Ryu AJ, et al. Automated echocardiographic detection of heart failure with preserved ejection fraction using artificial intelligence. JACC Adv. 2023;2(6):100452.

51. Salte I, Østvik A, Olaisen S, Karlsen S, Dahlslett T, Smistad E, et al. Deep learning for improved precision and reproducibility of left ventricular strain in echocardiography: a test-retest study. J Am Soc Echocardiogr. 2023;36(7):788–99.

52. Ambroise Grandjean G, Hossu G, Bertholdt C, Noble P, Morel O, Grange G. Artificial intelligence assistance for fetal head biometry: assessment of automated measurement software. Diagn Interv Imaging. 2018;99(11):709–16.

53. Matthew J, Skelton E, Day TG, Zimmer VA, Gomez A, Wheeler G, et al. Exploring a new paradigm for the fetal anomaly ultrasound scan: artificial intelligence in real time. Prenat Diagn. 2022;42(1):49–59.

54. Yang X, Yu L, Li S, Wen H, Luo D, Bian C, et al. Towards automated semantic segmentation in prenatal volumetric ultrasound. IEEE Trans Med Imaging. 2019;38(1):180–93.

55. Andreasen L, Feragen A, Christensen A, Thybo J, Svendsen M, Zepf K, et al. Multi-centre deep learning for placenta segmentation in obstetric ultrasound with multi-observer and cross-country generalization. Sci Rep. 2023;13(1):2221.

56. Ryou H, Yaqub M, Cavallaro A, Papageorghiou AT, Noble JA. Automated 3D ultrasound image analysis for first trimester assessment of fetal health. Phys Med Biol. 2019;64(18):185010.

57. Moratalla J, Pintoffl K, Minekawa R, Lachmann R, Wright D, Nicolaides KH. Semi-automated system for measurement of nuchal translucency thickness. Ultrasound Obstet Gynecol. 2010;36(4):412–6.

58. Akkus Z, Cai J, Boonrod A, Zeinoddini A, Weston AD, Philbrick KA, et al. A survey of deep-learning applications in ultrasound: artificial intelligence-powered ultrasound for improving clinical workflow. J Am Coll Radiol. 2019;16(9 Pt B):1318–28.

Dr Martin Weber Kusk Radiography diploma in 1998. Masters in Medical Imaging, University of Southern Denmark 2013. PhD in radiography from University College Dublin 2024. Employed as research radiographer at Esbjerg & Grindsted Hospitals, University Hospital of Southern Denmark and Associate Professor at University of Southern Denmark, Department of Regional Health Research. Primary areas of research in CT focusing on cardiac imaging, photon counting CT as well as clinical implementation and user/machine AI interaction. Besides considerable teaching experience he is also the author a Danish-language textbook on CT technology, used in radiography education.

Simon Lysdahlgaard is a Danish radiographer and researcher specialising in radiography and radiology. He is affiliated with the University of Southern Denmark and the Hospital of South West Jutland, where he contributes to the research department. Lysdahlgaard's research focuses on the integration of artificial intelligence in medical imaging, aiming to enhance diagnostic accuracy and workflow efficiency. Notably, he co-authored a study on the use of AI for the segmentation of infarcts in brain MRI scans of acute ischemic stroke patients, which was awarded an international prize. His work reflects a strong commitment to advancing radiographic practices through technological innovation.

Dr. Malene Roland Vils Pedersen Dr. Malene Roland Vils Pedersen holds a PhD in diagnostic ultrasound, an MSc in Public Health, and a BSc in Radiography. She is head of research at the Department of Radiology at Vejle Hospital – part of Lillebaelt Hospital and is Denmark's first radiographer in such a role. She has authored or co-authored more than 90 peer reviewed scientific papers within medical science and radiography. She serves as an adjunct associate professor at University College Cork, Ireland. She is affiliated with the University of Southern Denmark, where she contributes to research and teaching. To support her growing leadership responsibilities, she recently began a master's degree in public management. In addition, she is an experienced mentor and supervisor and have a great interest in supporting early-career researchers.

AI Applications in Nuclear Medicine and Hybrid Imaging

10

Lefteris Livieratos, Christoph Jan Trauernicht, and Mélanie Champendal

10.1 Introduction

This chapter provides an overview of AI in nuclear medicine and hybrid imaging applications. It refers to nuclear medicine with its widest definition, as the medical specialty that uses radioactive tracers (radiopharmaceuticals) to assess bodily functions and to diagnose and treat disease. Hybrid imaging refers to the combination of any imaging modality that uses radioactive tracers, along with any other imaging modality, often one that focuses on anatomy, for simultaneous or sequential imaging such as with computed tomography (CT) in positron emission tomography (PET)/CT, single photon emission computed tomography (SPECT)/CT, or magnetic resonance

imaging (MRI) in PET/MR. Such hybrid imaging modalities have been increasingly used to diagnose disease with improved accuracy of anatomical localisation compared to the typically poorer spatial resolution in functional diagnostic findings revealed by the radiotracer. The widespread use of hybrid imaging has significantly empowered the role of nuclear medicine imaging in recent years. The co-registration of the images from the two modalities offers a unique combination of functional and anatomical information with advantages, such as more accurate localisation of focal metabolic abnormality, and the potential to use the X-ray imaging data for attenuation correction of the nuclear medicine imaging data.

Recent developments in radiochemistry have led to radiopharmaceuticals where the same molecular target can be labelled with either a predominately gamma photon emitting isotope to drive diagnosis, or a predominately particle emitting isotope such as beta or alpha, to drive a therapeutic intervention aiming at a common biological target. This combined diagnostic and therapeutic approach is often referred to as theranostics, or specifically for radioisotope applications as radio-theranostics. Radio-theranostics are a driving force in modern nuclear medicine and examples include ^{68}Ga-DOTATATE and ^{177}Lu-DOTATATE as a diagnostic (PET/CT) and therapeutic (with post-therapy imaging with SPECT/CT) complimentary pair. These are, respectively, used for the diagnosis and treatment

on behalf of Association of Healthcare Technology Providers for Imaging, Radiotherapy and Care (AXREM)

L. Livieratos (✉)
Guy's & St Thomas' Hospitals, London, UK

King's College London, London, UK
e-mail: lefteris.livieratos@kcl.ac.uk; Lefteris.Livieratos@gstt.nhs.uk

C. J. Trauernicht
Tygerberg Hospital, Cape Town, South Africa

Stellenbosch University, Stellenbosch, South Africa
e-mail: cjt@sun.ac.za

M. Champendal
HES-SO University of Applied Sciences and Arts Western Switzerland, Lausanne, Switzerland
e-mail: melanie.champendal@hesav.ch

© The Author(s), under exclusive license to Springer Nature Switzerland AG 2026
C. Malamateniou et al. (eds.), *Artificial Intelligence for Radiographers*,
https://doi.org/10.1007/978-3-032-05080-9_10

of neuro-endocrine tumours (NET) [1, 2] and ^{68}Ga-PSMA and ^{177}Lu-PSMA as a diagnostic (PET/CT), and therapeutic (with post-therapy imaging with SPECT/CT) complementary pair, respectively, for the diagnosis and treatment of metastatic castration-resistant prostate cancer (mCRPC) [3].

Nuclear medicine and hybrid imaging techniques are affected by common challenges and limitations as in other medical imaging modalities, such as patient motion, variability of contrast-defining biological parameters, variability of equipment specifications and imaging protocols, data size, data handling, and reviewer subjectivity. The use of radiotracers often involves additional burdens related to minimising radiation dose, control of image noise (often as a result of limiting injected activity and/or shortening acquisition times), the biological variability of tracer uptake and tracer availability. As with all other healthcare applications and imaging modalities, various computer algorithm methodologies have been employed over the years in nuclear medicine to mitigate those limiting factors and optimise radiotracer imaging, diagnostic outcomes, resource allocation, and personalised patient care. These include statistical analysis, factor analysis, compartmental modelling, image classification techniques, all of which are based on pre-defined assumptions or models, and applied to numerous tasks in image segmentation, noise reduction, tracer kinetic analysis, and data corrections, as discussed further in this chapter.

The emergence of artificial intelligence (AI) in nuclear medicine has occurred over the last 50 years [4] and the integration of AI can be a disruptive addition to offer novel solutions in image acquisition, reconstruction, processing, segmentation, and analysis. AI supports specific tasks, rather than entire processes, and its use has increased rapidly over the past few years. Here we refer to AI as a collective term for machine learning techniques with a deep learning approach based on convolutional neural networks (CNNs) as the forefront of development in the field, as outlined in Chaps. 1 and 2. The introduction of AI approaches in nuclear medicine and hybrid imaging extends to a wide range of applications with potential impact to all stages of the diagnostic

process and the patient's journey [5, 6]. These may range from detector level for image acquisition to correction for physics-related processes, for example, photon attenuation and scatter, to image reconstruction, image processing, and analysis including denoising, segmentation, and hybrid image fusion. In addition, AI can be applied in the construction of models to derive diagnosis-specific metrics to aid the clinical decision-making and to pursue further optimisation of the diagnostic or therapeutic process, such as automated feature (lesion) detection or predictive internal radiation dosimetry for personalised therapy. Finally, AI is transforming nuclear medicine by optimising exam planning, reducing costs and resource usage, while also enhancing the patient experience and contributing to more sustainable waste and energy management [7, 8].

10.2 Data Acquisition and Image Formation

10.2.1 Data Acquisition

In data acquisition, the introduction of AI approaches at detector level includes the use of CNNs for sorting PET data into sinograms for large, pixelated crystal arrays to mitigate blurred coarse sampling and large parallax errors [9], thus potentially improving spatial resolution. In the context of PET, the position of a positron annihilation event can be determined more precisely along the line of response if the difference in the timing of the detection of the two photons is used, a methodology referred to as time-of-flight or TOF PET. AI tools can be used to predict the TOF differences from the detector signals themselves, resulting in a 23% increase in timing resolution in one study [10]. In PET imaging, thin-pixelated crystal designs have been proposed to provide higher spatial resolution images, but at the cost of sensitivity. One group proposed an approach to enhance PET image resolution and noise from scanners with large pixelated crystals [9], with potential of achieving comparable image resolution with the larger crystals. Whilst these approaches have been proposed by research-led teams, such advances have been rapidly explored by scanner manufacturers and may be seamlessly incorporated into future system designs and clinical scanning routine in the new generation of scanners. Another area of impact to routine scanning aims at ensuring reproducibility and standardisation of the image acquisition process, involves the introduction of deep learning AI algorithms to apply a specific protocol to both disease and patient characteristics and enable the scanner to define relevant protocol ranges; an example in hybrid imaging being the automated landmarking technology for setting up a patient scan [11]. AI enhances the optimisation of acquisition protocols by selecting the most appropriate settings for the patient, considering factors such as positioning, CT dose modulation, and contrast product injection [12, 13].

10.2.2 Spatial Alignment

Hybrid imaging relies on the co-registration of two datasets from different imaging modalities. Usually, a fixed set of spatial transformation parameters is defined during installation of a hybrid imaging system such as PET/CT or SPECT/CT scanner and periodically checked as part of a quality control program. Whilst such co-registration parameters are expected to show minimal variation with time, unless significant structural changes are introduced in the system, voluntary and involuntary patient motion can affect the spatial alignment between images of the two modalities [14–16]. Furthermore, images from separate imaging sessions may often be required to be co-registered to assist with feature localisation or assessment of progression. Machine learning models can be employed to address the image registration problem. This can be done by estimating the similarities between images, for example, through better intensity correspondences between the two imaging datasets, by comparing corresponding anatomy in the two datasets, by speeding up the optimisation of existing image registration algorithms, or by learning how to approximate the transformations directly [17].

10.2.3 Attenuation Correction (AC)

The CT dataset in hybrid imaging lends itself to attenuation correction of the photons emitted from the PET or SPECT radiotracer as they pass through tissues, because an X-ray image is an indication of how photons are attenuated through different parts of the body. Differences in attenuation properties between the energies of SPECT or PET imaging and the CT X-ray photons are typically addressed by (bi-linear) scaling of these values to match the appropriate energy. However, MR images cannot directly be used for attenuation correction purposes as these are formed by physical processes not related to the electron density in tissues, which would reflect the probability of photon interaction with the matter. Deep learning tools have successfully been used to transform MR images into pseudo-CT images that can be used for attenuation correction [18–20]. Deep learning trained with paired CT and PET/MR images was proposed for pseudo-CT synthesis for the generation of attenuation maps based on Dixon MRI [21] or multiparametric MRI consisting of Dixon and proton-density–weighted zero echo-time (ZTE) MRI [22] and applied to whole-body abdominal or pelvic PET/MR with only minimal bias compared with the CT-based approach, the current standard for attenuation correction.

In fact, current research is being done to investigate whether it is possible to create pseudo-CT images from PET or SPECT images alone. This can potentially be done by using the structural information from the non-attenuation corrected images themselves, which in turn could also lead to a radiation dose reduction. Additionally, if the CT component of a PET/CT is no longer required, it could be speculated that such a new generation of PET scanners could potentially be cheaper to acquire [18]. However, it is probably worth noting that the anatomical component in hybrid imaging, such as the CT in SPECT/CT and PET/CT, typically serves far more than the need for data corrections, such as attenuation and scatter correction, and the impact of anatomical localisation of the radiopharmaceutical uptake often is the dominant requirement for hybrid imaging. Therefore, a departure from the current hybrid imaging model is rather unlikely.

While the above focus on the generation of attenuation maps describes the distribution of the photon attenuation properties across the object, such attenuation maps are typically used as part of iterative image reconstruction in order to apply the actual attenuation correction. As we will see in a section below, the step of attenuation map generation can be incorporated in the image reconstruction step, with an AI approach, which can be expanded to include other corrections such as image registration. As an example of this approach, the use of CNNs trained with whole-body [18] F-FDG PET/CT data has been proposed to simultaneously reconstruct activity and attenuation maps as part of a maximum-likelihood image reconstruction scheme [23], see Fig. 10.1.

10.2.4 Scatter Correction

In the context of PET or SPECT imaging, the result of photon interactions with the tissues may contribute to either photon attenuation, that is, the removal of the photons from the line of site to the detector, or to erroneous entries of photons into the line of site of the detector in the case of photon scattering. Scatter correction methodologies include indirect measurements or modelling of a scatter distribution to estimate the amount of scatter in an image. Images can be obtained in one or several lower energy windows on the energy spectrum to measure the scatter compo-

nent, typically applicable to SPECT where detector energy resolution is appropriate for this approach. Monte Carlo models of the estimated scatter distribution are often used in both SPECT and PET imaging and tend to be computationally intensive and time-consuming.

Deep learning models can be used to obtain the total scattering distribution. Such models can be trained on Monte Carlo simulated data, which makes the training process initially quite time-consuming [19, 25]; however, they may offer processing time savings to the end-user. As with attenuation correction, scatter correction can lead not only to better quantification of the activity distribution but also to an overall higher accuracy as a result of an improved image reconstruction. This is because the inclusion of all the physical processes involved from the photon emission to its detection will result to a more accurate system matrix, which describes the activity-to-image relationship within the image reconstruction algorithm [26, 27].

10.2.5 Image Reconstruction

Traditional image reconstruction techniques include filtered back-projection (FBP) and iterative reconstruction algorithms. In FBP, the projection data acquired at each imaging angle are back-projected into an empty matrix to obtain images of the activity distribution which can be

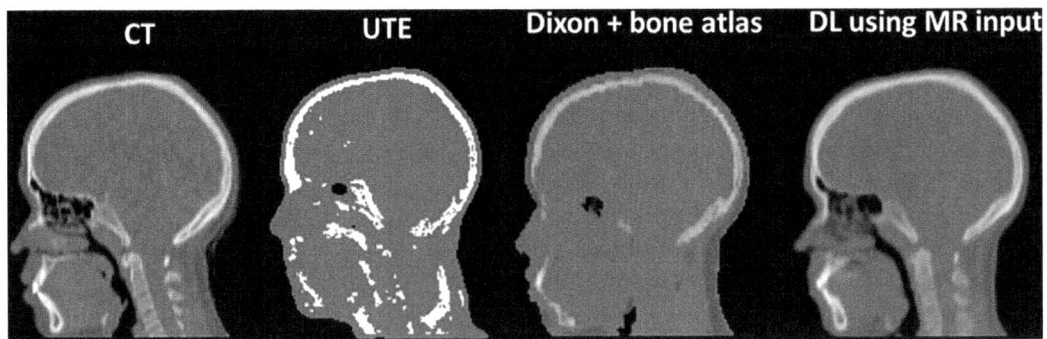

Fig. 10.1 Example of a patient scanned on both PET/CT and PET/MR. Shown from left to right are a sagittal view of the CT image, UTE image, Dixon image with atlas-based bone structure, and an image from a deep learning (DL) model [24] trained using 106 patients to predict a CT from T1 and T2 images. The current MR-based attenuation correction (MRAC) images provided from the scanner for comparison are the Dixon with a bone atlas and UTE. (Data courtesy Dr. Georgios Krokos, The Clinical PET Centre, King's College London)

viewed at transverse, coronal, or sagittal orientation. Inherently, any noise in the projection data is also back-projected, and thus amplified into the final image. To reduce this, a filter can be applied to each projection before the back-projection step. The filter can be modified based on the clinical task, for example, to obtain optimal images of the myocardium or the skeleton, with the applied filter optimised for the specific clinical application.

In iterative reconstruction, the acquired projections of an object or a patient are compared to projections of an estimate of the object or the patient. Corrections are applied to the estimate until the projections of the estimate closely match the acquired projections. Iterative reconstruction techniques are more computationally intensive than FBP, but also much more versatile, as various corrections for physical effects such as photon attenuation, scatter, or spatial resolution can be incorporated into the image reconstruction algorithm [26, 27].

Several AI approaches to image reconstruction for emission tomography have been described in literature [28, 29], see also Fig. 10.2. It is possible that a deep learning algorithm can

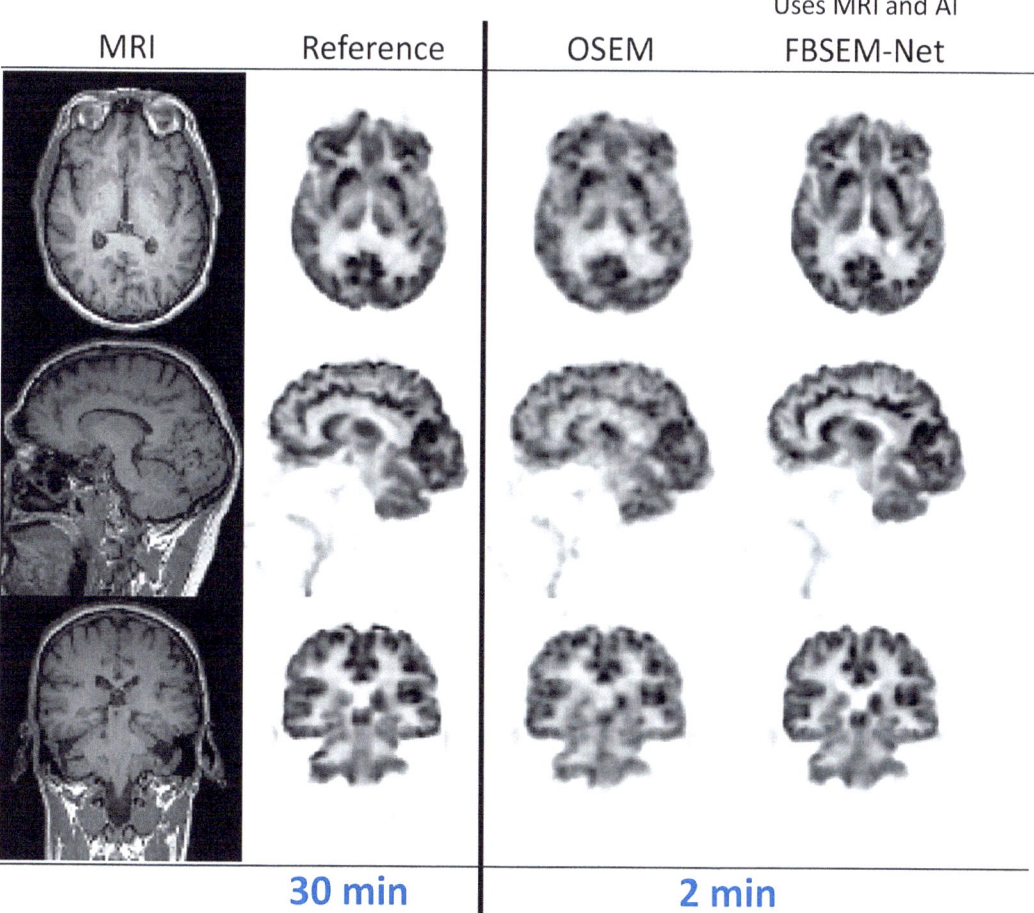

Fig. 10.2 Example of AI-based image reconstruction in PET from FBSEM-Net [28, 33, 34], which offers improved image quality at shorter acquisition times. The images demonstrate this in reconstructing data equivalent to just 2 min of scanning time, with image quality competitive to the reference reconstruction from 30 min of data. OSEM: ordered subsets expectation maximisation; FBSEM: forward backward splitting expectation maximisation

learn the iterative reconstruction process directly, without any intermediate steps describing in detail the system matrix. This can lead to vastly reduced processing times (potentially 100-fold) [18] and reduced image noise [30]. AI technology cannot solve the inverse problem, which is encountered in image reconstruction, but can provide a mapping relationship to solve problems in reconstruction. One such example is the transformation between the sinogram (projection data) domain and the image domain that can be achieved through AI technology [19]. While the training of a model that does this is very time-consuming, the direct AI reconstruction afterwards is very efficient for the end-user.

It should be noted that, independently of the exact approach used, the responsibility of performance assessment, quality assurance, and optimisation remains with the end-user. Consequently, AI approaches in data corrections and image reconstruction remain subject to the same rigorous quality control and optimisation as defined by the latest standards, regulations, or professional best practices, though approaches specific to AI performance may also be pursued [31, 32].

10.3   AI in Image Processing and Analysis

10.3.1 Radiation Dose Reduction and Signal-to-Noise Improvements

Reduction of noise, or improvements in signal to noise as part of the imaging optimisation process, can lead to improvements in image quality, which may be translated to reduction of radiation dose or image acquisition times. This has been an area of development for AI approaches, for example, to generate full-dose PET images from low-dose data [35] or to directly filter reconstructed PET images [36]. Similar AI approaches for noise control have been proposed in SPECT imaging [29]. It is possible to train a deep learning algorithm on how to create higher-count images from lower-count images. Intuitively, this can be explained using two matched datasets of the same object – one with lower counts (and thus lower image quality) and one with more counts (and thus less noise). Once the deep learning algorithm is trained on an adequate number of matched datasets, this information can then be used to create images of higher quality from images of lower quality [37]. In real terms, this means that one can either (a) reduce image acquisition time, particularly for patients who are unable to tolerate the full scanning process due to factors such as pain, claustrophobia, or specific populations like paediatric patients, individuals with dementia, and others who may struggle with the procedure or (b) reduce the injected activity, since it is possible to obtain good quality images from a lower quality acquisition. This has led to extreme dose reductions of up to 99% having been reported [38]. This approach is particularly valuable for paediatric patients, or when there are problems with radiotracer availability, as well as in terms of economic and environmental sustainability. See Case Study 10.1 and Fig. 10.3 for more information and insight.

Without Denoising   Denoised

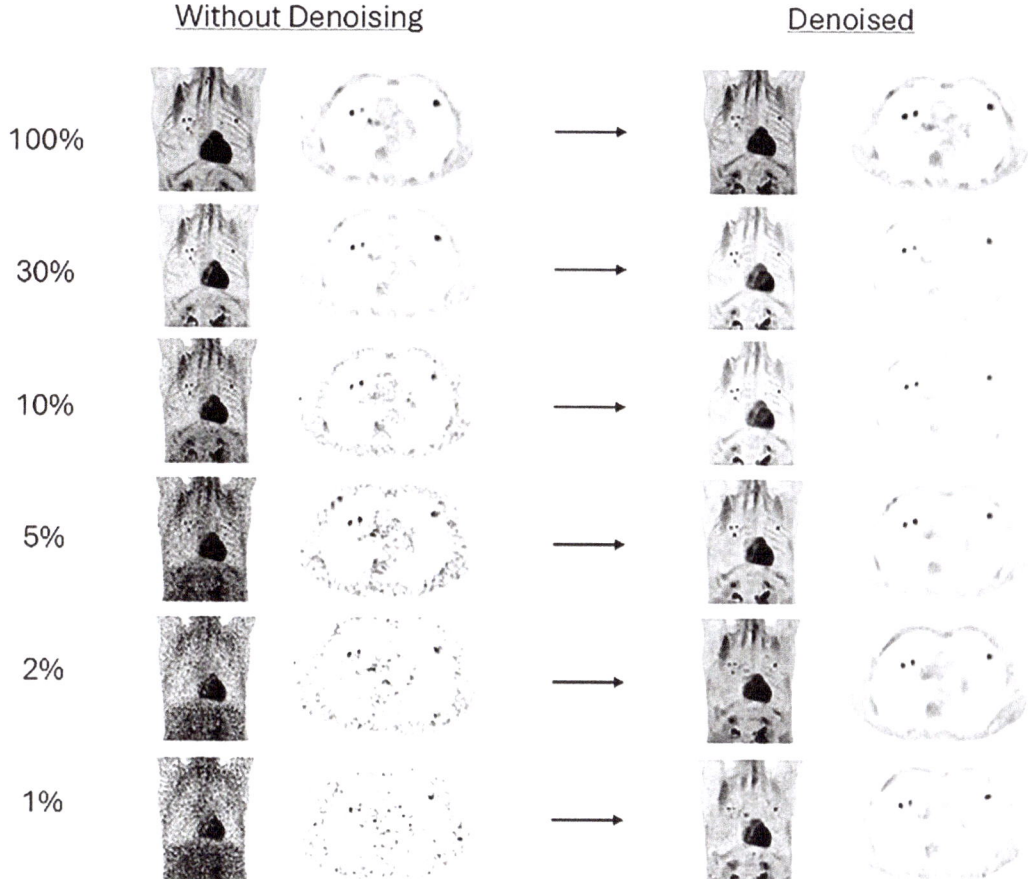

Fig. 10.3 Use of AI denoising in PET imaging. (Images courtesy Prof John Olivier Prior & Dr. Daphné Faist, Department of Nuclear Medicine and Molecular Imaging, Lausanne University Hospital and University of Lausanne, Lausanne, Switzerland)

10.3.2 Image Segmentation— Automated Lesion Detection

Case Study 10.1

Clinical challenge: Use of F-18 FDG PET/CT for lung cancer screening. In this context, a reduction in the injected activity is essential. This reduction will have a negative effect on the quality of the PET image, with a lower signal-to-noise ratio (SNR) [39].

AI-enabled solution: To address this issue, a 3D convolutional neural network (CNN) is employed to enhance the quality of FDG PET images through denoising [40]. A simulation of the reduction in injected activity from 100% to 1% was carried out (Fig. 10.3, left). The CNN was then used to reconstruct the degraded images (on the right side). The ground truth, framed in green, represents the PET acquired with 100% of the injected activity.

Benefits: In this scenario, the detectability of pulmonary nodules is maintained while simultaneously reducing the dose received by the patient. This approach can be applied to other clinical situations where a reduction in injected activity is necessary, such as in paediatric patients or during

(continued)

radiopharmaceutical shortages. Additionally, it is possible to shorten the acquisition time, which would also require the use of a denoising algorithm. This is particularly beneficial for patients with claustrophobia, those suffering from painful conditions, or children who have difficulty staying still.

Challenges: In the case of small nodules and very noisy images, AI -elated hallucinations may occur, as the nodule fades into the noise and is detected as such. As a result, it may disappear from the image reconstructed by the denoising AI. In the literature, cases of reverse hallucinations have been documented, with the apparition of false lesions in the reconstructed images that were not present in the original ground truth [41]. Additionally, denoised images tend to appear smoother compared to the ground truth.

One area where AI has shown to be extremely beneficial is in automated organ or lesion detection and segmentation. Fast and accurate lesion identification may be critical for an appropriate intervention [42, 43]. Image segmentation and automated definition of regions-of-interest (ROIs) to specify a volume or for organ delineation on a single or hybrid modality may have a significant impact in efficiency of applications such as the calculation of standardised uptake value (SUV), lesion evaluation, or radiation dosimetry derived from radionuclide imaging and therapy.

Numerous medical image segmentation tools have been developed for use on nuclear medicine and the functional, anatomical, or combined modalities of hybrid images [44–47] usually developed around the U-NET architecture [48], while V-Net, a volumetric network, uses 3D slices as input, unlike U-Net, which uses 2D slices. AI approaches previously proposed for image segmentation are often based on a CNN requiring a large amount of input data to be able to create an accurate segmentation model. U-NET-based algorithms aim to achieve accurate segmentation with smaller training datasets. This

is particularly applicable to medical images where there is often limited access to well-characterised image datasets, and memory, storage, and processing requirements may be demanding. U-NET architecture consists of a contracting path, as moving through the CNN layers, information is lost via down-sampling. A symmetric expanding path mirrors the encoding part of the algorithm but replaces convolutions with up-convolutions resulting to the output segmentation map. The addition of an up-sampling path gives information to the decoding part on where in the image a feature is extracted from by the use of skip connections [49] allowing for features present in the contracting path to be passed to the expanding path, which recovers the initially lost spatial information from down-sampling [48]. This architecture achieves a higher resolution output whilst maintaining an accurate and robust outcome. In hybrid imaging, the use of both modalities improves segmentation performance by using both anatomical (CT) and physiological (PET or SPECT) information [50].

Automated approaches to image segmentation can have a significant efficiency impact to organ and lesion delineation for applications related to the extraction of clinical image metrics and indices, such as SUV calculation [51], tumour characterisation, or the derivation of organ time activity curves as in internal radiation dosimetry applications in theranostics [52], which could considerably contribute towards personalised therapy [53]. See further information presented in Case Study 10.2 and Fig. 10.4. In radiation oncology, some of these AI approaches have already been commercialised and clinically approved for contouring of organs at risk in radiotherapy [54, 55]. See Chap. 11 for more information.

Further uses of AI-based automated segmentation and classification techniques include the clinical evaluation and automated identification of Parkinson's disease from I^{123}-Ioflupane (FP-CIT) or DaTSCAN SPECT imaging where machine learning approaches have been used to train models based on well-characterised data [56–58]. In such cases, authors have pointed out the use of training datasets that sufficiently reflect

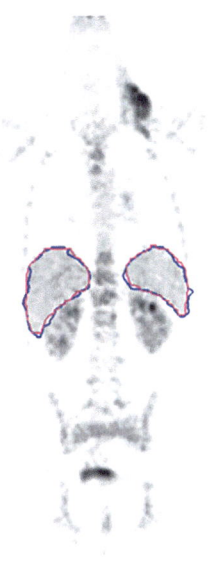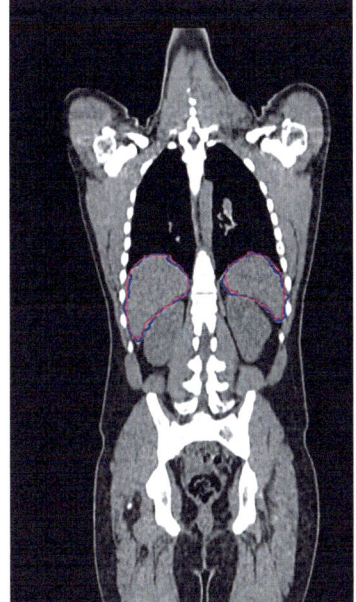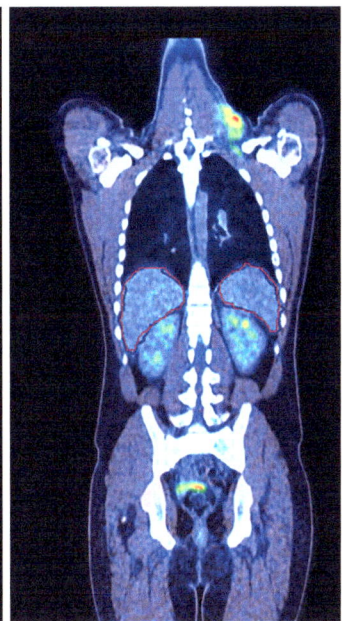

Fig. 10.4 Examples of manually defined liver and spleen regions on CT (blue line) and by AI model (red line) trained on 40 patients [51] to predict those regions. Regions shown on PET (left), CT (middle), and PET/CT (right) modalities. (Data courtesy Dr. Georgios Krokos, The Clinical PET Centre, King's College London)

the variability of scanning protocols, such as gamma cameras, collimators, and reconstruction parameters, to achieve robust and accurate outcomes.

Case Study 10.2: (Fig. 10.4) Use of Deep Learning-Based Image Segmentation in PET/CT

Clinical challenge: Organ segmentation is often required in order to report quantitative metrics, such as SUV (standardised uptake value) in PET and SPECT to express the level of radiopharmaceutical uptake normalised for the injected activity and patient body weight. In hybrid imaging, such as PET/CT and SPECT/CT, the availability of a spatially aligned anatomical modality allows the definition of organs with good anatomical accuracy; however, this manual process can be very time-consuming due to organs extending over many image slices and its accuracy may be subject to variability across different users.

AI-enabled solution: Use of deep learning-based image segmentation by an AI model (red line) trained on 40 patients [51] of manually segmented regions (blue line) to predict liver and spleen regions. Regions shown on PET (left), CT (middle), and PET/CT (right) modalities (Fig. 10.4).

Benefits: Organ segmentation can be achieved at significantly shorter times compared to manual organ delineation, for example, in seconds rather than several minutes (>20 min when organs extend to several image slices). The automated segmentation process is likely to avoid variability of the operation across multiple users [59].

Challenges: The accuracy of the results can vary depending on the complexity of the anatomy presented. Cases which might differ significantly from those used to train the

(continued)

model may lead to unexpected results. Cohorts of cases, for example, patient groups with differences in pathophysiology, compared to the training dataset, due to disease, ethnicity, etc., may lead to biased results such as those reported in other modalities [46]. These can be mitigated by carefully balanced training datasets and careful consideration of the required testing and quality assurance for the implementation of AI in the context of the application intended.

10.4 AI in Theranostics

Internal radiation dosimetry is a key aspect to personalised treatments in nuclear medicine theranostics. Individual dose estimates may contribute to reducing the risk of radiation-related toxicities. Whilst Monte Carlo simulations or other voxel-based dosimetry methods may be the gold standard for internal dosimetry [53] moving away from standard geometry pre-calculated dosimetric estimates of the MIRD (medical internal radiation dosimetry) model [60], these techniques are very time-consuming and often not clinically feasible. Furthermore, current clinical practice with molecular radiotherapy suggests that only limited imaging is performed as part of patient treatment planning. This imposes restric-

tions on the ability to provide dosimetric estimates, given the typically insufficient imaging time points. Therefore, there is a role for machine learning approaches that go beyond the automation of organ segmentation discussed in the previous section, in order to achieve accurate dosimetric estimates under current clinical limitations [52, 53]. Furthermore, a number of steps in the dosimetry estimation process can potentially be enhanced by AI methodologies. These include multi-modality image registration, multiple time-point image registration, segmentation of organs and tumours, curve fitting of time-activity curves, and conversion of time-integrated activity into absorbed dose. This will lead to comprehensive patient dose profiling [53, 61]. See Case Study 10.3 and Fig. 10.5 to explore this AI application further.

In applications of radio-theranostics outside dosimetry, there have been a number of AI approaches in focusing on diagnostic ability or prediction of therapy outcomes; for example, in thyroid cancer where there is a well-established use of radionuclides at diagnostic and therapeutic stages, data from fine-needle aspiration biopsy samples [62], or imaging [63] together with other approaches have been used in machine learning methodologies to improve diagnosis of thyroid cancer [64].

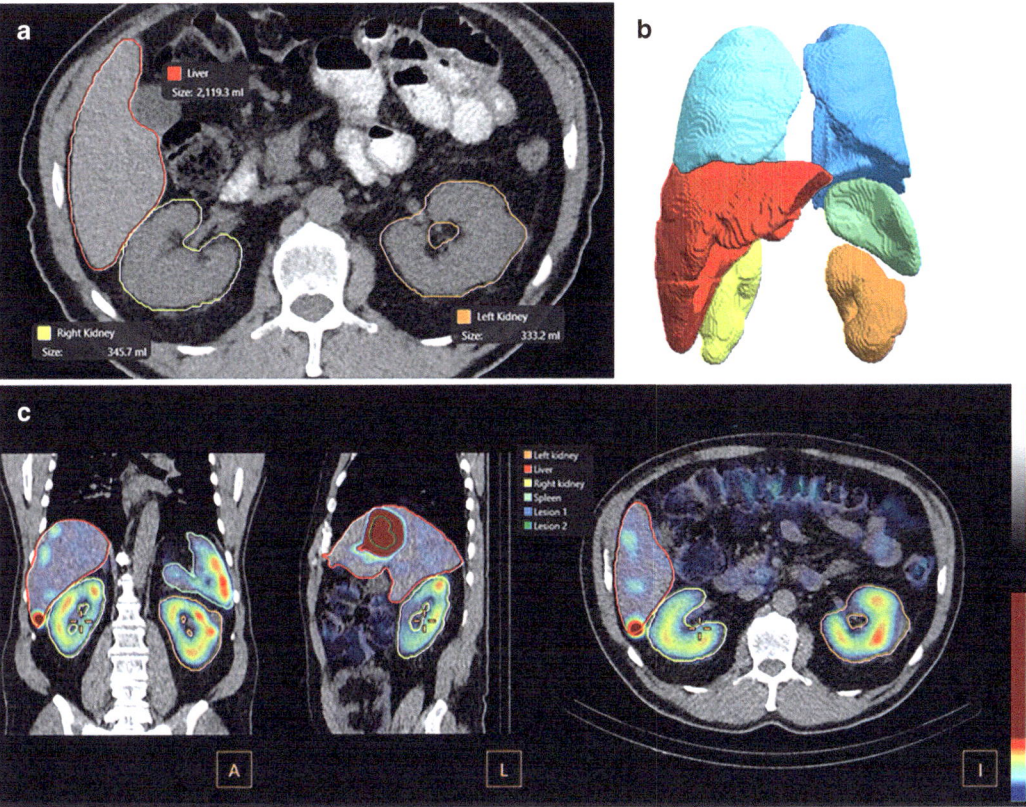

Fig. 10.5 Example of organ segmentation for dosimetry applications in molecular radiotherapy. (**a**) CT-based segmentation of liver, spleen, and left and right kidney shown on a transverse CT slice and (**b**) as 3D rendered volumes. (**c**) Segmentations applied onto a radiation dose map for ^{177}Lu-DOTATATE peptide receptor radiotherapy (PRRT) to derive personalised organ-level radiation dose metrics. Application implemented on the HERMIA (Hermes Medical Solutions, Sweden) software platform based on a CNN deep learning model, substantially expediting the image analysis process (<1 min on a regular current system) compared to the manual segmentation which remains significantly time-consuming due to its requirement to define several regions over a number of slices. Images courtesy Hermes Medical Solutions, Sweden

Case Study 10.3: (Fig. 10.5) Deep Learning-Based Organ Segmentation for Dosimetry in Molecular Radiotherapy

Clinical challenge: Organ segmentation is often required as part of internal radiation dosimetry to define absorbed radiation doses, for example, as part of molecular radiotherapy. Various organs should be defined in order to determine the radiopharmaceutical uptake throughout the course of the therapy, based on SPECT/CT or PET/CT imaging. Organs may have to be defined multiple times, for example, when a series of images is acquired at various time points. As discussed already, this manual process can be very time-consuming and subject to inter-operator variability.

AI-enabled solution: A CNN deep learning model trained on appropriate datasets can substantially expedite the volume of interest (VOI) definition part of the data analysis process for radiation dosimetry. As an example, Fig. 10.5 shows AI-based

(continued)

automated segmentation of organs (liver, spleen, kidneys) as part of the dosimetry workup for ^{177}Lu-DOTATATE peptide receptor radiotherapy (PRRT) to derive personalised organ-level radiation dose metrics. Organ VOIs can be applied to the images or directly to dose maps (Fig. 10.5).

Benefits: Organ segmentation in radiation dosimetry is a particularly time-consuming process, so, expediting this stage, from >1 h to <1 min with automated segmentation, may allow the implementation of personalised therapy within clinically relevant time frames and without excessive additional requirements in expert resources. Furthermore, automated organ segmentation may contribute to lower variability in the dosimetric calculations due to reduced intra-operator variability.

Challenges: As stated, the accuracy of results can vary depending on the complexity of the anatomy and the presence of 'outliers' from the datasets used for training the model. Careful consideration of the appropriate testing and on-going quality assurance of AI in the context of its clinical use is crucial for the successful implementation of the application.

10.5 AI in Other Nuclear Medicine Applications

10.5.1 Radiopharmaceutical Development

The prediction of drug-target interactions can inform the application of a radiotracer in nuclear medicine. Usually, the development of a new tracer is a time-consuming and expensive undertaking, but AI-based methods are being used to assist with this process [65–67]. This can be done, for example, by predicting the binding affinity of a new radiopharmaceutical for its target, or by predicting its pharmacokinetics [68].

10.5.2 Workflow Optimisation

One study showed the feasibility of predicting non-shows in an imaging department by training a model on 16 data elements from the electronic medical record system [69]. AI may help in patient scheduling and resource use [70], as well as device monitoring to detect errors [71]. It should be noted that the various AI solutions discussed above can significantly impact workflow optimisation. For instance, the use of denoising AI to reduce acquisition time, or AI solutions that automate time-consuming tasks, can streamline different stages of the process, thereby improving overall workflow efficiency.

10.5.3 Clinical Trials

AI can be used to observe clinical trial pipelines, including a wide variety of aspects, ranging from reasons for regulatory approval or refusal, safety issues, or strategic and financial aspects [72]. The potential of human error in data collection can be reduced. Data consistency affects the performance of machine learning algorithms, and therefore hospitals have to be very vigilant to ensure consistent data collection, curation and safe storage. Clear protocols are especially helpful in this regard. Machine learning has also been investigated for detecting centre-level irregularities in randomised controlled trials [73].

10.5.4 Education and Training

Aspects of the use of artificial neural network (ANN)-based tools were proposed early on in nuclear medicine and their role in training was envisaged as support systems in clinical decision-making. Examples include early applications in myocardial perfusion SPECT [74], where AI tools were proposed in clinical decision support as part of a semi-supervised training framework for reporting.

10.5.5 Sustainability

Artificial intelligence offers the potential to improve the sustainability of nuclear medicine in its various pillars. AI can promote social sustainability by reducing inequality and improving patient care. In human terms, it can increase efficiency and reduce practitioner burnout. Economic sustainability is addressed by optimising resources and reducing costs. In terms of ecological and environmental sustainability, AI can help to reduce waste and the use of energy in the production of radiotracers and the production of images [75]. However, the development of AI tools should consider actions to reduce the carbon footprint, energy consumption, and the use of computational resources [76].

10.6 Considerations for AI Implementation

As with other automated techniques, the introduction of machine learning methodologies may pose challenges. The clinical implementation of AI algorithms requires, similar to other new technologies introduced into clinical routine, appropriate testing and the knowledge of its limitations and shortcomings. As examples from AI applications in nuclear medicine and hybrid imaging emerge, some areas of potential concern have been reported in the literature. The potential introduction of artefacts has been reported in AI-based image reconstruction, which might cause false-positive and false-negative results [77]. AI-based denoising may 'remove' lesions [78], and AI-based lesion segmentation may wrongly identify healthy tissue as a lesion [79]. Such examples suggest that there may still be a need for further optimisation and refinement of the newly developed deep learning methodologies. Furthermore, AI algorithms trained on one dataset and performing well on similar data cohorts may perform worse on a new, unseen dataset, such as from a different scanner, population group, or one that experienced a change in patient demographics and imaging protocols [80–82].

Strategies should be developed for rigorous evaluation of AI algorithms in nuclear medicine and hybrid imaging. Key best practices were published by the Society of Nuclear Medicine and Molecular Imaging AI Task Force Evaluation team and are known as the RELAINCE guidelines (Recommendations for EvaLuation of AI for NuClear medicinE) [83]. The authors propose a framework to evaluate AI algorithms for promise, technical task-specific efficacy, clinical decision-making, and post-deployment efficacy. These include, amongst others, checking that the ground-truth quality is reasonable, that the training and testing datasets for the algorithm do not overlap, that appropriate clinically relevant tasks are chosen, that the collected clinical data represents the target population, and that data drift should be regularly monitored (see Chap. 4 for more information about post-market surveillance).

The generalisation of AI requires large amounts of data, which raises ethical questions around consent and data anonymisation. Regulatory pathways are also lagging behind the developments in the field [84]. Some of these aspects may particularly affect applications in nuclear medicine as an area often endemic to limited access to clinical trial data and a variability of scanners and protocols. For these reasons, standardisation of data and protocols and wider availability of open access data may be important for future developments, both in innovation and clinical implementation and testing of AI. More generic information on AI implementation considerations in medical imaging can also be found in Chap. 4.

It is also essential to consider the impact on healthcare professionals, particularly nuclear medicine technologists and radiographers. One study [85] showed that the implementation of an AI denoising algorithm for PET/CT faces barriers such as workflow challenges, professional resistance and lack of education. Facilitating factors include clear explanations and support, such as a 'local AI champion'. Thinking through procedures, workload, and resources, together with appropriate training and support to overcome these barriers, is crucial to success.

10.7 Chapter Summary

There is a wide range of AI in nuclear medicine to support both imaging-related tasks such as acquisition, analysis and therapeutic planning, and tasks relating to the optimisation of patient care processes. However, regulatory pathways are also lagging behind the developments in the field and standardisation of data and protocols and wider availability of open access data may be important for future developments, both in innovation and clinical implementation and testing of AI. Additionally, considering the needs and concerns of users during the implementation of these AI solutions is crucial to facilitate their adoption.

References

1. de Jong M, Breeman WA, Kwekkeboom DJ, Valkema R, Krenning EP. Tumor imaging and therapy using radiolabeled somatostatin analogues. Acc Chem Res. 2009;42(7):873–80.
2. Fani M, Nicolas GP, Wild D. Somatostatin receptor antagonists for imaging and therapy. J Nucl Med. 2017;58(Suppl 2):61s–6s.
3. Kratochwil C, Fendler WP, Eiber M, Hofman MS, Emmett L, Calais J, et al. Joint EANM/SNMMI procedure guideline for the use of (177)Lu-labeled PSMA-targeted radioligand-therapy ((177)Lu-PSMA-RLT). Eur J Nucl Med Mol Imaging. 2023;50(9):2830–45.
4. Currie G, Rohren E. Intelligent imaging in nuclear medicine: the principles of artificial intelligence, machine learning and deep learning. Semin Nucl Med. 2021;51(2):102–11.
5. Visvikis D, Cheze Le Rest C, Jaouen V, Hatt M. Artificial intelligence, machine (deep) learning and radio(geno)mics: definitions and nuclear medicine imaging applications. Eur J Nucl Med Mol Imaging. 2019;46(13):2630–7.
6. Nensa F, Demircioglu A, Rischpler C. Artificial intelligence in nuclear medicine. J Nucl Med. 2019;60(9):29S–37S.
7. Sarchosoglou A, Couto JG, Khine R, O'Donovan T, Pisoni V, Bajinskis A, England A, EFRS Executive Board. A European Federation of Radiographer Societies (EFRS) position statement on sustainability for the radiography profession. Radiography (Lond). 2024;30(Suppl 1):19–22.
8. Currie GM, Hawk KE, Rohren EM. The potential role of artificial intelligence in sustainability of nuclear medicine. Radiography (Lond). 2024;30(Suppl 1):119–24.
9. Hong X, Zan Y, Weng F, Tao W, Peng Q, Huang Q. Enhancing the image quality via transferred deep residual learning of coarse PET Sinograms. IEEE Trans Med Imaging. 2018;37(10):2322–32.
10. Berg E, Cherry SR. Using convolutional neural networks to estimate time-of-flight from PET detector waveforms. Phys Med Biol. 2018;63(2):02lt1.
11. Shah V. White Paper: Automatic landmarking and parsing of human anatomy (ALPHA) for innovative and smart MI applications: Siemens Healthineers; 2021. Available from: siemens-healthineers.com.
12. McCollough CH, Leng S. Use of artificial intelligence in computed tomography dose optimisation. Ann ICRP. 2020;49(1_suppl):113–25.
13. Haubold J, Hosch R, Umutlu L, Wetter A, Haubold P, Radbruch A, Forsting M, Nensa F, Koitka S. Contrast agent dose reduction in computed tomography with deep learning using a conditional generative adversarial network. Eur Radiol. 2021;31(8):6087–95.
14. Kyme AZ, Fulton RR. Motion estimation and correction in SPECT, PET and CT. Phys Med Biol. 2021;66(18):18TR02.
15. Livieratos L. Technical pitfalls and limitations of SPECT/CT. Semin Nucl Med. 2015;45(6):530–40.
16. Xie C, Gnanasegaran G, Mohan H, Livieratos L. Assessment of inter-modality spatial alignment accuracy in hybrid single photon emission computed tomography in patients with hand and wrist pain. World J Nucl Med. 2013;12(3):87–93.
17. Chen M, Tustison NJ, Jena R, Gee JC. Image registration: fundamentals and recent advances based on deep learning. In: Colliot O, editor. Machine learning for brain disorders. New York: Springer US; 2023. p. 435–58.
18. Zaharchuk G, Davidzon G. Artificial intelligence for optimization and interpretation of PET/CT and PET/MR images. Semin Nucl Med. 2021;51(2):134–42.
19. Cheng Z, Wen J, Huang G, Yan J. Applications of artificial intelligence in nuclear medicine image generation. Quant Imaging Med Surg. 2021;11(6):2792–822.
20. Papachristou K, Panagiotidis E, Makridou A, Kalathas T, Masganis V, Paschali A, et al. Artificial intelligence in nuclear medicine physics and imaging. Hell J Nucl Med. 2023;26(1):57–65.
21. Torrado-Carvajal A, Vera-Olmos J, Izquierdo-Garcia D, Catalano OA, Morales MA, Margolin J, et al. Dixon-VIBE deep learning (DIVIDE) pseudo-CT synthesis for pelvis PET/MR attenuation correction. J Nucl Med. 2019;60(3):429–35.
22. Leynes AP, Yang J, Wiesinger F, Kaushik SS, Shanbhag DD, Seo Y, et al. Zero-echo-time and Dixon deep pseudo-CT (ZeDD CT): direct generation of pseudo-CT images for pelvic PET/MRI attenuation correction using deep convolutional neural networks with multiparametric MRI. J Nucl Med. 2018;59(5):852–8.
23. Hwang D, Kang SK, Kim KY, Seo S, Paeng JC, Lee DS, et al. Generation of PET attenuation map for whole-body time-of-flight (18)F-FDG PET/MRI

using a deep neural network trained with simultaneously reconstructed activity and attenuation maps. J Nucl Med. 2019;60(8):1183–9.

24. Krokos G, MacKewn J, Dunn J, Marsden P. A review of PET attenuation correction methods for PET-MR. EJNMMI Phys. 2023;10(1):52.

25. Qian H, Rui X, Ahn S. Deep learning models for PET scatter estimations. In: 2017 IEEE nuclear science symposium and medical imaging conference (NSS/MIC). IEEE; 2017.

26. Shcherbinin S, Celler A, Belhocine T, Vanderwerf R, Driedger A. Accuracy of quantitative reconstructions in SPECT/CT imaging. Phys Med Biol. 2008;53(17):4595–604.

27. Bailey DL, Willowson KP. Quantitative SPECT/CT: SPECT joins PET as a quantitative imaging modality. Eur J Nucl Med Mol Imaging. 2014;41(Suppl 1):S17–25.

28. Reader AJ, Pan B. AI for PET image reconstruction. Br J Radiol. 2023;96(1150):20230292.

29. Shao W, Rowe SP, Du Y. SPECTnet: a deep learning neural network for SPECT image reconstruction. Ann Transl Med. 2021;9(9):819.

30. Kim K, Wu D, Gong K, Dutta J, Kim JH, Son YD, et al. Penalized PET reconstruction using deep learning Prior and local linear fitting. IEEE Trans Med Imaging. 2018;37(6):1478–87.

31. Kortesniemi M, Tsapaki V, Trianni A, Russo P, Maas A, Källman HE, et al. The European Federation of Organisations for Medical Physics (EFOMP) White Paper: Big data and deep learning in medical imaging and in relation to medical physics profession. Phys Med. 2018;56:90–3.

32. Bosmans H, Zanca F, Gelaude F. Procurement, commissioning and QA of AI based solutions: an MPE'S perspective on introducing AI in clinical practice. Phys Med. 2021;83:257–63.

33. Mehranian A, Reader AJ. Model-based deep learning PET image reconstruction using forward–backward splitting expectation–maximization. IEEE Trans Radiat Plasma Med Sci. 2020;5(1):54–64.

34. Reader AJ, Schramm G. Artificial intelligence for PET image reconstruction. J Nucl Med. 2021;62(10):1330–3.

35. Kaplan S, Zhu YM. Full-dose PET image estimation from low-dose PET image using deep learning: a pilot study. J Digit Imaging. 2019;32(5):773–8.

36. Gong K, Guan J, Liu CC, Qi J. PET image Denoising using a deep neural network through fine tuning. IEEE Trans Radiat Plasma Med Sci. 2019;3(2):153–61.

37. Shiyam Sundar LK, Muzik O, Buvat I, Bidaut L, Beyer T. Potentials and caveats of AI in hybrid imaging. Methods. 2021;188:4–19.

38. Xu J, Gong E, Ouyang J, Pauly J, Zaharchuk G. Ultra-low-dose 18F-FDG brain PET/MR denoising using deep learning and multi-contrast information. In: Medical imaging 2020: image processing. SPIE; 2020.

39. Xu J, Gong E, Pauly J, Zaharchuk G. 200x low-dose PET reconstruction using deep learning. 2017. ArXiv. http://arxiv.org/abs/1712.04119.

40. Schaefferkoetter J, Yan J, Ortega C, Sertic A, Lechtman E, Eshet Y, Metser U, Veit-Haibach P. Convolutional neural networks for improving image quality with noisy PET data. EJNMMI Res. 2020;10(1):105.

41. Weyts K, Lasnon C, Ciappuccini R, Lequesne J, Corroyer-Dulmont A, Quak E, et al. Artificial intelligence-based PET denoising could allow a two-fold reduction in [18F]FDG PET acquisition time in digital PET/CT. Eur J Nucl Med Mol Imaging. 2022;49:3750–60.

42. Gheisari F. Nuclear medicine's integral role in the dynamic landscape of infectious diseases. Mathews J Cardiol. 2024;8(1):1–12.

43. Jalili A, Ghaderzadeh M, Gheisari M. AI in nuclear medical applications: challenges and opportunities. Front Biomed Technol. 2024;11(2):158–61.

44. Kawauchi K, Furuya S, Hirata K, Katoh C, Manabe O, Kobayashi K, et al. A convolutional neural network-based system to classify patients using FDG PET/CT examinations. BMC Cancer. 2020;20(1):227.

45. Shiyam Sundar LK, Yu J, Muzik O, Kulterer OC, Fueger B, Kifjak D, et al. Fully automated, semantic segmentation of whole-body (18)F-FDG PET/CT images based on data-centric artificial intelligence. J Nucl Med. 2022;63(12):1941–8.

46. Lee SB, Cho YJ, Yoon SH, Lee YY, Kim SH, Lee S, et al. Automated segmentation of whole-body CT images for body composition analysis in pediatric patients using a deep neural network. Eur Radiol. 2022;32(12):8463–72.

47. Kondo S, Kasai S. Automated lesion segmentation in whole-body FDG-PET/CT with multi-modality deep neural networks. arXiv preprint arXiv:230212774. 2023.

48. Ronneberger O, Fischer P, Brox T. U-net: convolutional networks for biomedical image segmentation. In: Medical image computing and computer-assisted intervention–MICCAI 2015: 18th international conference, Munich, Germany, October 5–9, 2015, proceedings, part III 18. Springer; 2015.

49. Drozdzal M, Vorontsov E, Chartrand G, Kadoury S, Pal C. The importance of skip connections in biomedical image segmentation. In: International workshop on deep learning in medical image analysis, international workshop on large-scale annotation of biomedical data and expert label synthesis. Springer; 2016.

50. Li L, Zhao X, Lu W, Tan S. Deep learning for variational multimodality tumor segmentation in PET/CT. Neurocomputing (Amst). 2020;392:277–95.

51. Krokos G, Kotwal T, Malaih A, Barrington S, Jackson P, Hicks RJ, et al. Evaluation of manual and automated approaches for segmentation and extraction of quantitative indices from [(18)F]FDG PET-CT images. Biomed Phys Eng Express. 2024;10(2):025007.

52. Belge Bilgin G, Bilgin C, Burkett BJ, Orme JJ, Childs DS, Thorpe MP, et al. Theranostics and artificial intelligence: new frontiers in personalized medicine. Theranostics. 2024;14(6):2367–78.

53. Brosch-Lenz J, Yousefirizi F, Zukotynski K, Beauregard J-M, Gaudet V, Saboury B, et al. Role of artificial intelligence in theranostics: toward routine personalized radiopharmaceutical therapies. PET Clin. 2021;16(4):627–41.

54. Court LE, Kisling K, McCarroll R, Zhang L, Yang J, Simonds H, et al. Radiation planning assistant—a streamlined, fully automated radiotherapy treatment planning system. J Vis Exp. 2018;134:57411.

55. Court LE, Aggarwal A, Jhingran A, Naidoo K, Netherton T, Olanrewaju A, et al. Artificial intelligence-based radiotherapy contouring and planning to improve global access to cancer care. JCO Glob Oncol. 2024;10:e2300376.

56. Taylor JC, Fenner JW. Comparison of machine learning and semi-quantification algorithms for (I123) FP-CIT classification: the beginning of the end for semi-quantification? EJNMMI Phys. 2017;4(1):29.

57. Kim DH, Wit H, Thurston M. Artificial intelligence in the diagnosis of Parkinson's disease from ioflupane-123 single-photon emission computed tomography dopamine transporter scans using transfer learning. Nucl Med Commun. 2018;39(10):887–93.

58. Loh HW, Hong W, Ooi CP, Chakraborty S, Barua PD, Deo RC, et al. Application of deep learning models for automated identification of Parkinson's disease: a review (2011–2021). Sensors (Basel). 2021;21(21):7034.

59. Lee T, Puyol-Antón E, Ruijsink B, Shi M, King AP. A systematic study of race and sex bias in CNN-based cardiac MR segmentation. In: Camara O, et al., editors. Statistical atlases and computational models of the heart. Regular and CMRxMotion challenge papers. STACOM 2022, Lecture notes in computer science, vol. 13593. Cham: Springer; 2022. https://doi.org/10.1007/978-3-031-23443-9_22.

60. Howell RW, Wessels BW, Loevinger R, Committee M. The MIRD perspective 1999. J Nucl Med. 1999;40(1):3S–10S.

61. Saboury B, Bradshaw T, Boellaard R, Buvat I, Dutta J, Hatt M, et al. Artificial intelligence in nuclear medicine: opportunities, challenges, and responsibilities toward a trustworthy ecosystem. J Nucl Med. 2023;64(2):188–96.

62. Dov D, Kovalsky SZ, Assaad S, Cohen J, Range DE, Pendse AA, et al. Weakly supervised instance learning for thyroid malignancy prediction from whole slide cytopathology images. Med Image Anal. 2021;67:101814.

63. Zhang X, Lee VCS, Rong J, Liu F, Kong H. Multichannel convolutional neural network architectures for thyroid cancer detection. PLoS One. 2022;17(1):e0262128.

64. Lee KS, Park H. Machine learning on thyroid disease: a review. Front Biosci (Landmark Ed). 2022;27(3):101.

65. Wen M, Zhang Z, Niu S, Sha H, Yang R, Yun Y, et al. Deep-learning-based drug-target interaction prediction. J Proteome Res. 2017;16(4):1401–9.

66. Chen R, Liu X, Jin S, Lin J, Liu J. Machine learning for drug-target interaction prediction. Molecules. 2018;23(9):2208.

67. Webb EW, Scott PJH. Potential applications of artificial intelligence and machine learning in radiochemistry and radiochemical engineering. PET Clin. 2021;16(4):525–32.

68. Ataeinia B, Heidari P. Artificial intelligence and the future of diagnostic and therapeutic radiopharmaceutical development:: in silico smart molecular design. PET Clin. 2021;16(4):513–23.

69. Harvey HB, Liu C, Ai J, Jaworsky C, Guerrier CE, Flores E, et al. Predicting no-shows in radiology using regression modeling of data available in the electronic medical record. J Am Coll Radiol. 2017;14(10):1303–9.

70. Beegle C, Hasani N, Maass-Moreno R, Saboury B, Siegel E. Artificial intelligence and positron emission tomography imaging workflow:: Technologists' perspective. PET Clin. 2022;17(1):31–9.

71. Ullah MN, Levin CS. Application of artificial intelligence in PET instrumentation. PET Clin. 2022;17(1):175–82.

72. Delso G, Cirillo D, Kaggie JD, Valencia A, Metser U, Veit-Haibach P. How to design AI-driven clinical trials in nuclear medicine. Semin Nucl Med. 2021;51(2):112–9.

73. Petch J, Nelson W, Di S, Balasubramanian K, Yusuf S, Devereaux PJ, et al. Machine learning for detecting centre-level irregularities in randomized controlled trials: a pilot study. Contemp Clin Trials. 2022;122:106963.

74. Ohlsson M. WeAidU-a decision support system for myocardial perfusion images using artificial neural networks. Artif Intell Med. 2004;30(1):49–60.

75. Currie GM, Hawk KE, Rohren EM. Challenges confronting sustainability in nuclear medicine practice. Radiography (Lond). 2024;30(Suppl 1):1–8.

76. Jobin A, Ienca M, Vayena E. The global landscape of AI ethics guidelines. Nat Mach Intell. 2019;1:389–99.

77. Yang J, Sohn JH, Behr SC, Gullberg GT, Seo Y. CT-less direct correction of attenuation and scatter in the image space using deep learning for whole-body FDG PET: potential benefits and pitfalls. Radiol Artif Intell. 2021;3(2):e200137.

78. Yu Z, Rahman MA, Schindler T, Gropler R, Laforest R, Wahl R, et al. AI-based methods for nuclear-medicine imaging: need for objective task-specific evaluation. Soc Nuclear Med. 2020.

79. Leung KH, Marashdeh W, Wray R, Ashrafinia S, Pomper MG, Rahmim A, et al. A physics-guided modular deep-learning based automated framework for tumor segmentation in PET. Phys Med Biol. 2020;65(24):245032.

80. Reuzé S, Orlhac F, Chargari C, Nioche C, Limkin E, Riet F, et al. Prediction of cervical cancer recurrence using textural features extracted from 18F-FDG PET

images acquired with different scanners. Oncotarget. 2017;8(26):43169–79.

81. Noor P. Can we trust AI not to further embed racial bias and prejudice? BMJ. 2020;368:m363.

82. Finlayson SG, Subbaswamy A, Singh K, Bowers J, Kupke A, Zittrain J, et al. The clinician and dataset shift in artificial intelligence. N Engl J Med. 2021;385(3):283–6.

83. Jha AK, Bradshaw TJ, Buvat I, Hatt M, Kc P, Liu C, et al. Nuclear medicine and artificial intelligence: best practices for evaluation (the RELAINCE guidelines). J Nucl Med. 2022;63(9):1288–99.

84. Tamam MO, Tamam MC. Artificial intelligence technologies in nuclear medicine. World J Radiol. 2022;14(6):151–4.

85. Champendal M, Ribeiro RST, Müller H, Prior JO, Sá dos Reis C. Nuclear medicine technologists practice impacted by AI denoising applications in PET/CT images. Radiography. 2024;30(4):1232–9.

Dr Lefteris Livieratos Dr Livieratos is a Clinical Scientist (Medical Physicist) in Nuclear Medicine at Guy's & St Thomas' Hospitals and adjunct Reader in Medical Physics at King's College London. He has over 25 years work experience in diagnostic and therapeutic radionuclide applications and worked previously in PET methodology at Hammersmith Hospital, Imperial College. He served as program director for the MSc Clinical Sciences—Medical Physics at King's and is actively involved in undergraduate and postgraduate teaching and the supervision of post-graduate students and trainee clinical scientists. His research interests include radio-theranostics, multi-modality and translational imaging and patient-specific dosimetry in molecular radiotherapy.

Professor Christoph Jan Trauernicht Chris Trauernicht is the head of the medical physics division at Tygerberg Hospital, as well as an Associate Professor at Stellenbosch University. Chris is the past-president of the Federation of African Medical Physics Organizations (FAMPO) and the current chairperson of the South African Medical Physics Society. Chris' research focuses on three different areas: (1) Medical physics staffing, education, and training in Africa; (2) The use of machine learning in the automation of radiotherapy treatment planning; (3) Operational research in a clinical medical physics division; He was elected as a Fellow of the International Organization for Medical Physics in 2023.

Mélanie Champendal Mélanie is an expert radiographer in nuclear medicine and a member of the Nuclear Medicine Committee of the European Federation of Radiography Societies (EFRS). She worked for nine years in a clinic in the nuclear medicine department of the CHUV in Lausanne. She is currently a lecturer at HESAV School of Health Sciences-Vaud, HES-SO University of Applied Sciences and Arts, Western Switzerland, where she oversees nuclear medicine and bachelor's theses. She holds a master's degree in health sciences. Mélanie is pursuing a PhD in the development of an eXplainable Artificial Intelligence (XAI) tool for PET/CT image denoising.

AI in Radiotherapy

11

Caitlin Gillan, Yannie Lai, Brian Liszewski, and Anita Vloet

11.1 Introduction

Radiation therapy (RT), or radiotherapy (RT), is an integral and uniquely technologically reliant cornerstone of cancer care. Artificial intelligence (AI) is poised to transform many aspects of the RT patient trajectory, with impact already being demonstrated as data and related solutions are being harnessed in novel ways to inform care. In the therapeutic setting, AI empowers precision medicine by leveraging advanced computational techniques to analyse large-scale biomedical data, extracting actionable insights, and tailoring healthcare interventions to individual patient characteristics, leading to more effective, efficient, and personalised healthcare delivery.

AI can inform care at multiple points across the patient journey within the RT care path. In each step, there is an abundance of patient data ranging from demographic, imaging, clinical, temporal, and dosimetric data (Fig. 11.1), each requiring assurance of high-quality data and responsible data management. The scope of existing and emerging AI applications in RT ranges from radiomics [1], clinical decision support systems [2, 3], dose prediction and adjustments [4], predictive modelling and outcome predictions [5], treatment planning and optimisation [6, 7], automated contouring and segmentation [8, 9], adaptive radiation therapy [10, 11], and quality assurance [7, 12].

In this chapter, the basic principles and key applications of AI will be explored across a number of domains, to paint a picture of the role of big data in informing AI innovation, specific use cases to highlight the nature of impact on RT care, and the importance of considering potential impact to practice scopes of RT professionals. Given the central part of medical imaging in many aspects of RT, a number of the innovations and solutions defined in earlier imaging-focused chapters (such as Chaps. 6, 7, or 10) are also pertinent to the evolution of therapeutic applications of radiation. Linkages with other chapters will thus be made where relevant, expanding on use cases specific to the RT context.

on behalf of Association of Healthcare Technology Providers for Imaging, Radiotherapy and Care (AXREM)

C. Gillan (✉)
University of Toronto, Toronto, ON, Canada
e-mail: Caitlin.gillan@bccancer.bc.ca

Y. Lai
Sunnybrook Health Sciences Centre, North York, ON, Canada
e-mail: wingyan.lai@sunnybrook.ca

B. Liszewski
University of Toronto, Toronto, ON, Canada

Ontario Health, Toronto, ON, Canada

A. Vloet
Princess Margaret Cancer Centre, Toronto, Canada
e-mail: Anita.Vloet@uhn.ca

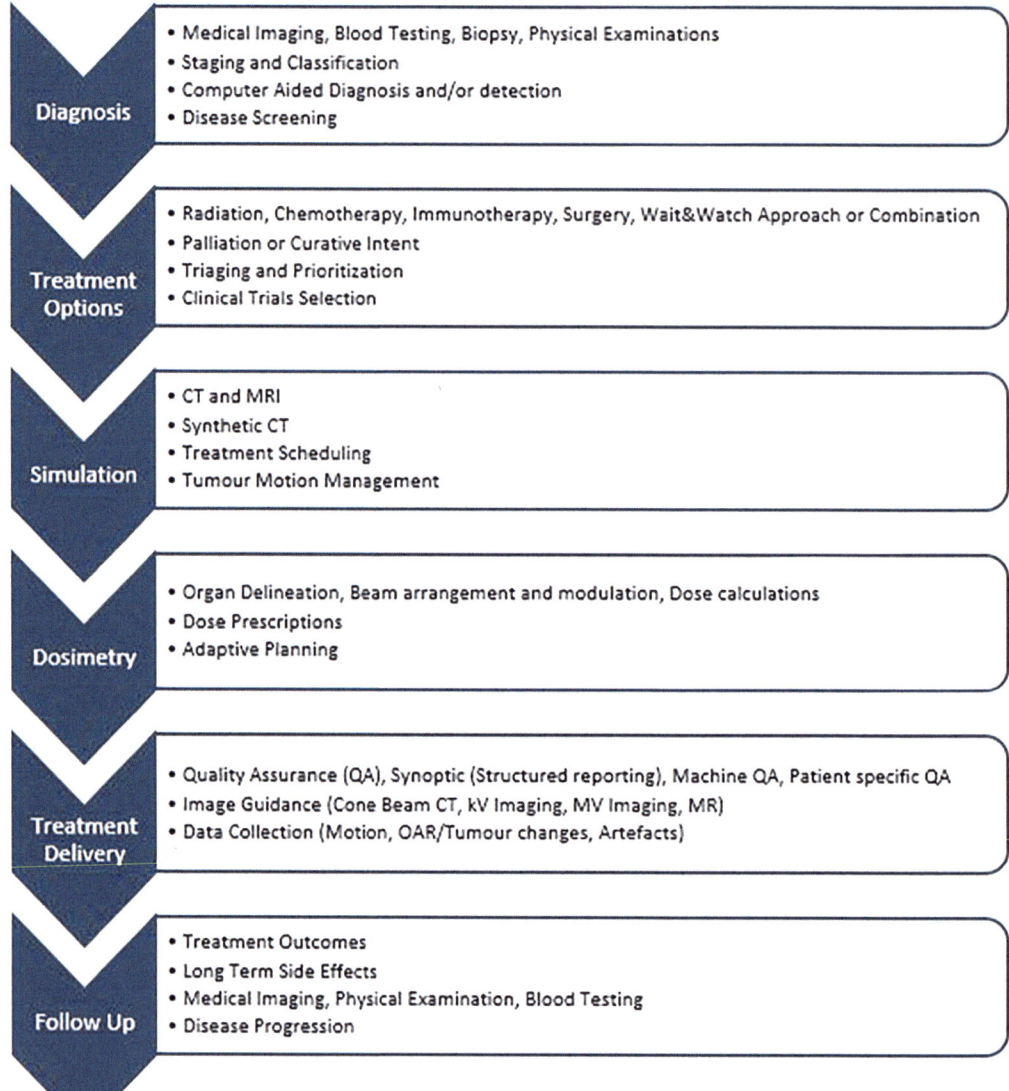

Fig. 11.1 The patient goes through a variety of steps during their cancer journey leading to the potential decision for radiation treatment planning. In each step of their journey, a variety of tests and procedures may be done that all have the potential for data extraction and analysis

11.2 The Role of Big Data and Standardisation in Realising AI-Enabled Practice

In the 1990s, John Mashey introduced the concept of 'big data', highlighting the vast volumes of data that exceed the capabilities of traditional analysis tools [13]. This term has become increasingly relevant as computational advancements, particularly the advent of cloud computing, have transformed our capacity to gather, store, and analyse data. Before, gathering data was done manually and not very often. However, with the growth of smartphones, social media, and smart devices, there is now an abundance of data from many different sources. This is also true in healthcare, where a lot of data are created during a patient's care plan. These data can be characterised using the five Vs of big data:

1. *Volume*: An RT department produces a significant volume of data, including demographics, history, image datasets, planning metrics, and technical details regarding treatment.
2. *Velocity*: As RT has become more digital in practice, the velocity of data has accelerated, become almost instantaneously available and transferable.
3. *Variety*: RT data includes images, planning metrics, and patient records consisting of different types of data including structured, unstructured, and semi-structured data.
4. *Veracity*: Given the complexity of RT, ensuring the accuracy of data is crucial to ensure safe and high-quality treatment to patients.
5. *Value*: The usefulness of the data produced in RT lies in its ability to provide insights and the ability to improve patient outcomes.

Leveraging big data is becoming increasingly important in RT, as it provides valuable insights that can improve patient outcomes and optimise treatment, leading to better value for both patients and healthcare providers. In the following sections, we will explore the importance of big data in RT and how it can be leveraged to improve patient care.

11.2.1 Data Standardisation in Radiation Therapy

Software-based RT planning requires consideration of the dose given to the organs at risk in the treated volume. When planning for a structure such as the kidney, how programmes name these volumes may vary, with one defining the dose delivered to 10% of the 'RT_Kidney' volume, another 10% of the 'Right Kidney' volume, and yet another defining 10% of the 'Kidney-Rt' volume. Although the measures of dose were standardised, it was recognised that the uncoordinated nomenclature used to describe the organs would become a challenge when linking data across populations. The American Association of Physicists in Medicine's (AAPM) *TG-263 Standardising Nomenclatures in Radiation Oncology* initiative [14], launched first in 2018, has been pivotal in standardising radiation oncology nomenclature. TG-263 tackles naming inconsistencies in anatomical structures and treatment parameters. Uniformity of data is crucial for facilitating data linkage, sharing, and analysis. Standardisation of data enables the comparison and aggregation of data, thereby enriching insights into treatment effectiveness and patient care. Furthermore, standardisation supports collaborative research and advances in quality within the field of RT.

While the use of big data as it relates to specific AI solutions will be revisited throughout this chapter, a number of key applications are presented briefly here to reinforce the underlying importance of concerted efforts towards data standardisation – both to inform AI and as part of broader RT care optimisation.

11.2.1.1 Facilitation of Re-irradiation Planning

As people are increasingly living longer with cancer, the need for re-irradiation is projected to continue to increase over time [15]. Standardised nomenclature enhances re-irradiation planning by ensuring consistent data sharing and interpretation across treatment centres, critical for addressing the complex needs of cancer patients undergoing subsequent treatments.

11.2.1.2 Emergency Preparedness

Standardised nomenclature is essential for emergency preparedness, such as with unanticipated RT department downtimes [16]. Related system level efforts can enable clear communication, swift response coordination, and effective resource allocation across agencies to efficiently manage and mitigate crises. As described in the article 'A National Cyberattack Affecting Radiation Therapy: The Irish Experience' [16] in May 2021, Ireland's public health services experienced a significant cyberattack, and without access to treatment records the radiation treatment for several patients was put on hold. Relying on agreements with the private sector facilities allowed for the resumed treatment for the impacted patients. However, common nomenclature and plan sharing tools could have mitigated the impact, ensuring rapid recovery and minimising treatment disruptions.

11.2.1.3 Support for Integration of Patient-Reported Outcomes (PROs)

TG-263 [14] standardises nomenclature, crucial for integrating patient-reported outcomes (PROs), offering insights into patient well-being, quality of life, and real-time feedback for symptom monitoring, thereby harmonising practices and enabling data-sharing for improved patient-centered care, and system-level consistency [17].

11.2.1.4 AI-Driven Treatment Planning

Standardised nomenclature is critical for AI-driven treatment planning in RT, ensuring data consistency and interoperability, which enhances AI model training, accuracy, and personalised treatment decision-making [18] (see Case Study 11.2 for more insight to this application).

11.2.1.5 Role in Research and Clinical Trials

Standardised nomenclature streamlines research and clinical trials by ensuring uniform data collection, analysis, and reporting, facilitating cross-study comparisons, enhancing data quality, and accelerating scientific discovery and clinical advancements.

11.2.1.6 Support for Quality Assurance Processes

Standardised nomenclature is essential for quality assurance in radiation therapy, enabling consistent procedure documentation, performance evaluation, and outcome measurement, ensuring high standards of patient care and safety [19].

Having articulated the importance of data and their standardisation as the foundational ingredient to fuel AI solutions, the next few sections will highlight a diverse, though not exhaustive, set of four individual applications of AI; medical imaging solutions in AI (Sect. 11.3, Case Study 11.1),

AI in RT treatment planning (Sect. 11.4, Case Study 11.2), AI applications in RT business operations (Sect. 11.5, Case Study 11.3), and PROs (Sect. 11.6 below).

11.3 Leveraging Medical Imaging AI Solutions

AI technologies have the potential to augment the capabilities of medical professionals in the field of radiation oncology, providing them with advanced tools for image analysis and decision support. The two topics of this section describe radiomics in radiation therapy and the potential of synthetic CTs for radiation treatment simulation and planning.

11.3.1 Radiomics in Radiation Therapy

Radiomics has emerged as a promising avenue to enhance clinical decision-making in RT. It can assist clinicians in a variety of checkpoints during a patient's journey from disease diagnosis through to treatment delivery and follow up processes. The gold standard approach to treatment decisions in both medical and radiation oncology is the use of biomarkers. Biomarkers are a measurable physical property that represents a phenomenon, serving as an indicator for a medical state [20]. Examples of biomarkers are genetic mutations, tumour factors, disease stage, and disease grading. These biomarkers will guide clinicians in the decisions for a patient's treatment regimen, treatment prescription, and urgency of treatment. Leveraging computational techniques, radiomics involves the extraction and analysis of quantitative features from medical images which can be used as biomarkers. This approach goes beyond visual assessment of images, diving into the intricate details within data that might not be readily perceptible to humans.

11.3.1.1 Extractable Data

Different imaging modalities will provide different types of data that could be extracted and analysed for potential biomarkers. Various imaging modalities include medical resonance imaging (MRI), computed tomography (CT), radiography, positron-emission tomography (PET), and even clinical photographs. The potential to assess data across different modalities introduces the opportunity to unlock more correlations as certain patients could have standard multimodality diagnostic scans. Quantifiable imaging parameters from those images include two-dimensional and three-dimensional elements, as well as temporal information, uniquely important in assessing response to RT. Parameters include regions or interest (ROI), volume of interest (VOI), surface area, flatness, voxel, or pixel intensity distribution [21]. Information can also be extracted by comparison of those parameters, such as differences in intensity levels in neighbouring pixels or voxels, or considering the time of data acquisition. In summary, radiomics can offer spatial and temporal information that traditional biomarkers may not provide. More on radiomics from a technical perspective can be found in Chap. 2.

11.3.1.2 Radiomics Workflows

Creating a radiomics solution is a multi-step process that involves several key stages [21–24]. Firstly, the acquisition of images of the patient will need to be carefully planned to consider the appropriate quality of the image acquired given the study objectives. For example, ensuring minimal patient motion or image artefacts that may skew data, thus producing false results. Any necessary image preprocessing can then be done to enhance image quality. For example, motion correction can be used to correct for misregistration or blurring, or image filtering can be used to increase or decrease sensitivity of radiomic features that may be of importance to the study objectives. Image segmentation will be the next step to define regions of interest or volume of interest as guided by study objectives, in which the model will focus during feature extraction steps. Feature extraction can be categorised into first-order features or second-order features, which can provide more information. First-order features are the simplest of features and are also

known as histogram features (such as mean and standard deviations). Second-order features, also known as grey-level co-occurrence matrix, which can provide spatial information about information regarding adjacent pixels.

Once radiomic features and clinical end points are identified, the process of modelling can commence. Radiomics can be combined with AI because of its better capability of handling the amount of data compared with traditional statistical methods [22]. If AI is used for feature extraction, then the imaging data will be split into a training set and a validation set, as it would be biased to test the model based on the same data used to train it. Once modelling is complete with the training set, the validation set is used to assess model performance.

Case Study 11.1: Detection of Interstitial Lung Disease on CT Imaging Using AI-Enabled Analysis Before Radiotherapy

Clinical challenge: Undetected underlying lung diseases can increase the risk of toxicity or even put patients at risk for fatal side effects of radiotherapy.

AI-enabled solution: Using a novel algorithm (MIRACLE-ILD) [29], each patient planned for lung radiotherapy was automatically screened for interstitial lung disease (ILD) by classifying the treatment planning CT as high or low risk. This prospective project had two phases. Initially, MIRACLE-ILD was deployed either in a 'silent mode', where the output of the algorithm was recorded but no notifications were sent. After validating the algorithm in the clinical workflow, the notification mode ('live mode') was activated, which sent a message to the attending physician in charge of the patient to let them know there was a potential risk of ILD detected on the planning CT. The algorithm threshold was tuned to accept a relatively high rate of false positive notifications (~15%) but was relatively sensitive and caught and flagged nearly 75% of all patients with ILD including nearly 50%

(continued)

of patients that were unknown to have ILD by their treating physician.

Benefits: Tan et al. [29] demonstrated the utility of AI algorithmic analysis of treatment planning imaging to detect underlying lung disease in a prospective clinical deployment. The system performed well regardless of the underlying malignant diagnosis and the overall performance of the algorithm in this environment had an AUROC of 0.76. This system now monitors every patient planned for thoracic radiotherapy at the centre where it was developed and continues to help identify patients who may be at risk from their planned radiotherapy.

Challenges: Improved versions of the algorithm are being developed that will hopefully increase both the sensitivity and specificity of the system, which will reduce the false positive rate. Related external validation work was published in 2024 [29].

11.3.1.3 Leveraging Radiomics Correlations and Information

Radiomics uses large scale data in medical imaging to find correlations, such as correlations with clinical endpoints. In the field of RT, radiomics has shown promise in a variety of applications. By deciphering subtle patterns and characteristics in medical images, clinicians can gain valuable insights into tumour heterogeneity, treatment response, and potential prognostic indicators. Studies have shown promise in predictingnd MRIs [25, 26], which allows clinicians to make timely decisions on treatment options. As well, during pre-treatment assessment of critical organs, prediction of onset of radiation-induced side effects has facilitated timely intervention [27]. Post-RT, clinicians are often challenged with assessing response and recurrence given radiation-induced tissue scarring or necrosis. Feature extraction of MRI brain images can unlock potential for a non-invasive approach to more reliably assess potential disease progression [28].

The strength of a correlation can be quantified by something called the area under the receiver operating characteristic curve (ROC), or AUROC. The ROC is a probability curve, assessing how well the classification performs at various thresholds, in terms of distinguishing between true positives and false positives. The AUROC is a number that represents the proportion of cases that fall under the curve. An AUROC of 0.5 suggests that the algorithm cannot distinguish presence of disease, being no better than chance, while an AUROC of 0.7–0.8 is generally considered to represent strong performance.

In summary, the integration of radiomics into RT workflows and care plans opens avenues for more personalised and precise treatment and care planning, enhancing therapeutic outcomes while minimising adverse effects.

11.3.2 Synthetic CTs in Radiation Therapy

Synthetic CT (sCT) refers to a method used in medical imaging where a CT-like image is generated from another imaging modality, typically from MRI. This technique is particularly useful in RT planning, where CT features (such as Hounsfield units to characterise tissue density) have traditionally been necessary for dose calculation and treatment planning [30].

The current standard RT planning requires the acquisition of CT scan in a specific positioning appropriate for treatment, with physicians occasionally requesting supplemental MRI to inform delineation of certain organs or targets of interest. CT scans are required for electron density information and geometric information that allows for the modelling of radiation attenuation for dose calculations, which is not possible with MRI. However, MRI provides unique soft tissue delineation and functional information. These additional imaging requirements can be cumbersome for patients and contribute to increased workload and resource utilisation, including time spent on the subsequent image fusion of CT and MRI scans. Using an AI algorithm to generate sCT from MRI images can mitigate some of those steps and allow for an MR-only workflow. Changes to the key steps in the simulation of radiation treatments come with advantages and disadvantages, outlined in Table 11.1 [31].

The process of generating sCT images involves registering MRI images with corresponding CT images from a database or by training a machine learning model to predict CT-like images directly from MRI data. This can involve a variety of different methods including classic machine learning methods or deep learning methods [32]. While sCT images may not perfectly replicate true CT images, research has demonstrated adequacy for treatment planning purposes (Fig. 11.2), including for intracranial tumours [33] and pelvic tumours [34, 35], with achievable dosimetry [36, 37] and acceptable daily pre-treatment CBCT image registrations [34].

Generating sCTs offers a non-invasive and efficient alternative to acquiring CT images, particularly beneficial in scenarios where MRI is the preferred imaging modality or when reducing radiation exposure is a priority. An example of MR only workflow for a site with scan preparations is outlined in Table 11.2, which compares the changes in steps compared to conventional CT simulation. However, MR is not the only

Table 11.1 Advantages and disadvantages of MR-only workflow with the introduction of sCTs [31]

Advantages	Disadvantages
Clinical	Reconsideration of
Reduced radiation exposure to patients	workload for different professions
Reduction in systematic registration errors, for example, bladder filling over time	Consideration of cases that may be complex and novel for accurate generation of sCT
Soft tissue delineation with MRI	
Operational	
Fewer appointments to schedule	
Resource utilisation (CT scanner is freed up)	
Greater efficiency with fewer scans and reduced need for fusion	

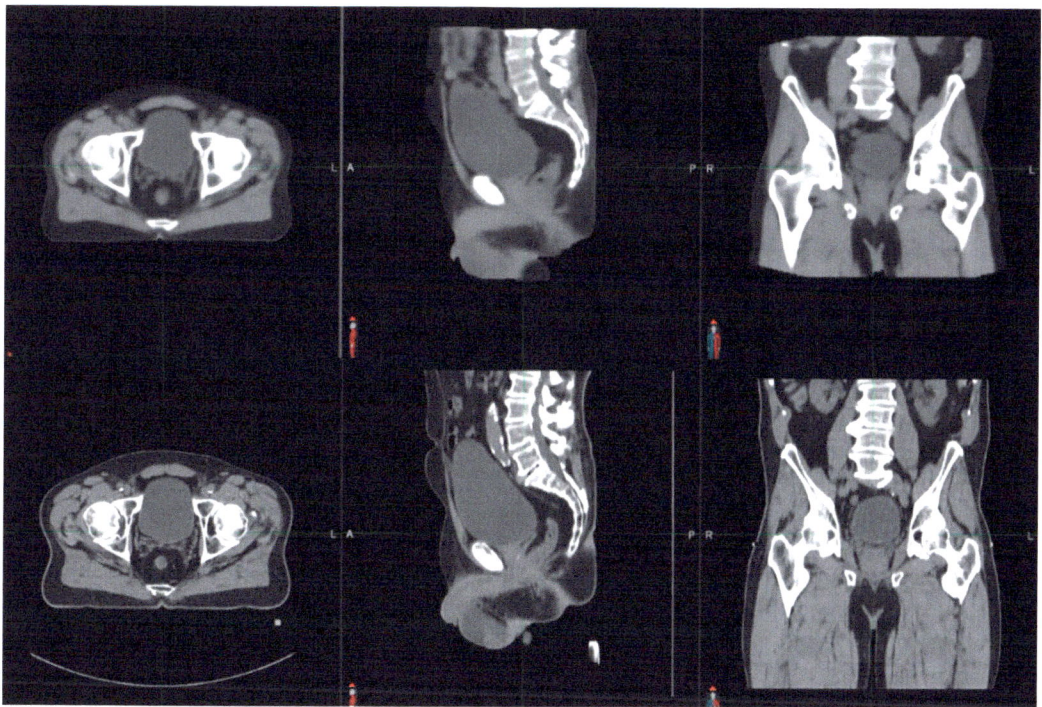

Fig. 11.2 MRI-based sCT (top) and conventional CT (bottom) of the same patient [31]

Table 11.2 Workflow considerations for traditional CT simulation compared to MRI-only workflow for a patient with scan preparations. The underlined steps from conventional CT simulation are not required for MRI only workflow simulation, providing efficiencies

Conventional CT simulation	MRI-only workflow simulation
Patient preparation (full bladder, empty rectum)	Patient preparation (full bladder, empty rectum)
Patient positioning	Patient positioning
CT scan	MRI scan
Tattooing	Tattooing
MRI scan	Contouring
Contouring	Dosimetry
Registration of CT and MRI scans	
Dosimetry	

modality from which sCT can be generated. Studies have explored generating sCT from cone beam CTs (CBCT). CBCTs are acquired during treatments to assess patient positioning and organ motion. CBCT is a low dose imaging option that can cause artefacts and provide inaccurate Hounsfield units, making this type of imaging inferior to diagnostic scans for treatment planning purposes. By generating sCT from CBCT, image corrections can be made exploring the potential for adaptive replanning, clinical evaluation of tumour shrinkage and organ shifts [38].

The application of sCT derived from an image modality frequently used for treatment delivery can have an impact on assessing temporal relationships of clinical parameters, especially in the abdominal site where organ motion is a concern [39, 40].

11.4 Treatment Planning

The traditional workflow in RT begins with segmentation of a CT image set, followed by optimisation of a RT treatment plan. Advancements in AI and automation technologies have resulted in the creation of new tools for automated segmentation and treatment plan generation. These tools can offer many potential benefits such as enhanced consistency, quality and efficiency compared to manual segmentation and treatment planning [41].

11.4.1 Auto-segmentation

Segmentation of tumour volumes and organs at risk is a critical step in RT planning. Manual image segmentation involves clinicians delineating regions of interest by hand. This process is time-consuming, taking up to several hours for complex cases [42]. The time spent contouring and the associated peer review required reduces the time clinicians have for direct patient care [43]. In addition to being extremely labour-intensive, manual delineation is also a subjective process affected by inter- and intra-observer variability, which can ultimately impact treatment precision and patient outcomes [44].

Automating segmentation of human anatomy can greatly reduce the amount of human time required to generate contours, while improving standardisation and quality. Automatic segmentation of human anatomy has been an active area of research and development since the introduction of 3D planning systems in RT [45].

There are four broad generations of auto-segmentation [45]:

1. *Intensity analysis* (voxels are assigned to a region of interest based on Hounsfield unit) and shape modelling (deformable shape models)
2. *Atlas-based methods* (based on manually segmented reference images)
3. Early (non-deep) *machine learning* (random forests, support-vector machines)
4. *Deep learning approaches* (convolutional neural networks)

Atlas-based and deep learning approaches are the most commonly used AI methodologies in commercially available auto-segmentation software packages [46]. These tools are being integrated into RT treatment planning systems, which allow clinicians to incorporate AI generated segmentations directly into their workflows [47]. Figure 11.3 illustrates the results of auto-segmentation in commercially available vendor software.

Overall, auto-segmentation can improve the accuracy and consistency of contours, particularly

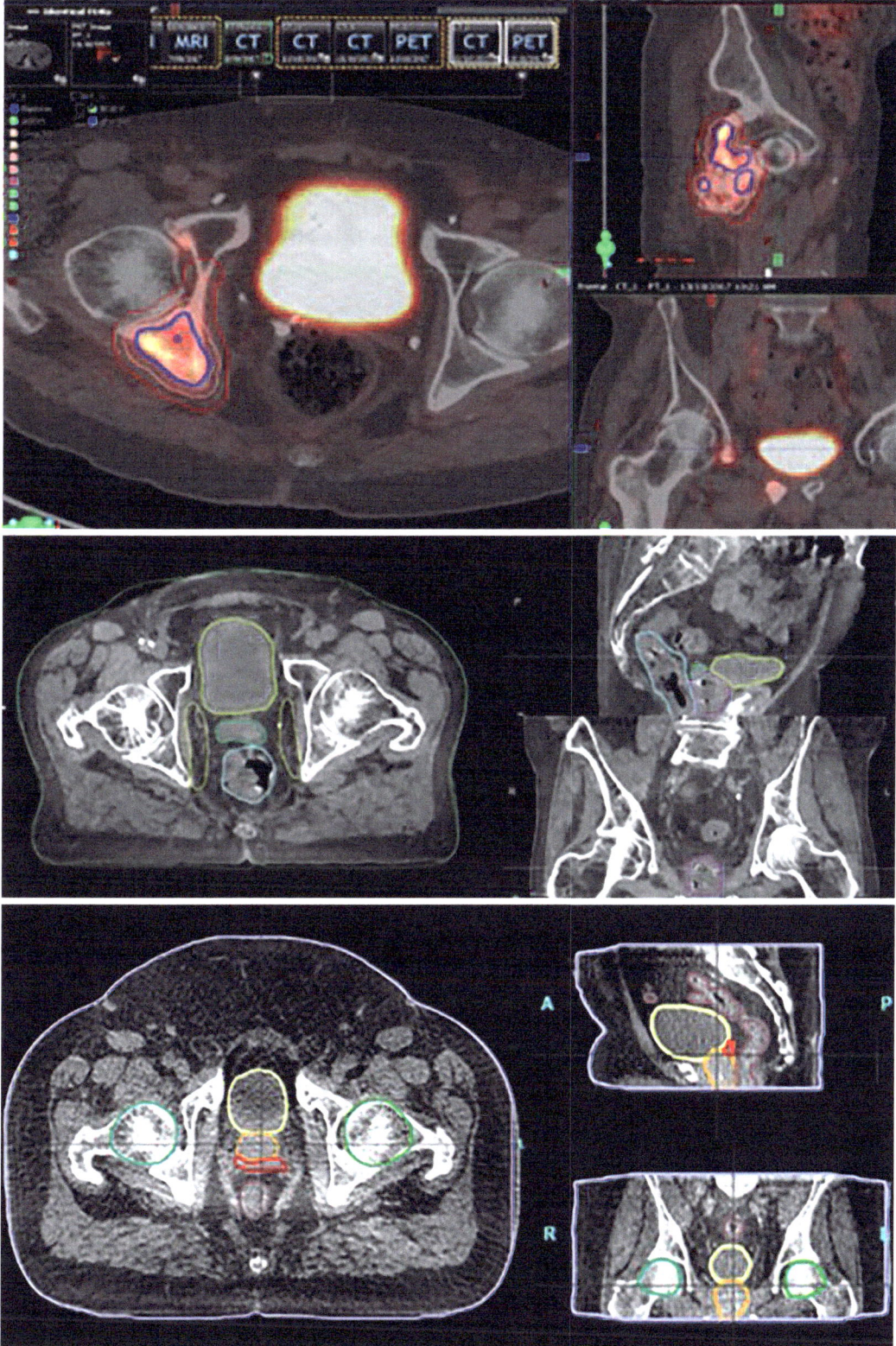

Fig. 11.3 Auto-segmentation precision examples on PET-CT, CT, and CBCT-guided contouring accuracy for pelvis organs at risk and targets using three current vendor software products [46]

when the structures are complex or difficult to distinguish. However, clinicians often refer to additional imaging studies and the health history of the patient when generating contours for planning. An optimal workflow may be a combination of auto-segmentation with clinician oversight (manual editing), which will ensure accuracy and clinical relevance of auto-generated contours [41].

11.4.2 Auto-planning

The objective of radiation treatment planning is to deliver prescribed radiation to a target to maximise tumour control with minimal damage to surrounding organs at risk. Trade-offs between tumour control and organ at risk protection are challenging to maintain, because each patient has a unique set of anatomical geometries and unique medical implications. These complexities cause treatment planning to be an iterative, time-consuming, and manual process.

Its complex nature can lead to significant variation in final treatment plans despite the identification of specific planning objectives [48]. Differences in experience and skill level of the clinicians involved in plan generation have been shown to contribute to plan quality variations, with greater levels of planning experience translating to improved plan quality [49]. These variations in plan quality can ultimately lead to poor patient outcomes by increasing the risks of normal tissue complications [50, 51]. Therefore, it is essential to ensure that all treatment plans are of consistently high quality.

Automated RT treatment planning can aid in creating time efficiencies and improve standardisation of plan optimisation. The evolution of automation in treatment planning began with user-defined scripts and templates, which enabled repetitive tasks such as beam arrangement and objective creation to be automated and based on defined protocols. Current automated treatment planning methodologies include non-knowledge based planning (non-KBP), which uses heuristic rules to mimic the manual planning process and knowledge-based planning (KBP) methods, which leverage planning information from prior

patients to train mathematical models [52]. Future developments will likely use more complex deep learning methods that utilise neural networks to determine optimal dosimetric predictions [53]. Irrespective of the approach utilised, automated treatment planning has demonstrated its ability to enhance the consistency and efficiency of the radiotherapy treatment planning process [54–56].

Case Study 11.2: Treatment Planning AI Algorithms

Clinical challenge: At present, so many algorithms and AI strategies exist only in very controlled non-clinical test environments. Research compares decisions and interpretations made by AI retrospectively to those that were actually made and implemented clinically, but rarely are the AI-derived outputs actually guiding care as yet.

AI-enabled solution: McIntosh et al [18] recognised the importance of demonstrating AI in a real-world application, where they 'prospectively deployed and evaluated a random forest algorithm for therapeutic curative-intent radiation therapy (RT) treatment planning for prostate cancer in a blinded, head-to-head study with full integration into the clinical workflow'. This work had two phases. In each phase, 50 prostate plans were generated by an AI algorithm previously built using high quality prostate treatment plans. In Phase 1, these plans were done for patients who had already been treated using human generated treatment plans, and physicians were asked to assess both plans for each patient in a blinded process against established review criteria. Following completion of this phase, a second phase applied the AI algorithm prospectively, such that 50 patients had both an AI-generated and a human-generated plan created prior to treatment, and each was reviewed in the same way as in Phase 1.

(continued)

Benefits: Overall, across both phases, in 72% of cases, physicians who were blinded to the origin of the plan selected the AI-generated plan over the human-generated plan as the most clinically appropriate for treatment (with 89% of plans being clinically acceptable). As well as being deemed to be of higher quality, the median time for the entire treatment planning process was also reduced by 60.1% when using AI over human treatment planners.

Challenges: Interestingly, though there was little difference in the percentage of AI plans deemed acceptable for treatment between Phase 1 (retrospective) and Phase 2 (prospective, implementation), a significantly lower percentage of AI-generated plans were ultimately selected for treatment in Phase 2 (61%) as compared to those that would have theoretically been preferred in Phase 1 (83%). The authors highlighted this as an important consideration in implementing AI—that even when preferring an AI plan over a human-generated plan in a blinded review, there may be other factors at play that lead to a human generated plan ultimately being implemented.

11.5 Optimisation of Operations

As noted earlier in this chapter, in the discussion of the logistical benefits of standardising RT big data at a system level, there are applications of AI that extend outside of the technical planning and delivery of care. As an increasing population and increased cancer incidence is placing a burden on limited radiation treatment resources, the system can be plagued with long waiting lists and delays in treatment [57]. Excessive delays in RT are associated with detrimental oncological outcomes, psychological distress for patients, and an increased eco-

nomic burden of cancer as a result of higher costs due to advanced stages of the disease [58, 59].

AI has emerged as a powerful tool in operations research (OR), which is a field of study that uses mathematical modelling, statistical analysis, and optimisation techniques to solve complex decision-making problems. All healthcare systems, including cancer care, face challenges such as resource allocation, scheduling, patient-flow optimisation, and decision-making processes. OR methods, such as computer simulation and mathematical programming, can be used to provide optimisation solutions for cancer care [60, 61].

RT is a complex workflow as previously described in this chapter, which requires the coordination of several different appointments (CT Sim, MR Sim, multiple fractions for treatment). There are many technical and clinical constraints that need to be considered for each patient (specific start date, allocation to a particular machine, coordination with other treatment modalities) when creating a patient schedule. Additionally, individualised needs of patients and their caregivers must also be accounted for to provide optimal patient care and experience [62]. All of these factors in conjunction with human resource constraints and resource scarcity create a complex scheduling problem, which is amenable to an AI enabled solution. Clinically deployed auto-scheduling solutions have shown improvements in patient waiting times, linear accelerator (Linac) utilisation, schedule consistency, and administrative burden [63].

Figure 11.4 is an example of an automated scheduling system which can be deployed in a radiation oncology department. Machine learning (ML) and statistical modelling (SM) can be utilised to predict patient flow. Operational research algorithms can then be applied to optimally align resources with the incoming patient flow. An automated schedule created with human oversight is able to optimally address the issues of patient flow, resource utilisation, and patient-specific factors.

AI POWERED AUTO-SCHEDULING PLATFORM

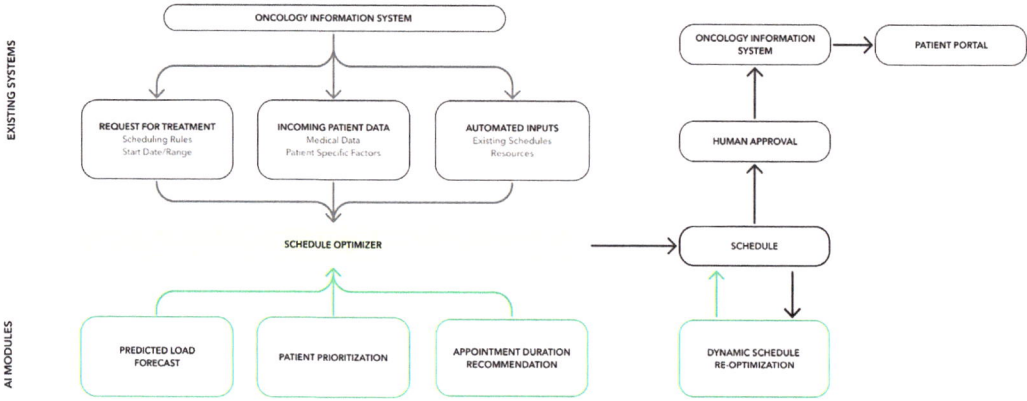

Fig. 11.4 Example of automated scheduling system

11.6 Patient-Reported Outcomes (PROs)

Case Study 11.3: Patient Auto-scheduling System in Radiotherapy

Clinical challenge: Healthcare systems struggle with long waiting lists, delays, staffing shortages and lack of resources. Delays impact patient outcomes, their well-being, and create healthcare costs for more complex cases, where disease has advanced, as discussed above. RT is a complex process that requires fine coordination which considers many parameters for each patient treated and equipment used.

AI-enabled solution: GRAY OS is a commercially available auto-scheduling platform that can be integrated with any radiation oncology information system (ROIS) [64]. Its main features are standardised radiation oncology care plan templates, automated patient appointment scheduling, and operational dashboards. The patient appointment scheduling algorithm consists of an initial integer program (IP), which assigns appointments to resources/days followed by a constraint programming model which selects specific time slots for appointments.

Benefits: Standardised care templates enable automation and allow users to customise their clinical protocols. Lastly, operational dashboards provide live monitoring of patient volumes so managers can optimise resources.

Challenges: Future developments will utilise ML and SM to build a prediction model based on consultation appointments with radiation oncologists. This predictive model will be directly integrated into the existing platform to provide managers with predicted patient loads on resources that can guide informed decision-making.

The integration of patient reported outcomes (PROs) into radiation oncology marks a transformative approach in delivering personalised and effective RT. By standardising these outcomes, healthcare providers can adopt a big data approach, leveraging vast datasets to gain insights into patient experiences and treatment efficacy [65]. To do this effectively, standardised reporting of outcome data is necessary. The operational ontology for oncology (O3) [66] is an initiative of the American Association of Physicists in Medicine's (AAPM) Big Data Science Committee that standardises PROs, describing standard instruments, questions, and responses. This standardisation not only enables a uniform method of assessing patient feedback, but also facilitates the aggregation and analysis of data across diverse patient populations and diagnoses. By analysing patterns in PRO and clinical data, AI can identify the most effective treatment approaches, tailoring therapies to individual patient needs [67].

The concept of predictive analytics employs a future-looking application of PRO data [68]. AI models can predict potential challenges in patient outcomes, enabling pre-emptive adjustments to treatment plans. This predictive capability allows healthcare providers to address issues before they escalate, potentially improving patient experience and treatment outcomes. The utilisation of real-time monitoring tools further enhances this approach, allowing for the continuous collection of PROs. These tools, integrated with predictive artificial intelligence (AI) algorithms, can anticipate patient needs, forecast potential health deteriorations, and recommend preventive measures, thus ensuring timely and proactive interventions [68].

The integration of patient reported outcomes (PROs) and the application of AI in radiation oncology represent significant advancements in personalising and improving patient care. These innovations allow for a more proactive, predictive, and patient-centered approach to treatment, ultimately aiming to enhance outcomes and patient satisfaction in radiation therapy.

11.7   Role of Collaboration in Responsible Implementation of AI in RT

The impact or value of an innovation cannot be assessed in a vacuum [69]. Optimal responsible use of AI solutions can only be achieved when practice is adjusted to best leverage their potential. This requires concerted reflection and planning within individual professional groups [70, 71], including specialty-level decisions about priorities in how AI should be implemented, and to what end. Priorities within one profession or for one aspect of practice must then also be considered in light of those defined by other professions

or broader stakeholder groups, ideally requiring collaborative consideration of common goals and implementation. This has been demonstrated in the implementation of other innovations in RT, such as intensity-modulated RT (IMRT) [72], CT-based planning [73], and image guided RT (IGRT) [74, 75], and may be of unique importance in as potentially disruptive and far-reaching an innovation as AI is proving to be.

From the AI solutions outlined throughout this chapter, it can be appreciated that for each solution, there is no single path to implementation, in terms of level of autonomy assigned to AI automation [76], how to harness AI-generated efficiencies in care [77], and other related considerations. It is incumbent on stakeholders across the RT practice environment, especially related professional groups, to assign concerted effort to defining optimal implementation as it relates to highest quality patient care. The risk of not doing so is that haphazard solution-specific implementation will prioritise the interests of whoever is positioned to make decisions about that individual technology, without needed consideration of the broader practice and care picture.

The concept of how to assign newfound time savings as a result of AI efficiencies provides a good example of higher order decisions that might inform implementation. In broad strokes, efficiencies can be leveraged to either allow more patients to be advanced through the radiation therapy care journey (reduce wait times), or to assign more time or resources to existing patients (adaptive RT, individual counselling) [77], or, as may be most likely, a balance between the two priorities. Dedicated consideration of an optimal balance, made in consultation with all relevant stakeholders (including patients themselves) may be indicated to ensure the most responsible realignment of practice alongside AI implementation.

Related considerations cannot be agnostic of professional identities and values [70, 77], as professions will inherently contextualise decisions through their professional lens, which includes protecting their own interests as part of advocating for responsible implementation. For radiation therapists, this may involve reflection on whether AI should shift their practice more towards technical skills or towards person-focused tasks, which would inform consideration of future competencies and scopes of practice in an AI-enabled world. This requires not only that professional groups facilitate related discussions, but that a critical mass of the professional community equip itself to appreciate AI and its potential impact. The work of various professional groups in RT (and medical imaging) to consider education, advocacy, and leadership in this space has been elucidated in the literature [78–81] and is further addressed in this book in Chaps. 4 and 14.

Comprehensive attention to AI development and implementation efforts, especially to the associated evolution of practice and related competencies, requires consideration of the inter-relatedness of professional roles and scopes. This can be accomplished through collaborative education, research, sharing of resources, consensus-building, and coordinated advocacy work, but doing so in more than a perfunctory manner can be challenging. There are nonetheless an increasing number of multi-stakeholder, cross-jurisdictional, interprofessional collaborations emerging that can serve to ensure an ideally-informed path forward. These include some of the initiatives acknowledged earlier in the chapter, both at the local level in individual research and development initiatives, but also larger system-level initiatives such as TG-263 [14] and O3 [66], described earlier in this chapter. A unique collaboration between radiation therapists, medical physicists, and radiation oncologists at a national level was launched in 2023 in Canada as the Canadian Artificial Intelligence and Big Data in Radiotherapy Alliance (CADRA) [82]. CADRA has a mandate to leverage relevant expertise and networks across disciplines and jurisdictions to inform innovation, standardisation, and knowledge exchange in AI and big data.

CADRA is a collaborative committee formed between three national partner organisations representing the radiation medicine landscape in Canada. The Canadian Association of Medical Radiation Technologists (CAMRT), the Canadian Association of Radiation Oncology (CARO), and the Canadian Organisation of Medical Physicists (COMP) recognise AI and big data as invaluable tools in the continued evolution of the interprofessional practice of radiation oncology. CADRA serves to provide a pan-Canadian lens to innovation, standardisation, and practice considerations with respect to big data and AI as they relate to radiation oncology. By leveraging relevant expertise and networks from across disciplines and jurisdictions, CADRA acts as a convenor to accelerate and amplify relevant initiatives in the optimisation of big data linkages and leveraging this data in the implementation of AI initiatives across Canada. When it comes to developing infrastructure to facilitate data pooling across institutions to feed algorithms, to establish mechanism to allow patients to move between radiation treatment centres (either for emergency downtimes or future re-irradiation), innovation and planning cannot be siloed within individual centres, research teams, or professions. It is only through true system level collaboration that solutions of the scale required and made possible by AI can be fully realised.

11.8 Chapter Summary

AI is increasingly exhibiting impact across the RT care trajectory and within the involved professions. Strategies developed and leveraged in other areas of healthcare and broader society, including systems level harnessing of big data, radiomics, automation, and predictive analytics, are all poised to transform the ability to deliver high-quality, patient-centered precision medicine.

The technical AI-driven strategies themselves are only one piece of the puzzle. It is up to human professionals to determine how AI will be responsibly applied; tasks that might be transitioned, the level of oversight assigned to AI in care decisions, and how the healthcare workforce will reposition itself to optimise workflows, scopes of practice, and interfacing with technology, other professionals, and our patients.

References

1. Arimura H, Soufi M, Kamezawa H, Ninomiya K, Yamada M. Radiomics with artificial intelligence for precision medicine in radiation therapy. J Radiat Res. 2019;60(1):150–7.

2. Steiner DF, Nagpal K, Sayres R, Foote DJ, Wedin BD, Pearce A, et al. Evaluation of the use of combined artificial intelligence and pathologist assessment to review and grade prostate biopsies. JAMA Netw Open. 2020;3(11):e2023267.

3. Chan JW, Hohenstein N, Carpenter C, Pattison AJ, Morin O, Valdes G, et al. Adv Radiat Oncol. 2022;7(2):100886.

4. Liu J, Zhang X, Cheng X, Sun L. A deep learning-based dose prediction method for evaluation of radiotherapy treatment planning. J Radiat Res Appl Sci. 2024;17(1):100757.

5. van Velzen SG, Gal R, Teske AJ, van der Leij F, van den Bongard DH, Viergever MA, et al. AI-based radiation dose quantification for estimation of heart disease risk in breast cancer survivors after radiation therapy. Int J Radiat Oncol Biol Phys. 2022;112(3):621–32.

6. van de Sande D, Sharabiani M, Bluemink H, Kneepkens E, Bakx N, Hagelaar E, et al. Artificial intelligence based treatment planning of radiotherapy for locally advanced breast cancer. Phys Imaging Radiat Oncol. 2021;20:111–6.

7. Ng F, Jiang R, Chow JC. Predicting radiation treatment planning evaluation parameter using artificial intelligence and machine learning. IOP SciNotes. 2020;1(1):014003.

8. van Velzen SG, Bruns S, Wolterink JM, Leiner T, Viergever MA, Verkooijen HM, Išgum I. AI-based quantification of planned radiation therapy dose to cardiac structures and coronary arteries in patients with breast cancer. Int J Radiat Oncol Biol Phys. 2022;112(3):611–20.

9. Zabel WJ, Conway JL, Gladwish A, Skliarenko J, Didiodato G, Goorts-Matthews L, et al. Clinical evaluation of deep learning and atlas-based auto-contouring of bladder and rectum for prostate radiation therapy. Prac. Radiat Oncol. 2021;11(1):e80–9.

10. Sibolt P, Andersson LM, Calmels L, Sjöström D, Bjelkengren U, Geertsen P, Behrens CF. Clinical implementation of artificial intelligence-driven cone-beam computed tomography-guided online adaptive radiotherapy in the pelvic region. Phys Imaging Radiat Oncol. 2021;17:1–7.

11. Mao W, Riess J, Kim J, Vance S, Chetty IJ, Movsas B, Kretzler A. Evaluation of auto-contouring and dose distributions for online adaptive radiation therapy of patients with locally advanced lung cancers. Pract Radiat Oncol. 2022;12(4):e329–38.

12. Li X, Wu QJ, Wu Q, Wang C, Sheng Y, Wang W, et al. Insights of an AI agent via analysis of prediction errors: a case study of fluence map prediction for radiation therapy planning. Phys Med Biol. 2021;66(23):23NT01.

13. Diebold FX. On the origin(s) and development of the term 'Big Data' (September 21, 2012). PIER Working Paper No. 12-037, Available at SSRN: https://ssrn.com/abstract=2152421.

14. American Association of Physicists in Medicine. TG-263: Standardising nomenclatures in radiation oncology. [PDF] 2018. Retrieved from https://www.aapm.org/pubs/reports/RPT_263.pdf.

15. Nieder C, Andratschke NH, Grosu AL. Increasing frequency of reirradiation studies in radiation oncology: systematic review of highly cited articles. Am J Cancer Res. 2013;3(2):152–8.

16. Flavin A, O'Toole E, Murphy L, Ryan R, McClean B, Faul C, McGibney C, Coyne S, O'Boyle G, Small C, Sims C, Kearney M, Coffey M, O'Donovan A. A national cyberattack affecting radiation therapy: the Irish experience. Adv Radiat Oncol. 2022;7(5):100914.

17. Howell D, Li M, Sutradhar R, et al. Integration of patient-reported outcomes (PROs) for personalised symptom management in "real-world" oncology practices: a population-based cohort comparison study of impact on healthcare utilisation. Support Care Cancer. 2020;28:4933–42.

18. McIntosh C, Conroy L, Tjong MC, et al. Clinical integration of machine learning for curative-intent radiation treatment of patients with prostate cancer. Nat Med. 2021;27:999–1005.

19. Chan MF, Witztum A, Valdes G, et al. Integration of AI and machine learning in radiotherapy QA. Front Artif Intell. 2020;3:577620.

20. Strimbu K, Tavel JA. What are biomarkers? Curr Opin HIV AIDS. 2010;5(6):463–6.

21. van Timmeren J, Cester D, Tanadini-Lang S, et al. Radiomics in medical imaging—"how-to" guide and critical reflection. Insights Imaging. 2020;11:91.

22. Koçak B, Durmaz EŞ, Ateş E, Kılıçkesmez Ö. Radiomics with artificial intelligence: a practical guide for beginners. Diagn Interv Radiol. 2019;25(6):485–95. https://doi.org/10.5152/dir.2019.19321. PMID: 31650960; PMCID: PMC6837295.

23. Shur JD, Doran SJ, Kumar S, Ap Dafydd D, Downey K, O'Connor JPB, Papanikolaou N, Messiou C, Koh DM, Orton MR. Radiomics in oncology: a practical guide. Radiographics. 2021;41(6):1717–32.

24. Ardakani AA, Bureau NJ, Ciaccio EJ, Acharya UR. Interpretation of radiomics features-a pictorial review. Comput Methods Prog Biomed 2022;215:106609.

25. Hirose TA, Arimura H, Ninomiya K. et al. Radiomic prediction of radiation pneumonitis on pretreatment planning computed tomography images prior to lung cancer stereotactic body radiation therapy. Sci Rep 2020;10:20424.

26. Fang M, Kan Y, Dong D, Yu T, Zhao N, Jiang W, Zhong L, Hu C, Luo Y, Tian J. Multi-habitat based Radiomics for the prediction of treatment response to concurrent chemotherapy and radiation therapy in locally advanced cervical cancer. Front Oncol. 2020;10:563.

27. Tran WT, Suraweera H, Quiaoit K, DiCenzo D, Fatima K, Jang D, Bhardwaj D, Kolios C, Karam I, Poon I, Sannachi L, Gangeh M, Sadeghi-Naini A, Dasgupta A, Czarnota GJ. Quantitative ultrasound delta-radiomics during radiotherapy for monitoring treatment responses in head and neck malignancies. Future Sci OA. 2020;6(9):FSO624.

28. Peng L, Parekh V, Huang P, Lin DD, Sheikh K, Baker B, Kirschbaum T, Silvestri F, Son J, Robinson A, Huang E, Ames H, Grimm J, Chen L, Shen C, Soike M, McTyre E, Redmond K, Lim M, Lee J, Jacobs MA, Kleinberg L. Distinguishing true progression from Radionecrosis after stereotactic radiation therapy for brain metastases with machine learning and Radiomics. Int J Radiat Oncol Biol Phys. 2018;102(4):1236–43.

29. Tan VS, Wang E, Chong J, Hope AJ, Tadic T, Kandel S, McIntosh C, Warner A, Palma DA, Lang P. External validation of an artificial intelligence screening tool for interstitial lung disease in patients receiving lung stereotactic ablative radiotherapy. Int J Radiat Oncol Biol Phys. 2024;120(2 Supp):E657–8.

30. Price RG, Kim JP, Zheng W, Chetty IJ, Glide-Hurst C. Image guided radiation therapy using synthetic computed tomography images in brain cancer. Int J Radiat Oncol Biol Phys. 2016;95(4):1281–9.

31. Hoesl M, Corral N, Mistry N. MR-based synthetic CT reimagined [White Paper]. 2022. Siemens Healthineers https://marketing.webassets.siemens-healthineers.com/4db6e75384fa9081/5832cae0e472/siemens-healthineers_syngo-via_white-paper-MR-based-Synthetic-CT.PDF.

32. Boulanger M, Nunes JC, Chourak H, Largent A, Tahri S, Acosta O, De Crevoisier R, Lafond C, Barateau A. Deep learning methods to generate synthetic CT from MRI in radiotherapy: a literature review. Phys Med. 2021;89:265–81.

33. Wang CC, Wu PH, Lin G, Huang YL, Lin YC, Chang YE, Weng JC. Magnetic resonance-based synthetic computed tomography using generative adversarial networks for intracranial tumor radiotherapy treatment planning. J Pers Med. 2022;12(3):361.

34. Chen S, Quan H, Qin A, Yee S, Yan D. MR image-based synthetic CT for IMRT prostate treatment planning and CBCT image-guided localisation. J Appl Clin Med Phys. 2016;17(3):236–45.

35. Young T, Dowling J, Rai R, Liney G, Greer P, Thwaites D, Holloway L. Clinical validation of MR imaging time reduction for substitute/synthetic CT generation for prostate MRI-only treatment planning. Phys Eng Sci Med. 2023;46(3):1015–21.

36. Tang B, Wu F, Fu Y, Wang X, Wang P, Orlandini LC, et al. Dosimetric evaluation of synthetic CT image generated using a neural network for MR-only brain radiotherapy. J Appl Clin Med Phys. 2021;22(3):55–62.

37. Kazemifar S, McGuire S, Timmerman R, Wardak Z., Nguyen, D., Park, Y., … & Owrangi, A. MRI-only brain radiotherapy: assessing the dosimetric accuracy of synthetic CT images generated using a deep learning approach. Radiother Oncol. 2019;136:56–6337.

38. Rossi M, Cerveri P. Comparison of supervised and unsupervised approaches for the generation of synthetic CT from cone-beam CT. Diagnostics. 2021;11(8):1435. https://doi.org/10.3390/diagnostics11081435.

39. Szmul A, Taylor S, Lim P, Cantwell J, Moreira I, Zhang Y, D'Souza D, Moinuddin S, Gaze MN, Gains J, Veiga C. Deep learning based synthetic CT from cone beam CT generation for abdominal paediatric radiotherapy. Phys Med Biol. 2023;68(10):105006.

40. Liu Y, Lei Y, Wang T, Fu Y, Tang X, Curran WJ, Liu T, Patel P, Yang X. CBCT-based synthetic CT generation using deep-attention cycleGAN for pancreatic adaptive radiotherapy. Med Phys. 2020;47(6):2472–83.

41. Baroudi H, Brock KK, Cao W, Chen X, Chung C, Court LE, El Basha MD, Farhat M, Gay S, Gronberg MP, et al. Automated contouring and planning in radiation therapy: what is 'clinically acceptable'? Diagnostics. 2023;13:667.

42. Teguh DN, Levendag PC, Voet PW, Al-Mamgani A, Han X, Wolf TK, et al. Clinical validation of atlas-based auto-segmentation of multiple target volumes and normal tissue (swallowing/mastication) structures in the head and neck. Int J Radiat Oncol Biol Phys. 2011;81:950e957.

43. Sherer MV, Lin D, Elguindi S, Duke S, Tan LT, Cacicedo J, et al. Metrics to evaluate the performance of auto-segmentation for radiation treatment planning: a critical review. Radiother Oncol. 2021;160:185e191.

44. Joskowicz L, Argenone A, Boboc GI, Cucciarelli F, De Rose F, De Santis MC, AIRO. Inter-observer variability of manual contour delineation of structures in CT. Eur Radiol. 2019;29:1391–9.

45. Cardenas CE, Yang J, Anderson BM, Court LE, Brock KB. Advances in auto-segmentation. Semin Radiat Oncol. 2019;29:185e197.

46. Jones S, Thompson K, Porter B, Shepherd M, Sapkaroski D, Grimshaw A, Hargrave C. Automation and artificial intelligence in radiation therapy treatment planning. J Med Radiat Sci. 2024;71:290–8.

47. Johnson CL, Press RH, Simone CB 2nd, Shen B, Tsai P, Hu L, Yu F, Apinorasethkul C, Ackerman C, Zhai H, Lin H, Huang S. Clinical validation of commercial deep-learning based auto-segmentation models for organs at risk in the head and neck region: a single institution study. Front Oncol. 2024;14:1375096. https://doi.org/10.3389/fonc.2024.1375096.

48. Nelms BE, Robinson G, Markham J, Velasco K, Boyd S, Narayan S, Wheeler J, Sobczak ML. Variation in external beam treatment plan quality: an inter-institutional study of planners and planning systems. Pract Radiat Oncol. 2012;2:296–305.

49. Batumalai V, Jameson MG, Forstner DF, Vial P, Holloway LC. How important is dosimetrist experience for intensity modulated radiation therapy? A comparative analysis of a head and neck case. Pract Radiat Oncol. 2013;3:e99–e106.

50. Moore KL, Schmidt R, Moiseenko V, Olsen LA, Tan J, Xiao Y, Galvin J, Pugh S, Seider MJ, Dicker AP, et al. Quantifying unnecessary Normal tissue complication risks due to suboptimal planning: a secondary study of RTOG 0126. Int J Radiat Oncol Biol Phys. 2015;92:228–35.

51. Peters LJ, O'Sullivan B, Giralt J, Fitzgerald TJ, Trotti A, Bernier J, Bourhis J, Yuen K, Fisher R, Rischin D. Critical impact of radiotherapy protocol compliance and quality in the treatment of advanced head and neck cancer: results from TROG 02.02. J Clin Oncol. 2010;28(18):2996–3001.

52. Meyer P, Biston MC, Khamphan C, Marghani T, Mazurier J, Bodez V, Fezzani L, Rigaud PA, Sidorski G, Simon L, Robert C. Automation in radiotherapy treatment planning: examples of use in clinical practice and future trends for a complete automated workflow. Cancer Radiother. 2021;25(6–7):617–22.

53. Momin S, Fu Y, Lei Y, et al. Knowledge-based radiation treatment planning: a data-driven method survey. J Appl Clin Med Phys. 2021;22(8):16–44. https://doi.org/10.1002/acm2.13337.

54. Kisling K, Zhang L, Shaitelman SF, Anderson D, Thebe T, Yang J, Balter PA, Howell RM, Jhingran A, Schmeler K, et al. Automated treatment planning of postmastectomy radiotherapy. Med Phys. 2019;46:3767–75.

55. Moore KL, Brame RS, Low DA, Mutic S. Experience-based quality control of clinical intensity-modulated radiotherapy planning. Int J Radiat Oncol Biol Phys. 2011;81:545–51.

56. Ouyang Z, Liu Shen Z, Murray E, Kolar M, LaHurd D, Yu N, Joshi N, Koyfman S, Bzdusek K, Xia P. Evaluation of auto-planning in IMRT and VMAT for head and neck cancer. J Appl Clin Med Phys. 2019;20:39–47.

57. World Health Organisation. Global cancer burden growing, amidst mounting need for services. Lyon; Geneva: World Health Organisation; 2024. Available from: https://www.who.int/news/item/01-02-2024-global-cancer-burden-growing%2D%2Damidst-mounting-need-for-services.

58. Chen Z, King W, Pearcey R, Kerba M, Mackillop WJ. The relationship between waiting time for radiotherapy and clinical outcomes: a systematic review of the literature. Radiat Oncol. 2008;87(1):3–16.

59. Mackillop WJ. Killing time: the consequences of delays in radiotherapy. Radiat Oncol. 2007;84(1):1–4.

60. Vieira B, Demirtas D, van de Kamer JB, Hans EW, van Harten W. A mathematical programming model for optimising the staff allocation in radiotherapy under uncertain demand. Eur J Oper Res. 2018;270(2):709–22.

61. Saville CE, Smith HK, Bijak K. Operational research techniques applied throughout cancer care services: a review. Health Syst. 2019;8(1):52–73.

62. Olivotto IA, Soo J, Olson RA, Rowe L, French J, Jensen B, et al. Patient preferences for timing and access to radiation therapy. Curr Oncol. 2015;22(4):279–86.

63. Vieira B, Demirtas D, van de Kamer JB, Hans EW, Jongste W, et al. Radiotherapy treatment scheduling: implementing operations research into clinical practice. PLoS One. 2021;16(2):e0247428. https://doi.org/10.1371/journal.pone.0247428.

64. Smart scheduling solution for optimal cancer care operations. https://www.gray-os.com/. Accessed 29 March 2025.

65. Bibault J-E, Giraud P, Burgun A. Big data and machine learning in radiation oncology: state of the art and future prospects. Cancer Lett. 2016;382(1):110–7.

66. Mayo CS, Feng MU, Brock K, et al. Operational ontology for oncology (O3): a professional society-based, multistakeholder, consensus-driven informatics standard supporting clinical and research use of real-world data from patients treated for cancer. Clin Invest. 2023;117(3):533–50.

67. Pillai M, Adapa K, Das SK, Mazur L, Dooley J, Marks LB, Thompson RF, Chera BS. Using artificial intelligence to improve the quality and safety of radiation therapy. J Am Coll Radiol. 2019;16(9, Part B):1267–72.

68. Ahmed Z, Mohamed K, Zeeshan S, Dong X. Artificial intelligence with multi-functional machine learning platform development for better healthcare and precision medicine. Database. 2020;2020:baaa010.

69. Gillan C, Giuliani M, Harnett N, Li W, Dawson LA, Gospodarowicz M, Jaffray DA. Image-guided radiation therapy: unlocking the future through knowledge translation. Int J Radiat Oncol Biol Phys. 2016;96(2):248–50.

70. Goto M. Collective professional role identity in the age of artificial intelligence. J Prof Organ. 2021;8:86–107.

71. Hardy M, Harvey H. Artificial intelligence in diagnostic imaging: impact on the radiography profession. Br J Radiol. 2020;93(1108):20190840.

72. Bak K, Dobrow MJ, Hodgson D, Whitton A. Factors affecting the implementation of complex and evolving technologies: multiple case study of intensity-modulated radiation therapy (IMRT) in Ontario, Canada. BMC Health Serv Res. 2011;11:178.

73. Kane GM. Step-by-step: a model for practice-based learning. J Contin Educ Health Prof. 2007;27(4):220–6.

74. White E, Kane G. Radiation medicine practice in the image-guided radiation therapy era: new roles and new opportunities. In: Seminars in radiation oncology. Elsevier; 2007.

75. Gillan C, Wiljer D, Harnett N, Briggs K, Catton P. Changing stress while stressing change: the role of interprofessional education in mediating stress in the introduction of a transformative technology. J Interprof Care. 2010;24(6):710–21.

76. Jaremko JL, Azar M, Bromwich R, Lum A, Alicia Cheong LH, Gibert M, et al. Canadian Association of Radiologists White Paper on ethical and legal issues related to artificial intelligence in radiology. Can Assoc Radiol J. 2019;70(2):107–18.

77. Gillan C, Hodges B, Wiljer D, Dobrow M. Health care professional association agency in preparing for artificial intelligence: a multiple-case study of radiation medicine and medical imaging in the Canadian context. Int J Rad Onc Biol Phys, epub ahead of print.

78. Tang A, Tam R, Cadrin-Chênevert A, Guest W, Chong J, Barfett J, et al. Canadian Association of Radiologists white paper on artificial intelligence in radiology. Can Assoc Radiol J. 2018;69(2):120–35.

79. American Society of Radiologic Technologists HCIAC Corporate Roundtable Subcommittee on Artificial Intelligence. The artificial intelligence era: The role of radiologic technologists and radiation therapists. 2020. 76.

80. International Society of Radiographers and Radiological Technologists & the European Federation of Radiographer Societies. Artificial intelligence and the radiographer/radiological technologist profession: a joint statement of the international society of radiographers and radiological technologists & the European Federation of Radiographer Societies. 2020.

81. The Society and College of Radiographers. The Society and College of Radiographers policy statement: artificial intelligence, 1st edition. 2020.

82. Canadian Artificial Intelligence and Data in Radiotherapy Alliance. https://www.cadra-acadr.ca/. Accessed 29 March 2025.

Dr. Caitlin Gillan is the Provincial Professional Practice Leader for Radiation Therapy for BC Cancer, in British Columbia, Canada. She practiced previously at the Princess Margaret Cancer Centre in Toronto before stepping into leadership, first as the Manager of Education and Practice at Toronto's Joint Department of Medical Imaging. She is an Associate Professor in the Department of Radiation Oncology at the University of Toronto and in the Division of Radiation Oncology for the University of British Columbia. Her research interests include advanced practice in radiation therapy and interprofessional education and practice approaches to the integration of novel technologies and innovations, namely image-guided radiation therapy and artificial intelligence.

Yannie Lai is a radiation therapist and practice-based researcher at Sunnybrook Health Sciences Centre. In her undergraduate studies, she enrolled in the Arts and Science Entrepreneurship Program at the University of Toronto Department of Computer Science where she opened her eyes to building solutions with a purpose whilst collaborating with computer science students. While working as a therapist, she then completed Michener's AI in Healthcare Certificate program in 2022 which allowed her to explore and understand the importance of AI enabled care to improve patient outcomes and patient experience.

Brian Liszewski is a radiation therapist and Advisor at Ontario Health, and a Lecturer at the University of Toronto's Department of Radiation Oncology. He holds a diploma in Radiation Therapy and a degree in Radiation Sciences from the Michener Institute and University of Toronto joint Medical Radiation Science Program. Brian has served in various roles including treatment, simulation, dosimetry, leadership, research, quality assurance, and education. Currently, he focuses on improving equitable access to care across Ontario through the administration of the radiation equipment grant, capacity planning, and supporting the provincial radiation treatment program.

Anita Vloet is a radiation therapist with over two decades of experience at the Princess Margaret Cancer Centre. She holds a certification in Artificial Intelligence in Health Care and has an interest in Operations Research. As an advocate for clinical research and innovation she has been involved in numerous clinical projects such as automated patient and staff scheduling throughout her career. She serves on the Canadian Association of Medical Radiation Technologists AI Professional Advisory Committee which aims to engage medical radiation technologists in developing, collaborating and integrating AI-enabled practice.

Person-Centred and Personalised Care for Radiography in the AI Era

12

Johnathan Hewis, Jae Hargan,
Ruth Mary Strudwick, and Cláudia Sá dos Reis

12.1   Introduction

The professional identity of both diagnostic and therapeutic radiographers consists of both technological expertise and patient-care competencies, as a requirement to meet the complex demands of this profession in a fast-changing world [1]. While technical skills enable radiographers to be experts in using advanced medical imaging and radiotherapy equipment, the humanistic values ensure they can effectively care for the different patients they work with at the radiology and radiotherapy departments. Person-centred care (PCC) has been evolving since the 1980s, building on the work of the Picker Institute [2], who strived to achieve their vision of:

> The highest quality person centred care for all, always.

The Picker Institute's eight patient-centred care principles can be found in Fig. 12.1.

The Health Foundation [3] built upon this work to develop their definition of person-centred care (PCC):

> Person-centred care supports people to develop the knowledge, skills and confidence they need to more effectively manage and make informed decisions about their own health and health care [3].

Within the United Kingdom (UK), there is an increased emphasis on national guidelines to define and ensure the quality of patient care provided by all health professionals. This can be found in publications such as the NHS Five Year Forward View [4], The Long-Term Plan [5], and the Health Foundation's Person-Centred Care Made Simple document [6]. These publications are driving forward changes in attitudes to patient care. The Francis Report [7] and 'Hello My Name is' campaign [8] also highlighted the need for improved communication skills from professionals to demonstrate care and compassion when providing healthcare services.

on behalf of Association of Healthcare Technology Providers for Imaging, Radiotherapy and Care (AXREM)

J. Hewis (✉)
Charles Sturt University,
Port Macquarie, NSW, Australia
e-mail: jhewis@csu.edu.au

J. Hargan
Service User and Carer Involvement Lead, University of Bradford, Bradford, UK
e-mail: j.hargan@bradford.ac.uk

R. M. Strudwick
University of Suffolk, Suffolk, UK
e-mail: r.strudwick@uos.ac.uk

C. Sá dos Reis
University of Applied Sciences and Arts Western Switzerland, Delemonte, Switzerland
e-mail: Claudia.sadosreis@hesav.ch

© The Author(s), under exclusive license to Springer Nature Switzerland AG 2026
C. Malamateniou et al. (eds.), *Artificial Intelligence for Radiographers*,
https://doi.org/10.1007/978-3-032-05080-9_12

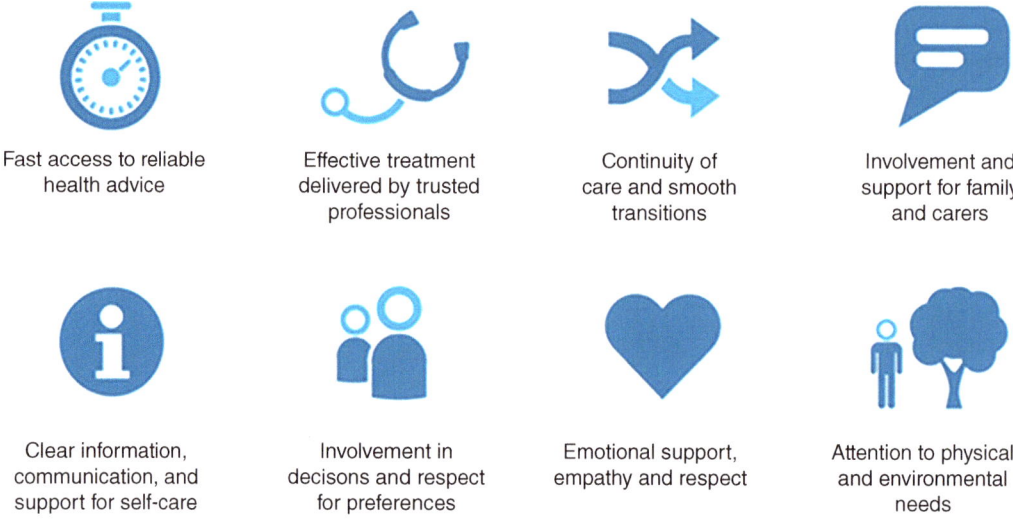

Fast access to reliable
health advice

Effective treatment
delivered by trusted
professionals

Continuity of
care and smooth
transitions

Involvement and
support for family
and carers

Clear information,
communication, and
support for self-care

Involvement in
decisons and respect
for preferences

Emotional support,
empathy and respect

Attention to physical
and environmental
needs

Fig. 12.1 The Picker Institute's patient-centred care principles [2]

12.2 What Matters to Patients

Personalised care takes this a step further and ensures that service users are given choice and control over their mental and physical health. A one-size-fits-all health and care system is not able to meet the increasing complexity of people's needs and expectations. Personalised care is based and driven by 'what matters' to people and their individual strengths and needs.

Within radiography practice, there can often be a tension between the highly technical nature of the professional role in either image production or treatment delivery, and the time, training and personal resources available for patient care. The COVID-19 pandemic has led to a greater focus on patient-care skills, and this highlighted the importance of the quality of the interaction between radiographer and patient to make a difference to their individual experiences. With more access to information and the emergence of the 'expert patient' [9], patients are now more empowered than ever before in managing their own health and they have a stronger 'voice' when evaluating clinical services involved in their care. They are not only the 'consumers of care, with their advocacy they can also become producers of health and wellbeing' [10]. Elements of person-centred care are also embedded within

professional body publications and guidance documents that underline radiographers' professional responsibilities [11]. Person-centred care is key to the interaction between the patient and radiographer, with the radiographer needing to avoid making assumptions, always consider the patient's values and prioritise what matters to them [12].

A qualitative study by Hyde and Hardy (2021) has shown that communication is at the centre of patient and practitioner interactions. Respectful and inclusive language, offering opportunity to ask questions, respecting their privacy, giving them choice and adopting a holistic approach to healthcare, all these matter to patients [13]. They have coproduced with patients a PCC audit tool customised for radiography, which can be found in Fig. 12.2.

Advances in imaging and radiotherapy technology are changing how services are delivered; this includes the use of artificial intelligence (AI) technology leading to greater automation. AI promises a new era of highly personalised medicine that is more accessible, providing faster, more accurate and potentially predictive medical diagnoses [14]. AI has the potential to free up healthcare practitioners from administrative tasks, increasing time for and with their patients through significant efficiency improvements

Pause & Check audit tool for measuring patient centred care in diagnostic radiography.

Element	Considerations to be made	Yes, No or Not Applicable
Pre Examination Checklist		
Patient	Have you ensured that the patient and/or carer understands what is going to happen during the examination?	
	Have you provided an opportunity for the patient and/or carer to ask questions about the examination?	
	Have you considered the role of the carer in the examination (if appropriate)?	
	Has communication been appropriate for the individual patient so far?	
Attire	Does patient need to change? If so, is there an appropriate gown size for them?	
	Have you explored the availability of dressing gowns?	
	Have you considered whether use of theatre scrubs or a tracksuit is appropriate?	
User needs	Does the patient have any specific needs which should be considered?	
& wellbeing	Does the patient need any assistance to change?	
	Has the patient been offered options to help support them during the examination, such as pads?	
	Could the patient benefit from a break midway through the examination?	
Safety & security	How can the patient be supported to maintain the position needed for the examination safely?	
	How will the patient's belongings be kept safe & secure for the duration of the examination?	
	Has the safety of the carer been considered (if appropriate)?	
	Have infection prevention and control measures been considered?	
Environment	Do the lighting levels need to be adjusted for the patient?	
	Have you offered a choice of music (if available)?	
	Have blankets or other ways to maintain warmth been offered?	
	Are examination aids available?	
During Examination Checklist		
Patient	Does the patient and/or carer understand what is happening during the examination?	
	Are there continued opportunities for the patient and/or carer to ask questions about the examination?	
	Does the carer have an appropriate role in the examination?	
	Has communication been appropriate for the individual patient so far?	
Attire	Is the patient appropriately covered by the clothing they are wearing for the examination?	
	Was there a dressing gown available for the patient?	
User needs	Have any specific needs the patient has been considered?	
& wellbeing	Has the patient been provided with options to help support them during the examination, such as pads?	
	Has the patient/carer been asked if a break is required midway through the examination?	
Safety & security	Has the patient been supported to maintain the position needed for the examination safely?	
	Are the patient's belongings safe & secure for the duration of the examination?	
	Has the safety of the carer been considered (if appropriate)?	
	Have infection prevention and control measures been followed?	
Environment	Are the lighting levels suitable for the patient?	
	Was a choice of music provided (if available)?	
	Were blankets or other ways to maintain warmth offered?	
	Were examination aids available?	
Post Examination Checklist		
Patient	Have you ensured that the patient and/or carer understands how to get the results?	
	Have you provided an opportunity for the patient and/or carer to ask questions about how the examination went?	
Attire	Does the patient need to change back into their own clothes now?	
	Does the patient need any assistance to change?	
User needs	Does the patient/carer know what the next steps are in the patients' diagnostic journey?	
& wellbeing	Does the patient have any specific needs which should be considered?	
	Does the patient need assistance to access their travel home?	
Safety & security	Is there any specific after care advice the patient/carer requires?	
	Can the patient eat and drink normally now?	
	Are there any infection prevention and control measures which need to be highlighted?	
Environment	Does the patient know the way out of the department?	

Fig. 12.2 A radiography-specific 'pause and check' audit tool for patient-centred care delivery [13]

[15]. The idea that AI can theoretically provide a solution to our lack of time with patients is highly appealing. However, the real-world role of AI in radiography is still emerging with heterogenous uptake and clinical implementation. There is no clear roadmap or linear pathway for AI adoption because every clinical context is unique and much exists only in the research realms. The direct clinical impact of AI on PCC at scale is currently uncertain and is yet to be fully realised [16]. Will the real-world implementation of AI enhance or hinder patient experience and care? We argue that any efficiency improvements should be used by radiographers and other clinical practitioners to also spend more time caring for patients. After all, the trust built by healthcare professionals with their patients is 'time-honoured' [17]. Given the emergence of more empowered patients, the shape person-centred care will take in the future will not only depend on policymakers; it can also be carved through the thoughts, intentions, behaviours and actions of healthcare practitioners, as patient advocates, and the patients themselves. More about the evolving relationship of radiographers and patients, and the ethical implications of AI in changing these interactions, can be found in Chap. 3.

12.3 The Care Journey in an AI World

For service users, radiography and radiotherapy already represents an intersection between high-level technology and a human, typically mediated by a radiographer. Our interactions with our patients are typically time limited, often highly task-orientated and can quickly become mechanistic in nature for the service user [18]. The adoption and implementation of AI tools adds a new opaque layer or black box aspect to an increasingly automated experience that needs to be carefully considered from the patient's perspective [19]. For service users and society more broadly, challenges for AI implementation in radiography include additional concerns around privacy, equity, and fairness [20]. The integration of advanced medical technologies can create greater distance between patients and healthcare practitioners, potentially leading to a loss of human connection, reduced empathy and compassion and even dehumanisation [21, 22]. The emergence of responsible AI is not just a tokenistic move; it is a necessary initiative to safeguard patient safety and patient-centredness [23].

Given we are in the nascency of AI implementation in radiography, it is hard to know the extent to which AI will permeate our daily clinical practice. Therefore, it is uncertain where AI tools will directly intersect with the patient pathway and how they will impact end user care or experience [24]. So far, large-scale real-world implementation of AI tools in radiography has predominantly focused on improving clinical tasks that are cognitive in nature, such as medical image analysis, augmenting human expertise to aid and improve decision-making [25]. But many more areas, such as the optimal communication of patient choices or personalisation of patient experience, require further development [26]. With the development and advances in deep learning and generative AI in particular, AI algorithms can already perform on a par or better than a human to analyse medical images thereby reducing diagnostic error [27]. Other recent clinical AI applications in radiography include solutions that can manage patient scheduling, optimise protocols and treatment planning, help reduce radiation dose and scan time and the provision of novel AI-assisted advanced reconstruction and post-processing tools [28]. More about AI implementation challenges and enablers can be found in Chap. 4.

There is significant hype and optimism that AI will enhance care and provide a more personalised healthcare model. Will service users be accepting of these new, rapidly emerging, disruptive AI tools, and will they empower individuals to better understand and take control of their own healthcare? Two of the Picker Institute's [2] core PCC principles include 'involvement in decisions and respect for preferences" and "involvement and support for family and carers' (Fig. 12.1). Therefore, engagement with service users is a critically important piece of the AI implementation jigsaw puzzle. An example of patient preferences, for those with chronic illness, and what matters to them can be seen in Fig. 12.3. This can vary between different patient populations.

AI is changing how patients think about their care. Studies about patient perspectives and acceptability of this new technology are divided. Some studies show enthusiasm about the potential of higher accuracy and service efficiency, while others discuss varied concerns. These concerns related to AI safety, risk to patient autonomy and choice, potential increases in healthcare costs, data bias, consent and data security [29]. This can impact patient trust to AI and their acceptability of these technologies to be used in their care. Radiographers can be central to this communication and reassurance of patients as human mediators, but before they do so, they need to ensure they understand AI well themselves. This is why AI training is not anymore a luxury but a central responsibility of radiographers' role: it becomes an integral part of who we are and what we do and our knowledge, skills and confidence in using AI ensure the safety and efficiency of our interactions with patients and other

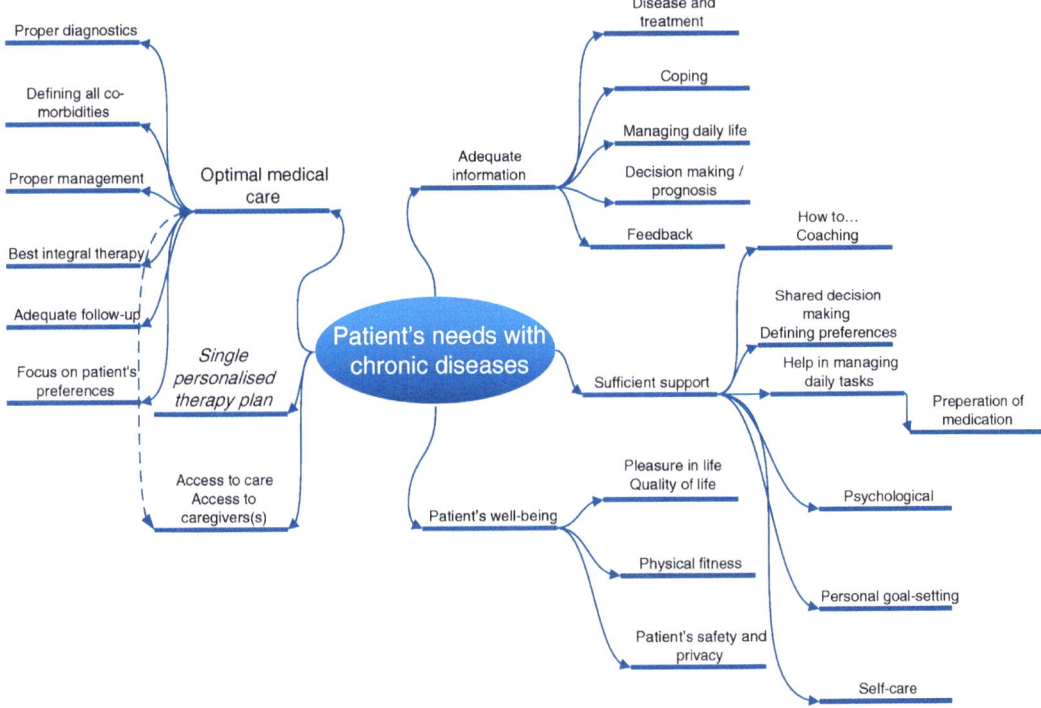

Fig. 12.3 Patient needs when having a chronic illness: A diagram that shows what patients with chronic illness prioritise: (**a**) optimal medical care, (**b**) personalised treatment plans, (**c**) enabling involvement of family/carer in their care, (**d**) clear information, (**e**) sufficient support and (**f**) attention to their well-being [30]

healthcare professionals in our clinical practice. Chapter 3 discusses further ethical concerns that are raised by the use of AI in radiography, impacting human interactions in healthcare.

12.4 Case Studies of Patient Care

The chapter will now explore four real-world case studies as exemplars where AI tools directly intersect with service user experience and impact on their care. The discussion draws upon consultation with service user group members and it is led by their perspectives. It illustrates how important it is to not make assumptions about what service users want, but to take into consideration their individual values and priorities each time [31, 32].

Case Study 12.1: AI to Provide Workflow Management/Exam Prioritisation
AI offers potential to automate administrative tasks and could be utilised to optimise the utilisation of hospital beds based on data and manage imaging referrals and waiting lists for imaging examinations [33]. Imaging protocols could also be managed via AI to reduce user error when setting up imaging examinations. Our service users were strongly in favour of this use of AI, as it could translate to better appointment systems, reduced patient waiting and more efficient use of resources.

Case Study 12.2: AI Assessing Social Determinants of Health to Predict Populations at Risk or Underutilised Care

AI can be utilised to review data about hospital admissions and to predict which members of the population and groups of people are more likely to access health or social care and would be admitted to hospital [27]. This represents a transition away from a reactive healthcare model to a more proactive approach [34]. An example of this can be found in the use of social determinants being used to predict cardiac outcomes in females with breast cancer [35]. In this study, it was found that AI machine learning models incorporating social determinants of health, demographics, risk factors, tumour characteristics and treatments were developed and compared. The results of the study showed that the inclusion of social determinants of health enhanced the performance of the machine learning model's performance in forecasting major adverse cardiac events within 2 years of breast cancer diagnosis.

This could be applied to other areas of healthcare, where AI could be utilised to predict vulnerable groups within society. Our service users were in favour of this as a development of AI, as they felt that anything that could help people access healthcare when needed would be beneficial to their outcomes and well-being. However, they also had some reservations; they were concerned about how all this information would be used, treated by governments, big pharmaceuticals, insurance companies and investors who have a vested interest in data sourcing that may detect personal vulnerabilities.

Case Study 12.3: Smart AI Chatbot for Healthcare Assistance

Smart AI chatbots are used in several commercial industries to provide online assistance for customers, for example, banks and insurance companies. Patient-care assistance technologies, such as the AI chatbot, can be 'trained' to respond to different questions and provide help to frequently asked questions or provide virtual health assistants to provide more personalised remote support [26]. Smart AI chatbots have the potential to be used in healthcare; this could be providing assistance to book imaging appointments, to prevent or minimise non-shows, to remind individuals to take required medications or to modify their diet prior to their examinations [27].

Our service users were not too convinced about the use of chatbots; they made the point that AI can only operate based on what solutions are put into their databank, whereas a human brain has the capacity to 'think outside the box'. They felt AI cannot replicate emotional intelligence and empathy. Therefore, this could create frustration for the service users. The use of AI for empathy was unheard of 5 years ago. However, recent AI tools using generative AI have shown that AI can produce text and speech, which can be seen as highly empathetic [36]. AI, though, remains unpredictable, and concerns remain about the impact of prolonged human interactions with AI-enabled chatbots on patients' mental health and the addiction to a digital reality that might isolate them from their real social life.

Case Study 12.4: AI for Disease Detection

AI has already been proven to provide accurate diagnosis of pathologies on radiographic images. Hwang et al. [37] carried out a study looking at AI reporting for chest images and found that AI was effective at detecting lung nodules. A variety of AI applications for disease detection is covered in the Chaps. 5, 6, 7, 8, 9, 10, and 11 dedicated to different medical imaging modalities in this textbook and beyond. The service users were really keen on this AI tool, stating that if AI was better than people at the diagnosis of pathology on images, then it should be used to improve patient outcomes.

12.5 Implementing AI to Enhance Person-Centred and Personalised Care

Digital technology plays a crucial role in healthcare and will continue to develop further. At the same time, it introduces barriers for certain patients, including those who have none or limited digital literacy, access or interest. Socioeconomic inequalities play a role in that those economically disadvantaged may be excluded [38]. People in rural communities may not have access to effective digital infrastructure [39], preventing them from accessing health information, medical records and telehealth services. Some patients have raised concerns about the decrease in interaction with healthcare professionals [22]. Patients can see AI as depersonalising care, especially if you value emotional support, rapport and reassurance or have concerns about the privacy of your data.

12.6 Values-Based Practice

We discussed above that patient preferences matter. When developing any AI tool to use in healthcare, the preferences of service users should always be considered. This can be done via coproduction and by incorporating values-based practice. Values-based practice (VBP) is the consideration of the individual service user's values in making decisions about their care [40]. By their values, we mean the unique preferences, concerns and expectations each person brings to a practice encounter, which must be integrated into any decisions about their care. VBP considers and highlights what matters, and is important to the patient [31]. We should not reflect our own values upon our service users. We need to learn to engage with service users and respect their choices.

We can do this by asking our service users to tell us what is important to them and providing them with enough information so that they can make informed choices. This is an important aspect of person-centred care and VBP [40]. We also need to be aware that different people have different values. Service users are likely to value very different things from practitioners. We also need to recognise that values can vary over time. For example, someone's values when commencing treatment may not reflect those towards the end of a course of treatment. In addition, one person's values may vary, depending on the situation, and how they are feeling. Values are variable and fluid.

When discussing with service users about AI, we need to bear this in mind. Patients generally support the use of health data for AI in radiology as it is perceived to benefit others with similar health needs and receive an earlier diagnosis and more accurate treatment [41]. Concerns are focused on the privacy of personal data, unintended or uncontrolled use of data and risk of discrimination due to bias of AI algorithms [42]. Research on AI systems has shown bias against certain community groups and protected characteristics including ethnicity and sex [43]. This can be mitigated by collecting more representative demographic data and involving patients in the design of AI technologies [37].

12.7 The Importance of Coproduction for Elevating Patient Voice and Choice

At the heart of patient-centred care is patient engagement in the decision-making of their care. A fundamental principle in the NHS is 'No decision about me, without me', a phrase encapsulated in the White Paper, 'Equity and Excellence; Liberating the NHS' [44]. This white paper outlines a vision for patient and public involvement. As the end users of AI in healthcare are patients, it seems appropriate and beneficial to use models of coproduction which go further than involvement [45]. Coproduction is where all stakeholders work in partnership and share power and decision-making, sustained over a long time so working relationships can develop [46]. To adopt a coproductive approach to involving patients and carers, a series of steps can help assess how you can work towards full coproduction. This is demonstrated in Fig. 12.4 through the concept of the ladder of coproduction [46].

Involvement and coproduction are not new concepts and practices, but are increasingly becoming the norm within healthcare education, research and service evaluation, yet currently there is limited information about patient involvement in the development and implementation of AI technologies. Despite this, involving patients with AI technologies will benefit all stakeholders, especially if conducted in an environment that enables everyone to reach value-driven collective outcomes.

Engaging members of the public will not just create technology that is useful; it will also help them to understand, embrace and trust the potential for current and future AI in healthcare [47]. At the same time, patients' unique insights and lived experiences have the potential to identify benefits and harm of AI [48], which healthcare professionals may not immediately recognise. Their involvement can also help improve AI on fairness and transparency of algorithms [49] and reduce mistrust in AI technologies [47].

The process of coproduction has the potential to change relationships between health providers, AI developers and patients [17]. Stakeholders

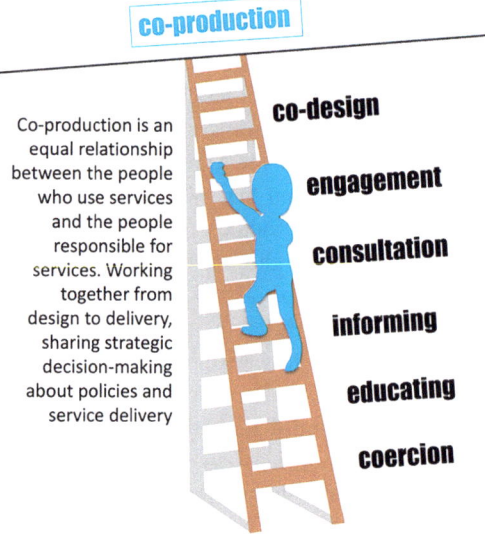

Fig. 12.4 The ladder of coproduction, adapted with permission from Think Local Act Personal and National Co-production Advisory Group [46]

need to be mindful that authentic coproduction can be a new way of working and may be difficult for those who are not used to working in a cooperative approach [50]. It is key that all knowledge sources are valued equally [51], recognising that patients do not provide extra knowledge that feeds into already formed epistemologies, but is welcomed as an alternative that contributes to the wider knowledge development [52].

To ensure patients feel safe and supported during coproduction, they have to draw on their lived experiences in healthcare; coproduction facilitators need to reflect on the possibility of triggering painful experiences [53]. McVey et al. [54] suggest discussing this at the start of a coproduction relationship and encouraging patients to explore how involvement could impact their mental well-being. Patients need to know they have the flexibility to opt in and out, as needed. Patients need to also be fully supported, therefore an inclusive environment from the outset is crucial. This could start with exploring what people already understand about AI, how algorithms could, for example, analyse medical images, impact diagnosis and aid radiological decisions. The discussion could then evolve into the basics on what AI applications in medical imaging can achieve or what other everyday applications used AI in daily life these patient coproducers have encountered, like apps on our phones or social media. Lay terms and explanations need to be used and jargon to be avoided, especially as some patients may have limited digital literacy or comprehension of how AI works. It is important to involve people with diverse lived experiences, protected characteristics and varying levels of digital or other literacy, including those with no knowledge of AI [55], but also to be mindful that diversity of coproduction groups may not be enough if accessibility to discussions is not ascertained through user-friendly platforms [52].

The discussion could explore patients' understanding around AI that may be unfounded and driven by mistrust, which is not helped by a culture of misinformation and multiple references to scaremongering by the media. There should be an exploration of common concerns including the perception that AI can misdiagnose conditions, personal data is lost or made public or will replace healthcare practitioners. This is all understandable, especially if people may fear the loss of empathy and rapport that digitalisation could bring upon healthcare. It is vital to discuss success stories about AI based on published peer-reviewed research evidence to ensure trust is reinstated for future healthcare visits.

12.8 Staff and Patient Education and Training

From the outset, student radiographers need to be adept at communicating with service users of different ages and from different backgrounds. They need to be able to demonstrate empathy and compassion. This is crucial to the role of the radiographer and, even more so, when the use of technology is increasing, service users need to feel valued and respected.

Recent research [19] identified a lack of knowledge and uncertainty amongst radiography professionals about AI implementation and its governance. This highlights that there is still a critical education and training gap that needs to be addressed. The perception and needs of service users should be included as a central compo-

nent of any AI education and training curriculum to include exploration of PCC, VBP and coproduction. Equally service users need to be educated, as discussed above, not only on the risks but, very importantly, on the benefits of AI for their diagnosis, treatment and well-being.

12.9 Top Tips for Implementing PCC in the AI Era

Our top five tips for implementing person-centred care in the era of AI:

1. Actively listen to each patient and understand what is important to them.
2. Look beyond the disease, test or intervention and see the whole person.
3. Treat each patient as an individual.
4. Do not trade-off efficiency over person-centred care. Caring needs time but saves time later down the patient pathway by avoiding miscommunications.
5. Involve service users in a coproductive way from the start of any research or service improvement project relating to their care, including the ones associated to AI. Patient-centred care in radiography does not stop in clinical practice. As we have seen, it also relates to how we do education and research.

12.10 Chapter Summary

AI as a disruptive technology must be harnessed to improve service user experience, increase autonomy and pivot towards greater person-centred and personalised care. PCC is a central consideration for any technological developments. Personalised care is based on 'what matters' to people and their individual strengths and needs. It is not a one-size-fits-all approach. Active engagement with service users through coproduction incorporating VBP is essential for the effective development and implementation of AI tools. Efficiencies gained through AI technologies should be judiciously used by radiographers to enhance and increase patient care, where possible.

References

1. Niemi A, Passivaara L. Meaning contents of radiographers' professional identify as illustrated in a professional journal – A discourse analytical approach. Radiography. 2007;13:258–64.

2. Picker Institute Europe. Principles of person centred care. 2019. Available at: https://www.picker.org/about-us/picker-principles-of-person-centred-care/. Accessed 11 Oct 2024.

3. The Health Foundation. Person-centred care made simple. 2014. Available at: http://www.health.org.uk/sites/health/files/PersonCentredCareMadeSimple.pdf. Accessed 29 Oct 2024.

4. NHS England. Five Year Forward View. 2014. Available at: https://www.england.nhs.uk/five-year-forward-view/. Accessed 29 Oct 2024.

5. NHS England. The NHS long term plan. 2019. Available at: https://www.longtermplan.nhs.uk/publication/nhs-long-term-plan/. Accessed 29 Oct 2024.

6. The Health Foundation. Person-centred care made simple – what everyone should know about person-centred care. 2016. ISBN 978-1-906461-56-0.

7. Francis R. Report of the Mid Staffordshire NHS Foundation Trust Public Inquiry. London: The Stationery Office; 2013. Available at: https://www.gov.uk/government/publications/report-of-the-mid-staffordshire-nhs-foundation-trust-public-inquiry/. Accessed 22 Nov 2024.

8. Granger K. Hello my name is Campaign. 2013. Available at : https://www.hellomynameis.org.uk/. Accessed 22 Nov 2024.

9. Donaldson L. Expert patients usher in a new era of opportunity for the NHS. BMJ. 2003;326(7402):1279–80. https://doi.org/10.1136/bmj.326.7402.1279.

10. Lorig K. Partnerships between expert patients and physicians. Lancet. 2002;359(9309):814–5. https://doi.org/10.1016/S0140-6736(02)07959-X.

11. Hyde E, Hardy M. Patient centred care in diagnostic radiography (part 1): perceptions of service users and service deliverers. Radiography. 2021;27(1):8–13. https://doi.org/10.1016/j.radi.2020.04.015. Epub 2020 Jun 13

12. Strudwick RM. Embedding values-based practice in day-to-day clinical practice. Synergy News, October 2019, p 11.

13. Hyde E, Hardy M. Patient centred care in diagnostic radiography (part 2): A qualitative study of the perceptions of service users and service deliverers. Radiography (Lond). 2021;27(2):322–31. https://doi.org/10.1016/j.radi.2020.09.008.

14. Poalelungi, et al. Advancing patient care: how artificial intelligence is transforming healthcare. J Pers Med. 2023;13(8):1214. https://doi.org/10.3390/jpm13081214.

15. Sauerbrei, et al. The impact of artificial intelligence on the person-centred, doctor-patient relationship: some problems and solutions. BMC Med Inform Decis Mak. 2023;23(73) https://doi.org/10.1186/s12911-023-02162-y.

16. Khera R, Simon M, Ross J, et al. Automation bias and assistive AI – risk of harm from AI-driven clinical decision support. JAMA. 2023;330(23):2255–7. https://doi.org/10.1001/jama.2023.22557.

17. Topol E. The topol review. Preparing the healthcare workforce to deliver the digital future. An independent report on behalf of the Secretary of State for Health and Social Care. 2019. Available at: http://topol.hee.nhs.uk.wp-content/uploads/HEE-Topol-Review-2019.pdf. Accessed 27 Feb 24.

18. Strudwick R. Labelling patients. Radiography. 2016;22(1):50–5.

19. Stogiannos N, Litosseliti L, O'Regan T, Scurr E, Barnes A, Kumar A, Malik R, Pogose M, Harvey H, McEntee M, Malamateniou C. Black box no more: a cross-sectional multi-disciplinary survey for exploring governance and guiding adoption of AI in medical imaging and radiotherapy in the UK. Int J Med Inform. 2024;186:105423. https://doi.org/10.1016/j.ijmedinf.2024.105423.

20. Koski E, Murphy J. AI in Healthcare. Stud Health Technol Inform. 2021;15:284:295–299. https://doi.org/10.3233/SHTI210726.

21. Haque O, Waytz A. Dehumanization in medicine: causes, solutions, and functions. Perspect Psychol Sci. 2012;7(2):176e86.

22. Temple S, Rowbottom C, Simpson J. Patient views on the implementation of artificial intelligence in radiotherapy. Radiography. 2023;29(1):S112–6.

23. Walsh G, et al. Responsible AI practice and AI education are central to AI implementation: a rapid review for all medical imaging professionals in Europe. BJR Open. 2023; https://doi.org/10.1259/bjro.20230033.

24. Malamateniou C. Technology-enabled patient care in medical radiation sciences: the two sides of the coin. J Med Radiat Sci. 2024;71(3):326–9.

25. Zsidai, et al. A practical guide to the implementation of AI in orthopaedic research – part 1: opportunities in clinical application and overcoming existing challenges. J Exp Orthop. 2023;10(117) https://doi.org/10.1186/s40634-023-00683-z.

26. Champendal M, Marmy L, Malamateniou C, Sá Dos Reis C. Artificial intelligence to support person-centred care in breast imaging – a scoping review. J Med Imaging Radiat Sci. 2023;54(3):511–44. https://doi.org/10.1016/j.jmir.2023.04.001.

27. Miller DD, Brown EW. Artificial intelligence in medical practice: the question to the answer? Am J Med. 2018;131(2):12933.

28. Hardy M, Harvey H. Artificial intelligence in diagnostic imaging: impact on the radiography profession. Br J Radiol. 2020;93(1108):20190840. https://doi.org/10.1259/bjr.20190840.

29. Richardson JP, Smith C, Curtis S, Watson S, Zhu X, Barry B, Sharp RR. Patient apprehensions about the use of artificial intelligence in healthcare. NPJ Digit Med. 2021;4(1):140. https://doi.org/10.1038/s41746-021-00509-1.

30. Barrett M, Boyne J, Brandts J, Brunner-La Rocca HP, De Maesschalck L, De Wit K, Dixon L, Eurlings C, Fitzsimons D, Golubnitschaja O, Hageman A, Heemskerk F, Hintzen A, Helms TM, Hill L, Hoedemakers T, Marx N, McDonald K, Mertens M, Müller-Wieland D, Palant A, Piesk J, Pomazanskyi A, Ramaekers J, Ruff P, Schütt K, Shekhawat Y, Ski CF, Thompson DR, Tsirkin A, van der Mierden K, Watson C, Zippel-Schultz B. Artificial intelligence supported patient self-care in chronic heart failure: a paradigm shift from reactive to predictive, preventive and personalised care. EPMA J. 2019;10(4):445–64. https://doi.org/10.1007/s13167-019-00188-9.

31. Fulford KWM, Newton-Hughes A, Strudwick R, Handa A. Values-based practice for imaging and therapy professionals: an introduction. Imaging Oncol. 2018:26–33.

32. Busch et al. Multinational attitudes towards AI in healthcare and diagnostics among hospital patients. medRxiv 2024.09.01.24312016.

33. Potocnik J, Foley S, Thomas E. Current and potential applications of artificial intelligence in medical imaging practice: a narrative review. J Med Imaging Radiat Sci. 2023;54:376–85.

34. Hewis J. A salutogenic approach: changing the paradigm. J Med Imaging Radiat Sci. 2023;54(2):s17–21. https://doi.org/10.1016/j.jmir.2023.02.004.

35. Stabellini N, Cullen J, Moore JX, Dent S, Sutton AL, Shanahan J, Montero AJ, Guha A. Social determinants of health data improve the prediction of cardiac outcomes in females with breast cancer. Cancers (Basel). 2023;15(18):4630. https://doi.org/10.3390/cancers15184630. PMID: 37760599; PMCID: PMC10526347.

36. Ayers JW, Poliak A, Dredze M, Leas EC, Zhu Z, Kelley JB, Faix DJ, Goodman AM, Longhurst CA, Hogarth M, Smith DM. Comparing physician and artificial intelligence Chatbot responses to patient questions posted to a public social media forum. JAMA Intern Med. 2023;183(6):589–96. https://doi.org/10.1001/jamainternmed.2023.1838.

37. Hwang SH, et al. Clinical outcomes and actual consequence of lung nodules incidentally detected on chest radiographs by artificial intelligence. Sci Rep. 2023;13:19732. https://doi.org/10.1038/s41598-023-47194-6.

38. Holmes H, Burgess G. Digital exclusion and poverty in the UK: how structural inequality shapes experiences of getting online. Digit Geogra Soc. 2022;3:100041. https://doi.org/10.1016/j.diggeo.2022.100041.

39. Hadjiat Y. Healthcare inequity and digital health – A bridge for the divide, or further erosion of the chasm? PLoS Digit Health. 2023;2(6) https://doi.org/10.1371/journal.pdig.0000268.

40. Strudwick RM, Harvey-Lloyd JM, Bleiker J, Gooch J, Hancock A, Hyde E, Newton-Hughes A. Person-centred care in radiography: skills for providing effective patient care. Wiley; 2023.

41. Aggarwal R, Farag. S, Martin G, Ashrafian H, Darzi A. Patient perceptions on data sharing and applying artificial intelligence to health care data: cross-sectional survey. J Med Internet Res. 2021;23(8):e26162.

42. Ueda D, Kakinuma T, Fujita S, Kamagata K, Fushimi Y, Ito R, Matsui Y, Nozaki T, Nakaura T, Fujima N, Tatsugami F, Yanagawa M, Hirata K, Yamada A, Tsuboyama T, Kawamura M, Fujioka T, Naganawa S. Fairness of artificial intelligence in healthcare: review and recommendations. Jpn J Radiol. 2024;42 https://doi.org/10.1007/s11604-023-01474-3.

43. Zou J, Schiebinger L. AI can be sexist and racist – it's time to make it fair. Nature. 2018;559:324–6. https://doi.org/10.1038/d41586-018-05707-8.

44. Department of Health. Equity and excellence: liberating the NHS. White Paper July 2010. http://www.dh.gov.uk/prod_consum_dh/groups/dh_digitalassets/@dh/@en/@ps/documents/digitalasset/dh_117794.pdf. Accessed 6 Nov 2024.

45. Hickey G. The potential for coproduction to add value to research. Health Expect. 2018;21(4):693–4. https://doi.org/10.1111/hex.12821.

46. Think Local Act Personal and National Co-production Advisory Group. The ladder of co-production: where are you on the ladder towards co-production. 2021. Available at: thinklocalactpersonal.org.uk/Latest/Co-production-The-ladder-of-co-production/. Accessed 8 Apr 2024.

47. Banerjee S, Alsop P, Jones L, Cardinal RN. Patient and publice involvement to build trust in artificial intelligence: a framework, tools, and case studies. Patterns. 2022;3:100506. https://doi.org/10.1016/j.patter.2022.100506.

48. Donia J, Shaw JA. Co-design and ethical artificial intelligence for health: an agenda for critical research and practice. Big Data Soc. 2021:1–12. https://doi.org/10.1177/20539517211065248.

49. Aizenberg E, van den Hoven J. Designing for human rights in AI. Big Data Soc. 2020;7(2) https://doi.org/10.1177/2053951720949566.

50. Happell B, Gordon S, Roger C, Scholz B, Ellis P, Waks S, Warner T, Platania-Phung C. 'It is always worth the extra effort': organizational structures and barriers to collaboration with consumers in mental health research: perspectives of non-consumer research allies. Int J Ment Health Nurs. 2020;29(6):1168–80.

51. Lathlean J, Burgess A, Coldham T, Gibson C, Herbert L, Levett-Jones T, Simons L, Tee S. Experiences of service user and carer participation in health care education. Nurse Educ Today. 2006;26:732–7.

52. Donetto S, Cribb A. Research involvement in health care practices: interrupting or reproducing medicalization? J Eval Clin Pract. 2011;17(5):907–12.

53. Maguire K, Britten M. 'You're there because you are unprofessional': patient and public involvement as liminal knowledge spaces. Sociol Health Illness. 2019;40(3):473–7.

54. McVey L, Frost T, Issa B, Davison E, Abdulkader J, Randell R, Alvarado N, Zaman H, Hardiker N, Cheong V-L, Woodcock D. Working together: reflections on how to make public involvement in research work. Res Involv Engagem. 2023;9:14. https://doi.org/10.1186/s40900-023-00427-4.

55. Katirai A, Yamamoto BA, Kogetsu A, Kato K. Perspectives on artificial intelligence in healthcare from a patient and public involvement panel in Japan: an exploratory study. Front Digit Health. 2023;5:1229308. https://doi.org/10.3389/fdgth.2023.1229308.

Johnathan Hewis is a diagnostic radiographer with extensive clinical expertise spanning major trauma imaging, neuro-interventional radiology, specialising in MRI, performance and reporting of gastrointestinal studies and planar image interpretation. His research interests centre on service user lived experience, image interpretation, advanced practice, and the role of social media in healthcare research. He has expertise in qualitative research design including phenomenology, hermeneutics, content analysis, and ethnography. Johnathan is currently in the final stages of completing his PhD, which explores the phenomenology of distress during MRI.

Dr. Jae Hargan has been at the forefront of leading patient and public involvement in both research and teaching activities at the University of Bradford. Jae oversees the involvement of 125 experts by experience, each bringing diverse lived experiences within health and social care services. Jae's role is particularly focused on facilitating co-productive collaborations between experts by experience and researchers, prioritising consistent communication and inclusion approaches. With over two decades of experience in user-led voluntary organisations, Jae has developed a specialist in disability rights. Jae's doctoral research investigated the discourse surrounding mental health reasonable adjustments in nursing and midwifery education.

Professor Ruth Mary Strudwick is a diagnostic radiographer by background. She has been a lecturer since 2003, and before that worked as a clinical lecturer at The Ipswich Hospital NHS Trust and as a Diagnostic Radiographer at The Ipswich Hospital NHS Trust. Ruth completed her professional doctorate in 2011, entitled 'An ethnographic study of the culture in a Diagnostic Imaging Department'. She continues to be research active, and her funded research focuses on radiography professional practice and education, service evaluation, person-centred care and service user involvement.

Professor Cláudia Sá dos Reis is a radiographer by background working in academic field as full professor and dean at HESAV (Haute École de Santé Vaud), part of the University of Applied Sciences and Arts Western Switzerland. Holding a PhD in Biomedical Engineering from Universidade Católica Portuguesa, her research focuses on mammography, radiographers practice optimisation, and patient-centred care. She has held positions at institutions including Curtin University in Australia and ESTeSL/IPL in Portugal. She works actively to improve Radiography professions through education and research, promoting innovation in radiographer practice and AI integration in medical imaging. She got 5 projects, published more than 50 articles, 10 book chapters, and several oral communications.

AI for Radiographers: Industry Perspectives

13

Nicholas J. B. Spencer, Ken Sutherland, Graham King, and Daniel Farley Jones

13.1 Introduction

It is not that hard to create a working AI model that can identify features or patterns in a radiographic image and classify those features or even indicate where in the image they are. However, it is considerably harder to successfully create a reliable, robust, and warranted as a safe 'medical device' product which has wide acceptance from clinical practitioners.

The tools and a reasonable amount of labelled radiology data and computing power are available open source to the world for anyone who wishes to develop a model. But commercialising a model—going from an idea to widely deployed product—is a huge undertaking.

There are also many areas in radiographic workflow where AI can play a part other than image recognition or 'pixel AI', and in Fig. 13.1

below, we show three broad categories of AI in imaging and how many AI applications in radiology and medical imaging could span those categories.

Pixel AI These are computer vision applications that use image recognition techniques to classify different features and findings in medical images and drive detection. They may also segregate regions or areas of the images by bounding boxes or contoured lines to show anatomical structures or pathology.

This is the most common category of AI in imaging, and the most common sub-category is clinical decision support software. This highlights findings that an image interpreter would want to know about in the image, acting as a 'second pair of eyes' and a guard against missing clinically significant findings in an exam. Medical AI applications in this category are often termed CADe—Computer Aided Detection.

But pixel AI can be used for other tasks without providing clinical decision support.

Workflow and Productivity Pixel AI may be used to drive workflow; for example, to visually identify different types of X-rays or scans in order to properly route them for specialist reporting.

Pixel AI can also be used to drive workflow prior to a radiologist or interpreter opening up an exam so that reporting can be prioritised on the basis of clinically significant findings in an X-ray

on behalf of Association of Healthcare Technology Providers for Imaging, Radiotherapy and Care (AXREM)

N. J. B. Spencer (✉)
Mid Yorkshire Teaching NHS Trust, Menston, UK
e-mail: nicholas.spencer@agfa.com

K. Sutherland
Canon Medical Research Europe, Edinburgh, UK
e-mail: Ken.Sutherland@mre.medical.canon

G. King
AI Special Focus Group, London, UK
e-mail: graham.x.king@annalise.ai

D. F. Jones
Global Marketing, Gleamer, London, UK
e-mail: daniel.jones@gleamer.ai

© The Author(s), under exclusive license to Springer Nature Switzerland AG 2026
C. Malamateniou et al. (eds.), *Artificial Intelligence for Radiographers*,
https://doi.org/10.1007/978-3-032-05080-9_13

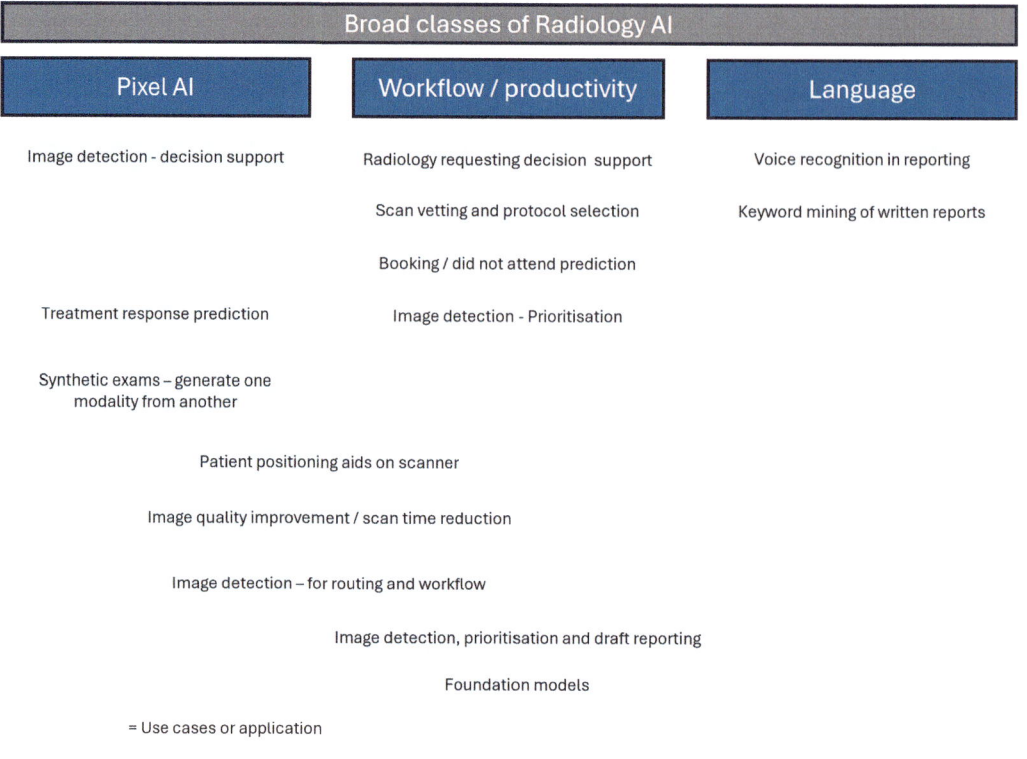

Fig. 13.1 Broad classes of AI applications in medical imaging, some spanning multiple categories

or scan. This is called 'triage' or 'prioritisation' and can be used to expedite the routing of patients with suspicious findings into treatment or the next stage in diagnosis.

AI applications performing prioritisation without detection are often referred to as CADt—Computer Aided Triage—but many applications perform CADt and CADe together.

Other applications in the workflow category include decision support for those requesting imaging procedures, automated booking, vetting/protocolling and AI-based scheduling software.

Language This includes speech-to-text voice recognition and keyword mining of reports, which can be used to identify cases for audit and research as well as potentially identify discrepancies between AI outputs and radiology reports.

The emerging class called 'foundation models' also spans all categories. These are models which can assess an image, produce text describing the image and potentially take in structured and unstructured data. Their outputs may include text, as well as producing coded data, which could then further drive workflow.

More about different AI models can be found in Chaps. 1 and 2.

13.2 Innovation in Imaging and Commercialisation of AI: Things to Consider

The healthcare industry across the globe, and especially in the field of diagnostic imaging, has an extraordinary track record of innovation and standard setting. It is unsurprising, therefore, that AI in radiology, and in particular 'pixel AI', is at the forefront of the application of artificial intelligence in medicine.

Technology creation, or development of an algorithm, is just the beginning of a complex and potentially convoluted journey aiming to get a product on the market. The process in any medical innovation would usually have many phases. But, in the relatively novel space of artificial intelligence, the challenges of new or emergent regulation—and the absence of a tried and tested model for product development—mean that the hurdles are potentially greater and much less well defined.

We use real-world case studies to demonstrate how challenging commercialisation can be. One is focused on development in an academic-commercial partnership context, and the other is a model built from the outset to commercialise into a deployable product, ready to insert new capability into existing clinical workflow. This chapter also outlines the likely phases and related constraints in product development and identifies some of the current challenges of regulation (as of mid-2025, when this book was sent to press). It also considers the major issue of funding AI innovation, as significant investment is required to support AI innovations getting to market and being adopted in clinical practice. Other potential issues, such as those related to procurement, adoption, and evaluation, will also be explored.

Anyone with solid knowledge of clinical challenges and understanding of AI implementation can innovate. Radiographers and radiologists could be at the forefront of this wave if they have customised AI training. For any reader who believes they have a great idea for an AI algorithm able to elegantly and safely solve a clinical problem, it is highly likely that, in its simplest form, someone else may already be on the same development journey in a different (or similar) geography, academic discipline, or clinical setting. As product development has a level of industrial secrecy, there may be no way of finding that out unless disclosed in patent applications or presented at a conference. However, do not be deterred! Even if another AI solution is launched before you have completed the development process, there will be space for adaptation and potential complementary application.

13.3   Case Study 1: Academic Research Enabled AI Solution for Mesothelioma Prediction

In an academic setting, the meeting of minds between clinical and technical experts has been at the heart of creating a model for mesothelioma detection and quantification. Like much academic research, idea generation needs to be supported by a successful grant application to fund the work. In this environment, partnership with industry becomes the catalyst for success. Stimulated by the Cancer Innovation Challenge from the Scottish Funding Council, Canon Medical worked with the University of Glasgow, NHS Greater Glasgow and Clyde and three of Scotland's Innovation Centres to develop a novel AI algorithm for the detection and measurement of mesothelioma [1].

13.3.1   The Clinical Challenge

Mesothelioma is commonly termed 'the asbestos cancer' and Scotland currently has the highest incidence of mesothelioma in the world, reflecting the historical use of asbestos in many industries, including shipbuilding and construction.

Existing techniques for measurement of mesothelioma use a modified RECIST criteria to estimate volume and growth changes, but techniques for applying them are subject to inter- and intra-observer variability. Guidance suggests that measurements of nodules on scans acquired at different times should ideally be done by the same individual [2].

In Glasgow, patients receiving treatment for mesothelioma are now being assessed with AI as part of a prototype imaging system which could improve how treatment response is measured and, hence, help identify which treatments are most beneficial. The long-term aim of the research work is to support the development of a novel treatment regime that will improve patient outcomes and enhance care plans for people with the disease.

Clinical leadership was critical in identifying the problem and determining the clinical utility of the solution proposed.

The iterative nature of innovation of this kind in medical sciences is somewhat obscure. Simplistically put, the clinical expert is less likely to understand the technical details of state of the art in AI or machine learning systems unless they also have a related degree in computer science or biomedical engineering. Similarly, a data/AI scientist is not necessarily skilled in the clinical domain. Consequently, it is only when these two groups and disciplines collaborate to solve a single problem that a joint vision of potential innovative solutions can be created.

13.3.2 Use Case for AI

Assessment of suspected mesothelioma is difficult due to its form being a multifocal rind around the lungs within the chest cavity (Fig. 13.2). Evaluation with computed tomography (CT) is time-consuming to assess and measure, with significant inter-observer variation. Accordingly, the study team's aim was to create a prototype AI system able to automatically find and measure mesothelioma tumour volume on CT, which is also used to assess patient's response to systemic treatments like chemotherapy.

The first task of the team was to find data from a representative cohort of patients who could be used to train the AI. Retrospective CT data sets were collected from three separate sites in Scotland and England to reduce bias. This also guards against AI 'overfitting' [4]—where a model is based too closely on one particular dataset but then does not accurately predict when it encounters new unseen data. Testing with these three different datasets helped check that the model didn't overfit the training data.

13.3.3 Training and Testing Datasets

The overall datasets used were in three groups, a training set, an internal validation set, and an external validation set. The training and internal validation set comprised 123 de-identified CT scans from 108 patients. A technique called k-fold cross-validation [5] (see [5] for a clear explanation with diagram) was used to train multiple 'folds' of the AI model (seven in this case), so that each fold is trained on a subset of the data and the remainder is used for internal validation. This is a common technique in machine learning which makes the best use of scarce data and usually also improves a model's prediction accuracy.

All CT scans were annotated by an expert clinician who drew around all areas of the tumour in the images of the CT scan—called 'segmentation'—and created measurements. More about segmentation in cross-sectional imaging can be found in Chaps. 6 and 7. Some patients had MRI exams too, and these were used as a reference to refine the boundary drawings on the CT scan. Eighty of the annotated (or 'labelled') scans were pre-treatment scans, and 43 out of the 123 labelled scans were post-treatment.

The convolutional neural network (CNN) AI model was then trained with the training set and tested with the internal validation set. The external validation dataset comprised 60 CT scans from 30 patients, with each patient having one pre-chemotherapy scan and one post-chemotherapy scan. Each of the three centres in the study therefore contributed data for 10 patients with mesothelioma. The trained AI model was then confirmed to be accurate and effective using the external validation set, which comprised CT scans that had not been used to train the model. The metrics used to assess accuracy—the degree of agreement—were Bland-Altman plots and Dice region overlap [3]. Performance metrics for AI models can be found in Chap. 2.

This case study highlights a research-led approach to AI, and the published results [3] are encouraging, but they are just the first step in getting an AI solution adopted in clinical practice. The volume of training and validation datasets needs to be increased to refine and reinforce this AI model and increase confidence in its accuracy and readiness for clinical application. At this stage, the tool will have the

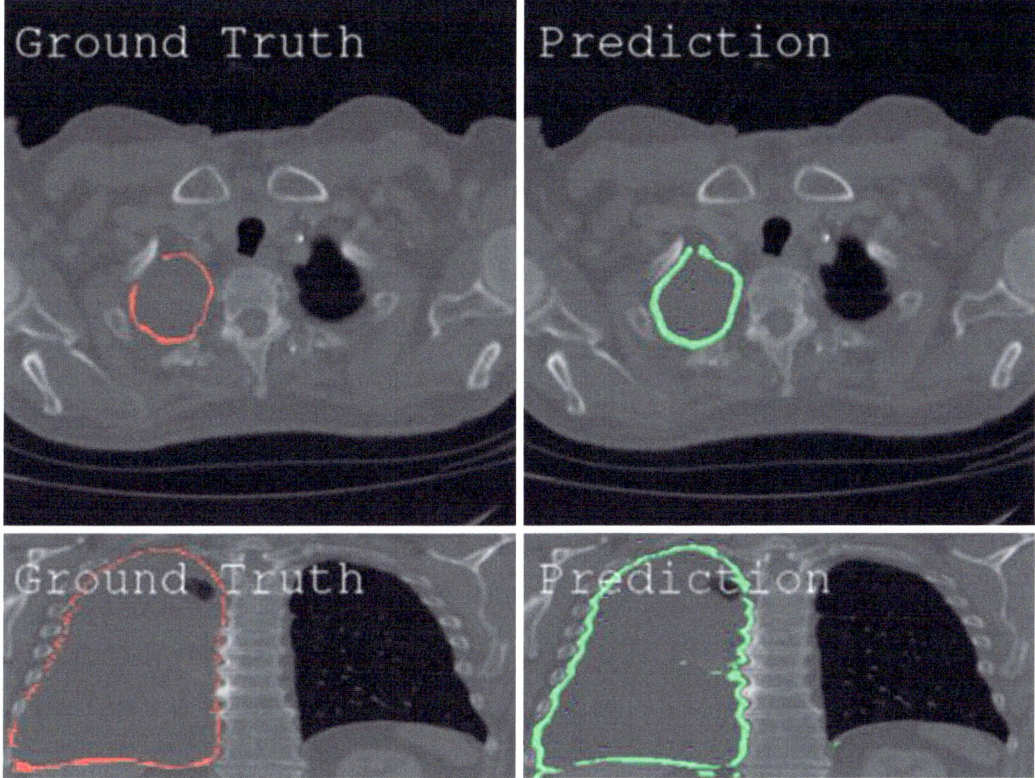

Human Annotation (Ground Truth) in RED

AI Annotation (Prediction) in GREEN

Fig. 13.2 Examples of annotated mesothelioma tumour volume by humans (in the two images on the left) and volume annotations performed by AI (from the same case, at the same slice position) (in the two images on the right). The AI volumes were generated by automatic segmentation without any user prompts [3]. (Image courtesy of Prof. Kevin Blythe, University of Glasgow)

potential to be commercialised with the expectation that this technology will be deployed at scale to improve patient treatment and outcomes for those diagnosed with mesothelioma in the future.

13.3.4 Key Success Factors for the Project

1. A well-defined clinical challenge that needed a solution.
2. Access to a leading academic and clinician who was ready to collaborate with a commercial partner.
3. Adequate financial support through a research grant to minimise the risk of what was essentially an exploratory research project.
4. Curation and access to representative and diverse data from multiple sites.
5. Expert support for image annotation. This may not always be required—a labelled dataset may already exist, or unsupervised learning is being used.
6. Support from data science experts to design the study effectively and take care of AI training and testing.

The second case study looks at how a model is developed to be commercialised from the outset.

We examine the scaling necessary to ensure sufficient training and validation data and other solid foundations, which must be built if a commercial solution is to be robust enough to fit into clinical workflows.

13.4 Case Study 2: From Training to Commercialisation; a Comprehensive Chest X-ray AI Solution

13.4.1 The Clinical Challenge

The chest X-ray (CXR) remains the world's most-performed medical imaging examination [6]. In some geographies, there have been lengthy delays for the provision of radiology reports for CXR to referrers. At one hospital in London, England, there was a backlog of over 22,000 unreported images, and 55 cases among the unreported backlog had positive findings, though a review of notes showed that the reporting delay had not led to patient harm [7]. In another hospital on England's South Coast, delays in getting an X-ray examination were found to have led to significant harm for three patients with lung cancer [8]. This is mainly due to services being understaffed to tackle the load of examinations for the given population and clinical load [9].

Both examples above pre-date the 2020 global COVID-19 pandemic, which saw a pause in most non-urgent treatment and caused a build-up of latent health issues and waiting lists in most health systems. Surveys performed since then confirm that radiology reporting backlogs are now observed in many countries [9], with radiologist burnout, reporter fatigue, and shortages of reporting clinicians all causing serious concern [10].

13.4.2 Use Case for AI

An AI application in CXR that only supports detection of a few findings has limited clinical value, purely because of the complexity of anatomy and diversity of clinical findings that could appear on a chest X-ray. The founders of annalise.ai had a vision to create a comprehensive AI clinical decision support model which would deal with time-sensitive findings, like pneumothorax, and broad classes, like 'nodule', 'mass', 'opacity', and 'foreign body', but cover everything that a thoracic radiologist would want to be notified of in a chest X-ray. In the end product, the supported findings include granular classes for nodules, lesions, and masses; pneumothoraxes; different types of lines and tubes; and the presence of various implants in addition to findings on the CXR image periphery such as clavicle, rib, and shoulder fractures as well as abdominal findings like gallstones.

In common with the previous case study, the founders recognised that robust clinical collaboration with industry was necessary to address this use case. One of the founders' comments was 'Healthcare is too broad and too complex for any startup to claim to disrupt or innovate' [11]. Annalise.ai was established as a joint venture between I-MED Radiology Group and harrison.ai in Australia, bringing together large-scale radiology and clinically focused AI and machine-learning expertise.

13.4.3 Assembling a Training Dataset

Chest X-ray images and associated reports and subsequent imaging from a diverse population were ethically sourced and de-identified. Machine learning (ML) models require large amounts of diverse data for training, with diversity consisting of several dimensions. These are shown below in Fig. 13.3.

To learn, medical imaging ML models must be fed with labelled (or annotated) data. Today, commercial packages exist for labelling images [12, 13], but in 2020, the most effective strategy was to build an in-house labelling tool, viewer, and associated data storage. The clinical and machine-learning development teams knew that robust data labels and a large training dataset were going to be essential for success.

A labelling classification scheme (called an 'ontology tree') and clinical inclusion-exclusion

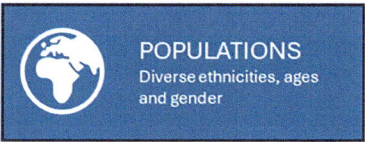
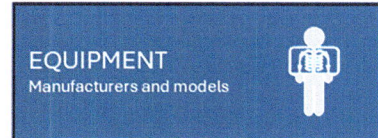
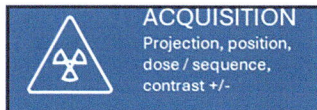
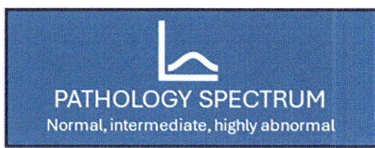
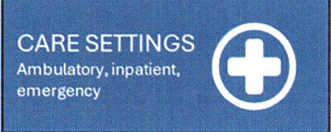

Fig. 13.3 Dimensions of data diversity required for adequate AI model training

criteria for each finding were created. Each CXR image was independently labelled by three expert radiologists, who marked each clinical finding as present or absent. The consensus findings for each triple-read case were generated mathematically as a score between 0 and 1 for each finding using the Dawid–Skene consensus algorithm [14].

Finally, a single radiologist outlined the edges of a subset of findings on each image so that segmentation overlays could be generated by the model. Segmentation, which can be shown as a box, polyline or—in this case—a colour wash, can aid explainability by showing the clinician viewing or reporting the image exactly which region(s) of an image triggered the prediction of a finding.

All of the above had to be encapsulated in standard operating procedures, plus training and assessment activities for radiologist labellers to ensure consistent standards of labelling [15].

Most medical image ML applications use open-source convoluted neural network (CNN) technologies, such as the TensorFlow framework [16]. So, it is actually the training data, labelling and model-tuning processes that make each product unique and influence how successful it will be when used in the clinical environment.

13.4.4 Model Training

Once the training data is labelled, it is fed into the model training pipeline. Model training requires investment in computing power to access the graphical processing units (GPUs) which ensure timely machine learning. The known outputs in the labelled data are vital for the model to learn from, as the model effectively adapts itself backwards, using many repeated 'epochs' of learning to do so.

As well as the pitfall of overfitting, described in the previous case study, machine learning experts must avoid risks during model learning, including hidden stratification [17]. In hidden stratification, a model learns to make inferences using two or more image features that may often appear together but do not have a causal connection.

A simple example of hidden stratification from the reference above is where an animal image classification application model calls any canine in snow a wolf and any canine on grass a dog by incorrectly associating the image background colour with the type of canine.

This is avoided by using large, diverse datasets and designing granular labelling with subclassification (see Fig. 13.4). As in the previous case

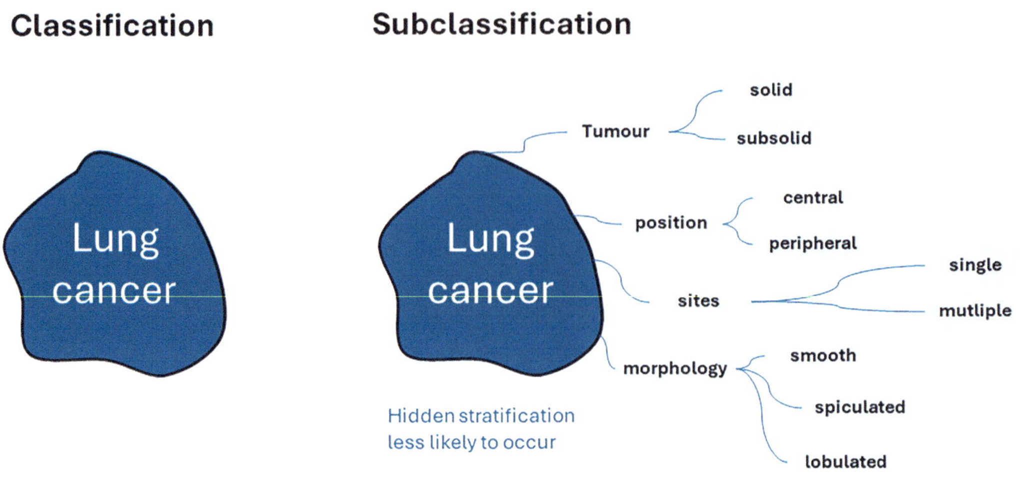

Classification   **Subclassification**

Fig. 13.4 A hypothetical example of subclassification—a technique which reduces the risk of hidden stratification

study, the K-fold validation technique was also used for the annalise.ai model training and initial validation [5]. This used data efficiently and improved how well the model generalises to unseen data.

13.4.5 Creating a Usable Application

A medical imaging AI detection model is not useful until it can convey results to a user. The model output must be visualised and presented alongside the original images and other supporting data like previous imaging for the patient.

A user interface must convert the numerical prediction values into a finding present/finding absent indicator. Segmentation coordinates may also be overlaid onto the original image as outline boxes, colour washes, or polygons. Some method of communicating 'prediction confidence' as a score or indicator may be used to help an image interpreter with explainability by communicating whether a prediction had a strong score or a borderline one.

User interface (UI) and user experience (UX) designers are software development experts. They work with clinical experts to help create applications that are intuitive, visually clear, and use a predictable visual 'language' for any interaction and which can convey important clinical

information with minimal risk of misunderstanding or miscommunication.

An interactive viewer application (Fig. 13.5) was created and installed on the diagnostic workstation and synchronised to display the same exam as shown in the PACS and RIS.

Alternatively, static DICOM Secondary Capture (SC) images could be returned to the PACS to appear as an additional image series alongside the original examinations. This technique is used by many AI radiology applications, as it uses standard capabilities present in all PACS.

Other applications, especially with a limited set of findings, may display these as DICOM Greyscale Softcopy Presentation State (GSPS) overlays. These are returned to the PACS from the AI application and are presented as a 'layer' on top of the original image in PACS. They may contain text, outlines/arrows or both and can be toggled on or off directly in the PACS.

An emerging area of standards-based communication is the use of a DICOM Structured Report (SR), particularly using Template ID (TID) 1500. This format can contain multiple data types in its payload, including a structured or coded list of findings, the segmentation 'overlays' and unique IDs for the images that have been analysed. In this way, AI findings can be displayed directly in a PACS viewer alongside the original images,

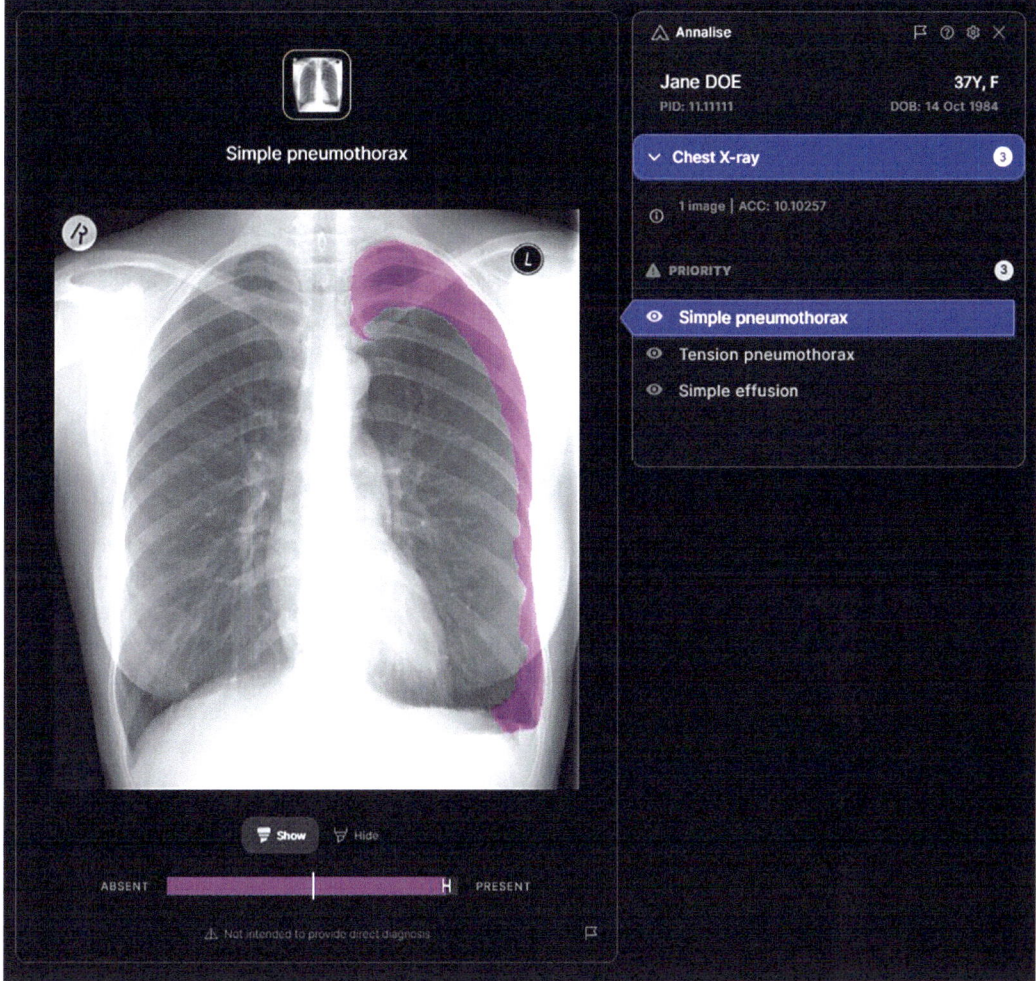

Fig. 13.5 AI findings and segmentation overlay display in Annalise Viewer. (Courtesy: Annalise.ai)

toggled on and off and potentially made available for integration into the radiology report. There are still open issues with this approach. For example, there is no industry standard means to convey a consistent confidence level or score. And this technique involves the PACS application (a medical device) taking responsibility for visualising outputs from the AI algorithm, which is usually a separate medical device.

No matter how a finding (or set of findings) is communicated to a user, the determination of whether it is shown as present or absent requires a threshold (or 'operating point') to be set for each finding. This is the score above which a finding is deemed present, and below it, absent.

Determining optimal thresholds is a multidisciplinary task, involving statisticians, clinical researchers, and machine learning experts, as well as the clinical practitioners involved in the project.

Furthermore, efficacy and safety of the AI model have to be proven. For this CXR model, a multireader, multicase (MRMC) study sought to answer both questions of model performance at different operating points and also demonstrate safety and efficacy. The resulting study was published open-access in a peer-reviewed journal [15].

Lastly, a commercial product must integrate into interpretation workflows. We have already described the ways that AI prediction results can be visualised, but to drive workflow, a prioritisation instruction message may also be sent to the main reporting worklist application. The reporting worklist could be contained within a PACS, RIS or even separate reporting and transcription software. Prioritisation sets a reporting urgency value for the exam and orders an interpreter's worklist based on the predicted severity of findings. This is often called 'triage' (from the French *trier*, to sort). Typically, deploying organisations will use three or four categories, but this is often configurable in many systems. The prioritised worklist enables the interpreter to commence immediate reporting of exams with the highest priority predictions.

Annalise.ai supports the generation of prioritisation messages in a range of formats, allowing the instruction to be received and processed by many different systems. To do this required creating a flexible workflow engine, which is used by integration specialists from both system providers to generate messages and convey structured prioritisation messages in an agreed format.

13.4.6 Legally Marketing the Product

If the AI/ML application is a medical device (and most triage/prioritisation and detection applications are), it requires approval or clearance from national regulators before it can be marketed. Company regulatory specialists work with external regulators and auditors (such as Notified Bodies). Every lifecycle stage used to build the product must have documented processes and evidence that the processes have been followed. Quality management processes were established before any data was labelled and before any design took place and continue throughout design, build, test, and the ongoing product lifecycle. For more information about AI implementation, the AI model lifecycle and AI regulations, see Chapter 4.

Approval of the software requires independent certification of the manufacturer's quality management system (usually to the ISO13485 standard) and the presentation of clinical evidence

and technical information about the product itself. The Annalise.ai CXR model's evidence included the MRMC study referred to above and the company obtained ISO13485 certification and sought and received regulatory clearance for the product in Australia, EU/EEA, the United Kingdom, the United States, and other territories. The evidence required and who assesses it varies; see this comparison of United States and EU/EEA approval pathways for more details [18].

13.4.7 Additional Compliance

Each healthcare organisation has individual compliance requirements. Because AI/ML applications are new to many adopters, as they use data at scale and may use cloud computing hosted outside the health organisation's network, developers must expect to describe what data they handle and supply reassurances about data privacy and cybersecurity. Evidence of meeting medical device and clinical safety requirements is also often required. Increasingly, sites are developing AI application questionnaires to enable them to fully understand the scope of an AI technology, the data it uses and how it is managed and supported. The National Health Service in England *AI Buyer's Guide* [19] is a useful resource which gives AI developers examples of the kinds of questions that are asked and helps buyers understand what to look for. Although created in the UK, many of the requirements and questions apply globally.

A pioneer or 'early adopter' health organisation will often be essential to prove that the AI model can function in a particular country or health system. These are typically organisations that are willing to collaborate closely and have a track record in clinical and digital transformation. A vendor will usually find having adopters like this invaluable for maturing the software in non-AI areas such as user interface, integration with other systems and workflow. Such adopters may also help with evidence generation for the product and act as a reference for future customers. Annalise.ai has benefitted from several early adopter organisations in various countries.

13.4.8 Getting the Message Out

Successful product release also involves marketing professionals creating material that aligns with any medical device claims made, as well as educational material to allow sales and technical staff to talk about the product, its evidence, and limitations.

Members of a company's clinical research and regulatory teams may also work to provide the AI model to external, independent validation initiatives which compare AI products using regional or national benchmark datasets. These initiatives build confidence that a product can generalise well in a region or country. Example initiatives which have included validation and cross-comparison of CXR models have included the Smart Chest study (Denmark) [20] and Project AIR (Netherlands) [21].

User training is required before clinical adoption, with ongoing support after go-live. Training is often delivered by a vendor's clinical staff, who typically have previous frontline clinical experience, often as radiographers. This complements academically accredited training courses that are increasingly available to different medical imaging and oncology professionals in the UK, Europe, and globally and are delivered either in person, online, or in a hybrid format [22, 23]. Finally, the application will need to provide analytical data about how it is functioning, both to demonstrate to the clinical setting that it is working well and to iron out any initial issues, and to meet medical device regulation requirements for post-market monitoring. This will involve the vendor's data analysts working with clinical applications staff. Data from these feeds back into regulatory, clinical research, and product development departments within the company.

13.4.9 Key Success Factors for the Product

1. Decision at the very start to design the product and label training data under a quality management system

2. Ethically obtaining a large and diverse dataset to label

3. Building a robust, in-house labelling process and platform, with a granular 'ontology tree' designed with subclasses to minimise hidden stratification

4. Creating the quality management system and clinical evidence needed to obtain regulatory clearance for the product

5. Designing a solution which could integrate seamlessly into existing reporting workflow, including support of standards like DICOM for image ingestion, synchronised viewer to display AI prediction results and standards-based messaging to enable reporting prioritisation

6. Marketing the product and early adoption case studies; also, being willing to undergo external validation by independent researchers to build confidence in the product's real-world use

7. Funding—For any AI application vendor, labelling/annotating the training data is a significant upfront investment. Creating the documents, investing in systems and processes, and generating the evidence make up the quality management system. Teams will be working on model training, software development, research, regulatory submissions, and integration with other systems for a period of time before the application receives medical device clearance and can start being sold in a market.

Finally, we have demonstrated that any model commercialisation, as in the previous case study, requires a multidisciplinary approach involving collaboration between clinical experts and many specialists within a company. Company specialists may be full-time company employees or part-time consultants or freelancers. Flexible use of consultants is often particularly helpful when a company is growing and when there may not be enough work in a specialist area to justify full-time employees in every role. Not all companies are the same, though, and different budgets and competencies can allow different team compositions and roles.

13.5   The Future: An Industry View

In 2016, the now Nobel Prize winner Geoffrey Hinton—often considered the godfather of deep learning—made a bold statement about the transformative potential of AI in diagnostic radiology. He exhorted the research community to equip clinicians with the knowledge they need to navigate the evolving landscape of AI, asserting that clinicians must remain at the forefront of innovation but must also be prepared to adapt and thrive in this ever-changing environment.

Alongside the detection and analysis of medical images, there is burgeoning growth in foundational, or generative, technologies highlighted by innovations like OpenAI's ChatGPT and Google's Gemini. Unlike traditional AI models, these generative systems are trained on vast unlabelled datasets, enabling them to produce novel content, ranging from text and images to music and code. Their expansive learning capability sets the stage for groundbreaking applications in healthcare, where the potential of AI extends beyond interpreting pixel data through conventional convolutional neural networks. In the future, we will leverage foundational AI for analysing an array of data types, including text and numerical data from electronic health records (EHR), alongside imaging, to enhance diagnostic precision and patient care. Chapter 2 discusses the different AI models extensively, with references to future AI model developments.

One of the most promising applications of generative AI in radiology lies in its ability to process and integrate this multi-modal data. We envisage an AI model that not only examines X-rays or CT exams but also sifts through patient histories, lab results, and genetic information to provide a holistic view of a patient's health. This approach could significantly improve diagnostic accuracy by contextualising findings in an image to other data points about the patient's current condition and medication. This also opens the door to treatments that are tailored to individual patient needs, heralding a new era of personalised medicine. See more about this in Chaps. 7 and 12.

Moreover, the ability of foundation models to analyse vast amounts of data could revolutionise operational aspects of radiology departments. For example, by mining clinical reports for insights, AI could help manage resources more effectively, reducing overbookings and optimising scheduling to address the imbalance between the growing demand for imaging services and limited supply.

However, the integration of such advanced AI technologies into healthcare raises important questions about data privacy, bias mitigation, and the ethical use of AI. Ensuring that these systems are transparent, equitable, and respectful of patient confidentiality will be crucial as we navigate the transition towards an AI-enhanced future in radiology. For more information about ethical AI, see Chap. 3.

As we consider AI's ability to reshape healthcare, we risk redrawing the regulatory boundaries. The future of AI applications in medicine is not just about technological advancement; it is equally about navigating the complexities of the regulations that govern these innovations. Medical technologies cannot scale impact without regulation, yet one size does not fit all. Globally, there is no single medical-technology compliance; rather, there are a myriad of regional clearances and regulations administered by the UK Medicines and Healthcare Products Regulatory Agency (MHRA), the US Food and Drug Administration (FDA), Therapeutic Goods Administration (TGA), Health Canada and the component authorities of EU and EEA member states on whose authority CE marks are issued. There are also emerging international standards for AI in healthcare, such as BS30440 for validation [24], ISO42001 for AI management systems [25], and evidence evaluation standards such as DECIDE-AI [26]. More information about AI regulation can be found in Chap. 4.

The challenge with medical AI regulation lies in its inherent nature: AI is not static. Unlike surgical implants, AI applications are dynamic, evolving over time in performance and functionality. They are not yet learning from data in real time, but their iterative improvement poses difficulty for regulators. This continuous evolution calls for a balance: On one side, there is the risk of stifling innovation with over-regulation; on the other, a concern for compromised safety due to under-regulation, see Fig. 13.6. The solution, like AI, is not static and must evolve.

As we edge closer to even more powerful AI systems that have been trained with unsupervised learning or which even may be unsupervised in operation and decision-making, regulation is a hotly debated topic on the international stage.

Nations are beginning to come together to publish their policies on wider AI regulation, such as the EU AI Act [28] and the US AI Bill of Rights [29]. These are not healthcare-specific, yet they affect medical AI by addressing risk classification, data governance, and human oversight. In the case of the EU AI Act, the requirement for organisations deploying AI to ensure 'AI literacy' among their staff has already come into effect, with further obligations for providers of high-risk

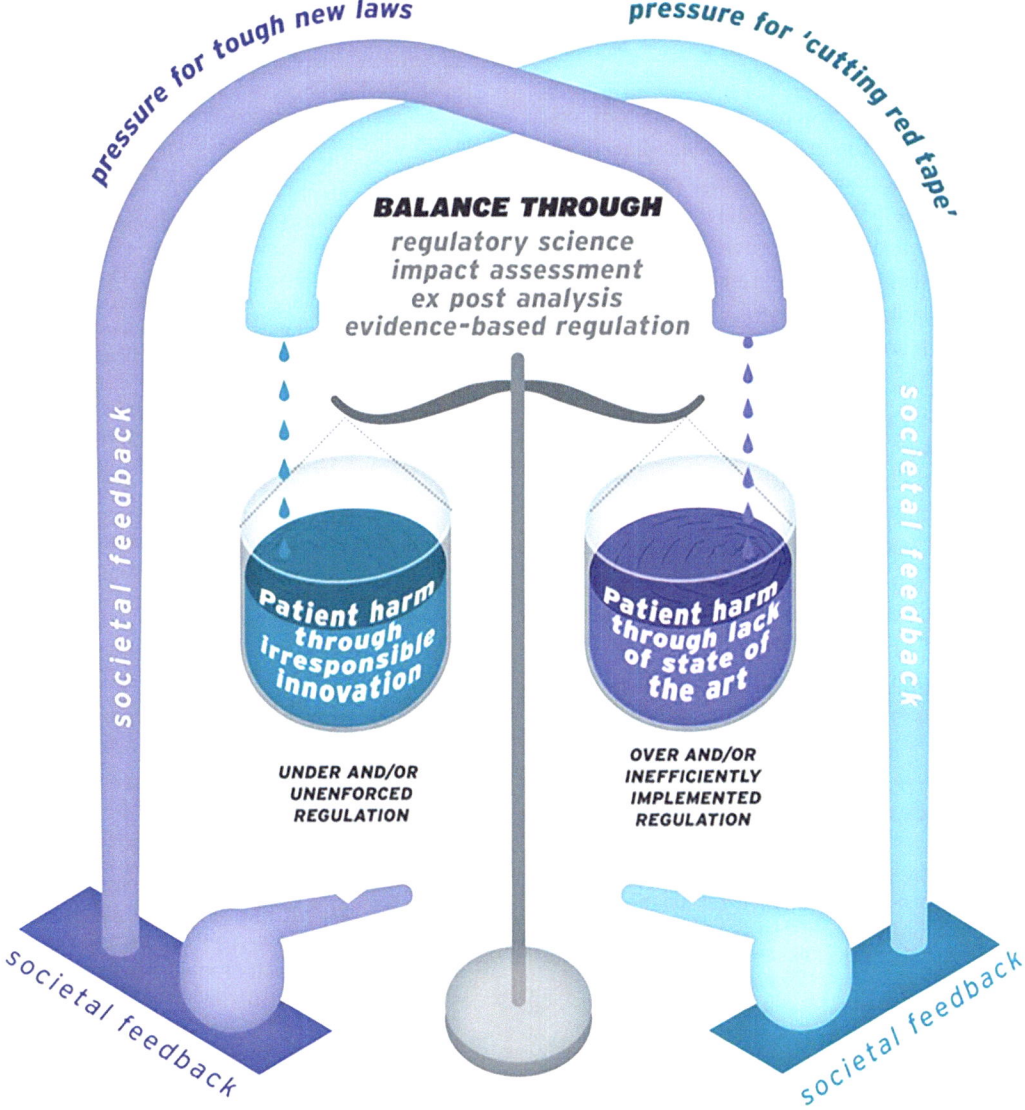

Fig. 13.6 Balance illustrates the tension between regulation and innovation. (Figure concept developed by Stephen Gilbert, Figure graphic design by Andrew Berry, shared with permissions from [27]

systems coming into effect during 2026 and 2027.

For developers, evaluators and commissioners of medical-AI technologies, ongoing monitoring of how AI regulation intersects with existing Medical Device Regulation (MDR) will be crucial. At present, many jurisdictions do not distinguish between AI as a Medical Device (AIaMD) and the more general class of Software as a Medical Device (SaMD), though this will change soon.

13.6 Chapter Summary

Today, the AI we encounter in radiology excels at specific tasks, for example lesion detection or image enhancement. These are powerful tools that have the potential to increase our accuracy and speed and thus improve clinical care and patient outcomes. Yet we are navigating an era of rapid technological growth, where the capabilities of AI are expanding at an unprecedented pace. Instead of dwelling on the debate between 'augmentation versus automation', whether AI will assist or replace human tasks, perhaps our focus should shift towards how we can adapt to and integrate these changes, envisioning a future where AI doesn't just automate tasks but also enhances our expertise, enabling us to provide even better care to our patients. The future of radiology AI is still taking shape, but staying informed and flexible is our best strategy for riding the wave of change.

References

1. University of Glasgow. Artificial Intelligence used to automate assessment of mesothelioma [Internet]; posted 13 Apr 2021, cited 3 Apr 2024, accessed at https://www.gla.ac.uk/news/archiveofnews/2021/april/headline_788451_en.html.
2. Tsao AS, Garland L, Redman M, Kernstine K, Gandara D, Marom EM. 2008, a practical guide of the Southwest Oncology Group to measure malignant pleural mesothelioma tumors by RECIST and modified RECIST criteria. J Thorac Oncol. 2011;6:598–601. https://doi.org/10.1097/JTO.0b013e318208c83d. Accessed 20 Dec 2024.
3. Kidd AC, Anderson O, Cowell GW, Weir AJ, Voisey JP, Evision M et al. Fully automated volumetric mea-surement of malignant pleural mesothelioma by deep learning AI: validation and comparison with modified RECIST response criteria. Thorax. 2022;77:1251–9. Cited 3 Apr 2024 from https://thorax.bmj.com/content/77/12/1251.abstract.
4. Amazon Web Services. Machine learning resources: what is overfitting? Cited 3 Apr 2024 from https://aws.amazon.com/what-is/overfitting/.
5. Amazon Web Services Inc. Cross-validation, Amazon machine learning developer's guide, cited 18 March 2025 from https://docs.aws.amazon.com/machine-learning/latest/dg/cross-validation.html.
6. United Nations, United Nations Scientific Committee on the Effects of Atomic Radiation (UNSCEAR), 208 Report on sources and effects of ionizing radiation. 2008, United Nations, New York, United States, ISBN 978-92-1-142274-0, cited 3 Apr 2024 from http://www.unscear.org/docs/publications/2008/UNSCEAR_2008_Annex-A-CORR.pdf Table B41a.
7. Care Quality Commission. A national review of radiology reporting within the NHS in England, Radiology Review, 2018 Newcastle-upon-Tyne, UK. Document reference CQC-418-072018.
8. Care Quality Commission, Portsmouth Hospitals NHS Trust must review backlog of X-rays, CQC News release, 1 Dec 2017, cited 20 Dec 2024 from https://www.cqc.org.uk/news/releases/portsmouth-hospitals-nhs-trust-must-review-backlog-X-rays.
9. Omofoye TS, Vlahos I, Marom EM, Bassett R, Blasinska K, Ye X, et al. Backlogs in formal interpretation of radiology examinations: a pilot global survey. Clin Imaging. 2024;106:110049. ISSN 0899-7071, cited 3 Apr 2024 from https://doi.org/10.1016/j.clinimag.2023.110049.
10. Royal College of Radiologists, Clinical Radiologists Census Report 2022, published 2023, Royal College of Radiologists, London, UK, cited 3 Apr 2024 from https://www.rcr.ac.uk/media/qs0jnfmv/rcr-census_clinical-radiology-workforce-census_2022.pdf.
11. Interview with Dimitry Tran, Annalise.ai co-founder, Ausbiz.tv, broadcast 9 Jun 2021, cited 3 Apr 2024 from https://vimeo.com/576603062
12. V7 Labs (www.v7labs.com)
13. Flywheel (https://flywheel.io)
14. Nguyen AT, Wallace BC, Li JJ, Nenkova A, Lease M. Aggregating and predicting sequence labels from crowd annotations. Proc Conf Assoc Comput Linguist Meet. 2017;2017:299–309. https://doi.org/10.18653/v1/P17-1028.
15. Seah JCY, Tang CHM, Buchlak QD, Holt XG, Wardman JB, Aimoldin A, et al, Effect of a comprehensive deep-learning model on the accuracy of chest X-ray interpretation by radiologists: a retrospective, multireader multicase study Lancet Digit Health. 2021;3:e496–506, cited 3 Apr 2024 from https://doi.org/10.1016/S2589-7500(21)00106.
16. https://www.tensorflow.org/about
17. Oakden-Rayner L, Dunnmon J, Carneiro G, Re C. Hidden stratification causes clinically meaningful failures in machine learning for medical imaging, CHIL '20: Proceedings of the ACM Conference on Health, Inference, and Learning, April 2020,

pp. 151–159, cited 3 Apr 2024 from https://doi.org/10.1145/3368555.3384468.

18. Muehlematter UJ, Daniore P, Vokinger KN. Approval of artificial intelligence and machine learning-based medical devices in the USA and Europe (2015–20): a comparative analysis. Lancet Digit Health. 2021;3:e195–203, cited 3 Apr 2024 from https://doi.org/10.1016/S2589-7500(20)30292-2.

19. Joshi I, Cushnan D, A buyer's guide to AI in health and care, NHS England, London UK, Version 1.3, November 2022, accessed 20 Dec 2024 at https://transform.england.nhs.uk/ai-lab/explore-all-resources/adopt-ai/a-buyers-guide-to-ai-in-health-and-care/.

20. Plesner LL, Müller FC, Brejnebøl MW, Laustrup LC, Rasmussen F, Nielsen OW, et al. Commercially available chest radiograph AI tools for detecting airspace disease, pneumothorax, and pleural effusion. Radiology. 308 (3):e231236 cited 3 Apr 2024 from https://doi.org/10.1148/radiol.231236.

21. Van Leeuwen KG, Schalekamp S, Rutten MJCM, Huisman M, Schaefer-Prokop CM, de Rooij M, et al. Comparison of commercial AI software performance for radiograph lung nodule detection and bone age prediction. Radiology. 2024;310(1):e230981, cited 3 Apr 2024 from https://doi.org/10.1148/radiol.230981.

22. van de Venter R, Skelton E, Matthew J, Woznitza N, Tarroni G, Hirani SP, Kumar A, Malik R, Malamateniou C. Artificial intelligence education for radiographers, an evaluation of a UK postgraduate educational intervention using participatory action research: a pilot study. Insights Imaging. 2023;14(1):25. https://doi.org/10.1186/s13244-023-01372-2.

23. Doherty G, McLaughlin L, Hughes C, McConnell J, Bond R, McFadden S. A scoping review of educational programmes on artificial intelligence (AI) available to medical imaging staff. Radiography (Lond). 2024;30(2):474–82. https://doi.org/10.1016/j.radi.2023.12.019.

24. BSI standards, BS 30440:2023: Validation framework for the use of artificial intelligence (AI) within healthcare. Specification, 2023, BSI Standards Limited, ISBN 978 0 539 17160 0, ICS 11.020; 35.240; 35.240.80, Limited preview accessed 19 Mar 2025 at https://knowledge.bsigroup.com/products/validation-framework-for-the-use-of-artificial-intelligence-ai-within-healthcare-specification.

25. International Standards Organisation. ISO/IEC 42001:2023 - Information technology — Artificial intelligence — Management system, 2023. Edition 1, ISO, Geneva, Switzerland. Preview accessed 19 Mar 2025 at https://www.iso.org/standard/81230.html.

26. Vasey B, Nagendran M, Campbell B, et al. Reporting guideline for the early stage clinical evaluation of decision support systems driven by artificial intelligence: DECIDE-AI. BMJ. 2022;377:e070904. https://doi.org/10.1136/bmj-2022-070904.

27. Gilbert S, Anderson S, Daumer M, Li P, Melvin T, Williams R. Learning from experience and finding the right balance in the governance of Artificial Intelligence and digital health technologies. J Med Internet Res. 2023;25:e43682. https://doi.org/10.2196/43682.

28. European Parliament, EU Artificial Intelligence Act. 2024. Final Draft text, cited 3 Apr 2024 at https://data.consilium.europa.eu/doc/document/ST-5662-2024-INIT/en/pdf.

29. The White House: Office of Science & Technology Policy, Blueprint for an AI Bill of Rights: Making Automated Systems Work for the American People, 2022. The White House, United States, cited 3 Apr 2024 from https://www.whitehouse.gov/ostp/ai-bill-of-rights/.

Dr. Nicholas JB Spencer is an experienced radiologist and PACS expert. He was a past president of UKIO and previously held several UK healthcare sector roles as a clinical and governance expert and medical director. His current roles include Appointed Trustee at the UK's College of Radiographers, and Chief Clinical Information Officer at AGFA HealthCare.

Dr. Ken Sutherland is President of Canon Medical Research Europe and is also Assistant to the Chief Technology Executive of Canon Medical Systems in Japan. He is responsible for Canon Medical's AI Centre of Excellence in Edinburgh and the collaboration with Prof Sotos Tsaftaris at the University of Edinburgh. Ken studied Electronics and computer science at University of Edinburgh and gained a PhD in image analysis and four years postdoctoral research experience in medical image analysis. He is a Fellow of the Royal Society of Edinburgh and was recently elected as a fellow of the Royal Academy of Engineering.

Graham King has worked in mission-critical IT since graduating with a degree in Biology in 1997 and in various NHS and vendor roles since 2003. He has worked for Lexmark Healthcare (now Hyland), DesAcc and IBM Watson Health Imaging. He is a leading UK health interoperability practitioners and has worked with AI and data-driven technologies since 2018. He currently works for Annalise.ai as a Solution Architect, helping customers and prospective customers understand and use AI technology in clinical practice. He also represents AXREM's AI members' interests to national stakeholders and has strong interest in health policy and its intersection with technology.

Daniel Farley Jones is an expert in AI and digital health, specialising in the application and commercialisation of artificial intelligence in medical imaging and healthcare informatics. With extensive industry experience, Daniel led the implementation of Gleamer's AI technologies across healthcare systems, including the NHS. His research focuses on the use and development of machine learning software for early chronic condition diagnosis. With a background in both Business Management and Data Science, he is committed to advancing ethical AI adoption and ensuring its safe, effective integration into global healthcare systems, believing in AI's transformative potential to improve patient outcomes worldwide.

Radiographer Professional Body Contributions

14

Christina Malamateniou, Maryann Hardy, Karen M Knapp, and Aarthi Ramlaul ⓘ

14.1 Introduction

This chapter provides an overview of the guidance, training and support offered by radiographer professional bodies and AI multidisciplinary learned societies in medical imaging and radiotherapy around the world. The resources are wide-ranging and include position statements, white papers, guidance, webinars/podcasts, publications, awards, study and training events for members. We are grateful to the following pro-

The authors of each professional body are stated below their contribution. The editors have been named as chapter authors to comply with publication requirements due to the number of contributors to this chapter.

on behalf of Association of Healthcare Technology Providers for Imaging, Radiotherapy and Care (AXREM)

C. Malamateniou (✉)
Division of Radiography, Department of Allied Health Sciences, School of Health and Medical Sciences, City St George's University of London, London, UK
e-mail: Christina.Malamateniou@citystgeorges.ac.uk

M. Hardy
Faculty of Health Studies, University of Bradford, Bradford, UK

K. M. Knapp
Faculty of Health and Life Sciences, University of Exeter, Exeter, UK

A. Ramlaul
College of Health and Society, Buckinghamshire New University, High Wycombe, UK

fessional bodies who have contributed to this chapter and are presented in alphabetical order:

- Australian Society of Medical Imaging and Radiation Therapy (ASMIRT, Australia)
- American Society of Radiation Technologists (ASRT, USA)
- British Institute of Radiology (BIR, UK)
- Canadian Association of Medical Radiation Technologists (CAMRT, Canada)
- European Federation of Radiographer Societies (EFRS, Europe)
- European Society of Medical Imaging Informatics (EusoMII, Europe)
- International Society of Radiographers and Radiological Technologists (ISRRT, Global)
- Irish Institute of Radiography and Radiation Therapy (IIRRT, Ireland)
- Radiographers Society of Emirates (RASE, UAE)
- Society and College of Radiographers (SCoR, UK)
- Society of Radiographers of South Africa (SORSA, SA)

14.2 Australian Society of Medical Imaging and Radiation Therapy (ASMIRT, Australia)

Mr Yasas Botenne, ASMIRT AI Reference Group Member

Mr Jens Loberg, ASMIRT AI Reference Group Member

Mr Nick Gatehouse, ASMIRT AI Reference Group Member

Dr. Christopher Hayre, ASMIRT AI Reference Group Member

Mr Andrew Murphy, ASMIRT AI reference group chair

Mr Ajesh Singh, ASMIRT AI reference group member

The Australian Society of Medical Imaging and Radiation Therapy (ASMIRT) is the peak body representing medical radiation practitioners in Australia. We aim to promote, encourage, cultivate and maintain the highest principles of practice and proficiency of medical radiation science, always mindful that the welfare of the patient should be at the centre of everything we do.

Artificial intelligence (AI) within medical imaging is not an emerging technology, but rather a reality in contemporary Australian healthcare. As AI tools are implemented within clinical settings, medical radiation professionals have a role in advocating for the safe, justified use of new technology [1].

Regulatory bodies such as the Medical Radiation Practice Board of Australia (MRPBA) have begun work on position statements to help guide medical radiation practitioners; in 2022, the MRPBA published the *Statement on artificial intelligence in medical radiation practice* [2]. The statement provided a brief comment on the need for medical radiation practitioners to be more educated and active in the safe rollout of AI tools in a clinical setting.

As an adjunct to the MRPBA statement, the artificial Intelligence reference group of the ASMIRT has authored the following set of principles to help assist medical radiation practitioners in considering and monitoring AI technology in healthcare. The principles should be used in conjunction with local, state and national regulatory guidelines for medical devices.

14.2.1 Justification

- AI systems should be justified in the context of the proposed environment, that is, the prod-

uct proposed should aim to solve or improve a current workflow or healthcare matter that is specific to the practice. *Example: a fracture detection algorithm developed on an adult data set would not be appropriate in a paediatric setting.*

The proposed AI system should demonstrate a clear benefit to healthcare outcomes from either a staff or patient perspective. *Example: an automated stroke detection tool that does not communicate with the local PACS infrastructure may pose less of a benefit than one that does.*

14.2.2 Evidence-Based

- AI systems should be evidence-based and demonstrated to perform safely in a clinical environment similar to the proposed setting. *Example: a brain haemorrhage detection system that has published evidence demonstrating efficacy in a similar hospital setting including commentary on potential pitfalls would be more beneficial than a system with no evidence attached.*

If the AI system is only tested within a company's data set without clinical evidence of intended concept, the vendor should declare it as such.

14.2.2.1 Transparency

- Whilst maintaining commercial confidence, AI developers should disclose their testing populations, including how the system would perform on specific demographics based on the local clinical setting.
  - Example: an algorithm tested on a homogenous population group within a certain age range or habitus may not perform as advertised in a trauma hospital setting servicing a wide population group
- AI manufacturers must declare how data is handled and how local data retention standards are met to ensure appropriate privacy and data protection.

14.2.2.2 Accountability

- AI systems should undergo an auditing phase during initial installation to ensure results are comparable to the proposed outcomes.
- If possible, a 90-day trial should be undertaken to allow clinical sites to audit and feedback on AI systems.
  - AI manufacturers should provide assistance if failures or anomalies are noted during an audit period.

14.3 American Society of Radiation Technologists (ASRT, USA)

Mr Craig St. George, Director of Education, ASRT

The mission of the American Society of Radiologic Technologists (ASRT) is to advance and elevate the medical imaging and radiation therapy profession and to enhance the quality and safety of patient care. Achieving this means being an innovator of knowledge and a resource for radiologic technologists seeking guidance about emerging technologies and changes in clinical practice.

Annually, ASRT Foundation hosts the Corporate Roundtable Summit, a group of industry partners who identify critical issues in radiology and share strategies to educate and prepare R.T.s for the future of the profession. In 2018, the group elected to study artificial intelligence (AI) and machine learning (ML). A roundtable subcommittee created a survey to evaluate U.S. R.T.s' knowledge and experience of AI and ML integration into medical imaging and radiation therapy practices. ASRT collected and analysed data to develop a white paper, The Artificial Intelligence Era: The Role of Radiologic Technologists and Radiation Therapists. Following the release of the 2019 Artificial Intelligence Survey results, the ASRT surveyed individuals who design and develop imaging and therapeutic equipment for six of the largest equipment manufacturing companies in the world. The purpose was to compare vendor attitudes of AI and ML to the R.T. population surveyed in 2019. Results were analysed for the 2021 Artificial Intelligence Survey: Comparing Vendors with the General Population executive summary. Though their usage of everyday technology and software skills aligned, the significant difference is vendors reported being more confident in their knowledge and attitudes of AI and ML than the general population. In 2022, ASRT produced another report to gather a post-COVID pandemic analysis of familiarity and comfort with AI and ML among working R.T.s and released the 2022 Artificial Intelligence Follow-up Survey. Little changed between the 2019 and 2022 cohorts in daily AI use and the familiarity and attitudes of AI and ML concepts. ASRT then launched a study about AI and ML use in the classroom. The 2023 AI Educator Survey [3] demonstrated that though 84.5% of educators believe these concepts are important to teach, only 23.7% currently include lessons in their course curriculum. ASRT's research demonstrated a need to provide AI and ML education for R.T.s. Using the ASRT Live platform, ASRT developed 'Medical Imaging Using Artificial Intelligence' and 'AI for Radiologic Technologists: Moving Beyond the Basics'. Course access is an ASRT member exclusive. Educators can show the lectures to their students through the Archived Webcasts site, and members can receive continuing education (CE) credit via their CE Library. Other CE Library resources include the articles 'Applications of Artificial Intelligence in Breast Imaging', 'Artificial Intelligence in Diagnostic Imaging and Radiation Therapy', and 'Artificial Intelligence in Medical Imaging'. Lastly, during the current 5-year revision cycle of ASRT's 10 curricula revision projects (2022–2026), artificial intelligence and machine learning will be included in each document.

ASRT's vision is to be the premier professional association for the medical imaging and radiation therapy community through education, advocacy, research and innovation. To that end, the ASRT will continue to offer CE, educational resources and research on AI and ML for the profession. Courses are available to non-members in the ASRT Store at www.asrt.org/store.

14.4 British Institute of Radiology (BIR, UK)

Dr Amrita Kumar, AI Advisor, British Institute of Radiology & Royal College of Radiology

The British Institute of Radiology (BIR) has played a pivotal national role given its multidisciplinary approach, in the last 5 years in the AI space, from education to addressing the multiple challenges in AI implementation (Fig. 14.1).

The BIR's work in this arena has been spearheaded by its Artificial Intelligence & Innovation Special Interest Group (AI SIG), which is a forum for those with an interest in the latest digital health technologies affecting imaging and oncology, including, but not limited to, AI and generative AI systems, supporting radiological diagnostic and therapeutic practices, and how the data generated by these systems may be better harnessed to improve clinical outcomes.

SIG members represent the breadth of the BIR community including radiologists, radiographers, radiation oncologists, academics, medical physicists, trainees and industry partners. This gives the SIG a unique membership and overview of the entire imaging pathway making its contribution multidisciplinary with a global overview of the landscape.

SIG members have been involved in the following:

1. BIR AI Congress: 2-day annual flagship in-person national and international event bringing together all stakeholders involved in AI implementation in Imaging, including healthcare workers, academics, industry, policymakers and government bodies. https://www.bir.org.uk/get-involved/special-interest-groups/bir-ai-and-innovations.aspx
2. BIR Annual Congress: With a regular AI-dedicated stream, providing the BIR multidisciplinary membership of over 4000 members, an overview of the latest AI technologies being implemented in the NHS. Non-members can also attend.
3. AI in Scotland and other events throughout the year.
4. BIR AI Essentials educational webinar series launched in March 2023 to provide free access to AI education for all healthcare workers, to aid in AI implementation, in partnership with Health Education England and NHS Digital Academy. This webinar series follows the competency framework from Health Education England and covers the following sections:
   - Introduction to AI
   - Governance
   - Implementation
   - Clinical use
   - Bias
   - Additional topics of interest

   Additional resources and access can be found at https://www.bir.org.uk/education-and-events/ai-essentials-webinar-series.aspx
5. Setting up *AI roundtables* bringing together key opinion leaders, clinicians, data experts and clinical stakeholders for a frank and in-depth discussion about the challenges of AI implementation, capturing the learnings through white paper publications and webinars. This has allowed the group to share valuable insights, provide expert advice, problem-solve, and explore how data can be better harnessed to improve clinical outcomes.

   The first roundtable article was published in *BJR|Artificial Intelligence* in 2024 entitled 'Adoption, orchestration, and deployment of artificial intelligence within the National Health Service—facilitators and barriers: an expert roundtable discussion', and can be accessed here: https://doi.org/10.1093/bjrai/ubae009. The free recording of the roundtable can be viewed here: https://www.mybir.org.

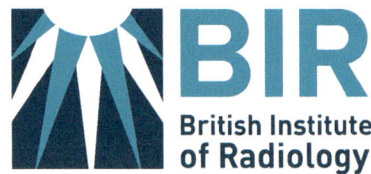

Fig. 14.1 BIR Artificial Intelligence Journal

uk/l/s/library-video-detail?recordId=a3LQC0 00005SK5l.

6. Multiple *AI-related publications* from members of the SIG contributing to AI governance, workforce challenges and AI implementation.

7. *AI Fellowship* launched at the BIR AI Congress 2024. Through this scheme, the BIR help connect interested trainees with industry partners to advance knowledge and training.

8. *Proactively forging links* with the Royal College of Radiologists (RCR), Institute of Physics & Engineering in Medicine (IPEM), Society College of Radiographers (ScoR), medical equipment vendors and the data analytics industry.

9. *Providing evidence and opinions* in official contributions to the National Institute for Health & Care Excellence (NICE), Medicines & Healthcare products Regulatory Agency (MHRA), British Standards Institution (BSI) and in development of the Multi Agency Advice service.

In 2023, the BIR launched a new open access journal, *BJR|Artificial Intelligence*, with the remit to publish high-quality, cutting-edge research and other original content focused on AI within imaging, radiation oncology and all the underpinning sciences. The journal has a multidisciplinary, international, expert Editorial Board to oversee the robust peer review process and publishes work by authors based all over the world for its global readership. *BJR|Artificial Intelligence* has published numerous high-quality articles and is currently in its second volume: https://academic.oup.com/bjrai/issue/2/1.

14.5 Canadian Association of Medical Radiation Technologists (CAMRT, Canada)

Ms Megan Brydon, Past President of the CAMRT Board of Directors
Dr Caitlin Gillan, Past Board Director and Co-founder of the CAMRT-AI Professional Practice Advisory Council

As we prepare for continued and evolving integration of AI with the medical radiation technology (MRT) environment, it can at times seem as though we are building the bridge as we cross it. In Canada, we have a relatively small population (~38 million) given our size (9,984,670 km^2), with a healthcare system funded by the federal government, with health legislation and regulation governed at the provincial level. To that end, we have a mix of jurisdictions as well as urban and very remote communities where MRTs provide care. Nationally, the Canadian Association of Medical Radiation Technologists (CAMRT) represents magnetic resonance imaging technologists, nuclear medicine technologists, radiation therapists and radiological technologists.

Since 2018, CAMRT has collaborated with MRTs, vendors and thought leaders to engage, educate and lead initiatives related to AI and MRT practice at all levels. The CAMRT leadership established an AI Advisory Council (AIAC) consisting of AI experts and change agents that have championed education for membership, established principles for CAMRT in responsible AI implementation and highlighted opportunities for collaboration.

CAMRT is a key founding partner of the Canadian Artificial intelligence and big Data in Radiotherapy Alliance (CADRA), established in 2023 in collaboration with Canadian Association of Radiation Oncology), and Canadian Organisation of Medical Physicists (COMP). Recognising the role and impact of big data and AI on the interprofessional practice of radiation oncology, CADRA is the global first profession-led collaboration in AI and big data [4].

Empowering MRTs to strategically combine their knowledge, skills and expertise with AI opportunities, CAMRT provides AI resources for, and by, MRTs. Each year, the CAMRT Annual General Conference hosts AI content as a regular/standing offering, available in-person and virtually, with on-demand options following the conference [5]. CAMRT-sponsored *Journal of Medical Imaging and Radiation Sciences* commissioned a special issue on AI, highlighting MRT-led original research, primarily arguing for the need for collaboration, attention to education and data governance considerations and initial perspectives on the potential scope of AI-enabled practice [6]. CAMRT offers a full-length self-directed continuing education course, AI and its Application in Medical Radiation Technology [7]. Designed for practicing MRTs interested in AI as it applies to their field, it covers basic concepts relevant to machine learning and big data, and how emerging AI strategies will impact MRT practice, including practical, ethical, regulatory and professional considerations.

The CAMRT webinar bank has several AI offerings: Asserting the MRT voice in championing a responsible AI-enabled future through the Canadian Artificial intelligence and Big Data in Radiotherapy Alliance (CADRA); CAMRT 2024: Generative AI: Implications for Medical Imaging Education (Among Other Things); CAMRT 2024: Population-Based Mammography Quality Using AI (2) Enhancing Breast Cancer Detection: The Impact of Breast Tomosynthesis on Screening Programs;Ethics and AI; Digital & AI 101—Webinar for Healthcare Professionals; Digital 101 Cloud & AI—Webinar for Healthcare Professionals; Snapshots of AI Innovation in Practice; There is an 'I' in AI: How do I fit into an AI-enabled future?; with more to come [8].

CAMRT is committed to proactively build capacity through a variety of mechanisms, principles and initiatives to ensure MRTs play a meaningful role in the implementation of AI in healthcare in Canada.

14.6   European Federation of Radiographer Societies (EFRS, Europe)

Dr. Patrizia Cornacchione, EFRS President
Prof. Mark F. McEntee, EFRS Vice-President
Dr Andrew England, EFRS Immediate Past-President
Mr Altino Cunha, EFRS CEO

The growth of artificial intelligence (AI) over recent years has been exponential and continues to have huge potential to revolutionise many industries, including healthcare, finance, education and many more [9] in healthcare, AI has demonstrated potential to improve disease diagnosis, treatment selection, service efficiency and patient safety [10]. Europe, through organisations such as the European Federation of Radiographer Societies (EFRS), plays a significant role in addressing the challenges and opportunities presented by AI. While there are clear advantages from AI, concerns have risen regarding its potential ethical implications [10] and safety issues [11]. Furthermore, reports of the potential for job losses [12] also continue to dominant mainstream media.

While there is much interest and debate on AI, there is no doubt that this technology is here to stay and will impact on how we practise diagnostic imaging and radiotherapy. Questions rightly exist regarding the role of a multi-professional body in this domain. The EFRS represents over 110,000 radiographers across 51 national societies and 61 affiliate members in 39 countries (www.efrs.eu). Pursuit of the optimum role for AI within radiography has been a focus of the EFRS for many years (see Fig. 14.2). This ongoing commitment underscores the EFRS's recognition of the transformative potential of AI to shaping its integration to enhance the practice of radiography.

In 2020, the EFRS in partnership with the International Society of Radiographers and Radiological Technologists (ISRRT),published a *Joint Statement* on AI in the journal *Radiography* [13]. This work identified that radiographers must play a critically important role in the planning, development, implementation, utilisation and use and validation of AI applications within their field. The *Joint Statement* also advocated that AI development should focus around the most pressing clinical and technical challenges and that appropriate education of the current and future workforce is required.

The EFRS advocates that implementation of AI must follow an evidence-based approach. Europe is paving the way in this area; since 2020, there have been over 26 peer-reviewed publications on AI within *Radiography (official journal*

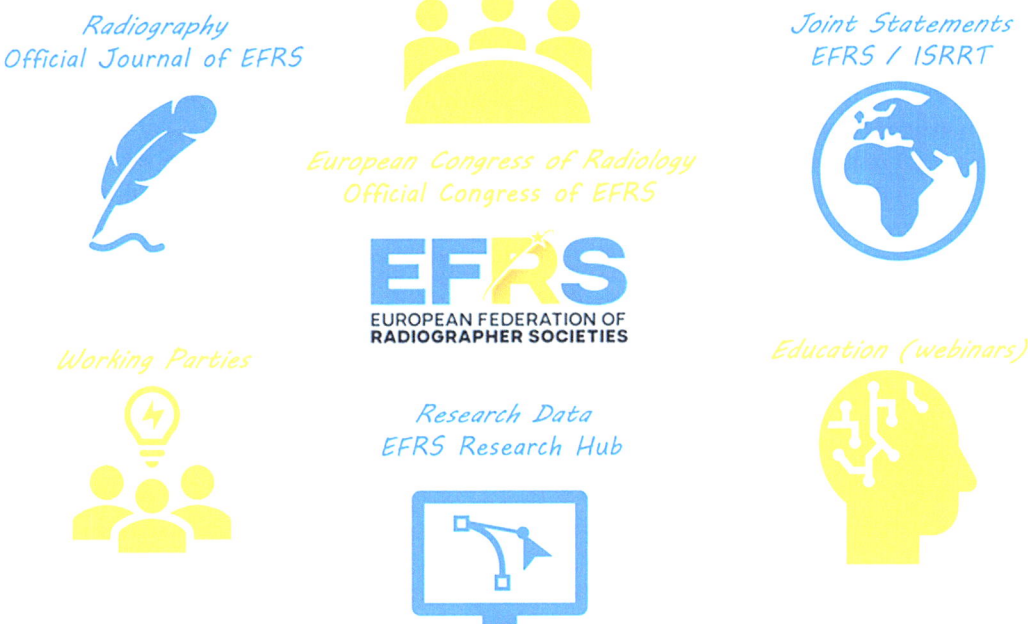

Fig. 14.2 Illustration of EFRS activities in the field of AI

of the EFRS). Topics span the full breadth of the profession, including education, radiotherapy, justification and MRI, to name only but a few. The EFRS is also contributing to debate on AI through its *Expert Network*. Nominated EFRS experts sit on several European working groups which have a focus on AI. The EFRS, through its position within the European Congress of Radiology (*official congress of the EFRS*) Programme Planning Committee, also ensures that AI remains a core component of annual congresses.

The EFRS published a leading white paper on the *Future of the Profession (Radiographer Education, Research, and Practice—RERP 2021–2031)*. Within this, AI was again a prominent feature, and this was reiterated at the EFRS Summits in Dubrovnik (2023) and Athens (2024).

The EFRS maintains its commitment to maintaining a robust and well-balanced stance on AI. As the field continues to evolve, the organisation remains vigilant, echoing the sentiments of thought leaders like Elon Musk, advocating for thoughtful regulatory oversight at both national and international levels. The EFRS stands firm in

its dedication to actively contribute to shaping responsible practices in the integration of AI within the realm of diagnostic imaging and radiotherapy. The EFRS looks forward to a future where AI contributes positive to clinical outcomes, healthcare efficiency and the development of our profession.

14.7   European Society of Medical Imaging Informatics (EuSoMII, Europe)

Prof. Erik Ranschaert, Past President EuSoMII
Prof. Peter van Ooijen, EuSoMII Past President

The European Society of Medical Imaging Informatics (EuSoMII) has a long tradition as an interdisciplinary society where professionals from various backgrounds come together based on their shared interest in Medical Imaging Informatics. As a subspecialty society of the European Society of Radiology (ESR), EuSoMII has historically been composed mainly of radiologists, medical physicists, biomedical engineers and computer scientists.

In recent years, the society has recognised the increasing role of radiographers in medical imaging informatics.

Initially, radiographers played a crucial role in digitising radiology workflows. More recently, the growing adoption of artificial intelligence (AI) in medical imaging has encouraged radiographers to engage more actively in this evolving field.

To strengthen collaboration, since 2023, EuSoMII has established an agreement with the European Federation of Radiographer Societies (EFRS), ensuring that EFRS representatives are included in the EuSoMII board and the scientific and educational subcommittees. This initiative aims to ensure that the voice of radiographers is heard and that EuSoMII's efforts in education and research align with their needs.

Under this agreement, cooperation will be intensified in the areas of both scientific research and education. EFRS members are encouraged to submit scientific papers for the EuSoMII annual meeting and are also allowed to seek collaboration from other members of the association to participate in research projects. In terms of training, all EFRS members can also make use of the material made available on the EuSoMII website, consisting of webinars and podcasts. This cooperation also includes a greater focus on the profession of radiographers in such educational platforms. Finally, the EuSoMII will also increase the involvement of the radiographer's viewpoint in publishing white papers and other recommendations for the radiological community.

14.7.1 Joint Initiatives

EuSoMII and EFRS have jointly launched several collaborative initiatives in recent years, emphasising the importance of interdisciplinary engagement and the evolving role of radiographers in the era of artificial intelligence (AI).

One notable outcome of their cooperation is the co-authored paper titled 'Responsible AI practice and AI education are central to AI implementation: a rapid review for all medical imaging professionals in Europe'. This publication high-lights key themes such as the necessity of ethical AI practices, interdisciplinary collaboration, tailored educational efforts and the cultivation of trust in AI among both healthcare professionals and patients.

In addition to joint publishing efforts, the two societies organised a webinar entitled 'Framing in the Fourth Research Paradigm: An Educational Perspective', delivered by Robin Decoster on 27 June 2023. This session explored how the Fourth Research Paradigm reshapes healthcare research by fostering collaboration, promoting data-driven methodologies, supporting patient-centred approaches and reinforcing ethical considerations in educational practices.

Radiographer engagement in EuSoMII's activities has also grown steadily. At the EuSoMII Annual Meeting 2023 and 2024, radiographers represented 15% of participants, while 9% took part in the 2023 AI Contest and 15% in the 2024 edition.

A further joint effort is the AIMIROE project, a collaborative initiative funded and endorsed by EuSoMII, with support from EFRS and the European Society of Radiology (ESR). AIMIROE aims to establish a comprehensive register of AI-related educational programs in medical imaging and radiotherapy (MIRO) across Europe. Developed in collaboration with experts, the project uses survey-based data collection to map existing AI training initiatives. The findings will be presented at the EuSoMII Annual Meeting 2025, themed 'Prompting the Future', in Heraklion, Crete. The outcome of this initiative will be a searchable platform to be published on the EuSoMII website, providing a valuable resource for radiographers and other professionals seeking AI education opportunities.

In support of advanced AI training, EuSoMII has also contributed to the development of the AI Masterclass, which is now part of ESR's premium education package. This course, designed by international experts and coordinated by EuSoMII, covers both foundational AI concepts and real-world clinical applications through engaging e-learning modules.

Finally, in early 2025, following formal elections, EuSoMII renewed its Core Board. Peter van Ooijen handed over the presidency to Daniel Pinto dos Santos. Among the five elected Members at Large, one represents EFRS, reinforcing the ongoing partnership. Additionally, the Education and Scientific Committees now each include a member appointed by the EFRS, further solidifying the role of radiographers in shaping EuSoMII's educational and research agendas.

14.8   International Society of Radiographers and Radiological Technologists (ISRRT, Global)

Mr Hakon Hjemly, Vice President of the Europe and Africa Region, ISRRT
Mr Lars Henriksen, Member, ISRRT
Prof Naoki Kodama, Director of the Asia and Australasia Region, ISRRT
Dr Yudthaphon Vichianin, Director of Public Relations and Communication, ISRRT
Mr Edward HT Chan, Director of Professional Practice, ISRRT

For the development of AI in radiography, ISRRT made one joint position statement with EFRS, two FB webinars (https://www.youtube.com/watch?v=vKOpm3tYNq8) and https://www.youtube.com/watch?v=xNAZJlDP_ZM) and one special edition of the WRD publication in 2020. (https://www.isrrt.org/wp-content/uploads/2023/07/WRD-2020-special-edition_N.pdf)

• The Summary of Joint Position Statement [14]

'Artificial Intelligence and the Radiographer/Radiological Technologist Profession is a joint statement by ISRRT & EFRS. (https://www.isrrt.org/proffesional-practice/artificial-intelligence/)

The International Society of Radiographers and Radiological Technologists (ISRRT) and the European Federation of Radiographer Societies (EFRS) made a joint statement, 'Artificial Intelligence and the Radiographer/Radiological Technologist Profession' in 2020. The statement addresses the role of radiographers and radiological technologists in relation to artificial intelligence (AI) in the field of medical imaging and radiotherapy.

Radiographers and radiological technologists are responsible for the well-being of patients during imaging investigations and therapy procedures. They play a crucial role in ensuring patient safety, justification and optimisation of medical imaging procedures and radiation safety in accordance with relevant legislation.

The document highlights the increasing integration of AI and machine learning algorithms in medical imaging and radiation therapy, emphasising the need for radiographers and technologists to adapt their practices to ensure the appropriate implementation and regulation of AI technologies. They should rely on high-quality research evidence and undergo appropriate education and training to maximise the benefits of AI for patients.

The statement provides several key points regarding the use of AI in radiography:

1. Validated Implementation: AI should only be implemented in clinical practice after being validated and proven beneficial to patients through robust research evidence.
2. Clinical Decision Support: Radiographers should utilise AI as a tool for clinical decision support, particularly in justifying examinations and communicating relative benefit/risk discussions of radiation dose to patients.
3. Workflow optimisation: AI has the potential to optimise imaging and radiotherapy workflows, including streamlined appointments, prioritisation of examinations and shorter examination times. Radiographers must ensure that care is patient-centred, prioritise equitable healthcare, and minimise potential biases within AI systems.
4. Dose reduction and quality assurance: AI can contribute to dose reduction and optimisation in modalities involving ionising radiation. It may also play a role in automated quality assurance and indicate the need for repeat examinations in case of equivocal or poor-quality images. Clear protocols and quality

standards should be developed for the implementation of AI systems.

5. Immediate results and triage: AI-supported image interpretation can enable radiographers to provide immediate results to patients, facilitating triage for additional imaging examinations or referral to other specialties.

The document also emphasises the role of radiographers and radiological technologists in optimising the use of AI:

1. Evidence-based practice: Radiographers should embrace and adapt technology based on evidence and patient needs. AI should be used as a support tool, not a replacement for clinical judgement.

2. Collaboration and education: Radiographers should collaborate with industry and healthcare professionals to develop AI solutions for current and future medical imaging challenges. They should have a broad understanding of AI algorithms and their limitations, as well as actively maintain and develop core skills and competencies.

3. Advocacy and leadership: Radiographers should advocate for the adaptation of legislation to maximise the benefits of AI for patients and professionals. They should work at national and international levels with policymakers and ensure investment in AI research and workforce development.

In conclusion, the joint statement emphasises the active involvement of radiographers and radiological technologists in the planning, development, implementation, use and validation of AI applications in medical imaging and radiation therapy. It underlines the importance of appropriate education and engagement to achieve optimal integration of AI technologies while addressing the pressing clinical problems in the field.

Two AI-related webinars are on Facebook for a rerun, viz. 'Overview of the current status of AI surrounding the field of radiological medical technology' (https://www.youtube.com/watch?v=xNAZJlDP_ZM) and (https://www.

youtube.com/watch?v=vKOpm3tYNq8) and 'AI in radiography practice: International Perspectives'. (https://www.youtube.com/watch?v=vKOpm3tYNq8)

On the other hand, both organisations agreed to review the statement in 2025 to address the advancements in AI technology.

ISRRT released a special edition of newsletters titled 'Elevation Patient Care with AI' in 2020. It includes perspectives and ideas from various stakeholders of radiography around the world on AI applications and their impact on the profession. (https://www.isrrt.org/communication/world-radiography-day/special-edition-2020/)

14.9 Irish Institute of Radiography and Radiation Therapy (IIRRT, Ireland)

Dr. Jennifer Grehan, IIRRT President
Liam Downey, IIRRT Vice-President

The Irish Institute for Radiography and Radiation Therapy (IIRRT) is the professional body for radiographers and radiation therapists in Ireland. Regarding the evolution of artificial intelligence (AI), a set of computer algorithms capable of undertaking tasks traditionally performed by humans and given the speed of introduction and potential for challenge to conventional work practices, as a professional body, we are committed to ensuring that our members are as supported as possible in becoming familiar with the fundamentals before integrating AI into their everyday practice. While no strangers to advances in digital imaging and its' impact on service provision, given the potential impact of AI to diagnostic imaging modalities and radiation therapy services, the IIRRT have implemented a range of initiatives to optimise knowledge on the benefits of AI while upholding the highest standards of patient care.

The IIRRT has ongoing collaborations with academic and industry partners to develop and endorse comprehensive CPD packages focused on AI applications in radiography. These packages range from single online introductory talks, to face-to-face offerings on the topic, to bespoke online CPD events focused on the integration of AI into the clinical space. Webinars are further offered as a post-event member resource through the IIRRT website. This has culminated in building the central theme of the most recent IIRRT National Conference around AI, ethical considerations, opportunities and boundaries.

With the imminent arrival of the European AI Act [15] and ongoing guidance from working groups and professional bodies working in the area [16, 17], the IIRRT are in the process of establishing guidelines and standards for the ethical and responsible use of AI in radiography and radiation therapy in Ireland. Through collaboration with academic and clinical colleagues, regulatory bodies and industry experts, the framework will address key considerations such as patient privacy, data security and transparency. These best practice guidelines will serve as a reference for radiographers and radiation therapists to navigate ethical and legal implications surrounding AI implementation in clinical practice.

The IIRRT provides a range of online resources to support members in understanding AI. These include access to professional journals, best practice toolkits and guides and materials developed by affiliated organisations offering practical insights into the implementation of AI in clinical settings. Additionally, facilitated face-to-face events offer networking opportunities for knowledge exchange, and to share experiences.

Through research, and collaborative partnerships with academic institutions, the IIRRT fosters a culture of innovation and inquiry within the professional community. In this way, we advance the evidence base for AI integration and contribute to the development of evidence-based practices.

The IIRRT is dedicated to supporting radiographers and radiation therapists in Ireland in their adoption of AI into clinical practice. Through education, guidelines, resource provision and research support, we continue to empower radiographers to embrace these technologies appropriately, while upholding the highest standards of patient care and professional excellence.

By providing and facilitating necessary support and resources, we ensure that radiographers and radiation therapists are well-prepared to harness AI benefits and contribute to the advancement of both professions in Ireland.

14.10 Radiographers Society of Emirates (RASE, UAE)

Mrs   Samar   El-Farra,   Vice   President, Radiographers Society of Emirates

The field of radiography has undergone significant transformation in recent years largely due to advancements in AI technology, and the Radiographers Society of Emirates (RASE) plays an important role in advancing and embracing artificial intelligence (AI) education and training in medical imaging. AI applications have the potential to revolutionise radiographic practices, enhancing accuracy, efficiency and accessibility, ultimately improving patient care, concentration and communication. However, the successful integration of AI relies not only on technological innovation but also on the active involvement of our society in educating its members. This pivotal role that our society plays in incorporating AI applications into radiography is evident through our annual educational conferences.

AI in radiography encompasses a wide range of applications, including image interpretation, diagnosis, workflow optimisation and predictive analytics. These applications have the potential to streamline workflows, reduce human errors, alleviate radiographers' burnout and enhance patient care. However, to realise these benefits, radiographers must be equipped with the knowledge and skills required to effectively integrate AI into their daily practice. Our annual educational conferences serve as crucial platforms for disseminating knowledge, sharing best practices and fostering professional development among radiographers. These conferences bring together experts, researchers and practitioners from the field to discuss the latest advancements and challenges. In the context of AI, these conferences are instrumental in providing radiographers with the tools and insights needed to harness this technology effectively.

Our society plays a pivotal role in disseminating knowledge about AI applications in radiography. Through lectures, workshops and panel discussions, these conferences provide radiographers with an opportunity to learn about the latest AI algorithms, tools and techniques. Experts from both academia and industry share their insights and experiences, helping radiographers stay updated on the rapidly evolving AI landscape. Education conferences also prioritise skills development. Radiographers can participate in hands-on workshops where they can practice using AI tools and software for image analysis and interpretation. These practical sessions empower radiographers to develop the necessary skills to seamlessly integrate AI into their clinical workflows. Ethical and regulatory considerations are crucial when it comes to AI in radiography, including patient data privacy, liability and algorithm transparency. Our society uses these conferences as platforms to discuss these issues and provide guidance to its members. This ensures that radiographers are not only proficient in using AI but also knowledgeable about the ethical and legal aspects of its implementation. Collaboration and networking opportunities abound at our annual education conferences. Radiographers can connect with AI developers, researchers and industry representatives to explore potential partnerships and collaborations. These interactions can lead to the development of AI solutions tailored to the specific needs of radiography. Conferences also serve as forums for radiographers to provide feedback on AI tools and technologies. This feedback loop is essential for AI developers to refine their solutions and address any issues that may arise in real-world clinical settings. Our society plays a crucial role in incorporating artificial intelligence applications into radiography through its annual education conferences. These conferences serve as hubs for knowledge dissemination, skill development, ethical discussions, collaboration and feedback. A link to the conference platform is provided here https://radiologyuae.com/. This is the 10th meeting and showcases the early integration of AI sessions. As AI continues to evolve and become increasingly integrated into radiography, the active engagement of our society in educating its members will be paramount in ensuring that AI enhances patient care while maintaining the highest standards of quality and ethics. The ongoing commitment of our society to AI education will ultimately shape the future of radiography and healthcare as a whole.

14.11 Society and College of Radiographers (SCoR, UK)

Dr Tracy O'Regan, Professional Officer Clinical Imaging and Research

The UK Society of Radiographers (SoR) is a trade union and professional body for diagnostic and therapeutic radiographers, sonographers and associated professionals. The SoR takes a proactive role towards artificial intelligence (AI), which includes a focus on clinical practice, research, education, guidance, collaboration and advocacy.

The SoR aims to empower its members to embrace and navigate the safe and effective integration of AI into clinical practice. The actions taken by SoR to date have been informed by the initial 2020 publication of The Society and College of Radiographers policy statement: Artificial Intelligence | SoR.

With the recognition of the extensive philosophical, ethical, professional and legal debate present in a range of fields, the SoR set up an AI Working Party to develop guidance for members. In 2021, the working party developed Artificial intelligence: Guidance for clinical imaging and therapeutic radiography workforce profess | SoR, which provided recommendations based on clinical practice, education, research and stakeholder partnerships. Recommendations from the SoR guidance have since been incorporated into SoR publications including Education and Career Framework for the Radiography Workforce | SoR The AI Guidance will be reviewed and updated in 2025.

The SoR Artificial Intelligence Advisory Group | SoR was formed following publication of the guidance. The AI advisory group is supported by a SoR Professional Officer, has terms of reference and an annual work plan to support their remit. Members have authored a range of peer-review publications in relevant international journals. To date, the group have undertaken collaborations with multiprofessional teams on national and international basis (see Fig. 14.1). SoR therefore engage with government bodies, regulatory agencies and other stakeholders to shape policies that promote the safe and effective use of AI in radiography. SoR Patient Advisory Group (PAG) | SoR provide comment and suggestions for ongoing work and publications.

Alongside that partnership work, the SoR AI Advisory Group have provided members with a series of educational resources Recorded Artificial Intelligence Webinars | SoR including general introduction to AI for radiographers, uses of AI in radiography, and AI implementation challenges and opportunities with planned updates to the series, see Fig. 14.3. The college of radiographers (CoR) and NHS England e-learning for clinical imaging programme has also published an online session *Introduction to AI for healthcare professionals* e-LfH.

SoR host Artificial Intelligence Webinar Series Hub | SoR, which has links to additional online resources and also provide an online workspace and discussion board for digital, informatics and artificial Intelligence, which is open to all SoR members by contacting pande@sor.org

With respect to research, the CoR held two calls for AI Radiography Research Gran vts to date, with awards made to SoR members for 8 projects covering a range of AI topics related to diagnostic and therapeutic radiography. The intention is to foster innovation by providing grants, funding or resources for healthcare professionals to develop and implement AI solutions in their practice. SoR members are kept up to date with information, calls for research and developments in SoR AI work via monthly Synergy | SoR newsletter updates and social media accounts.

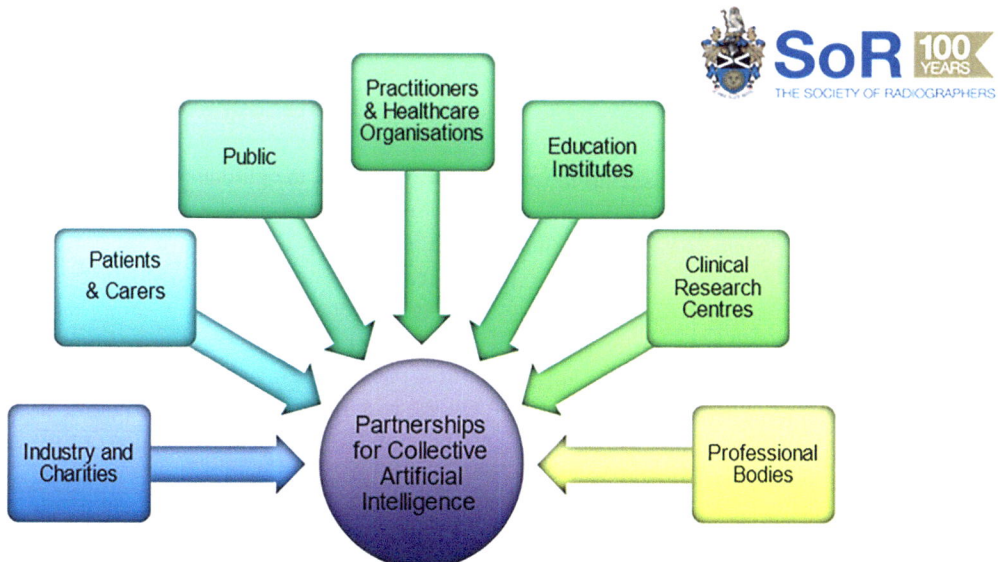

Fig. 14.3 The Society of Radiographers Artificial Intelligence Advisory Group

14.12 Society of Radiographers of South Africa (SORSA, SA)

Dr Riaan van de Venter, SORSA Executive Committee Member
Dr Fozy Peer, SORSA Executive Committee Member
Mrs Ferial Isaacs, SORSA Executive Committee Member
Mrs Leonie Munro, SORSA Executive Committee Member
Mr Selvan Govindsamy, SORSA Executive Committee Member
Ms Taahirah Mookrey, SORSA Executive Committee Member

Since 2018 the Society of Radiographers of South Africa (SORSA) has been proactive in raising awareness about artificial intelligence (AI) and its impact on the medical imaging and radiation sciences professions. There are three open-access publications that cover AI-related topics in *The South African Radiographer*: the emerging role of AI in imaging, informed consent in the use of patient data in AI, and challenges of the use of AI by authors and peer reviewers in scientific publications. From 2019 to 2023, AI papers were presented at continuing professional development events. SORSA also submitted comments pertaining to the scope of the profession, and shared AI documents with the higher education institutions (HEIs) that offer radiography programmes. The scientific programme of the SORSA-IAFR 2025 congress in September includes a session on AI in imaging.

The RSSA-SORSA August 2019 Imaging Congress included presentations on AI in imaging as well as a 2 h congress course on ethical issues pertaining to AI in imaging and health and its use in medical devices. In 2020, SORSA hosted a virtual symposium in September and one in November. Six speakers at the September event discussed elevating patient care with AI; AI and emotional intelligence was discussed at the November event. SORSA participated in the ISRRT Facebook webinar on 8 November 2020 in terms of how AI may impact radiography practice.

SORSA's 7th virtual symposium in July 2022 included a presentation on the legal principles pertaining to the use of AI in radiology service in South Africa. At SORSA's hybrid congress in August 2023, the chairperson of the International Bioethics Committee, UNESCO presented a paper on an ethical perspective of the UNESCO AI guidelines.

In August 2020, SORSA submitted comments to the National Minister of Health underscoring that the profession of radiography is constantly adopting technological advances including the impact of AI and machine learning. SORSA recommended that AI should be included in the proposed amendments to the regulations of the scope of the profession. In May 2022, SORSA submitted a recommendation to the Professional Board of Radiography and Clinical Technology (PBRCT), Health Professions Council of South Africa, to consider the development of guidelines for HEIs in terms of inclusion of AI in radiography programmes. The proposed amendments to the scope of the profession, and the above recommendation, are work in progress.

In 2022 and 2023, SORSA shared the World Health Organisation (WHO) AI guideline documents with the HEIs offering radiography in South Africa, as well as the PBRCT.

14.13 Chapter Summary

In this chapter, the guidance and support offered to radiographers has been provided by 11 radiographer professional bodies worldwide. There is a range of helpful resources already being implemented for the training and education of radiographers on AI worldwide. Information is being updated as AI tools become more widely embedded into routine practice. The professional bodies presented outlined their supportive approaches and commitment to the ongoing training and development of radiographers in their countries. Radiographers are practicing at the forefront of advances in medical imaging and it is imperative that their training and education keep pace with the evolving advancements in AI technology.

References

1. Murphy A, Liszewski B. Artificial Intelligence and the medical radiation profession: How our advocacy must inform future practice. J Med Imaging Radiat Sci. 2019;50(4). https://doi.org/10.1016/j.jmir.2019.09.001.

2. Statement on Artificial Intelligence (AI) [Internet]. [cited 2024 Jan 8]. Available from: https://www.medicalradiationpracticeboard.gov.au/Registration-Standards/Statementon-Artificial-Intelligence.aspx.

3. Stogiannos N, et al. The American Society of Radiologic Technologists (ASRT) AI educator survey: a cross-sectional study to explore knowledge, experience, and use of AI within education. J Med Imaging Radiat Sci. 2023;55(4):101449.

4. Canadian Artificial Intelligence & Data in Radiotherapy Alliance. 2023. Available from https://www.cadra-acadr.ca/.

5. CAMRT Conferences and Events. 2024. Available from https://www.camrt.ca/conferences-and-events/.

6. Artificial Intelligence in Medical Radiation Sciences: Special Issue. J Med Imaging Radiat Sci. 2019;50(4):Supplement 2.

7. CAMRT Professional Development. 2024. Available from https://www.camrt.ca/professional-development/.

8. CAMRT CPD At your fingertips; A national repository. 2024. Available from https://repository.camrt.ca/

9. Devlin H. AI 'could be as transformative as Industrial Revolution'. The Guardian, 3rd May 2023. Available at: https://www.theguardian.com/technology/2023/may/03/ai-could-be-as-transformative-as-industrial-revolution-patrick-vallance.

10. Alowais SA, Alghamdi SS, Alsuhebany N, Alqahtani T, Alshaya AI, Almohareb SN, Aldairem A, Alrashed M, Bin Saleh K, Badreldin HA, Al Yami MS, Al Harbi S, Albekairy AM. Revolutionising healthcare: the role of artificial intelligence in clinical practice. BMC Med Educ. 2023;23(1):689.

11. Da Silva M, Flood CM, Goldenberg A, Singh D. Regulating the safety of health-related artificial Intelligence. Healthc Policy. 2022;17(4):63–77.

12. Khogali HO, Mekid S. The blended future of automation and AI: examining some long-term societal and ethical impact features. Technol Soc. 2023;73:102232.

13. The European Federation of Radiographer Societies. Artificial Intelligence and the Radiographer/Radiological Technologist Profession: A joint statement of the International Society of Radiographers and Radiological Technologists and the European Federation of Radiographer Societies. Radiography. 2020;26(2):93–5.

14. The International Society of Radiographers & Radiological Technologists (ISRRT) & EFRS. Artificial Intelligence and the Radiographer/Radiological Technologist Profession- A Joint Statement of the International Society of Radiographers and Radiological Technologists and the European Federation of Radiographer Societies [document on the Internet]. 2020. [cited 2024 Jan 8]; Available from: https://www.isrrt.org/proffesional-practice/artificial-intelligence/.

15. European Union. AI Act (Regulation (EU) 2024/1689). Available via https://eur-lex.europa.eu/legal-content/EN/TXT/?uri=CELEX%3A32024R1689. Accessed 17 Mar 2025.

16. Kotter E, D'Antonoli TA, Cuocolo R, Hierath M, Huisman M, Klontzas ME, Martí-Bonmatí L, May MS, Neri E, Nikolaou K, Pinto dos Santos D. Guiding AI in radiology: ESR's recommendations for effective implementation of the European AI Act. Insights into Imaging. 2025;16(1):33. Available via https://insightsimaging.springeropen.com/articles/10.1186/s13244-025-01905-x. Accessed 17 Mar 2025.

17. The Royal College of Radiologists. Clinical Radiology: AI deployment fundamentals for medical imaging. Nov 2024. Available via https://www.rcr.ac.uk/media/sbdhwnfl/ai-deployment-fundamentals-for-medical-imaging-2024.pdf. Accessed 17 Mar 2025.

Preparing for a Future with AI

15

Maryann Hardy, Karen M Knapp, Aarthi Ramlaul ⓘ,
and Christina Malamateniou

15.1 Introduction

While this book has focussed on currently deployed AI applications in radiography and the potential of AI for the present and immediate future, we should also consider the longer-term impact of AI on radiography education, research and practice, some of which is also touched upon in Chap. 4. Importantly, some of the changes explored below are already evident or in play, but our understanding of how they will change our professional roles and activities is still evolving [1]. To begin this perspective into the future, let us start at the very beginning of the radiographer's journey and the impact of AI on student learning.

on behalf of Association of Healthcare Technology Providers for Imaging, Radiotherapy and Care (AXREM)

M. Hardy
University of Bradford, Bradford, UK

Radiant Horizons Coaching Ltd, Bingley, UK

K. M. Knapp
Faculty of Health Studies, University of Exeter, Exeter, UK

A. Ramlaul
College of Health and Society,
Buckinghamshire New University, High Wycombe, UK

C. Malamateniou (✉)
Division of Radiography, Department of Allied Health Sciences, School of Health and Medical Sciences, City St George's University of London, London, UK
e-mail: christina.malamateniou@city.ac.uk

15.2 Radiography Education

AI is poised to significantly impact higher education in the United Kingdom across teaching, learning, administration and research. While we have read about the potential of AI platforms to streamline clinical workflows (Chaps. 4, 5, 6, 7, 8, 9, 10 and 11), AI also has the potential to streamline higher education admissions processes from virtual open days and advertisements supported by chatbots, targeted advertisements to interested candidates, through to candidate selection based on pre-set criteria predicting likely success and enhancing enrolment processes through automation. After admissions, digital coaches may also be able to support students in their learning by responding to questions or directing students to relevant resources, for example, for well-being of academic support, saving administrative workload from professional service and academic staff and offering prompt student support 24/7. Through the analysis of individual student learning patterns, areas of strength and area in need of greater development, AI systems could create customised student learning experiences with educators being supported to tailor learning content to meet student learning needs, moving away from the 'one lecture suits all' mindset of the past and helping all students to fulfil their academic potential. Adaptive learning platforms, intelligent tutoring systems and learner analytics systems to identify students who are struggling and suggest interventions have all been developed in different settings, but the future adoption of such systems, combined with an internationally agreed knowledge and skills threshold learning framework for radiography, could revolutionise radiography education and pave the way for a truly global workforce [2]. Without doubt, AI can help make education more accessible for students with disabilities, learning differences or other barriers to learning [3, 4]. For example, speech-to-text and text-to-speech tools are already in use for students with hearing or visual impairments, but for international students or students for whom English is a second language, AI-powered translation tools may be advantageous. Similarly, for those impacted by dyslexia or other neurodivergence, AI-based tools like Grammarly can assist in assignment writing or note taking and screen readers support engagement with wider resources [5, 6].

But it is not just students who may benefit from chatbot coaches. Lecturers and academic staff can use AI coaching systems to improve lesson plans, create engaging learning activities and provide student feedback. These tools can support advancements in personalised learning and adaptive teaching making radiography education within the university setting more inclusive and person centred [7]. To provide a globally inclusive system then, we need to consider the accessibility of AI. Support for the use of such systems varies between learning institutions but forward-thinking organisations are planning for a student learning experience vastly different from the past [8]. AI advancements are prompting educators to rethink curricula to prepare students for an AI-driven world. As university structures, facilities and student cohorts are uniquely diverse, the issue of equity of access must be considered, as unequal access to AI technologies could potentially widen digital inequalities and educational opportunities.

The potential future changes in education are not without ethical and pedagogical challenges, most notably the rise in the use of generative AI systems and concerns over plagiarism and the authenticity of student work [9]. This is a challenge for educators today without currently an agreement or a solution, but perhaps the way forward could be for AI platforms to initially mark and assess submitted work (as a first-pass quality control), flagging work where high levels of plagiarism or lack of adherence to assignment guidelines are determined, much like a clinical triage AI-enabled system in chest interpretation. In this way, educators could become the second marker, reducing assessment marking burden and freeing academic time to support student learning more actively. However, a major issue yet to be resolved is the potential bias within AI algorithms or AI resources that may inadvertently bias training materials and data, and discriminate against certain student demographics or groups, or suggest unbalanced or flawed interpretations and summaries. Hence, humans will continue to be the mediators for some time, until these systems are trialled and tested under different conditions. Some academic publishers have already paved the way, as they started using AI for triage of submitted academic papers, as a way to minimise the load to editors and reviewers and streamline the review process, increasing consistency and minimising delays [10]. It is a matter of time before this can be transferred to other areas of academic publishing and quality assessment, such as academia.

We are at the beginning of the AI education revolution for radiography, with many exciting developments lying ahead; but learning in radiography does not just take place in the University setting and AI-assisted learning within the clinical setting has additional challenges we are yet to explore fully. What is clear is that the knowledge and digital skills of everyone involved in radiography education, from clinical radiographers who support practice learning in the clinical environment to experienced academic educators, will need to be developed if they are to be ready for the changes ahead. Significant debate has arisen on whether we need to rid of old knowledge, skills and competencies in favour of new ones; this is to ensure the taught curriculum remains manageable within the allocated time. Also, the fear or deskilling because of AI automation remains significant. However, as Ai has yet to prove its ability to solved real problems with accuracy across different contexts, human intelligence remains central. The old ways will still serve us well, while we try to master the new requirements.

15.3 Skills Development for Education: Training the Trainers

Preparing radiography educators within both university institutions and clinical departments for a future with AI requires a multifaceted and collaborative approach combining professional development, technical training, ethical awareness and organisational support for change. However, it is not without significant psychological and cultural challenges as academic and clinical radiographers alike may feel threatened by AI and vulnerable in terms of understanding their role in the new AI-driven educational environment. Such concerns might be overcome by highlighting the importance of human-AI collaboration and emphasise that AI is a tool to enhance teaching and learning and not replace educators. Additionally, organisations might encourage and foster a culture that values innovation and experimentation with AI in teaching and provide counselling or peer support networks for those struggling with the transition. However, central to enabling AI-supported education is assuring all educators have a foundational level of knowledge in AI [11].

All educators need a solid understanding of AI concepts, tools and applications and how they might be applied to support learning. Such knowledge needs to be developed and supported through purposeful training and, in addition to AI concepts, should include the development of skills to explore and navigate AI-powered platforms aimed at streamlining and personalising the student experience; exploration of the use of AI in academic and practical assessments, ethical and pedagogical challenges, peer mentoring and contribution towards evolving strategic and operational policy in the use of AI for teaching and learning within different organisational settings. Finally, it may be necessary for the content of teaching qualifications, whether focussed on supporting learning in practice or in the academic setting, to be regularly reviewed and revised to ensure AI competencies are embedded and remain current as technology advances.

Developing clinical and academic radiography educators to confidently, competently and optimally use AI technologies requires a comprehensive approach that combines technical training, ethical awareness and support for ongoing continuous professional development. By equipping educators with these skills, we can ensure that radiography education continues to thrive as a person focussed process enriched by technological innovation. However, education must ensure it keeps up with changes in clinical practice and so the next question to consider is how might AI impact radiography clinical practice?

15.4 Clinical Practice

Without doubt, AI has the potential to revolutionise radiography clinical practice by enhancing efficiency, accuracy and patient outcomes as has been discussed in Chaps. 4, 5, 6, 7, 8, 9, 10 and 11. These chapters have already discussed opportunities for:

- *Workflow optimisation* by triaging appointments based on urgency of clinical history, patient demographics and staff or equipment availability to reduce bottlenecks in examination lists as well as adjusting reporting priority status based on AI findings.
- *Enhanced image acquisition processes* making it faster and more reliable by assessing acceptability of patient positioning and exposure parameters and making recommendations for additional or repeat imaging. AI may also provide real-time feedback within cross-sectional imaging modalities to detect motion artefact, optimise exposure parameters and suggest patient-centred imaging protocols dependent on clinical history, patient demographics and referral pathway.
- Support interventional imaging through *real-time procedural guidance*. For example, highlighting anatomical landmarks for catheter placement, predicting optimal needle trajectory for biopsies and analysing pre- and post-

procedural data to predict, mitigate and monitor procedural risks.

- *Improved image analysis* systems leading to higher diagnostic accuracy earlier in the patient pathway and reduction in reporting inconsistencies between image readers.
- *Potential provision of AI preliminary reporting services* being developed using language appropriate to the referral pathway, clinical question and to provide lay summaries understandable to patients.
- Provision of an *AI-driven comprehensive QA analysis* service based on equipment and radiographer operation to confirm compliance and inform interventions and continuing professional development enhancements.
- *Augmented patient care*, supporting radiographers in their interactions with patients, enabling tailored communication and care based on patient clinical history or preferences. As with education, the availability of AI-powered chatbots or virtual assistants to answer patient queries could ensure provision of person-centred wrap-around care.

While AI systems could provide excellent opportunities for improving radiography practice and patient experience, the transition to AI-driven practice also brings challenges related to implementation, ethics and professional adaptation and cost (see also Chap. 4). Acquiring, integrating and maintaining AI systems seamlessly into clinical practice in a vendor-neutral context, as within larger imaging equipment, remains someway off and is currently an expensive undertaking and therefore further work exploring cost-effectiveness, robust business cases and proportionate reimbursement is required.

There is also a concern that radiographers may become over-reliant on AI tools, potentially leading to deskilling in problem-solving in relation to both image acquisition and image evaluation practices. In contrast, some radiographers may be resistant to adopt AI due to fear of job displacement or lack of knowledge of or familiarity with the technology, resulting in inconsistent or suboptimal imaging practices and poorer patient experience. To address these concerns, radiographers need to be educated in AI functionality and create or accept the new roles, working collaboratively with AI systems and taking responsibility for validating AI outputs to ensure that decisions made with AI are accurate and clinically relevant. As with all AI systems, radiographer awareness of potential database bias that could result in disparities in care, and how to mitigate these, is essential.

AI is set to transform radiography clinical practice and radiographers will need to embrace AI as a tool to augment their expertise rather than replace it, focussing on tasks that require human judgement, empathy and ethical oversight. While challenges such as deskilling, ethical concerns and resistance to change exist, ongoing professional development and thoughtful integration of AI into workflows will ensure that radiographers continue to play a vital role in healthcare delivery, although professional identity and role may need to be revised to reflect the digital imaging environment.

15.5   Professional Identity

This has been discussed already in Chaps. 3 and 4, with brief references in Chap. 7. Advances in AI will undoubtedly impact the professional identity of radiographers, as AI technologies become increasingly capable of assisting or automating aspects of radiographic work. However, these advances also permit radiographers to reshape their roles, extend their impact on patient journey, redefine their clinical and research responsibilities and challenge traditional perceptions of the profession. Perhaps most fundamental of the changes that may occur is the change of radiographer role emphasis from image acquisition to clinical advice. AI systems can evaluate and analyse medical images with a high degree of accuracy leaving space for radiographers to transition from image acquisition and interpretation roles to acting as clinical advisors and AI experts, integrating AI findings at all stages of the patient imaging pathway, with clinical knowledge suitable to provide comprehensive patient care [12]. In addition, widespread AI adoption may drive radiographers towards more advanced technical responsibilities, requiring upskilling and professional transition. For example, radiographers may take on roles in training and managing AI systems, ensuring that these tools are properly calibrated, validated and interpreted [13]. Similarly, expertise in AI advanced analytics may provide opportunities for radiographers to collaborate more closely with other professions, becoming integral to multidisciplinary team (MDT) meetings and contributing data to inform treatment options, ultimately elevating radiographer status beyond imaging professional to healthcare strategist. This pathway may not be for everyone and tasks requiring empathy, communication and patient care, such as explaining procedures, addressing patient concerns and patient advocacy and tailoring imaging to patient needs, potentially guided by AI suggestions, will remain central to radiographers' roles, reinforcing the human element of their professional identity. Additionally, radiographers may play a key role in shaping the responsible use of AI in healthcare, influencing their professional identity as ethical leaders with expertise in AI governance, bias and fairness, data privacy, security and policy development. Furthermore, radiographers, with the right training and industry collaborations, may become AI innovators, as their native position, working on the interface between the patient, where clinical challenges may occur, and the technological equipment, where technical challenges may arise, is strategic for problem solving. Regardless of pathway taken, radiographers who can embrace and adapt to AI-enhanced workflows while excelling at tasks that AI cannot replicate (e.g. patient interaction, and ethical oversight) may find themselves becoming role models for the clinical radiographer practitioner and professional leaders of the future. By leveraging AI to deliver more accurate, efficient and ethical care, radiographers can position themselves as essential, forward-thinking healthcare professionals in an increasingly AI-driven world. However, without opportunities for upskilling and developing technological expertise, radiographers may face concerns over their future, particularly in areas where AI is viewed as a cost-saving alternative. It is therefore incumbent upon all in the radiography profession, but, in particular, clinical managers, practice and academic educators, to ensure that the current and future workforce are prepared for the AI responsibilities envisaged. One of those is the advancement of radiography research in the field of AI, which is discussed further below.

15.6 Revolutionising Radiography Research with AI

Artificial intelligence is set to revolutionise radiography and radiology research both now and in the future. There are a number of avenues where AI could both enhance our ability to undertake research but also require research which differs from the historical types of research undertaken by radiographers.

There are opportunities for radiographers to be involved in interdisciplinary research to develop AI tools. To achieve this, radiographers require enhanced skills in image processing and basic knowledge of AI models to work with mathematicians and computer scientists and support the development of new AI solutions. In this area of research, radiographers could provide the imaging expertise, understanding of clinical presentations, image acquisition, radiotherapy and patient needs, which are needed to carry product development forward.

Radiographers could also be involved in the implementation and testing of AI in practice (see Chap. 4). Therefore, they need to be familiar with performance metrics for AI tools (as discussed in Chap. 2) and in evaluating the sensitivity and specificity of AI in diagnostics but also be able to consider the accuracy of auto-segmentations in both diagnostics and therapeutic image processing situations. Familiarisation with common tools and methods to achieve this will be part of the role for some radiographers in the future.

As AI becomes further integrated into medical imaging and radiotherapy, radiographers will require at the least a basic understanding of how AI works and its potential limitations, so that they can remain vigilant to spurious results, image acquisition concerns, unexpected radiation doses or adverse events in radiotherapy. Extensive testing and research will be required to achieve this, and radiographers will need to work with a range of research methodologists in interdisciplinary teams to undertake this work and develop the evidence base that is currently missing. Radiographers will also need to understand how to measure reproducibility not only within the research setting, but also in clinical practice across image acquisition, therapeutic planning and delivery and image interpretation AI tools. Finally radiographers will need to understand and explore optimal ways in harnessing the capabilities of new, more comprehensive forms of AI models, like agentic AI and foundation models. (please add this reference https://www.sciencedirect.com/science/article/pii/S2211568425001858). Artificial intelligence may also help research and clinical radiographers more quickly identify relevant academic publications and to summarise findings for progressing the evidence base.

15.7 Post-Market Surveillance

Post-market surveillance will be a key requirement for radiographers using AI, as a natural legacy of quality assurance and quality control processes, which were traditionally performed by radiographers, so that any failures could be recorded and fed back to the manufacturers. For example, with the increasing use of AI in image acquisition, large gains in patient dose reduction, standardisation of imaging and image quality optimisation are a reality. However, this does not mean AI will be risk-free; Radiographers will need to be aware that some patient characteristics may have been unseen by the training data and could pose challenges for the AI decision-making pipelines, causing potential risk to the patient by contributing to a wrong diagnosis or treatment regime. It will be therefore essential that radiographers are aware of the benefits and risks associated with the AI they are using. Furthermore, as radiographers who train in the presence of AI

move into their careers, specific attention will need to be placed on ensuring that methods to recognise and address AI failures are taught and included in departmental protocols and standard operating procedures (SoPs). To identify potential problems, radiographers will need to be able to monitor patterns and recognise inconsistencies, particularly when new equipment is installed, which could result in images with subtle differences that may impact diagnosis and treatment decisions. Mechanisms for feeding back into AI tools when it does not work as intended will become an essential part of the future, and each new version of the AI algorithm should have these feedback loops included, to improve robustness for the longer term. Similarly, the governance to support this type of initiatives will need to be addressed and revisited as technology evolves, so radiographers can overtake and bypass AI in case it is needed, similar to how pilots can bypass the auto-pilot in cases where humans are at risk.

15.8 Risk Prediction and Clinical Decision Support Tools

Risk prediction tools are already widely used in healthcare, and these are modelled on epidemiological datasets, thus providing risk estimates for individuals based on their own clinical risk factors for various diseases. AI will also provide the opportunity to explore risk prediction and clinical decision support tools aligned to imaging and therapy, in a way that has previously been unachievable. At the moment, these include manual entry of data, often by box ticking, but it is possible in the future that AI research will support pre-population of these from general practice records to enable virtual health assessments, which can be considered in consultations with patients. Artificial intelligence will be able to be incorporated into some of the standard risk prediction models, which are used for various diseases and a growing field exploring causative AI will yield models, which are more refined and are able to help clinicians and patients to understand the impact of changing their lifestyle or drugs on their potential risks or outcomes. For example, QRISK3 is used to identify patients at risk of heart disease who may benefit from statins [14]. While smoking is a risk factor within QRISK3, it cannot currently indicate the impact of stopping smoking on a patient's risk. However, in the future, causative AI will aim to estimate how long a patient needs to stop smoking for before they risk will reduce and by how much it will reduce by. While this is an interesting and important field for research, data integrity to support such developments will be key.

Furthermore, the ability to use various biomarkers from CT scans as an indicator of glucose control in patients with diabetes [15] opens up the possibility for a greater emphasis on preventative medicine, empowering and supporting people to change their health outcomes through lifestyle and behavioural changes, or the opportunity for earlier pharmacological interventions. However, the ethical aspects of such opportunistic diagnoses require wide research, because any new diagnosis can have a negative impact on a patient's life in terms of anxiety, life or travel insurance and a person's quality of life. This is a large area where future research is needed.

Artificial intelligence will also enable more rapid analysis of large datasets, enabling epidemiological studies that will be able to identify associated comorbidities, providing greater insights into risk prediction for patients and potential treatments.

15.9 Data Collection and Access to Datasets

Data is the driver for AI. As we have seen in Chaps. 1 and 2, AI generally requires big data for training the machine learning algorithms. Curated datasets, which are clean datasets, are important for AI developers and researchers. Ensuring appropriate ground-truth images and cases for both developing and testing of AI is also essential but expensive; there is furthermore a need to anonymise datasets, provide storage for large volumes of data and to provide labels or segmentations of regions of interest. Radiographers and other clinical researchers collecting imaging data can assist in this process

by labelling data themselves or by consenting patients to be able to use anonymised study images in open-access datasets, to minimise duplication and reduce the time and financial burden of creating similar datasets across different centres and across the world. This will both enhance efficiency, but also provide diversity of data from different countries, different centres and from different populations, with diversity in age, sex ethnicity and geographical locations. This will further enable the development of truly inclusive and reproducible AI, since it is developed on a multitude of images from different scanners using potentially different pulse sequences in MRI or exposure factors in CT and planar radiography. It is essential that the community works together to reduce the cost of creating AI, so more useful AI tools can become clinically available in the future.

15.10 Medical Imaging Plus

As AI becomes integrated in supporting the analysis of imaging data, there is the potential to integrate multimodal data beyond imaging, such as genomic data, metabolomics, proteomics and more. Existing large datasets, such as the Biobank [16] in the United Kingdom and 'All of Us' [17] in the United States, among other similar datasets across the world, hold health and genomic data on tens of thousands of volunteers and are providing useful insights into normal development, treatment monitoring and disease progression. In the future, it is probable that for some patients using AI could help combine genomics with radiomics and other imaging assessments, and provide greater insights into pathologies, disease progression, prognosis and treatments, leading the way to personalised precision medicine.

15.11 Interpretable AI

Current machine learning algorithms are largely a "black box", with data input and an output, but no understanding of what happens in the background to form the decision. There are two areas for the future, which will be important for increasing our understanding of how AI works. Explainable (XAI)AI provides explanations for AI model decisions, while interpretable AI looks to create understandable models, which describe how they make the prediction. The latter field is likely to be key in medical imaging and radiotherapy, providing users with the information they desire to understand how the AI has come to the decision they are presented in the output. More on AI explainability is discussed in Chaps. 2 and 4 but also in chapter 10.

15.12 Impacts of AI Deployment on Staff Cognitive Load and Well-Being

There will need to be a significant body of research undertaken into the impacts of AI implementation on staff. It is essential that AI reduces burden, makes environments safer and supports healthcare delivery, working in harmony with staff. However, as AI removes some of the lower-level more repetitive tasks that radiographers and other professionals undertake, the cognitive load and physical burdens on radiographers have the risk of increasing. Research will need to be undertaken to explore impact on safety and effectiveness, without the risk of unintended consequences of AI, such increasing the risk of burnout. For example, if AI screens out all of the normal cases for a review and verification, reporting lists for radiographers and radiologists may become ever more complex and challenging. This will not only deskill them in the recognition of normality, but will, in turn, increase the cognitive load required for reporting and it is possible that current reporting patterns will become unsustainable. Research is therefore essential to explore the impacts on radiographer and other health professionals work flows and working patterns from the introduction of AI. The way AI is implemented in each area (AI model, staff expertise, technical infrastructure and human factors) will also influence how staff is impacted each time, so will be largely contextual.

15.13 Service Redesign

The implementation of AI needs to be considered within the context of the service or patient pathway. Research into the redesign of medical imaging and radiotherapy services with AI to maximise the benefit to patients, radiographers and other healthcare professionals and to facilitate cost-effectiveness of services will need to be modelled. This will require more data scientists, implementation scientists and operational research methodologists working with radiographers and the multidisciplinary team to ensure that the benefits of AI are maximised while any risks or unintended consequences are minimised or mitigated [18].

15.14 Recommendations for Radiographers As Healthcare Professionals that Need to Embrace AI for Public Benefit

The below recommendations focus on skills and strategies that complement the opportunities presented by AI rather than competing with AI. These can help increase readiness of the radiography workforce for an AI-enabled world.

1. *Understand the role of AI in healthcare*

   - Stay informed: Learn how AI is being integrated into healthcare (e.g. diagnostic tools, predictive analytics, personalised medicine and administrative automation).
   - Follow new trends: Keep track of emerging AI solutions in healthcare through journals, webinars, courses and industry reports.

2. *Develop your digital literacy*

   - Learn about AI basics and theoretical principles: Understand AI concepts like machine learning, natural language processing and data analytics.
   - Use AI tools in practice to acquire intuition: Familiarise yourself with AI-powered

tools in your field (e.g. imaging software and virtual assistants).

3. *Focus on human skills*

- Empathy and communication: AI can process data, but human interaction remains essential for building trust with and emotional support of patients.
- Critical thinking and reasoning: Develop the ability to interpret AI-generated results critically and make informed decisions. Recognise and address AI errors.
- Ethics in AI: Understand ethical implications, such as bias in AI algorithms and patient data privacy, to advocate for responsible AI use.

4. *Embrace new technology*

- Work with IT teams: Build relationships with data scientists, IT experts, and technologists to better understand AI implementation challenges and opportunities and become part of the solution, not the problem.
- Participate in technical training: Attend workshops and seminars to develop new skills and keep skills current.
- Advocate for usability: Provide feedback on AI tools to ensure they meet healthcare professionals' needs effectively, from a workflow, operational but also occupational health perspective.

5. *Work within multidisciplinary teams*

- Learn about data science working with computer and data scientists: Gain a basic understanding of how AI algorithms are trained, tested and validated.
- Understand healthcare analytics: Learn how AI is used for population health management, predictive modelling and operational efficiencies. Understand the financial implications of AI working with health economists and implementation experts or operation research scientists

6. *Engage in continuous learning*

- Qualifications: Pursue qualifications and certifications in healthcare informatics or AI in medicine. Accredited learning is better for skills and learning.
- Professional groups: Join networks or forua focussed on AI in healthcare to share insights, learn from others and lead on future developments.

7. *Advocate for patient-centric AI*

- Prioritise patients: Ensure AI tools are used to enhance patient care, not replace human interaction.
- Educate patients: Help patients understand AI's role in their care, addressing their concerns and misconceptions.

8. *Prepare for new roles*
   AI will create new opportunities, such as:

- AI system trainers: Professionals who help train AI systems with healthcare expertise.
- AI interpreters: Specialists who analyse AI outputs and explain them to patients and teams.
- Data-driven decision-makers: Leaders who integrate AI insights into strategic healthcare decisions.

15.15 Chapter Summary

There will be significant changes to radiography in education, practice and research over the next decades as AI develops and is widely implemented into healthcare settings. AI will transform radiography by enhancing image and data analysis, driving innovation in imaging techniques, enabling personalised medicine and fostering interdisciplinary collaboration. While challenges such as ethical considerations, dataset limitations and algorithm transparency remain, AI offers unprecedented opportunities to advance and reimagine the field. By embracing AI research, radiography researchers can accelerate discoveries, improve patient care and shape the future of medical imaging. Radiographers, including those in clinical, educational and research roles, will need to work collaboratively together with interdisciplinary teams to ensure they maximise the benefits of AI in radiography for everyone.

References

1. Malamateniou C, Knapp KM, Pergola M, Woznitza N, Hardy M. Artificial intelligence in radiography: where are we now and what does the future hold? Radiography (Lond). 2021;27(Suppl 1):S58–62. https://doi.org/10.1016/j.radi.2021.07.015.

2. Janumpally R, Nanua S, Ngo A, Youens K. Generative artificial intelligence in graduate medical education. Front Med (Lausanne). 2025;11:1525604. https://doi.org/10.3389/fmed.2024.1525604.

3. Panjwani-Charania S, Zhai X. AI for students with learning disabilities: a systematic review. In: Zhai X, Krajcik J, editors. Uses of artificial intelligence in STEM education. Oxford: Oxford University Press; 2024. p. 469–93.

4. Mitra S. AI-powered adaptive education for disabled learners [Internet]. 2024 Dec 03 [cited 2025 Apr 28]. Available from: https://ssrn.com/abstract=5042713 or https://doi.org/10.2139/ssrn.5042713.

5. Barua PD, Vicnesh J, Gururajan R, Oh SL, Palmer E, Azizan MM, Kadri NA, Acharya UR. Artificial intelligence enabled personalised assistive tools to enhance education of children with neurodevelopmental disorders: a review. Int J Environ Res Public Health. 2022;19(3):1192.

6. Pontikas CM, Tsoukalas E, Serdari A. A map of assistive technology educative instruments in neurodevelopmental disorders. Disabil Rehabil Assist Technol. 2022;17(7):738–46.

7. Quality Assurance Agency. How can generative AI be used in learning and teaching? [Internet]. 2025. [cited 27 April 2025]. Available from: https://www.qaa.ac.uk/membership-areas-of-work/generative-artificial-intelligence/how-can-generative-ai-be-used-in-learning-and-teaching-external.

8. BERA. Dyslexia and artificial intelligence [Internet]. 29 September 2003. [cited 27 April 2025]. Available from: https://www.bera.ac.uk/blog/dyslexia-and-artificial-intelligence.

9. Amedu C, Ohene-Botwe B. Harnessing the benefits of ChatGPT for radiography education: a discussion paper. Radiography (Lond). 2024;30(1):209–16. https://doi.org/10.1016/j.radi.2023.11.009.

10. Springer Nature. AI tool to help streamline integrity and ethics checks [Internet]. 7 Jan 2025. [cited 27 April 2025]. Available from: https://group.springernature.com/gp/group/media/press-releases/ai-tool-to-help-streamline-integrity-and-ethics-checks/27730892.

11. Malamateniou C, O'Regan T, McFadden SL, Jackson M. Artificial intelligence (AI) in radiography practice, research and education: a review of contemporary developments and predictions for the future. Radiography (Lond). 2024;30(Suppl 2):56–9. https://doi.org/10.1016/j.radi.2024.09.062.

12. Rainey C, O'Regan T, Matthew J, Skelton E, Woznitza N, Chu KY, Goodman S, McConnell J, Hughes C, Bond R, Malamateniou C, McFadden S. An insight into the current perceptions of UK radiographers on the future impact of AI on the profession: a cross-sectional survey. J Med Imag Radiat Sci. 2022;53(3):347–61. https://doi.org/10.1016/j.jmir.2022.05.010.

13. Stogiannos N, Walsh G, Ohene-Botwe B, McHugh K, Potts B, Tam W, O'Sullivan C, Quinsten AS, Gibson C, Gorga RG, Sipos D, Dybeli E, Zanardo M, Sá Dos Reis C, Mekis N, Buissink C, England A, Beardmore C, Cunha A, Goodall A, John-Matthews JS, McEntee M, Kyratsis Y, Malamateniou C. R-AI-diographers: a European survey on perceived impact of AI on professional identity, careers, and radiographers' roles. Insights Imaging. 2025;16(1):43. https://doi.org/10.1186/s13244-025-01918-6. PMID: 39962024; PMCID: PMC11832980.

14. Hippisley-Cox J, Coupland C, Vinogradova Y, Robson J, May M, Brindle P. Derivation and validation of QRISK, a new cardiovascular disease risk score for the United Kingdom: prospective open cohort study. BMJ. 2007;335(7611):136.

15. Warner JD, Blake GM, Garrett JW, Lee MH, Nelson LW, Summers RM, et al. Correlation of HbA1c levels with CT-based body composition biomarkers in diabetes mellitus and metabolic syndrome. Sci Rep. 2024;14(1):21875.

16. UK Biobank. Imaging study [Internet]. 14 Feb 2025. [cited 27 April 2025]. Available from: https://www.ukbiobank.ac.uk/explore-your-participation/contribute-further/imaging-study.

17. All of Us Research Program. [Internet]. 2025. [cited 27 April 2025]. Available from: https://www.researchallofus.org/.

18. Stogiannos N, Gillan C, Precht H, Sá Dos Reis C, Kumar A, O'Regan T, Ellis V, Barnes A, Meades R, Pogose M, Greggio J, Scurr E, Kumar S, King G, Rosewarne D, Jones C, van Leeuwen KG, Hyde E, Beardmore C, Alliende JG, El-Farra S, Papathanasiou S, Beger J, Nash J, van Ooijen P, Zelenyanszki C, Koch B, Langmack KA, Tucker R, Goh V, Turmezei T, Lip G, Reyes-Aldasoro CC, Alonso E, Dean G, Hirani SP, Torre S, Akudjedu TN, Ohene-Botwe B, Khine R, O'Sullivan C, Kyratsis Y, McEntee M, Wheatstone P, Thackray Y, Cairns J, Jerome D, Scarsbrook A, Malamateniou C. A multidisciplinary team and multiagency approach for AI implementation: a commentary for medical imaging and radiotherapy key stakeholders. J Med Imaging Radiat Sci. 2024;55(4):101717. https://doi.org/10.1016/j.jmir.2024.101717. Epub 2024 Jul 26. PMID: 39067309.

Professor Maryann Hardy with over 30 years of experience in healthcare, radiography, and leadership, she is a recognised professional leader, educator, and coach. She specialises in empowering radiographers and wider healthcare professionals to thrive in high-pressure environments, build resilience, and navigate leadership challenges including embracing the opportunities that advancing technology and AI present. As a National Teaching Fellow and Principal Fellow of the Higher Education Academy, she has a proven track record of advancing professional development in radiography through education, research, and strategic leadership. She is passionate about empowering radiographers to fulfil their potential, ensuring that the future of radiography, and the next generation of practitioners and professional leaders is well-equipped for success.

Professor Karen M Knapp is a leading expert in musculoskeletal imaging and diagnostic radiography, with a notable research focus on osteoporosis and artificial intelligence in radiological practice. Currently Professor of Musculoskeletal Imaging and Head of Health and Care Professions at the University of Exeter, her work spans AI-driven imaging innovations, bone health diagnostics, is an experienced radiographer educator, and clinically, a DXA reporting radiographer. Professor Knapp has authored seminal publications, led research projects, and contributed to clinical guidelines. Her impactful research continues to shape clinical practice and advance radiographic sciences.

Professor Aarthi Ramlaul is an associate professor of Diagnostic Radiography at Buckinghamshire New University. Her primary research focused on the development of critical thinking in diagnostic radiography education and its impact on autonomous clinical decision-making. Her research interest lies in the ethicolegal aspects of professional practice and the implementation of AI in clinical decision-making. Aarthi is also an MSc and PhD supervisor and examiner and has edited and authored numerous publications, including five textbooks in medical imaging aimed at radiographers globally.

Professor Christina Malamateniou is an associate professor of technology-enabled care in radiography and the director of the CRRAG research group at City St George's University of London. She had held many AI leadership positions at national and international level (EFRS, SCoR, ECR, EuSOMII). She is a well-published author with more than 100 papers in peer reviewed journals and 7 published national and international guidelines, including the first guidance on AI for radiographers, and has delivered more than 150 keynote lectures, 60 of them on AI, at a global audience. She has total research funding as PI and Co-I of more than £3.7mi and has supervised many master's and PhD students. She has been researching AI education, governance, implementation, leadership and the impact of AI on the profession of radiography and on professional identities. She has established the first AI course for radiographers since 2019, which was the inspiration for this textbook.

Further Reading

The below list was put together by a group of AI experts in medical imaging and oncology and includes academic papers that can help build the learning of clinicians, academics and researchers, from trainee to consultant. It is organised by different categories as subheadings, arranged alphabetically in ascending order. This is by no means an exhaustive list, but a good start for learners and early adopters of AI.

*Agentic AI

Tzanis E, Adams LC, D'Antonoli TA, Bressem KK, Cuocolo R, Kocak B, Malamateniou C, Klontzas ME. Agentic systems in radiology: principles, opportunities, privacy risks, regulation, and sustainability concerns. Diagn Intervent Imaging. 2025; in press. https://doi.org/10.1016/j.diii.2025.10.002.

*AI Act

Kotter E, D'Antonoli TA, Cuocolo R, Hierath M, Huisman M, Klontzas ME, Martí-Bonmatí L, May MS, Neri E, Nikolaou K, Pinto Dos Santos D, Radzina M, Shelmerdine SC, Bellemo A, European Society of Radiology (ESR). Guiding AI in radiology: ESR's recommendations for effective implementation of the European AI Act. Insights Imaging. 2025;16(1):33. https://doi.org/10.1186/s13244-025-01905-x.

*AI Adoption

Kim JY, Boag W, Gulamali F, Hasan A, HDJ H, Lifson M, Mulligan D, Patel M, Raji ID, Sehgal A, Shaw K, Tobey D, Valladares A, Vidal D, Balu S, Sendak M. Organizational governance of emerging technologies: AI adoption in healthcare. In: Proceedings of the 2023 ACM conference on fairness, accountability, and transparency (FAccT '23). New York: Association for Computing Machinery; 2023. p. 1396–417. https://doi.org/10.1145/3593013.3594089.

*AI Data

Willemink MJ, Koszek WA, Hardell C, Wu J, Fleischmann D, Harvey H, Folio LR, Summers RM, Rubin DL, Lungren MP. Preparing medical imaging data for machine learning. Radiology. 2020;295(1):4–15. https://doi.org/10.1148/radiol.2020192224. Epub 2020 Feb 18.

*AI Evidence

Antonissen N, Tryfonos O, Houben IB, Jacobs C, de Rooij M, van Leeuwen KG. Artificial intelligence in radiology: 173 commercially available products and their scientific evidence. Eur Radiol. 2025. https://doi.org/10.1007/s00330-025-11830-8.

*AI and Human Interaction

Tejani A, Rajpurkar P. Human-Artificial Intelligence (AI) interactions: a conversation with Pranav Rajpurkar, From the AJR Video Series on AI in Radiology. Am J Roentgenol. 2025. https://doi.org/10.2214/AJR.25.34003.

Topol EJ. High-performance medicine: the convergence of human and artificial intelligence. Nat Med. 2019;25(1):44–56. https://doi.org/10.1038/s41591-018-0300-7.

Padhani AR, Papanikolaou N. AI and human interactions in prostate cancer diagnosis using MRI. Eur Radiol. 2025;35(9):5695–700. https://doi.org/10.1007/s00330-025-11498-0. Epub 2025 Mar 7. PMID: 40055229.

C. Malamateniou et al. (eds.), *Artificial Intelligence for Radiographers*,
https://doi.org/10.1007/978-3-032-05080-9

Vaccaro M, Almaatouq A, Malone T. When combinations of humans and AI are useful: a systematic review and meta-analysis. Nat Hum Behav. 2024;8(12):2293–303. https://doi.org/10.1038/s41562-024-02024-1. Epub 2024 Oct 28. PMID: 39468277; PMCID: PMC11659167.

*AI Reporting

Tejani AS, Klontzas ME, Gatti AA, Mongan JT, Moy L, Park SH, Kahn CE Jr, CLAIM 2024 Update Panel. Checklist for Artificial Intelligence in Medical Imaging (CLAIM): 2024 Update. Radiol Artif Intell. 2024;6(4):e240300. https://doi.org/10.1148/ryai.240300.

Kocak B, Akinci D'Antonoli T, Mercaldo N, Alberich-Bayarri A, Baessler B, Ambrosini I, Andreychenko AE, Bakas S, Beets-Tan RGH, Bressem K, Buvat I, Cannella R, Cappellini LA, Cavallo AU, Chepelev LL, Chu LCH, Demircioglu A, deSouza NM, Dietzel M, Fanni SC, Fedorov A, Fournier LS, Giannini V, Girometti R, Groot Lipman KBW, Kalarakis G, Kelly BS, Klontzas ME, Koh DM, Kotter E, Lee HY, Maas M, Marti-Bonmati L, Müller H, Obuchowski N, Orlhac F, Papanikolaou N, Petrash E, Pfaehler E, Pinto Dos Santos D, Ponsiglione A, Sabater S, Sardanelli F, Seebӧck P, Sijtsema NM, Stanzione A, Traverso A, Ugga L, Vallières M, van Dijk LV, van Griethuysen JJM, van Hamersvelt RW, van Ooijen P, Vernuccio F, Wang A, Williams S, Witowski J, Zhang Z, Zwanenburg A, Cuocolo R. METhodological RadiomICs Score (METRICS): a quality scoring tool for radiomics research endorsed by EuSoMII. Insights Imaging. 2024;15(1):8. https://doi.org/10.1186/s13244-023-01572-w.

Kocak B, Baessler B, Bakas S, Cuocolo R, Fedorov A, Maier-Hein L, Mercaldo N, Müller H, Orlhac F, Pinto Dos Santos D, Stanzione A, Ugga L, Zwanenburg A. CheckList for EvaluAtion of Radiomics research (CLEAR): a step-by-step reporting guideline for authors and reviewers endorsed by ESR and EuSoMII. Insights Imaging. 2023;14(1):75. https://doi.org/10.1186/s13244-023-01415-8.

Koçak B, Kӧse F, Keleş A, Şendur A, Meşe İ, Karagülle M. Adherence to the Checklist for Artificial Intelligence in Medical Imaging (CLAIM): an umbrella review with a comprehensive two-level analysis. Diagn Interv Radiol. 2025;31(5):440–55. https://doi.org/10.4274/dir.2025.243182. Epub 2025 Feb 10. PMID: 39937033; PMCID: PMC12417908.

Kocak B, Borgheresi A, Ponsiglione A, Andreychenko AE, Cavallo AU, Stanzione A, Doniselli FM, Vernuccio F, Triantafyllou M, Cannella R, Trotta R, Ghezzo S, Akinci D'Antonoli T, Cuocolo R. Explanation and

elaboration with examples for CLEAR (CLEAR-E3): an EuSoMII radiomics auditing group initiative. Eur Radiol Exp. 2024;8(1):72. https://doi.org/10.1186/s41747-024-00471-z.

*AI Risk

Gerigoorian A, Kloub M, Dembrower K, Engwall M, Strand F. Risk inventory and mitigation actions for AI in medical imaging-a qualitative study of implementing standalone AI for screening mammography. BMC Health Serv Res. 2025;25(1):998. https://doi.org/10.1186/s12913-025-13176-9.

*Bias in AI

Koçak B, Ponsiglione A, Stanzione A, Bluethgen C, Santinha J, Ugga L, Huisman M, Klontzas ME, Cannella R, Cuocolo R. Bias in artificial intelligence for medical imaging: fundamentals, detection, avoidance, mitigation, challenges, ethics, and prospects. Diagn Interv Radiol. 2025;31(2):75–88. https://doi.org/10.4274/dir.2024.242854.

Rouzrokh P, Khosravi B, Faghani S, Moassefi M, Vera Garcia DV, Singh Y, Zhang K, Conte GM, Erickson BJ. Mitigating bias in radiology machine learning: 1. Data handling. Radiol Artif Intell. 2022;4(5):e210290. https://doi.org/10.1148/ryai.210290.

Zhang K, Khosravi B, Vahdati S, Faghani S, Nugen F, Rassoulinejad-Mousavi SM, Moassefi M, Jagtap JMM, Singh Y, Rouzrokh P, Erickson BJ. Mitigating bias in radiology machine learning: 2. Model development. Radiol Artif Intell. 2022;4(5):e220010. https://doi.org/10.1148/ryai.220010.

Faghani S, Khosravi B, Zhang K, Moassefi M, Jagtap JM, Nugen F, Vahdati S, Kuanar SP, Rassoulinejad-Mousavi SM, Singh Y, Vera Garcia DV, Rouzrokh P, Erickson BJ. Mitigating bias in radiology machine learning: 3. Performance metrics. Radiol Artif Intell. 2022;4(5):e220061. https://doi.org/10.1148/ryai.220061.

*Deep Learning

Wu AN, Kulbay M, Cheng PM, Cadrin-Chênevert A, Létourneau-Guillon L, Chartrand G, Chong J, Montagnon E, Ben Ayed I, Tang A. Deep learning models connecting images and text: a primer for radiologists. Radiographics. 2025;45(9):e240103. https://doi.org/10.1148/rg.240103.

*Evaluation Metrics in AI

Klontzas ME, Groot Lipman KBW, Akinci, D' Antonoli T, Andreychenko A, Cuocolo R, Dietzel M, Gitto S, Huisman H, Santinha J, Vernuccio F, Visser JJ, Huisman M. ESR Essentials: common performance metrics in AI-practice recommendations by the European Society of Medical Imaging Informatics. Eur Radiol. 2025. https://doi.org/10.1007/s00330-025-11890-w.

Kocak B, Klontzas ME, Stanzione A, Meddeb A, Demircioğlu A, Bluethgen C, Bressem KK, Ugga L, Mercaldo N, Díaz O, Cuocolo R. Evaluation metrics in medical imaging AI: fundamentals, pitfalls, misapplications, and recommendations. Eur J Radiol Artif Intell. 2025;3:100030. https://doi.org/10.1016/j.ejrai.2025.100030.

*Foundation Models

Paschali M, Chen Z, Blankemeier L, Varma M, Youssef A, Bluethgen C, Langlotz C, Gatidis S, Chaudhari A. Foundation models in radiology: what, how, why, and why not. Radiology. 2025;314(2):e240597. https://doi.org/10.1148/radiol.240597.

Akinci D'Antonoli T, Bluethgen C, Cuocolo R, Klontzas ME, Ponsiglione A, Kocak B. Foundation models for radiology: fundamentals, applications, opportunities, challenges, risks, and prospects. Diagn Interv Radiol. 2025. https://doi.org/10.4274/dir.2025.253445.

*Generative AI

Fahrner LJ, Chen E, Topol E, Rajpurkar P. The generative era of medical AI. Cell. 2025;188(14):3648–60. https://doi.org/10.1016/j.cell.2025.05.018.

*Human Factors AI

Sujan M, Pool R, Salmon P. Eight human factors and ergonomics principles for healthcare artificial intelligence. BMJ Health Care Inform. 2022;29(1):e100516. https://doi.org/10.1136/bmjhci-2021-100516.

*Large Language Models (LLMs) in Radiology

Akinci D'Antonoli T, Stanzione A, Bluethgen C, Vernuccio F, Ugga L, Klontzas ME, Cuocolo R, Cannella R, Koçak B. Large language models in radiology: fundamentals, applications, ethical considerations, risks, and future directions. Diagn Interv Radiol. 2024;30(2):80–90. https://doi.org/10.4274/dir.2023.232417.

*Radiomics for Beginners

Santinha J, Pinto Dos Santos D, Laqua F, Visser JJ, KBW GL, Dietzel M, Klontzas ME, Cuocolo R, Gitto S, T AD'A. ESR essentials: radiomics-practice recommendations by the European Society of Medical Imaging Informatics. Eur Radiol. 2025;35(3):1122–32. https://doi.org/10.1007/s00330-024-11093-9. Epub 2024 Oct 25. PMID: 39453470.

Koçak B, Durmaz EŞ, Ateş E, Kılıçkesmez Ö. Radiomics with artificial intelligence: a practical guide for beginners. Diagn Interv Radiol. 2019;25(6):485–95. https://doi.org/10.5152/dir.2019.19321. PMID: 31650960; PMCID: PMC6837295.

van Timmeren JE, Cester D, Tanadini-Lang S, Alkadhi H, Baessler B. Radiomics in medical imaging—"how-to" guide and critical reflection. Insights Imaging. 2020;11(1):91. https://doi.org/10.1186/s13244-020-00887-2.

*Responsible AI

FUTURE-AI: international consensus guideline for trustworthy and deployable artificial intelligence in healthcare. BMJ. 2025;388:r340. https://doi.org/10.1136/bmj.r340.

Walsh G, Stogiannos N, van de Venter R, Rainey C, Tam W, McFadden S, McNulty JP, Mekis N, Lewis S, O'Regan T, Kumar A, Huisman M, Bisdas S, Kotter E, Pinto Dos Santos D, Sá Dos Reis C, van Ooijen P, Brady AP, Malamateniou C. Responsible AI practice and AI education are central to AI implementation: a rapid review for all medical imaging professionals in Europe. BJR Open. 2023;5(1):20230033. https://doi.org/10.1259/bjro.20230033.

Stogiannos N, Malik R, Kumar A, Barnes A, Pogose M, Harvey H, McEntee MF, Malamateniou C. Black box no more: a scoping review of AI governance frameworks to guide procurement and adoption of AI in medical imaging and radiotherapy in the UK. Br J Radiol. 2023;(1152):20221157. https://doi.org/10.1259/bjr.20221157. Epub 2023 Oct 3.

Sujan M, Smith-Frazer C, Malamateniou C, Connor J, Gardner A, Unsworth H, Husain H. Validation framework for the use of AI in healthcare: overview of the new British standard BS30440. BMJ Health Care Inform. 2023;30(1):e100749. https://doi.org/10.1136/bmjhci-2023-100749.

*Post-market Surveillance and Monitoring

Chow J, Lee R, Wu H. How do radiologists currently monitor AI in radiology and what challenges do they face? An interview study and qualitative analysis. J Imaging Inform Med. 2025. https://doi.org/10.1007/s10278-025-01493-8.

*Sustainability in AI

Kocak B, Ponsiglione A, Romeo V, Ugga L, Huisman M, Cuocolo R. Radiology AI and sustainability paradox: environmental, economic, and social dimensions. Insights Imaging. 2025;16(1):88. https://doi.org/10.1186/s13244-025-01962-2.

*Trust in AI

Prinster D, Mahmood A, Saria S, Jeudy J, Lin CT, Yi PH, Huang CM. Care to explain? AI explanation types differentially impact chest radiograph diagnostic performance and physician trust in AI. Radiology. 2024;313(2):e233261. https://doi.org/10.1148/radiol.233261.

Glossary

AI-assisted compressed sensing techniques AI-assisted compressed sensing (ACS) techniques combine traditional compressed sensing methods with advanced AI algorithms to enhance the speed and quality of medical imaging, such as MRI and CT scans. ACS works by reconstructing high-quality images from fewer samples than typically required, assuming the image has some level of sparsity or structure. When intergrated with AI, these techniques can significantly reduce scan times while maintaining or even improving image quality and diagnostic accuracy.

Aleatoric uncertainty Aleatoric uncertainty refers to the inherent noise in the data that cannot be reduced but can be modelled probabilistically.

Algorithm An algorithm is a set of rules or instructions given to an AI system to help it learn on its own. In radiography, algorithms are used to process and analyse medical images.

Alpha particle An alpha particle consists of two protons and two neutrons bound together, making it identical to a helium-4 nucleus. These particles are typically produced during alpha decay of heavy elements like uranium and radium.

Area under the curve The area under the curve (AUC) provides a summary of the performance of the receiver operating curve (ROC)

Artificial intelligence The simulation of human intelligence processes by machines, especially computer systems. In radiography, AI can assist in image analysis and diagnosis.

Artificial neural network Artificial neural network (ANN) is a computational model inspired by the way biological neural networks in the human brain process information. ANNs consist of interconnected nodes, or neurons, organised in layers. They are used in applications such as image recognition, natural language processing and predictive analytics.

Atlas-based learning Atlas-based learning refers to a technique used in image segmentation that involves using a reference image, known as an atlas, which contains prior knowledge about structures of interest. The 'atlas' guides the segmentation process by making it easier to identify and delineate specific regions within new images.

Attention U-Net Attention U-Net is an enhanced version of the classic U-Net, incorporating attention to focus on relevant regions while suppressing irrelevant ones. In this architecture, attention gates replace the traditional skip connections.

Attenuation correction Attenuation correction (AC) is a technique used particularly in positron emission tomography (PET) and single-photon emission computed tomography (SPECT) to improve image quality and accuracy by compensating for the loss of signal intensity caused by the absorption or scattering of photons as they pass through different tissues in the body.

Attenuation map Attenuation maps are generated using computed tomography (CT) or magnetic resonance imaging (MRI) to correct PET or SPECT images.

C. Malamateniou et al. (eds.), *Artificial Intelligence for Radiographers*, https://doi.org/10.1007/978-3-032-05080-9

Autoencoders Autoencoders are a type of unsupervised neural network designed to learn a compressed representation (encoding) of input data and then reconstruct the data from this representation.

AUTOMAP Automated transform by manifold approximation is a neural network that can learn from the raw MR data using the forward-encoding model. This approach can achieve real-time reconstruction of radial data and it can be used in MR-guided radiotherapy to adapt to anatomical changes.

Automated slice prescription Automated slice prescription refers to the use of AI and deep learning algorithms to automatically determine the optimal imaging planes for MRI scans. This technique aims to improve the consistency, accuracy and efficiency of MRI procedures by reducing the reliance on operator expertise and minimising variability between scans.

Automation bias Automation bias refers to the tendency for humans to favour suggestions from automated systems and to overlook or ignore contradictory information, even if it is correct; this can lead to errors.

Autonomy Autonomy refers to the ability of individuals to make their own decisions free from external control or influence.

Auto-segmentation Auto-segmentation refers to the use of AI and machine learning algorithms to automatically segment data into meaningful groups or clusters. Auto-segmentation accurately delineates anatomical structures or regions of interest within images, improving the efficiency and consistency of tasks like tumour detection and organ segmentation.

Average surface distance/Hausdorff distance The average surface distance is also known as Hausdorff distance is a surface-based metric that measures the maximum difference between the predicted boundary and the ground truth boundary, but can be sensitive to noise and outliers.

Back-projection Back-projection is a technique used to reconstruct images from raw data collected during scans, such as CT (computed tomography) scans. This method involves projecting the collected data back onto an image space to create a visual representation of the scanned area.

Bayesian neural networks Bayesian neural networks refer to weights that are treated as probability distributions rather than fixed values allowing them to quantify uncertainty in predictions by sampling from these distributions

Beneficence Beneficence refers to the ethical and moral principle of doing good and promoting the well-being of others.

Beta particle A beta particle is a high-energy, high-speed electron or positron emitted during radioactive decay of an atomic nucleus.

Bias Biases are systematic errors in AI algorithms that can lead to unfair outcomes. In radiography, it is important to ensure that AI tools do not introduce bias in medical diagnoses.

Biomarker A biomarker is a measurable indicator of a biological condition or process that can be detected through imaging techniques.

Black box (effect) The term 'black box' is used to describe complex machine learning models, such as deep neural networks, where the decision-making process is opaque and difficult to interpret; the more competent they get, the harder it is to work out how they do what they do.

Bland-Altman A Bland-Altman plot is a graphical method used to assess the agreement between two measurement methods by plotting the difference between the two methods against their average.

Computer-aided triage Computer-aided triage (CADt) involves the use of AI in assisting in the prioritisation and management of patient care.

Classification Classification is the process of identifying the category or class an input belongs to based on its features. It is a type of supervised learning, where the algorithm is trained on a labelled dataset.

Clustering In clustering, the aim is to partition the data into a predefined number of groups based on a criterion, such that there is good internal cohesion within the clusters, while also having good separation between the clusters.

Coincidence detection Coincidence detection involves neurons firing in response to the simultaneous arrival of multiple spikes. This mechanism helps in efficient information processing and mimics the way biological neurons operate. It is characterised by a low number of input spikes and short integration intervals.

Compressed Compressed AI refers to techniques used to reduce the size and computational requirements of AI models without significantly compromising their performance.

Computational simulations Computational simulations (CS) employ mathematical models to simulate cardiovascular interventions, generating patient-specific data that guides treatment strategy, stent placement and device selection.

Computer-aided detection Computer-aided detection (CAD) is the use of software systems to assist in interpreting medical images. CAD systems highlight suspicious areas that may require further investigation.

Computer vision Computer vision refers to a feature in AI that enables machines to interpret and make decisions based on visual data. Computer vision combines techniques from machine learning, deep learning and image processing to enable machines to understand and interact with the visual world.

Cone beam computed tomography Cone beam computed tomography (CBCT) uses a cone-shaped X-ray beam, which allows for the capture of volumetric data in a single rotation around the patient.

Connectionist AI Connectionist AI is an approach in AI that models mental processes using interconnected networks of simple units, often referred to as artificial neural networks (ANNs).

Connectivity patterns Connectivity patterns refer to how different components of an AI system are interconnected to facilitate efficient data processing, communication and decision-making.

Contours A contour is the outline or boundary of an object in an image. It helps in identifying the shape and structure of objects.

Convolutional neural network A convolutional neural network (CNN) is the most popular type of neural network for analysing images. CNNs are biologically inspired networks of convolutional and subsampling layers, including feature extraction (receptive fields that filter local features), feature mapping (weight sharing, which forces invariance) and subsampling (pooling).

Correlation Correlation refers to the statistical relationship between two or more variables; the relationship helps in identifying patterns and dependencies within data.

Data privacy The protection of personal data from unauthorised access and use. In radiography, maintaining data privacy is crucial when using AI tools that handle patient information.

Data preparation Data preparation refers to the process of cleaning, transforming and organising raw data into a suitable format for analysis and model training to ensure that the data input into machine learning models is accurate, consistent and relevant.

Decision trees Decision trees are a type of model used for both classification and regression tasks that is structured as a tree, where each node represents a decision based on a feature, and each branch represents the outcome of that decision.

Decision hygiene Decision hygiene refers to practices aimed at improving the quality and consistency of decision-making processes by minimising biases and unwanted variability, often referred to as 'noise'.

Deep Learning Deep learning (DL) is a subset of ML that uses neural networks with many layers (deep neural networks) to analyse various types of data. In radiography, DL is often used for image recognition and classification.

Deep learning techniques Deep learning techniques are methods used to train deep neural networks, a subset of machine learning models that are designed to simulate the way the human brain processes information

DeepMind's AlphaGo AlphaGo was a self-taught AI system, which, in addition, showed creativity in executing unexpected winning movements. It must be noted that Go is much more complex than chess. At the opening move in chess, there are 20 possible moves. In Go, the first player has 361 possible moves.

Denoising Denoising refers to the process of removing noise from data, particularly images, to improve their quality and clarity. Noise in images refers to random variations in brightness or colour that can obscure the image details; denoising aims to eliminate these unwanted artefacts while preserving features like edges and textures.

Dice similarity coefficient The Dice similarity coefficient, also known as a 'Dice score,' measures similarity between two sets of data, often represented as a binary x, y array. Dice scores are often used to compare similarities in image segmentation, where one segmentation area or outline has been created as ground truth by a human and the other segmentation has been created by AI.

DICOM Digital Imaging and Communications in Medicine is a standard for handling, storing, printing and transmitting information in medical imaging. AI tools in radiography often need to work with DICOM files.

Diffusion models Diffusion models are a powerful class of generative techniques, capable of creating high-quality synthetic data that work by adding noise to data and then learning to reverse the process, generating new samples.

Dixon MRI The Dixon MRI method, also known as the Dixon technique, is a specialised MRI sequence designed to achieve uniform fat suppression.

Domain A domain refers to the area or field of knowledge to which an AI system is applied and encompasses the subject matter, context and environment in which an AI system operates, including data types, tasks and problems the AI is designed to address.

Domain adaptation Domain adaptation is a subfield of transfer learning focused on adapting a model trained on data from one domain (the source domain) to perform well in a different, but related, domain (the target domain).

Dose creep Dose creep describes the gradual rise in radiation exposure levels during diagnostic radiography. This occurs as incremental adjustments to exposure settings are made to enhance image quality, without recognising the cumulative impact on patient radiation dose.

Dosimetric Dosimetric refers to the measurement and calculation of radiation dose.

Edge detection Edge detection refers to the process of highlighting the structural features of objects, making it easier to analyse and interpret images during image processing tasks, such as object recognition, image segmentation and feature extraction.

Epistemic uncertainty Epistemic uncertainty refers to uncertainty in the model and can be reduced with more data.

Epoch One complete pass of all the training data through a machine learning model or algorithm. Each pass alters the internal model parameters based on the model's prediction versus the truth in the labelled data. The number of epochs is traditionally large, often hundreds or thousands, allowing the learning algorithm to run until the error from the model has been sufficiently minimised.

Expert systems Expert systems are a type of AI designed to emulate the decision-making abilities of a human expert that is gained from a comprehensive knowledge base of facts, rules and heuristics about the domain.

Explainability The extent to which human reviewers can access, interpret and understand the decision-making processes of an AI system.

Explainable artificial intelligence Explainable artificial intelligence (XAI) is an enabler for AI implementation in medical imaging that aims to make AI-driven diagnostic decisions transparent and understandable for healthcare providers.

Explanation user Interface The explanation user interface (EUI) is the component of an AI system designed to provide users with understandable and interpretable details of the AI outputs. They typically comprise textual reports, heat 'salience' colour maps or region-of-interest annotations, thereby augmenting image data visualisation and diagnostic accuracy

Extractable data Extractable data involves the process of selecting and retrieving data from various sources to store, transform, integrating and analysing it.

Feature engineering Feature engineering is the process of using domain knowledge to create new features or modify existing ones in a dataset to improve the performance of machine learning models.

Feature extraction Feature extraction is the process of transforming raw data into a set of features that can be used for machine learning. In radiography, feature extraction is crucial for identifying relevant characteristics in medical images.

Feature mapping Feature mapping involves the process of transforming input data into a set of features that can be used for further analysis or decision-making. A feature map is the output of a convolutional layer in a convolutional neural network (CNN) and represents features such as edges, textures or patterns, in the input image.

Federated learning Federated learning is an approach that enables the transfer of knowledge between tasks or domains through model training across multiple decentralised devices or institutions without the need to share sensitive data. This approach allows models to learn from data stored locally on various devices, ensuring privacy and security of users' data while benefiting from diverse datasets.

Filtered back-projection Filtered back-projection (FBP) is a common variant used in CT imaging. It applies a convolution filter to the raw data before back-projecting it, which helps to reduce blurring and improve image quality.

Flagging Flagging refers to the process of identifying, marking or categorising data that requires further review.

Flatness Flatness refers to how smooth or flat the surface representing the loss or error of a model is. The loss landscape is a multidimensional surface where each point represents a specific configuration of the model's parameters and the corresponding loss value.

Foundation models Foundation models (FL) are large, deep-learning AI models that are trained on a broad spectrum of generalised and unlabelled data and can perform a wide variety of general tasks such as understanding language, generating text and images from prompts and conversing in natural language

Gamma radiation Gamma radiation is a form of electromagnetic radiation with the shortest wavelength and highest energy.

Gaussian mixture model A Gaussian mixture model (GMM) offers a more flexible approach by assuming data is generated from a mixture of Gaussian distributions (62)

Generative adversarial networks Generative adversarial networks are a popular deep learning paradigm known for their ability to generate new data. It consists of two networks – a generator (G) and a discriminator (D), where the generator aims to produce realistic looking images, while the discriminator tries to differentiate between real and generated samples.

Gray OS Gray OS is a commercially available auto-scheduling platform.

Grayscale Softcopy Presentation State A DICOM information type which is not an image in its own right but which can contain multiple types of reversible image transformations, linked back to one or more source applications.

Ground truth Ground truth refers to the accurate, real-world data used as a benchmark to train and evaluate models and serves as the reference point for validating the accuracy of AI models.

Hidden layer A hidden layer is a layer of neurons that lies between the input layer and the output layer within neural networks that process the inputs received from the previous layer and pass the processed information to the next layer.

Hidden stratification Where data contains unrecognised subsets that may affect model training and model performance. For example, a particular finding may have good overall accuracy measured by area under the curve (AUC), but subclasses of data (e.g. inpatient images or supine X-ray images) display poorer accuracy.

Hounsfield unit The Hounsfield unit (HU) is a unit of measurement used in computed tomography (CT) scans to quantify the radiodensity of tissues. It represents a linear transformation of the tissues' attenuation coefficients.

Hybrid imaging Hybrid imaging involves combining two or more imaging modalities to create a single, more comprehensive diagnostic tool that capitalises on the strengths of each modality to deliver detailed anatomical and functional information that may be challenging to obtain using just one imaging technique.

Hyperparameter tuning Hyperparameter tuning involves the process of optimising the parameters that govern the learning process of a model.

Image-guided radiation therapy Image-guided radiation therapy (IGRT) is a type of radiation therapy that uses imaging techniques to improve the precision and accuracy of treatment while minimising exposure to surrounding healthy tissues.

Image reconstruction Image reconstruction involves using advanced algorithms, such as convolutional neural networks (CNNs) and generative adversarial networks (GANs), to enhance or recreate images from incomplete, degraded or low-resolution data.

Intensity-modulated radiation therapy Intensity-modulated radiation therapy (IMRT) is an advanced form of radiation therapy that uses computer algorithms to deliver precise radiation doses to a tumour from multiple angles, allowing higher radiation doses to be concentrated on the tumour while minimising exposure to surrounding healthy tissue.

Independent component analysis Independent component analysis (ICA) is a dimensionality reduction technique that separates multivariate signals into additive, independent non-Gaussian components.

Input layer The input layer is the initial layer of a neural network where data enters the model. This layer accepts raw data, such as images, text or numerical values, and forwards it to the subsequent layers for further processing.

Intensity distribution Intensity distribution refers to the way pixel values are spread across an image.

Interpretable deep learning Interpretable deep learning is a model that seeks to address the opacity of deep learning models by providing explanations that highlight important features in the input data.

Intersection over union/Jaccard index Intersection over union, also known as the Jaccard index, is defined as the intersection between the predicted and ground truth class over their union.

Iterative reconstruction Iterative reconstruction refers to the process where algorithms repeatedly refine the image by comparing the current image with the original data and making adjustments.

Justice Justice refers to the principle of fairness and moral rightness, ensuring that individuals are treated equitably and that their rights are respected.

Kernel A kernel refers to a function used to transform data into a higher-dimensional space, enabling linear classifiers to solve non-linear problems, which allows complex data patterns to be more easily separated and analysed.

K-fold cross-validation Cross-validation is a resampling procedure used to train and evaluate machine learning models which makes efficient use of limited training data.

KIKI-Net KIKI-Net is an AI-assisted reconstruction approach that is named after its operation in the k-space, image domain.

k-means clustering k-means clustering is an unsupervised algorithm that partitions data into k clusters by minimising intra-cluster variance.

k-nearest neighbours k-nearest neighbours (kNN) algorithm is a simple, yet effective supervised machine learning method for classification.

Labelling Labelling refers to the process of identifying and tagging data samples with meaningful labels to provide context for machine learning models, such as in supervised learning, where models learn to make predictions based on labelled data.

Large language models Large language models (LLMs) are models trained on language data and used for natural language processing tasks (e.g. ChatGPT – a transformer-based generative LLM that predicts the next word in a sentence using autoregressive learning).

Large multi-model models Large multi-model models are models trained on multiple data types (e.g. language and vision) to manage both single- and multi-model tasks

Large vision models Large vision models are models trained on vision data and applied to image-based tasks.

Lasso regression A lasso regression model is a regularisation model that can perform feature selection by reducing some coefficients to zero.

Lesion segmentation Lesion segmentation involves precisely locating, quantifying and monitoring the progression or regression of lesions.

Linear models Linear models are models that assume a linear relationship between input features and target variables and are often used as baselines due to their simplicity and interpretability.

Linear regression A linear regression model predicts continuous outcomes.

Localisation Localisation refers to the process of adapting content, products or services to fit the cultural and linguistic context of different regions by translating text, adjusting elements like date formats, currencies, units of measurement and even cultural references to ensure the content is relevant and appropriate for the target audience.

Logic functions Logic functions refer to the use of logical operations to process and analyse data.

Logistic regression A logistic regression model handles classification tasks.

Machine learning Machine learning (ML) is a subset of AI that involves the use of algorithms and statistical models to enable computers to improve their performance on a task through experience. In radiography, ML can help in identifying patterns in medical images.

Machine learning algorithms These machine learning algorithms learn patterns from annotated medical images to classify and segment different structures.

Machine learning architecture Machine learning architecture refers to the design and structure of machine learning models and systems.

Medical ethics Medical ethics refers to the principles and values that guide healthcare and the conduct of healthcare professionals.

Medical internal radiation dosimetry Medical internal radiation dosimetry (MIRD) involves the assessment of the radiation dose absorbed by tissues and organs from radionuclides that have been introduced into the body.

MIRACLE-ILD algorithm The MIRACLE-ILD algorithm is a diagnostic tool designed to systematically evaluate interstitial lung diseases (ILDs) by integrating clinical, radiographic and pathological data, aiding clinicians in the accurate assessment and diagnosis of these conditions.

Molecular radiotherapy Molecular radiotherapy is a type of radiation therapy that uses radiopharmaceuticals to treat cancer and other medical conditions.

Monoenergetic beams Monoenergetic beams consist of a single energy level, and when using high-energy X-rays, they help reduce beam-hardening artefacts and improve image quality by providing clearer contrast in dense areas, while also mitigating secondary artefacts associated with conventional or projection-based methods.

Monte Carlo modelling Monte Carlo modelling is a computational technique that uses repeated random sampling to obtain numerical results to understand the impact of risk and uncertainty in prediction and forecasting models.

Morbidity Morbidity refers to the disease rate within a population.

Mortality Mortality refers to the death rate within a population.

Multi-reader multi-case A multi-reader multi-case study (MRMC) design is used to assess the ability of readers using specific imaging methods to detect, locate and characterise disease (in other words, measure diagnostic accuracy). In AI/machine-learning, MRMCs are often used to compare the performance of human and AI-readers and sometimes the performance of human readers compared with human plus AI-assistance.

Multilayer perceptron Multilayer perceptrons (MLP) are made of an input layer, one or more fully connected hidden layers and one output layer. Connections between pairs of neurons from adjacent layers have a weight attached to them, signifying the strength of those connections.

Natural language processing Natural language processing (NLP) is a field of AI that focuses on the interaction between computers and humans through natural language. In radiography, NLP can be used to analyse radiology reports and extract relevant information.

Neurons Neurons are the fundamental units of artificial neural networks, also known as nodes and are designed to process and transmit information within the network.

Newell and Simon's physical symbol system hypothesis A symbol system has the necessary and sufficient means for general intelligent action, defined the symbolic approach in the first decades of AI, between the 1950s and the 1970s.

Noise Random or unpredictable fluctuations in data that disrupt the ability to identify target patterns or relationships. The result is decreased accuracy or reliability of a model's predictions or output.

Non-maleficence Non-maleficence is a medical ethics principle that means 'do no harm'.

Normalising Normalising refers to the process of adjusting values measured on different scales to a common scale to improve the performance and training stability of machine learning models.

Notified bodies Notified bodies are organisations designated to assess the conformity of certain products, including AI systems, with regulatory requirements.

Operational ontology for oncology The operational ontology for oncology (O3) is the initiative of the American Association of Physicists in Medicine's (AAPM) Big Data Science Committee that standardises Patient Reported Outcomes (PROs), describing standard instruments, questions and responses.

Operations/operational research (OR) Operations research (OR) refers to the practice of applying advanced analytical methods to find the best solution in complex decision-making.

Organ segmentation Organ segmentation involves outlining organs on images, enabling accurate volumetric measurements and providing insights into organ health.

Orientation Orientation refers to the alignment or positioning of data within a dataset.

Outlier data points Outlier data points refer to observations that are significantly different from other observations in the dataset, such as unusually high or low values that do not fit the general pattern.

Output layer The output layer is the final layer in the neural network that produces the predictions or results.

Overfitting Overfitting is where a machine learning model predicts well based on training data but does not generalise to data it has not seen before because it has been tuned too much to the training data, or because training data is not sufficiently diverse or because it has learned too much from 'noise' in the data.

Overlay Text or lines placed on top of a medical image. These may contain one or more segmentations, either as lines with transparent centres or semi-transparent colour regions.

Picture archiving and communication system The picture archiving and communication system (PACS) is a medical imaging technology used for storing, retrieving, presenting and sharing images. AI systems in radiography are often integrated with PACS to access and analyse images.

Patient reported outcomes Patient reported outcomes (PROs) refer to health data provided directly by patients, reflecting their subjective experiences, symptoms and quality of life.

Patient reporting outcome measures Patient reporting outcome measures (PROMs) are tools used to capture patients' perspectives on their health status, quality of life and the impact of treatments.

Peak signal-to-noise ratio The peak signal-to-noise ratio is commonly used to assess image quality, especially in image super-resolution and denoising tasks.

Perceptron A perceptron is a type of artificial neural network unit that serves as a building block for more complex neural networks.

Positron emission tomography Positron emission tomography (PET) is a type of nuclear medicine imaging technique that uses radioactive tracers to visualise and measure changes in metabolic processes and physiological activities in the body.

Positron emission tomography/computed tomography Positron emission tomography (PET) combined with computed tomography (CT) is a hybrid medical imaging technique that allows for the simultaneous acquisition of functional and anatomical images.

Positron emission tomography/magnetic resonance Positron emission tomography combined with magnetic resonance imaging (PET/MRI) is a hybrid medical imaging technique that combines the functional imaging capabilities of PET with the detailed anatomical imaging provided by MRI.

Photon A photon is a particle of light and other forms of electromagnetic radiation.

Photon counting Photon counting involves detecting and measuring individual photons to accurately determine the intensity and properties of light.

Pixel A pixel or 'picture element' is the smallest unit of a digital image or display.

Pooling Pooling involves reducing the spatial dimensions (width and height) of feature maps while retaining valuable information within convolutional neural networks.

Positive predictive value The positive predicted value, also known as precision, is the fraction of relevant instances (TP) among the retrieved instances (TP + FP).

Positron A positron is the antimatter counterpart of an electron, possessing the same mass but carrying a positive charge.

Principal component analysis Principal component analysis (PCA) is a dimensionality reduction technique that projects high-dimensional data into a lower-dimensional space while preserving as much variance as possible. It identifies principal components that capture the largest variance in the data.

Prioritisation Prioritisation refers to structured messages sent from an AI/ML application to prioritise exams for reading on a reporting worklist, which may be hosted in a RIS, PACS or third-party reporting application (such as Powerscribe).

Probabilistic models Probabilistic models estimate the probability of a voxel belonging to a particular structure, providing a more nuanced segmentation output.

PROST system The PROST system is an innovative robotic device designed to enhance the accuracy and efficiency of prostate biopsies.

Protocol optimisation Protocol optimisation involves enhancing parameters and settings to improve the quality, efficiency and performance and reduce latency.

Proton-density-weighted zero-echo time MRI Proton-density-weighted zero-echo time (ZTE) MRI is an imaging technique that combines proton density weighting with zero-echo time acquisition for high-contrast images with reduced artefacts.

Pseudo-CT Pseudo-CT refers to images that are created using advanced algorithms, often involving deep learning, to simulate CT images from MRI data.

qXR qXR AI is a deep learning-based (convolutional neural network) computer-aided detection software device trained on 9 million datasets to triage, detect and segment 30 findings in a CXR.

R2 score The R2 score is a statistical measure used to assess the performance of a linear regression model as the proportion of variance in the data explained by the model.

Radiogenomics Radiogenomics explores the relationships between imaging features and genomic or molecular data and can identify imaging-based biomarkers associated with specific genetic mutations or gene expression patterns.

Radiomics Radiomics is a field in medical imaging that involves extracting a large number of quantitative features from medical images using advanced data-characterisation algorithms. These features, known as radiomic features, can reveal patterns and characteristics of tissues and tumours that are not easily visible to the naked eye.

Radiopharmaceutical Radiopharmaceuticals are drugs containing radioactive isotopes used in nuclear medicine for diagnostic and therapeutic purposes.

Radio-theranostics Radio-theranostics is an advanced medical approach that combines diagnostic imaging and targeted therapy using radioactive substances.

Random forest A random forest is a machine learning algorithm that uses multiple decision trees to make predictions to improve accuracy, reduce overfitting and provide a more stable prediction compared to a single decision tree. It operates by constructing multiple decision trees during training and outputting the mode of the classes (classification) or mean prediction (regression) of the individual trees.

Raw input Raw input refers to unprocessed data that is fed into an AI model, system or algorithm, which has not been transformed, cleaned or altered.

Receiver operating characteristic curve The receiver operating characteristic curve is a graphical plot that illustrates the true positive rate against the false positive rate across different thresholds.

Recurrent neural networks Recurrent neural networks (RNNs) are neural networks that are designed to manage sequential data, with connections that allow them to retain memory of previous inputs.

Reinforcement learning Reinforcement learning is a unique paradigm within ML and DL whose goal is to achieve the maximum expected cumulative reward through interaction with the environment rather than from labelled datasets or patterns. In radiography, this can be applied to optimise imaging protocols.

ReLU function The ReLU (rectified linear unit) function is a non-linear activation function used in neural networks and deep learning models that helps models to learn complex patterns.

Ridge regression A ridge regression model is a regularisation technique that shrinks coefficients to mitigate multicollinearity

Radiology information system The radiology information system (RIS) is a networked software system for managing medical imagery and associated data. AI tools in radiography may interact with RIS to streamline workflows and improve efficiency.

Scaling Scaling refers to the process of expanding AI solutions to reach a wider scope and impact across different use cases by increasing the size of the models or infrastructure and integrating them widely across applications.

Scatter correction Scatter corrections refer to techniques used to reduce scatter in imaging systems.

Secondary capture A DICOM information type used by many AI/ML applications to return findings and predictions. Text, images and any segmentation outlines are converted into a two-dimensional matrix of pixels and presented to the interpreting reader as one or more images. Images are static, can support colour, but are not interactive.

Image segmentation In image recognition, partitioning an image into discrete groups or regions of pixels. A segmented area may be shown by a bounding box, contoured polyline or a colour wash. Within radiology and radiotherapy, the segmented area may be used to depict pathology, specific organs or anatomical features.

Semantic segmentation Semantic segmentation involves AI models performing pixel-level classification, labelling each pixel value (0, 1...255) on an image to a specific class (e.g. tissue type, blood vessel and lesion).

Sensitivity Sensitivity refers to a model's ability to correctly identify true positives.

Spatial information Spatial information involves data that details the location, position and spatial relationships of objects or events within physical or virtual environments.

Specificity Specificity refers to a model's ability to correctly identify true negatives

SPECT Single-photon emission computed tomography (SPECT) is a medical imaging technique that uses radioactive tracers to create 3D images of the body.

SPECT/CT SPECT-CT is a medical imaging technique that combines single-photon emission computed tomography (SPECT) and computed tomography (CT) scans to create 3D images of the body.

Standardising image resolution Standardising image data involves transforming images into a common range of values that affects the variability, complexity of the data, speed and efficiency of the algorithms and comparability and compatibility of the images.

Standardised uptake value Standardised uptake value (SUV) is a semiquantitative measure of the concentration of radiotracer uptake in tissues.

Statistical modelling Statistical modelling refers to using mathematical and statistical tools and methods to analyse and interpret the data.

Statistical shape modelling Statistical shape modelling refers to a technique using geometric models to analyse variations within a population having similar objects or shapes.

Structural similarity index The structural similarity index (SSIM) is a perceptual metric that evaluates the similarity between two images while considering local structures, making it more robust to small pixel shifts or intensity changes.

Subsampling layer A subsampling layer follows the convolutional layer in convolutional neural networks to reduce the height and width dimensions of input feature maps, helping to decrease computational load and control overfitting.

Supervised learning Supervised learning is a type of machine learning where the model is trained on labelled data. In radiography, supervised learning is used to train models to recognise specific features in medical images. The algorithm learns from a labelled dataset, meaning that each input has a corresponding output (the 'correct' answer).

Support vector machine A support vector machine is a versatile supervised ML algorithm used for classification and regression tasks.

Symbolic AI Symbolic AI focuses on representing knowledge in a formal language.

Synthetic CT Synthetic CT refers to the generation of a computed tomography (CT) image using data from another imaging modality, such as magnetic resonance imaging (MRI).

Temporal information Temporal information refers to data that details the timing, sequence and duration of events.

TG-263 TG-263 refers to the American Association of Physicists in Medicine (AAPM) Task Group 263 which convened to develop a standard nomenclature for radiation oncology.

Theranostics Theranostics is a medical approach that combines therapy and diagnostic imaging to enhance the treatment of diseases, particularly cancer.

Threshold Threshold refers to a numerical value that has been determined as the cut-off point for distinguishing between the presence and absence of a finding. The threshold value is compared with the prediction value output by a classification model. If the prediction value is above the threshold, the finding is deemed to be present. If the prediction value is below the threshold, the finding is deemed to be absent

Tissue segmentation Tissue segmentation in medical imaging involves dividing an image into distinct areas for studying anatomy, pinpointing specific regions of interest or gauging tissue volume.

Transfer learning Transfer learning is a machine learning technique that uses a pretrained model, that is, where a model developed for one task is reused as the starting point for a model on a second task. This is useful in radiography for applying pre-trained models to new but related imaging tasks. It is also known as 'knowledge transfer'.

Triaging Triaging refers to sorting tasks to prioritise the urgent ones first.

True positive rate The true positive rate (TPR), also known as sensitivity or recall, is defined as the fraction of correctly classified positive classes (TP) out of the total number of actual positive instances (TP + FN).

Turing test The Turing test conjectures that if a human cannot determine via exchanging messages in a computer console whether they are interacting with another human or a machine, they must acknowledge that, be it a machine, the machine would be intelligent.

Uncertainty estimation Uncertainty estimation and quantification are critical aspects of deep learning model deployment, particularly for assessing the reliability of models used in healthcare. By providing a measure of confidence in model predictions, uncertainty quantification enhances trust in AI-driven decisions and supports more informed clinical interpretations.

U-Net U-Net is a type of convolutional neural network (CNN) architecture designed primarily for image segmentation, characterised by its U-shaped structure.

Universal approximators A universal approximator is a system or model capable of accurately approximating any continuous function, provided it has sufficient resources and parameters.

Unsupervised learning Unsupervised learning is a type of machine learning where the model is trained on unlabelled data and must find patterns and relationships in the data on its own. This can be used in radiography to discover new patterns in imaging data. The algorithm is given data without explicit labels. The model must find patterns, structures, or relationships in the data on its own, without being told what the 'correct' output should be.

Variational autoencoders Variational autoencoders are a probabilistic extension of traditional autoencoders that encode the input data as a distribution over the latent space, sample from this distribution and pass it through the decoder to reconstruct the data.

Vector machines Vector machines refer to support vector machines (SVMs), which are supervised machine learning algorithms used for classification and regression tasks.

Voxel A voxel or 'volume pixel' is a unit of graphic information representing a point in three-dimensional space, analogous to a pixel in two-dimensional images.

Weight sharing Weight sharing refers to a method used in neural networks, such as convolutional neural networks (CNNs) and neural

architecture search (NAS), to enhance efficiency and performance.

XOFF input XOFF input (transmit off) refers to a component of software flow control in serial communication protocols like RS-232 that sends specific control characters to halt data transmission when the receiving device's buffer is full or nearly full.

XON input XON input (transmit on) refers to a component of software flow control in serial communication protocols like RS-232 that sends specific control characters to restart data transmission after it has been paused.

XOR functions XOR (exclusive OR) functions refer to a specific type of mathematical function.

XOR input XOR input refers to the signals fed into an XOR (exclusive OR) gate used in electronics and computing.

Index